Case Studies in Nephrology A Practical Approach

Editors

ASHISH NANDWANI

MD (Medicine), DNB (Nephrology), FASN
Consultant, Department of Nephrology and Transplant Medicine
Manipal Hospital, Dwarka, New Delhi, India

SHYAM B BANSAL

MD (Medicine), DM (Nephrology), FISN, FASN, FRCP (London)
Director, Department of Nephrology and Transplant Medicine
Medanta, The Medicity, Gurugram, Haryana, India

Co-Editors

SIDHARTH SETHI

MD (Pediatrics), FASN, FIAP
Senior Consultant, Pediatric Nephrology and Pediatric Kidney Transplantation
Medanta, The Medicity, Gurugram, Haryana, India

MANISH JAIN

MD (Medicine), DM (Nephrology), FISN, FICP, Clinical Fellow (UBC, Vancouver, Canada)
Director, Department of Nephrology and Transplant Medicine
Medanta, The Medicity, Gurugram, Haryana, India

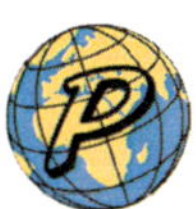

Peepee Publishers and Distributors (P) Ltd.®

Case Studies in Nephrology–A Practical Approach

Published by
Pawaninder P. Vij and Anupam Vij

Peepee Publishers and Distributors (P) Ltd.
Head Office: 160, Shakti Vihar, Pitam Pura, Delhi-110 034 (India)

Correspondence Address:

7/31, First Floor, Ansari Road, Daryaganj
New Delhi-110 002 (India)

Ph: 41512412, 23246245, 9811156083

e-mail: peepee160@yahoo.co.in

e-mail: peepee160@gmail.com

www.peepeepub.com

join us on facebook.com/pp.publishers

First Edition: 2022
Reprint: 2025

ISBN: 978-81-8445-294-5

DEDICATED TO

My parents for guiding and helping me to achieve whatever I could do in life, My wife and daughters for their continuous support, My teachers for all the guidance and My patients for improving my skills to be a better doctor.

Ashish Nandwani

Dedicated to all my patients without them it wouldn't have been possible to have quest for knowledge and try to be a better doctor.

Shyam B Bansal

Dedicated to our patients, who are our teachers.

Sidharth Sethi

My parents Late Dr Krishan Jain and Mrs Shobha Jain for making me who I am today, Dr Shalu Gupta, my wife and children Devyansh and Shreyansh for their patience, love and continuous support. To all my Teachers for their guidance and my friends, fellow Doctors and patients for always trusting me.

Manish Jain

ABOUT THE AUTHORS

Dr. Ashish Nandwani

Dr. Ashish Nandwani is Consultant, Department of Nephrology and Transplant Medicine at Manipal Hospital, Dwarka, New Delhi, India. Dr. Nandwani has done fellowship in Nephrology and Transplant from University of Ottawa, Ontario, Canada, after his post-graduation. He has keen interest in academics and is involved in teaching the nephrology fellows. His chief interests are Acute Kidney Injury, Critical Care Nephrology and Renal Transplantation. He has presented papers in various conferences and authored number of chapters in reputed books. He has been a faculty at multiple meetings on Acute Kidney Injury, Dialysis and Transplant Update. He is executive member of Delhi Nephrology Society and is involved in organizing various nephrology conferences. He was awarded Fellowship by American Society of Nephrology (FASN) for contributions to the field.

Dr. Shyam B Bansal

Dr. Shyam B Bansal is Director at Medanta's Institute of Nephrology and Kidney Transplant. He was accoladed with best oral paper award in 2005 at Indian Society of Nephrology Conference on 'Treatment of Hepatitis C Infection' in Kidney Transplant recipients. Dr. Bansal established Department of Nephrology at Medical College, Gwalior in 2006. Subsequently he has worked as consultant in Fortis Hospital and joined this institute since its inception in 2009. Apart from working, he has published extensively in field of kidney transplantation also has the honour of publishing first case report of kidney transplantation in an HIV positive patient in India. He is secretary at Delhi Nephrology Society and regularly organizes Transplant update. He has been awarded FASN and FRCP for his outstanding work.

Dr. Sidharth Sethi

Dr. Sidharth Sethi is currently Senior Consultant, Pediatric Nephrology and Renal Transplant Medicine, Kidney and Urology Institute, Medanta, The Medicity, Gurugram, India. His chief interests are Acute Kidney Injury, Dialysis and Pediatric Renal Transplantation. He was trained as a Fellow (International Pediatric Nephrology Association Fellowship) and Senior Resident in Pediatric Nephrology at All India Institute of Medical Sciences and Division of Pediatric Nephrology and Transplant Immunology, Cedars Sinai Medical Centre, Los Angeles, California. He has been a faculty at multiple meetings on Pediatric Acute Kidney Injury and Pediatric Dialysis nationally and internationally. He has been actively involved in the care of children with all kinds of complex renal disorders, including acute kidney injury, dialysis, nephrotic syndrome, tubular disorders, urinary tract infections, hypertension, chronic kidney disease and renal transplantation. He has been a part of 8-member writing committee for the Indian guidelines of Steroid Sensitive Nephrotic Syndrome and Expert Committee involved in the formulation of guidelines of Pediatric Renal Disorders including Steroid Resistant Nephrotic Syndrome and urinary tract infections. He has more than 50 indexed publications in Pediatric Nephrology and chapters in reputed nephrology textbooks. He is currently the Editor–Journal of Clinical Pediatric Nephrology. He was awarded in 2014 by Case Western Reserve University, for his outstanding contributions to the field.

Dr. Manish Jain

Dr. Manish Jain works as a Director at Medanta, The Medicity, Gurugram. He has expertise in renal disorders with special interest in Renal Transplantation and Peritoneal Dialysis. He has been awarded FICP and FISN for his outstanding work. He is DNB teacher and Faculty in many CMEs and Conferences. He has published and presented articles in various books, journals and various conferences including Chapter on Kidney Transplantation in elderly and those with diabetes published in prestigious Oxford Book on Renal Transplantation in Developing Countries. He did Clinical Fellowship from University of British Columbia, Vancouver, Canada after completing post-graduation. After finishing DM, he joined Meenakshi Medical College, Kanchepuram as an Assistant Professor where he established the Nephrology Department and started the Dialysis unit.

FOREWORD

It is pleasure to write a foreword for **Case Studies in Nephrology–A Practical Approach** edited by Drs. Ashish Nandwani, Shyam Bansal, Manish Jain and Sidharth Sethi.

I find this book to be different from other books in Nephrology as the approach and theme of this book is clinical, case based and topic based like you diagnose your patients in the clinics. This is going to be very useful to students of Internal Medicine, Nephrology, Critical Care, Emergency Medicines as well as to busy practising nephrologists to quickly brush up about the disease. I found the book pleasing to the eyes, with tables and pictures highlights and has features with bold headlines and colourful presentation which makes reading easy.

I am confident the readers will find this book interesting and useful. Do keep the editors informed about suggestions to improve and what needs to be included which they can do in the next edition.

Wishing the book a large readership.

Vijay Kher
MD, DM, FAMS, FRCPE
Chairman
Medanta Kidney and Urology Institute
Division of Nephrology and Kidney Transplant Medicine
Medanta, The Medicity
Gurugram, Haryana

PREFACE

Case Studies in Nephrology–A Practical Approach, is an attempt to present the commonly encountered diseases related to kidneys in a simple and practical way. Practical approach to diagnose a renal problem, along with differential diagnosis and management aspects have been discussed. It contains tables, flowcharts and concise text to understand the given problem. The book will benefit the nephrology fellows, postgraduate students, who are preparing for their exit examination. Apart from clinical cases often given for practical examination, chapters on renal histopathology, renal imaging, nuclear medicine, urodynamic studies, dialysis and renal transplant patient work up have been added to help to prepare for examination. This book will also be helpful for practising physicians for their day-to-day practice to understand better regarding the renal disease.

We are very thankful to all the authors, who have contributed to the book, giving their precious time for writing the chapter. We request you all to let us know regarding the shortcomings and give your valuable opinion regarding the improvements required to make this book more informative and practical.

Ashish Nandwani
Shyam B Bansal
Sidharth Sethi
Manish Jain

ACKNOWLEDGEMENTS

We thank the Almighty for giving us strength and guidance to complete this book.

We thank all the authors, who have put in their best efforts and helped us to complete the task.

We would like to express our gratitude to all our teachers, who have mentored us over years.

We are indebted to our family members, who supported us to realize this dream.

Special thanks to all our students, who inspired us to write this book.

Special gratitude to the publishers for helping us at each step to accomplish the task.

Last but not the least, we would like to acknowledge all our patients, who have been constant source of improving our knowledge.

CONTRIBUTORS

Abhijeet Kumar
Consultant, Nephrology
Medanta, The Medicity
Lucknow

Abhishek Garg
Consultant, Nephrology
Maharaja Agarsen Hospital
New Delhi

Abhishek Saini
Scientist, Molecular and Transplant Immunology
Medanta, The Medicity
Gurugram

Abhyuday Rana
Associate Consultant, Nephrology
Medanta, The Medicity
Gurugram

Aditi Sinha
Associate Professor
Division of Nephrology, Department of Pediatrics
All India Institute of Medical Sciences
New Delhi

Ajay Kher
Consultant, Nephrologist and Transplant Physician
Max Hospital, Vaishali, Vishwasth Healthcare
Noida

Aliza Mittal
Associate Professor
Department of Pediatrics
All India Institute of Medical Sciences
Jodhpur

Amit Gupta
Senior Consultant, Nephrologist and Transplant Physician
Apollomedics Super Specialty Hospitals
Lucknow

Amit Kumar Mahapatra
Consultant, Nephrology
Medanta, The Medicity
Gurugram

Aniket Hase
Consultant, Nephrologist and Renal Transplant Physician
Jupiter Hospital
Thane, Maharashtra

Arpana Iyengar
Professor, Department of Pediatric Nephrology
St John's Medical College Hospital
Bangalore

Arun Kumar S
Assistant Professor
Department of Nephrology
All India Institute of Medical Sciences
New Delhi

Arushi Nautiyal
Consultant, Nephrology
Jaipur Golden Hospital
Rohini, New Delhi

Aseem Kumar Tiwari
Director, Department of Transfusion Medicine
Medanta, The Medicity
Gurugram

Ashish Nandwani
Consultant, Nephrologist and Renal Transplant Physician
Manipal Hospital
Dwarka, New Delhi

Ashwini Gadde
Associate Consultant
Department of Nephrology
Medanta, The Medicity
Gurugram

Brig Ranjith K Nair
Professor and Head, Department of Nephrology
Command Hospital (EC)
Kolkata

Davinder Kundra
Consultant, Pulmonology
Manipal Hospital
Delhi

Deepanshu Gupta
Consultant, Urology
Dr RML Hospital and ABVIMS
New Delhi

Dhawal Khetia
Consultant, Nephrology
Bankers Heart Hospital
Vadodara

Dinesh Kumar Yadav
Senior Consultant, Nephrology
Medanta, The Medicity
Gurugram

Dipankar Bhowmik
Professor, Department of Nephrology
All India Institute of Medical Sciences
New Delhi

Gaurav Sagar
Senior Consultant, Interventional Nephrologist
Indraprastha Apollo Hospital
New Delhi

Gurinder Kumar
Pediatric Nephrologist
Sheikh Khalifa Medical City
Abu Dhabi
UAE

Harshal Joshi
Assistant Professor, Department of Nephrology
SBKS Medical Institute and Research Center
Pipariya, Vadodara

Hemanth Kumar MK
Consultant, Nephrology
Paras Hospital
Gurugram

Jammaludin
Fellow, Urology
Medanta, The Medicity
Gurugram

Joyita Bharati
Assistant Professor
Department of Nephrology
Postgraduate Institute of Medical Education and Research
Chandigarh

K Praveen Kumar
Professor and Head
Department of Nephrology
Narayana Medical College
Nellore

Kishore Kumar Ariga
Senior Resident
Department of Nephrology
All India Institute of Medical Sciences
New Delhi

Laxmikant Sharma
Fellow, Urology, Medanta, The Medicity
Gurugram

Manas Ranjan Patel
Assistant Professor, Nephrology
Sanjay Gandhi Post Graduate Institute of Medical Sciences
Lucknow

Manas Sahoo
Consultant, Department of Nuclear Medicine
Medanta, The Medicity
Gurugram

Manav Suryavanshi
Director
Endourology and Robotic Surgery
Medanta,The Medicity
Gurugram

Manish Jain
Director, Nephrology
Medanta, The Medicity
Gurugram

Manish Rathi
Professor
Department of Nephrology
Postgraduate Institute of Medical Education and Research
Chandigarh

Manoj Kumar Sharma
Professor, Hepatology
Institute of Liver and Biliary Sciences
New Delhi

Manoj Singhal
Director, Nephrology and Renal Transplant
Max Superspeciality Hospital
Vaishali, Ghaziabad

Mayank Bansal
Consultant
Ophthalmologist and Vitreo-Retinal Surgeon in Delhi and
Fortis Memorial Research Institute
Gurugram

Mayank Bharti
Consultant, Uro-Oncology and Robotic Surgery
Fortis Memorial Research Institute
Gurugram

Mohit Madken
Fellow, Nephrology
The Ottawa Hospital
Canada

Narayan Prasad
Professor and Head Nephrology
Department of Nephrology and Renal Transplantation
Sanjay Gandhi Postgraduate Institute of Medical Sciences
Lucknow

Nikhil Khattar
Consultant, Urology
Medanta, The Medicity
Gurugram

Pankaj Bansal
Professor of Medicine
Sharda University Hospital
Greater Noida

PN Gupta
Senior Consultant, Nephrology
Paras Hospital
Gurugram

Pranaw Kumar Jha
Senior Consultant
Division of Nephrology and Renal Transplant Medicine
Medanta Institute of Kidney and Urology
Gurugram

Prasad Dandekar
Associate Consultant, Nephrology
Fortis Hospital
Noida

Praveen Kumar Etta
Consultant, Nephrologist
Virinchi Hospitals
Hyderabad

Pulkit Nandwani
Senior Consultant
Obstetrics and Gynecology
Saroj Medical Institute
Delhi

Punit Gupta
Director and Head
Department of Nephrology and Organ Transplantation
Sharda University Hospital
Greater Noida

Rahul Grover
Senior Consultant, Nephrology
Max Super Speciality Hospital
Saket, New Delhi

Raj Kanwar Yadav
Associate Professor
Department of Nephrology
All India Institute of Medical Sciences
New Delhi

Rajan Duggal
Associate Director and Head
Histopathology and Cytopathology
BLK Super Speciality Hospital
Pusa Road, New Delhi

Rajiv Sinha
Professor and Head Division of Paediatric Nephrology
Institute of Child Health
Kolkata

Rajiv Yadav
Director and Head
Urologic Oncology and Robotic Surgery
Fortis Memorial Research Institute
Gurugram

Ramniwas Yadav
Senior Fellow Minimal Invasive Urology
Medanta, The Medicity
Gurugram

Rana Saha
Consultant, Paediatrician and Paediatric Nephrologist
Institute of Child Health
Kolkata

Rashmi Kavindram
Consultant
Department of Nuclear Medicine
Medanta, The Medicity
Gurugram

S Raghavendra
Assistant Professor
Department of Nephrology
Narayana Medical College
Nellore

Salil Jain
Director, Nephrology
Fortis Memorial Research Institute
Gurugram

Sanjiv Jasuja
Senior Consultant, Nephrologist
Indraprastha Apollo Hospital
New Delhi

Santosh Varughese
Professor and Head
Department of Nephrology
Christian Medical College
Vellore

Saurabh Pokhariyal
Head of Department, Nephrology
Manipal Hospital
Delhi

Saurabh Shukla
Consultant, Nephrologist
Arvy Hospital
Gurugram

Shailendra Singh
Consultant, Nephrology
Manipal Hospital
Dwarka, Delhi

Shalu Gupta
Consultant, Obstetrics and Gynecology
Cloudnine Hospital
Gurugram

Shyam Bihari Bansal
Director, Department of Nephrology and Renal Transplant
Medanta, The Medicity
Gurugram

Sidharth Kumar Sethi
Senior Consultant
Pediatric Nephrology and Pediatric Kidney Transplantation
Kidney and Urology Institute
Medanta, The Medicity
Gurugram

Somendra Bansal
Assistant Professor
SMS Medical College
Jaipur

Sree Bhushan Raju
Professor and Head
Department of Nephrology
Nizams Institute of Medical Sciences
Hyderabad, Telangana

Suceena Alexander
Professor, Department of Nephrology
Christian Medical College
Vellore

Sudhir Mehta
Assistant Professor, Nephrology
Maharishi Markandeshwar Institute of Medical Sciences and Research
Mullana, Ambala

Sulakshna Dahiya
Senior Resident
Sharda University Hospital
Greater Noida

Suman Lata
Director, Nephrology and Renal Transplant
Dharamshila Narayana Superspecialty Hospital
New Delhi

Suprita Kalra
Associate Professor
Pediatric Nephrology
Army Hospital R & R
Delhi Cantt

Sushma Yadav
Senior Resident
Department of Obst and Gynae
SHKM GMC
Nalhar

Tarun Jeloka
Director
Nephrology and Renal Transplant
Aditya Birla Memorial Hospital
Pune

Tarun Kaushik
Consultant, Nephrology
Dharamshila Narayana Superspecialty Hospital
New Delhi

Umapati Hegde
Vice Chairman, Department of Nephrology
Muljibhai Patel Urological Hospital
Nadiad, Gujarat

Varun Mittal
Senior Consultant
Uro-Oncology and Robotic Surgery
Fortis Memorial Research Institute
Gurugram

Vijay Kher
Chairman, Institute of Nephrlogy and Urology
Medanta, The Medicity
Gurugram

Vikas Makkar
Professor, Nephrology
Dayanand Medical College
Ludhiana

Vinay Malhotra
Senior Professor
Department of Nephrology
SMS Medical College and Hospital
Jaipur

Vivek Kute
Professor
Department of Nephrology and Clinical Transplantation
Institute of Kidney Diseases and Research Center
Dr HL Trivedi Institute of Transplantation Sciences
[IKDRC-ITS], Ahmedabad

CONTENTS

CHAPTER

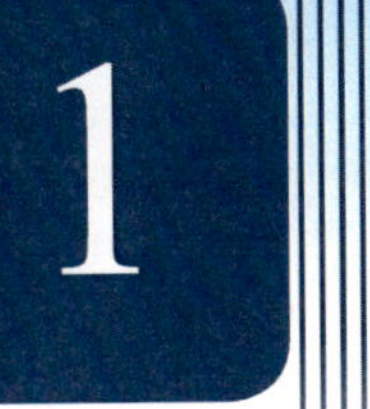

Clinical Approach to a Patient with Renal Disease

Ashish Nandwani[1], Manish Jain[2]

[1] *Consultant, Nephrology, Manipal Hospital, Dwarka, New Delhi*

[2] *Director, Nephrology, Medanta, The Medicity, Gurugram*

Patients with renal disease usually present with variety of non-specific complaints like malaise, fatigue, generalized weakness etc. and usually detected to have renal dysfunction during evaluation for the same. They may have symptoms directly related to renal disease or extra renal disorders. Some asymptomatic patients may get to know the renal disease during routine health checkups.

The various ways in which, renal diseases are detected:

- Non-specific symptoms due to anemia and uremia (e.g., nausea, vomiting, malaise, dyspnea, edema).
- Abnormal blood laboratory studies (e.g., deranged kidney function test).
- Asymptomatic urinary abnormalities (e.g., microscopic hematuria, proteinuria, microalbuminuria).
- Incidental discovery of anatomic kidney abnormalities on routine imaging studies.
- Symptoms of polyuria, oliguria, hematuria, dysuria, nocturia, urgency.
- New-onset hypertension especially in young.
- Facial and pedal edema/anasarca.
- Symptoms of urinary tract obstruction (e.g., ipsilateral flank pain in those with obstructing nephrolithiasis).
- Symptoms related to underlying systemic disease.

What are Signs and Symptoms Indicating Renal Dysfunction?

Symptoms

- Loss or decreased appetite.
- Nausea and vomiting, Dyspepsia.
- Generalized itching.
- Easy fatigability and Generalized weakness.
- Intractable hiccups (Uremia).
- Alterations in sensorium (e.g., lethargy, difficulty in concentrating, seizure).
- Breathlessness (Anemia, fluid retention, metabolic acidosis).
- Edema (fluid overload).
- Frothy appearance of urine (usually results from proteinuria).
- Decreased libido (e.g., erectile dysfunction).
- Restless legs syndrome.
- Bony pains.
- Flank pain/Gross Hematuria/Graveluria (Stone disease).
- Dysuria, frequency, urgency (Urinary tract infection).
- Polyuria/Nocturia (Loss of concentration ability of kidneys).
- Oliguria (< 400 ml urine in 24 hours), Anuria (< 50 ml urine in 24 hours)–(symptoms of acute kidney injury).

Signs

- Pallor.
- Dermatologic manifestation (Xerosis or dryness of the skin, changes in pigmentation, uremic frost, Lindsay nails, also known as "half and half nails").
- Hypertension.
- Asymmetric pulses (In large vessel vasculitis).
- Signs of volume overload (Jugular venous distention, peripheral edema, pulmonary edema, anasarca).
- Friction rub (Pericarditis).
- Neuropathy.
- Asterixis and myoclonus (Uremic encephalopathy).
- In children–bony abnormalities (Metabolic bone disorder).
- Features of cardiac failure (Anemia, fluid overload, Hypertension).
- Abdominal Bruit (Renal artery stenosis).
- Palpable kidneys (Polycystic kidneys, Mass lesions).
- Flank tenderness (Stone disease, Pyelonephritis).
- Urine analysis–various abnormalities.

What are Various Syndromes of Clinical Presentation of Renal Disease? (Table 1.1)

Table 1.1: Syndromic presentation in nephrology

S. No.	Syndromes
1.	Acute kidney injury
2.	Chronic kidney disease
3.	Nephrotic syndrome
4.	Acute nephritic syndrome
5.	Rapidly progressive renal failure
6.	Urinary tract obstruction
7.	Urinary tract infection
8.	Hypertension
9.	Asymptomatic urinary abnormalities
10.	Tubulointerstitial diseases

Acute Kidney Injury (AKI)

AKI is sudden and usually reversible loss of renal function caused by ischemic or nephrotoxic insult. KDIGO definition of AKI is increase in serum creatinine by 0.3 mg/dl; or more within 48 hours or increase in serum creatinine to 1.5 times baseline or more within the last 7 days or urine output less than 0.5 ml/kg/hour for 6 hours.The common causes are prerenal, obstructive nephropathy and intrinsic forms of AKI due to ischemic acute tubular necrosis and due to administration of nephrotoxic agents. It usually recovers in 4-12 weeks time. However, recovery may not be complete leading to chronic renal damage.

Chronic Kidney Disease (CKD)

CKD is defined as the presence of structural or functional abnormalities of kidney with or without decrease in glomerular filtration rate. It results from progressive and irreversible loss of nephrons from a number of causes. There are pathological abnormalities and decreased kidney function (defined as estimated glomerular filtration rate [eGFR] , <60 ml/min per 1.73 m^2) for 3 or more months (Table 1.2).

Table 1.2: Chronic kidney disease classification based on glomerular filtration rate and albuminuria

GFR Stages	eGFR (ml/ min/1.73 m^2)	Terms
G1	>90	Normal or high
G2	>60–<89	Mildly decreased
G3a	> 45–<59	Mildly to moderately decreased
G3b	>30–44	Moderately to severely decreased
G4	>15–<29	Severely decreased
G5	<15	Kidney failure (add D if treated by dialysis)
Albuminuria Stages	**Albumin/ Creatinine Ratio (mg/g)**	**Terms**
A1	<30	Normal to mildly increased
A2	30–<300	Moderately increased
A3	>300	Severely increased

Causes of Chronic Kidney Disease

- **Glomerular:** Focal and segmental glomerulosclerosis, IgA nephropathy, membranous nephropathy, diffuse proliferative glomerulonephritis, deposition diseases, diabetic nephropathy.
- **Tubulointerstitial:** Urinary tract infection, autoimmune disease, stones, obstruction.
- **Vascular:** Anti-neutrophil cytoplasmic antibody-associated renal limited vasculitis, Renal artery stenosis.
- **Cystic and congenital:** Kidney dysplasia, medullary cystic disease, polycystic diseases.

Nephrotic Syndrome

Nephrotic syndrome represents a cluster of abnormal findings. It comprises four distinct elements: One physical sign, edema; and three laboratory test abnormalities, massive proteinuria (>3.5 g per 1.73 m^2 body surface area per day, or > 40 mg per square meter body surface area per hour in children), hypoalbuminemia (<2.5 g/dl), hyperlipidemia. Edema usually begins in the face. Lipiduria (lipids in urine) can also occur, but is not essential for the diagnosis of nephrotic syndrome.

Nephrotic syndrome is classified into primary (or idiopathic) and secondary causes.

The principal primary etiologies of nephrotic syndrome include:

- Minimal change disease (MCD).
- Focal segmental glomerulosclerosis (FSGS).
- Membranous nephropathy (MN).
- Membranoproliferative glomerulonephritis (MPGN).

In adults, IgA nephropathy, fibrillary and immunotactoid glomerulonephritis can present with nephrotic syndrome.

The secondary causes of nephrotic syndrome include:

- Post-infectious glomerulonephritis.
- Systemic lupus erythematosus.

- Henoch-Schönlein purpura.
- Medications (e.g., Non-steroidal anti-inflammatory drugs, gold therapy, penicillamine, heroin, interferon-alfa, lithium and pamidronate).
- Infections (e.g., Hepatitis B, Hepatitis C, HIV).
- Malignancies (Hodgkin's diseases).
- Amyloidosis.
- Diabetes mellitus.

Acute Nephritic Syndrome

Acute glomerulonephritis is an acute kidney injury characterized by the sudden onset of edema and new-onset or worsening hypertension. Urinalysis demonstrates an active sediment, including abnormal proteinuria, hematuria, and red cell casts, elevated serum blood urea nitrogen and creatinine concentrations. The prototype of this disease is acute post infectious glomerulonephritis. This usually occur 10-20 days after infection. This is usually seen in children and resolves completely with time.

Rapidly Progressive Renal Failure (RPRF)

Rapidly progressive renal failure is characterized by insidious deterioration of renal function over days to weeks as compared to AKI, where renal function deteriorates abruptly over hours to days. The most important cause is rapidly progressive glomerulonephritis (RPGN). It is a glomerular disease (proteinuria, hematuria, and red cell casts) accompanied by rapid loss of kidney function over days to weeks. If untreated, RPGN often results in kidney failure. The pathologic hallmark of RPGN is the presence of crescents on kidney biopsy, and RPGN is also described as crescentic nephritis. The causes are Anti-GBM antibody disease (Goodpasture disease), Pauci immune glomerulonephritis and immune complex associated glomerulonephritis.The diagnosis requires renal biopsy along with serological markers such as Anti-neutrophil cytoplasmic antibodies (ANCA); Anti-glomerular basement membrane antibodies (Anti-GBM); anti-nuclear antibodies and complement levels.

Other causes of RPRF are acute interstitial nephritis, which can be secondary to infections or drugs, hemolytic uremic syndrome, malignant hypertension and other vasculitis syndromes.

Urinary Tract Obstruction

It is structural or functional interference of normal urine flow anywhere along the urinary tract. Obstructive nephropathy causes elevated pressures in the renal pelvis and calyces due to hydronephrosis and can lead to dilation and ischemia of the distal tubules of nephrons and subsequent interstitial fibrosis and renal parenchymal atrophy. The common causes of obstruction in the tract are stone disease, malignancy, congenital (pelvi-ureteric junction obstruction), bladder outlet obstruction in elderly. It can also be caused by extrinsic compression either due to malignancy or retroperitoneal fibrosis.

Urinary Tract Infection (UTI)

UTI is the presence of microorganisms in the urine or tissues of the normally sterile genitourinary tract. Infection may be localized to the bladder alone or involve the kidneys and, in men, the prostate. Acute uncomplicated UTI occurs in women with a normal genitourinary tract and usually manifests as acute cystitis (bladder infection or lower tract infection). These patients experience, less frequently, kidney (upper tract or kidney parenchymal) infection, referred to as acute uncomplicated or acute non-obstructive pyelonephritis. Complicated UTI occurs in individuals with structural or functional abnormalities of the genitourinary tract, including those with indwelling devices, such as urethral catheters. Recurrent urinary infection may be reinfection, with a new organism, or relapse, when the same organism is isolated post therapy. Asymptomatic bacteriuria is isolation of bacteria from the urine culture in quantitative counts consistent with infection but with no genitourinary signs or symptoms attributable to infection.

Hypertension

Renovascular hypertension, progressive loss of kidney function from ischemic nephropathy, and recurrent episodes of flash pulmonary edema are the clinical syndromes typically associated with renal artery stenosis. The two important causes of renal artery stenosis are atherosclerosis and fibromuscular dysplasia. Atherosclerotic renal artery stenosis is the more common cause and is often seen in older patients. It occurs in the setting of atherosclerotic disease affecting other vascular beds, such as the coronary, cerebral and peripheral arterial circulation. These patients often have other risk factors for atherosclerosis, such as diabetes, hypertension and smoking. In contrast, fibromuscular dysplasia is typically seen in younger female patients. Renal parenchymal disease also cause hypertension through renin angiotensin mechanism.

Asymptomatic Urinary Abnormality

Asymptomatic patients are diagnosed to have renal disease following routine evaluation during health checkups or for insurance purposes. The routine investigations such as urine analysis, biochemical analysis or USG abdomen for unrelated complaints may detect renal abnormalities. These asymptomatic patients may have proteinuria, hematuria, abnormal kidneys on USG examination, which requires further evaluation for diagnosis.

Tubulointerstitial Disease

Acute tubulointerstitial nephritis (ATIN) is characterized by inflammation and edema in the tubulointerstitium and can cause acute kidney injury. The most common causes of ATIN are drugs, infections and autoimmune disorders. Drugs account for most ATIN cases. Drug-induced ATIN is not dose dependent, but rather is an idiosyncratic reaction. Repeat exposure to the same drug or a closely related agent can lead to recurrence of the disease process. Chronic kidney disease secondary to tubulointerstitial disease is typically due to interstitial fibrosis and tubular atrophy. The common conditions are chronic infections, reflux nephropathy, stone disease and bladder disorders.

Tubular disorder such as renal tubular disorders, Fanconi's syndrome, familial disorders and disorders related to ADH require specific evaluation for tubular functions.

Genetic Syndromes

Kidneys may be involved in various genetic/familial disorders. These may be suspected in patients with positive family history and require high index of suspicion. These include cystic diseases of kidneys, Alport's syndrome, Fabry's disease and congenital nephrotic syndromes.Various tubular disorders are also familial and need genetic and biochemical evaluation of family members.

Suggested Reading

1. Davison AM, Grunfeld JP, Fitzpatrick M. History and clinical examination of the patient with renal disease. In: Ponticelli C, Ritz E, Winearls CG, van Ypersele CG, (Eds) New York, Oxford Textbook of Nephrology, Oxford University Press 2005;3-22.

CHAPTER 2

Urine Analysis

Brig Ranjith K Nair

Professor and Head, Department of Nephrology, Command Hospital (EC), Kolkata

Urinalysis

The urinalysis is a simple and inexpensive test which yields invaluable information about not just the health of the kidney; but also throws light upon a large number of diseases which could involve other organs of the body. Its contribution towards diagnosis of kidney diseases is so significant that certain nephrologists consider it equal to a "liquid kidney biopsy". A urinalysis consists of a detailed visual examination of the sample followed by multiple chemical investigations and finally a microscopic examination to detect cells and their fragments and other substances such as crystals or casts which are associated with various conditions, benign and pathologic.[1]

(a) **Collection:** It is very important to use an appropriately wide mouthed container with a tight screw cap, which is clean and dry, to collect the sample and store or transport it. A 'clean catch – mid stream' sample must always be insisted upon. This reduces the chances of perineal contamination of the sample. However, there is no advantage of perineal cleansing prior to collection.[2]

(b) **Storage and transport:** If the sample is not going to be analysed within an hour, then it must be stored at 4°C, or a preservative added until it can be processed.

(c) **Timing:** The first morning void is preferred when assessing for proteins, however, for most other tests a fresh void at any time can be used.

(d) **Physical appearance:**

(i) *Odour:* The normal smell of urine is described as "urinoid" and can vary with the concentration of the sample. A more pungent smell does not indicate an infection. Ketoacidosis can cause the urine to have a "fruity" odour. The sample can have a "fecal smell" in patients with enterovesical fistula. Cysteine decomposition can lead to a sulfuric smell. A large number of dietary products and drugs can alter the odour of urine.

(ii) *Colour:* The normal colour of urine is due to the urochromes present in it, which is a product of oxidation of urobilinogen absorbed from the gut. The urine can change colour due to the presence of chemicals derived from food, medication and other metabolic processes. The summary of various changes in urine colour are summarized in Table 2.1.

(e) **Specific gravity:** The specific gravity of urine indicates the osmolality of the urine sample and is a marker of hydration of the individual. The normal range of specific gravity of urine is 1.003 to 1.030. Patients with chronic kidney disease usually have a fixed specific gravity of 1.010, called "isosthenuria" as the osmolality of the urine is similar to that of plasma or the glomerular ultrafiltrate. Specific gravity declines in conditions such as diuretic use, diabetes insipidus, hyperaldosteronism, adrenal insufficiency and impaired renal function while it

Table 2.1: Abnormal urine colour and its cause

Colour	Chemical	Food
1. Red	Hemoglobin, Myoglobin	Beet root, phenolphthalein
2. Orange	Bile, Rifampicin, Phenothiazines	
3. Brown	Bile pigment, myoglobin, Nitrofurantoin, Metronidazole, Levodopa	Fava beans
4. Black	Melanin, methemoglobin, methyldopa	
5. Greenish - blue	Methylene blue, IV Amitryptiline, IV Cimetidine, IV Promethazine, Triamterene	Indigo carmine food colour
6. Yellowish	Urochromes	Carrot, Cascara

is increased in conditions leading to concentrated urine formation like dehydration or Syndrome of Inappropriate Antidiuresis (SIAD) or solvent diuretic states like diabetes mellitus and radiocontrast use.

(f) **Urine pH:** The normal urine pH can range from 4.5 to 8.0; however, it is usually acidic and varies from 5.5 to 6.5. Diets rich in animal protein and acidic fruits like cranberries can increase urinary acidity, while consumption of citrate causes alkaline urine. The inability of the kidney to acidify urine below 5.5 despite overnight fasting and acid loading is diagnostic of renal tubular acidosis (RTA). In type I RTA the serum is acidic while the urine is alkaline as a result of inadequate proton excretion in the distal tubules, while in type II RTA, excessive bicarbonate secretion from the proximal renal tubular epithelial cells initially leads to alkaline urine, which becomes acidic over time as the filtered load of bicarbonate reduces. The pH of urine is altered with urinary tract infections and calculus disease. Uric acid stones are more often seen with acidic urine. Urea splitting organisms like Proteus are associated with alkaline urine and can lead to the aggregation of triple phosphate crystals which lead to the formation of staghorn calculi.

(g) **Hematuria:** The presence of more than three red blood cells (RBCs) per high power field in two out of three urine samples is diagnostic of hematuria as per the American Urological Association.[3] Hematuria of glomerular origin is characterized by the presence in urine of significant proteinuria, dysmorphic RBCs and RBC casts. Non glomerular hematuria could occur from the kidney in conditions such as acute tubulointerstitial nephritis and certain renovascular or metabolic disorders. However, such conditions can be identified by the presence of proteinuria without associated dysmorphic RBCs or hematuria. Urological causes of hematuria do not have significant proteinuria, dysmorphic RBCs or RBC casts, while they may lead to the presence of clots in the urine.[4,5] Hematuria could be functional following exercise such as long distance running or fever. In such cases, a repeat urine examination after 48 to 72 hours would reveal complete clearance of hematuria.

(h) **Proteinuria:** The normal range for proteinuria is less than 150 mg/day (< 20 mg/dl), of which albumin is usually < 30 mg/day. The rest is made up by Tamm-Horsfall protein, filtered serum globulins and broken down proteins from enzymes etc. Proteinuria above this level is invariably pathological except in cases of functional proteinuria as happens in fever, post tonic clonic seizures, post exercise, hyperthyroidism and orthostatic proteinuria, which is usually transient and self-remitting.

Persistent proteinuria could be due to glomerular causes, tubular causes or overflow. Tubular proteinuria is usually restricted to < 2 gm/day and usually results from the inability of tubular cells to metabolise or reabsorb filtered protein. Overflow proteinuria occurs when low molecular weight proteins like globulins are filtered in quantities much larger than the absorptive and metabolic capacity of the tubules. Glomerular proteinuria on the other hand, predominantly consists of albumin and is the most common type. Protein in urine can be detected by simple heating test, in which case the protein coagulates. Quantitative assessment of proteinuria is usually done by nephelometry.

(i) **Glycosuria:** It may be due to either the inability of the kidney to reabsorb filtered glucose in the proximal tubule despite normal plasma glucose concentration or an overflow scenario related to high plasma glucose concentrations overwhelming the capacity of the renal tubules to reabsorb glucose. In patients with normal kidney function, significant glycosuria does not generally occur until the plasma glucose concentration exceeds 180 mg/dl. When glycosuria occurs with a normal plasma glucose, a primary defect of proximal tubule reabsorption needs to be examined. Benedict's solution can be used to test for the presence of glucose in urine.

(j) **Ketonuria:** Dipsticks detect acetoacetic acid alone, and hence remain positive despite the ketonemia subsiding in blood because of continued conversion of beta hydroxybutyrate to acetoacetate. Poorly controlled diabetes, starvation, excessive alcohol use are common causes of ketonuria.

(k) **Nitrites:** Nitrites are normally not present in urine. However, many Gram negative and a few Gram positive bacteria convert urinary nitrates to nitrites. Hence when positive, it suggests the presence of significant numbers ($>10^5$/ml) of bacteria in the urine. Unfortunately, it is a more specific than sensitive test, and a negative test does not rule out infection with confidence.[6] False negative reports can be obtained in case of non nitrite producing bacteria causing infection and patients consuming low nitrate diets. Exposure of the dipstick to air for prolonged duration leads to false positive results, with almost 75% of all sticks giving false positive reports if kept exposed to room air for more than two weeks.[7]

(l) **Leukocyte esterase:** This enzyme is found in neutrophils which are expected to be present in patients with UTI. However, in the absence of leukocyte esterase activity and persistent pyuria on microscopy with sterile cultures, other causes of pyuria such as Chlamydia and Ureaplasma urealyticum infection should be considered besides balanitis, urethritis, tuberculosis, bladder tumors, viral infections, nephrolithiasis, foreign bodies, exercise, glomerulonephritis, and corticosteroid and cyclophosphamide use.

(m) **Bilirubin:** Unconjugated bilirubin being albumin bound and water insoluble is not excreted in urine. Normally bilirubin in not present in urine. Conjugated bilirubin which is excreted via bile into the gut is converted into urobilinogen by bacterial proteases. More than 80% of this is excreted in the feces as stercobilin, while about 2% enters the circulation where it is oxidized to urobilin and excreted by the kidney (also called urochromes) which gives the urine its characteristic colour. Urobilinogen is a colourless substance and is usually excreted in urine in conditions where its production increases, like hemolysis and acute hepatitis. Urobilinogen is detected by its reaction with Ehrlich's reagent, which contains para-dimethylaminobenzaldehyde to give a pink-red color. In conditions which lead to obstructive jaundice lead to a decline in the amount of urobilinogen in the gut, while at the same time increasing the amount of conjugated bilirubin in the blood which then enters the urine, giving the typical appearance of high coloured urine with clay coloured stools.

Microscopic Analysis

10 to 15 ml aliquot of fresh urine sample is centrifuged at 1500 to 3000 rpm for five minutes. The supernatant is decanted and the left over sediment is then taken into a pipette. One drop of this sediment is placed on a glass slide and a cover slip placed on it. The specimen is now ready for observation under the microscope. The following structures can be seen/looked for:

(a) **Cells:** Transitional epithelial cells are usually seen. The presence of squamous cells suggests contamination. Leukocytes are usually seen in normal urine samples, upto 2/hpf in male and upto 5/hpf in females. RBCs can be seen under higher magnification. Upto three RBCs per high power field is considered normal. The presence of dysmorphic RBCs usually indicates a glomerular pathology. However, the quantum of dysmorphism in a urine sample to confirm the presence of glomerular etiology with confidence is widely variable in literature, with reports varying between 20% to 75% of all RBCs seen.[8-10] Dysmorphic RBCs are typically erythrocytes with odd shapes created due to their transit across the glomerular filtration barrier and are best identified under phase contrast microscopy.

(b) **Casts:** Casts are formed by the coagulation of the Tamm-Horsfall protein in the distal tubules during periods of low urine flow, stasis, excessive urinary concentration or very low urine pH. They trap whatever material is present in the distal tubule at that time and hence are representative of the location of the urinary tract where the injury has occurred. The various types of casts and their causes are summarised in Table 2.2.

(c) **Crystals:** Formed from the crystallisation of solutes which are present in the urine in appropriate conditions, crystals could be seen in the urine of normal individuals while certain crystals are pathognomonic of disease states. Crystals of uric acid, calcium oxalate, calcium phosphate, triple phosphate and calcium bicarbonate are seen in normal urine. While crystals of bilirubin, cholesterol, cysteine, leucine, tyrosine and drugs like sulfa, indinavir, acyclovir etc. are usually pathological. Triple phosphate crystals could be seen in UTI with proteus species and can suggest the formation of a stage horn calculus. Uric acid crystals which are rhomboid in shape and yellowish in colour can be seen in urate nephropathy and urate nephrolilthiasis. Dumbbell shaped monohydrate crystals of calcium oxalate can be seen in ethylene glycol toxicity.

Table 2.2: Various types of urinary casts and their causes

Type of cast	Contents	Cause of cast
Hyaline (Most common)	Mucoproteins	Pyelonephritis, chronic renal disease Could be a normal finding in dehydrated individuals
Granular (second most common)	Broken down cellular material	Chronic kidney disease, acute tubular necrosis
RBC	RBCs	Glomerulonephritis, post exertional, renal infarction, infective endocarditis
Leukocyte	WBCs	Pyelonephritis, glomerulonephritis, interstitial nephritis
Epithelial	Desquamated renal tubular cells	Acute tubular necrosis, interstitial nephritis, eclampsia, nephritic syndrome, allograft rejection, heavy metal ingestion
Waxy	Waxy	Advanced renal disease
Fatty	Lipid-laden tubular cells	Nephrotic syndrome, hypothyroidism
Broad	Various cells	End stage renal disease (ESRD)
Pigment	Hemoglobin, myoglobin, bilirubin, certain drugs	Hemolysis, rhabdomyolysis, conjugate hyperbilirubinemia, ingestion of drugs which colour the urine

Causes of false positive and false negative results with urine dipstick testing (Table 2.3).

The accuracy of urinalysis in the detection of renal disease (Table 2.4).

Table 2.3: Causes of false positive and false negative results with urine dipstic testing

Type of test	False positive	False negative
Specific gravity	Dextran solutions, iodinated radiocontrast, proteinuria	Alkaline urine
Protein	Alkaline or concentrated urine, phenazopyridine, quaternary ammonia compounds	Non albumin proteinuria, Acidic or dilute urine
Bilirubin	Phenazopyridine	Chlorpromazine, selenium
Blood	Dehydration, exercise, hemoglobinuria, menstrual blood, myoglobinuria	Captopril, concentrated urine, pH < 5.1, proteinuria, vitamin C
Glucose	Ketones, levodopa	Concentrated urine, uric acid, vitamin C
Ketones	Concentrated urine, pH < 5.1, Mesna Phenolphthalein, Levodopa	Delay in sample testing
Leukocyte esterase	Sample contamination	Concentrated urine, glycosuria, ketonuria, proteinuria, drugs like Vitamin C, Nitrofurantoin, Cephalexin, Tetracycline, Gentamicin
Nitrites	Exposure of dipstick to air, contamination of sample, phenazopyridine	Concentrated urine, elevated urobilinogen levels, nitrate reductase-negative bacteria, pH < 6.0, vitamin C

Table 2.4: The accuracy of urinalysis in the detection of disease

Condition	Result	Sensitivity	Specificity
Microscopic Hematuria	≥ 1+ Blood	91 – 100%	65 – 99%
Significant proteinuria	≥ 3+ protein	96%	87%
Culture positive UTI	Leukocyte Esterase +	72 – 97%	41 – 86%
	Nitrites +	19 – 48%	92 – 100%
	Both Leucocyte esterase and nitrites	46 – 100%	42 – 98%
	≥ 3+ protein	63 – 83%	50 – 53%
	≥ 1+ Blood	68 – 92%	42 – 46%
	>5 WBCs/hpf	90 – 96%	47 – 50%
	>5 RBCs/hpf	18 – 44%	88 – 89%

Commonly Encountered Urinary Abnormalities

(a) Dysmorphic red blood cells, RBC casts, and proteinuria is suggestive of a proliferative glomerular disease.

(b) Heavy proteinuria with oval fat bodies, lipid-laden casts, and absent or minimal hematuria is indicative of nonproliferative glomerular diseases including severe diabetic nephropathy.

(c) Presence of granular and/or epithelial cell casts with or without free renal tubular epithelial cells is strongly suggestive of acute tubular necrosis (ATN).

(d) Isolated pyuria is usually indicative of bacterial urinary tract infection.

References

1. Simerville JA, Maxted WC, Pahira JJ. Urinalysis: A comprehensive review. Am Fam Physician 2005 Mar 15, 71(6):1153-62.
2. Lifshitz E, Kramer L. Outpatient urine culture: Does collection technique matter? Arch Intern Med 2000; 160:2537-40.
3. Grossfeld GD, Litwin MS, Wolf JS, Hricak H, Shuler CL, Agerter DC, *et al.* Evaluation of asymptomatic microscopic hematuria in adults: The American Urological Association best practice policy – Part I: Definition, detection, prevalence and etiology. Urology 2001;57:599-603.
4. Grossfeld GD, Litwin MS, Wolf JS Jr, Hricak H, Shuler CL, Agerter DC, *et al.* Evaluation of asymptomatic microscopic hematuria in adults: The American Urological Association best practice policy – Part II: Patient evaluation, cytology, voided markers, imaging, cystoscopy, nephrology evaluation and follow-up. Urology 2001;57:604-10.
5. Ahmed Z, Lee J. Asymptomatic urinary abnormalities. Hematuria and proteinuria. Med Clin North Am 1997;81: 641-52.

6. Pels RJ, Bor DH, Woolhandler S, Himmelstein DU, Lawrence RS. Dipstick urinalysis screening of asymptomatic adults for urinary tract disorders for Bacteriuria. JAMA 1989;262:1221-24.
7. Gallagher EJ, Schwartz E, Weinstein RS. Performance characteristics of urine dipsticks stored in open containers. Am J Emerg Med 1990;8:121-23.
8. Pollock C, Liu PL, Györy AZ, Grigg R, Gallery ED, Caterson R, Ibels L, Mahony J, Waugh D. Dysmorphism of urinary red blood cells–value in diagnosis. Kidney Int 1989;36(6): 1045-49.
9. Gyory AZ, Kesson AM, Talbot JM. Microscopy of urine—now you see it, now you don't. Am Heart J 1980;99:537-38.
10. Shichiri M, Oowada A, Nishio Y, Tomita K, Shiquai T. Use of autoanalyser to examine urinary red cell morphology in the diagnosis of glomerular hematuria. Lancet 1986; 2:781-82.

CHAPTER 3

An Adult Patient with Nephrotic Syndrome

Praveen Kumar Etta[1], Narayan Prasad[2]

[1] Consultant, Nephrologist, Virinchi Hospitals, Hyderabad

[2] Professor and Head Nephrology, Department of Nephrology and Renal Transplantation, Sanjay Gandhi Postgraduate Institute of Medical Sciences, Lucknow

CASE

56 years old male, with no previous comorbidities presented with complaints of swelling feet for last 2 months duration, which gradually increased over last 7 days along with exertional shortness of breath. There was history of passing frothy urine, however there was no dysuria or hematuria. Over last 3 days, his urine output was also decreasing. On exam, he was edematous with pedal edema, BP 150/90 mm Hg, no pallor. He had bilateral pleural effusion as well. Lab evaluation revealed Hb 13 gm/dl, urine analysis showed 3+ proteinuria with no active sediments. 24-hour urine protein was 7 gm. Blood urea 50 mg/dl, serum creatinine 1.1 mg/dl, serum protein 4.2 gm/dl with albumin 1.9 gm/dl. Serum cholesterol 402 mg/dl. USG KUB showed bilateral normal sized kidney. With a diagnosis of nephrotic syndrome, renal biopsy was done, which showed evidence of membranous glomerulopathy (MGN) with staining for PLA2R positive. Secondary causes of MGN were ruled out.

Introduction

Proteinuria is a common urinary finding in adults. Massive proteinuria is most often glomerular in origin, comprising predominantly albumin. Glomerular diseases can manifest in a variety of ways like asymptomatic urinary abnormalities, nephrotic syndrome (NS), nephritic syndrome and renal dysfunction progressing to end-stage renal disease. A practical approach to an adult patient with NS is presented here.

Definitions

The 'nephrotic syndrome' (NS) refers to a distinct constellation of clinical and laboratory features characterized by heavy proteinuria [urine protein excretion of more than 3.5 g/day or random urine protein-to-creatinine ratio (UPr/Cr) of more than 3.0 g/g], hypoalbuminemia (serum albumin less than 3.5 g/dl), peripheral edema, hyperlipidemia, lipiduria, and usually a bland urine sediment. However, not all persons with this range of proteinuria are labeled as NS. In contrast, 'nephritic syndrome' is characterized by sub-nephrotic proteinuria, hematuria (gross or microscopic), hypertension, oliguria, sometimes leading to renal insufficiency with urine analysis showing leukocytes, dysmorphic red blood cells (RBC), acanthocytes and RBC casts. But many a times, these features may overlap in a variety of primary and secondary glomerular diseases leading to so-called 'nephritic-nephrotic syndrome'. Hence the clinical approach and evaluation of a suspected glomerulonephritis (GN) should follow an algorithm. A suggested algorithm for the clinical approach to adult NS is presented in Figure 3.1.

Overflow proteinuria is associated with increased production and filtration of abnormal low molecular weight proteins (e.g., light chains in multiple myeloma) that exceeds the reabsorption capacity of the proximal tubule. This can be easily identified by discordance between urine sulphosalicylic acid (SSA) testing or 24-hour urine protein and dipstick testing (where SSA is strongly positive and dipstick negative or low positive). This suggests the presence of non-albumin proteinuria.

Causes of Nephrotic Syndrome in Adults

NS may occur in association with a variety of primary (a disease specific to kidneys) and systemic diseases. The most common primary glomerular diseases leading to NS in adults are Membranous glomerulonephritis (MGN), Focal segmental glomerulosclerosis (FSGS), and Minimal change disease (MCD). FSGS is the most common cause in African-Americans and in Hispanics; while MGN is the most common in Caucasians. Up to 30% of NS in adults are due to systemic diseases like diabetes mellitus, infections, collagen vascular disorders, amyloidosis or paraproteinemias. Diabetes mellitus is the most common secondary cause of NS (Table 3.1).

Primary glomerular disorders usually present with acute onset of NS. Secondary cause for proteinuria can be suspected if there is slowly increasing proteinuria, non-nephrotic range, with absence of edema and hypoalbuminemia even when proteinuria is massive. Isolated heavy proteinuria without edema or other

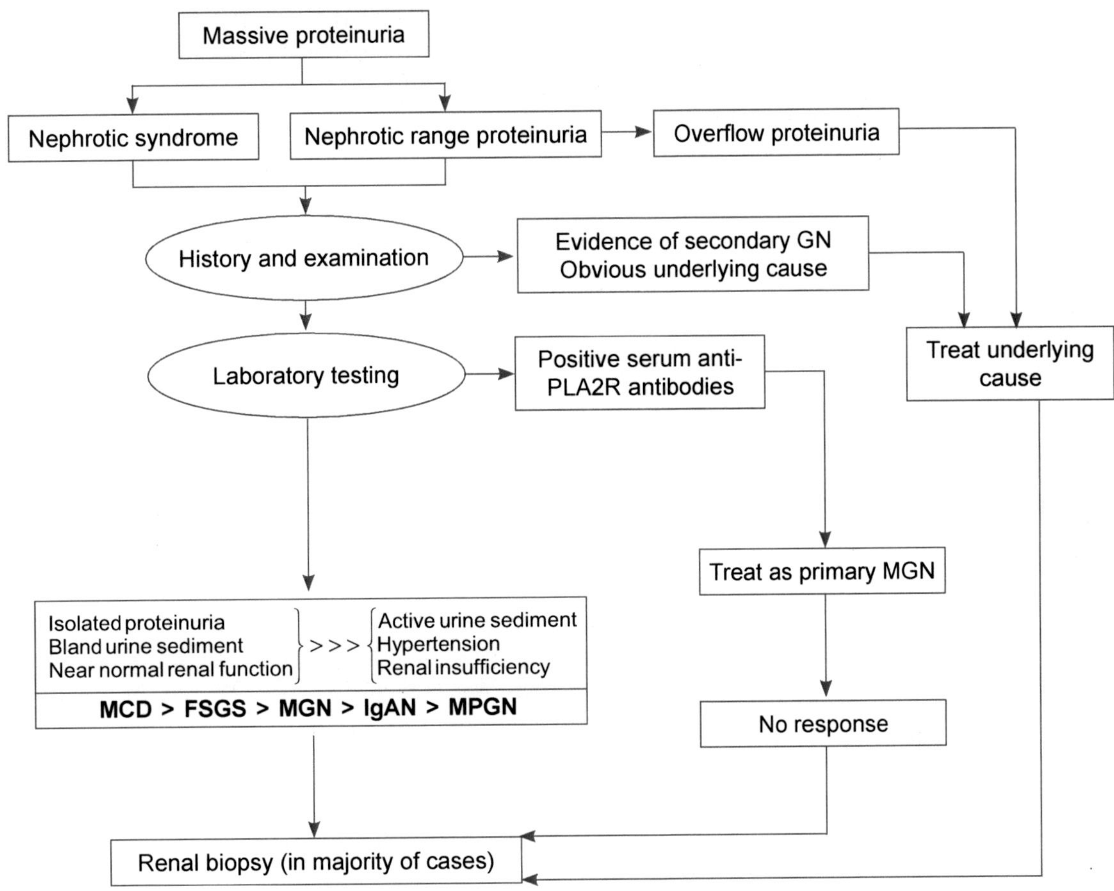

Figure 3.1: A suggested algorithm for the clinical approach to adult nephrotic syndrome

GN: Glomerulonephritis; MCD: Minimal change disease; FSGS: Focal segmental glomerulosclerosis; MGN: Membranous glomerulonephritis; IgAN: IgA nephropathy; MPGN: Membranoproliferative glomerulonephritis; PLA2R: Phospholipase A2 receptor

Table 3.1: Common causes of nephrotic syndrome in adults
• **Primary glomerulopathies** Membranous glomerulonephritis (MGN), Focal segmental glomerulosclerosis (FSGS), Minimal change disease (MCD), Membranoproliferative glomerulonephritis (MPGN), C3 glomerulopathy, IgA nephropathy (IgAN)
• **Secondary glomerular diseases** Diabetic nephropathy, Collagen vascular disorders (e.g., lupus nephritis), Amyloidosis, Preeclampsia, Infection (e.g., HIV, hepatitis B and C, poststreptococcal illness, syphilis, malaria and endocarditis), Solid organ malignancy, Lymphoma, Multiple myeloma
• **Drug induced** NSAIDs, Heroin, Gold, Penicillamine, Lithium, Heavy metals
• **Genetic or congenital** Alport syndrome, Nail-patella syndrome, Fabry's disease

features of the NS is more likely to be due to secondary FSGS.

Clinical Approach to Adult Onset Nephrotic Syndrome

Important clues in the history and examination are given in Table 3.2.

Table 3.2: History and physical examination
Age of onset of NS
Morbid obesity
Frothy urine
Edema–peripheral or periorbital edema, ascites, pleural or pericardial effusion, anasarca
Degree and duration of proteinuria
Rate of progression of proteinuria
Hematuria
Hypertension
Raised JVP
Azotemia
Dyslipidemia, Xanthelasma, Eruptive xanthoma
Leukonychia, Muehrcke's lines of finger nails
Treatment history and responsiveness/relapses
Exposure to drugs/toxins
Non-renal organ involvement – skin, musculoskeletal, pulmonary, GI tract, neurological, ocular, ENT
Systemic diseases leading to secondary NS – infection, collagen vascular disorders, malignancy
Family history
Assess for complications – deep vein/renal vein thrombosis, infections

Proper history and systemic examination can give clues to etiology of NS (e.g., hematuria, hypertension and renal insufficiency are more common in FSGS as compared to MCD; steroid resistance in a patient with presumed MCD should raise suspicion about FSGS).

Laboratory Tests

Laboratory tests required for diagnosis are given in Table 3.3.

Table 3.3: Laboratory test

Basic tests (for all cases)
Complete hemogram
Serum urea, creatinine, electrolytes, eGFR
Serum total protein, albumin
Lipid profile
Complete urine examination
24-hour urine protein level or Spot UPr/Cr ratio
Renal ultrasonography
Special tests (selected based on clinical suspicion)
Chest radiograph
ESR, CRP
Fasting blood glucose, HbA1c
Serum calcium, phosphorus, uric acid
Complement pathway analysis (complement C3 and C4)
ANA, Anti ds-DNA
APLA
Anti-PLA2R antibody
C and P – ANCA (IF)
PR3 and MPO – ANCA (ELISA)
ASO titer
Anti-GBM antibody
Hepatits-B and C, HIV
VDRL test
Blood culture
Serum cryoglobulins, Rheumatoid factor
LDH
SPEP, UPEP, SFLC, SIFE, urine for Bence-Jones proteins
Genetic studies

eGFR: Estimated glomerular filtration rate; UPr/Cr: Urine protein to creatinine ratio; ESR: Erythrocyte sedimentation rate; CRP: C-reactive protein; ANA: Antinuclear antibody; APLA: Antiphospholipid antibody; Anti-PLA2R: Anti-phospholipase A_2 receptor; ANCA: Antineutrophil cytoplasmic autoantibody; ASO: Antistreptolysin O; LDH: Lactate dehydrogenase; SPEP: Serum protein electrophoresis; UPEP: Urine protein electrophoresis; SFLC: Serum free light chain assay; SIFE: Serum immunofixation electrophoresis.

Urine Dipstick Analysis

It semiquantitatively measures the urine protein concentration. The results are graded as negative (less than 10 mg per dl), trace (10 to 20 mg per dl), 1+ (30 mg per dl), 2+ (100 mg per dl), 3+ (300 mg per dl) or 4+ (1,000 mg per dl). This method preferentially detects albumin.

Urine Microscopy

Microscopic analysis of urinary sediment is helpful. MCD usually has bland urine sediment. Active urine sediment (leukocytes, dysmorphic RBC and RBC casts) usually indicates a form of proliferative glomerulopathy, which can be mesangial proliferation, endocapillary hypercellularity or extracapillary proliferation (crescents). MPGN, IgAN, infection related GN (IRGN) can present with heavy proteinuria associated with 'nephritic' type of urinalysis with hematuria and cellular casts (nephritic-nephrotic picture). Lipiduria is identified by the fatty casts, free fat or oval fat bodies (within sloughed tubular cells). Fat droplets have a characteristic 'Maltese cross' appearance under polarized light.

The Sulfosalicylic Acid (SSA) Test

In SSA test, the degree of turbidity provides a semiquantitative method of estimating proteinuria. The advantage of this easily performed test is its greater sensitivity for proteins such as Bence Jones. The SSA method requires a few milliliters of freshly voided, centrifuged urine. An equal amount of 3% SSA is added to that specimen. Turbidity will result from protein concentrations as low as 4 mg/dl.

Urine Protein Quantification

24-hour urinary protein estimation: The patient should be instructed to discard the first morning void; a specimen of all subsequent voidings should be collected, including the first morning void on the second day. The urinary creatinine concentration should be included in the 24-hour measurement to determine the adequacy of the specimen.

An alternative to the 24-hour urine specimen is the UPr/Cr ratio determined in a random urine specimen. The spot UPr/Cr ratio correlates closely with daily protein excretion in g/1.73 m^2 BSA, except in patients whose creatinine generation varies greatly from 1g/day.

Genetic Studies

An increasing number of monogenetic defects have been found to cause neonatal or childhood NS, most of which affect genes critical to podocyte function. Mutations are increasingly being found in older patients with NS. The precise role of genetic screening in adults remains ill-defined. But it is reasonable to screen selected patients with the availability of next-generation sequencing.

Ultrasonography

It shows kidney sizes, shape and echogenicity. Individuals with a single kidney may prone to secondary FSGS. Solitary kidney is also a relative contraindication to kidney biopsy. Increased renal echogenicity is consistent with intrarenal fibrosis. Enlarged kidneys are sometimes seen in NS associated with diabetes, amyloid disease, myeloma HIV infection.

Other Tests

Serum complement levels may be useful in differentiating the underlying etiology of GN; complement levels are typically normal in anti-GBM disease and pauci-immune GN but low in immune complex-mediated GN (with the exception of IgAN). Low levels of complement C3 with normal C4 is found in few cases of IRGN, hemolytic uremic syndrome (HUS) and dense deposit disease (DDD). Low levels of both C3 and C4 are found in lupus nephritis, cryoglobulinemia and MPGN type 1.

Phospholipase A_2 receptor (PLA_2 R) is a cell surface transmembrane receptor expressed on the surface of podocytes. 70% of patients with idiopathic MGN have autoantibodies directed against PLA_2 R. Levels of this antibody have a strong correlation with clinical disease activity and thus help in monitoring disease activity and treatment efficacy. During treatment, the levels of the antibodies generally decline before remission of proteinuria.

ANCA mediated pauci-immune GN and anti-GBM diseases usually present as rapidly progressive GN, but can rarely result in massive proteinuria. Plasma cell dyscrasias can lead to proteinuria from amyloidosis, monoclonal immunoglobulin (Ig) deposition disease (MIDD), immunotactoid glomerulopathy, proliferative glomerulonephritis with monoclonal IgG deposits (PGNMID) and cryoglobulinemic GN.

Kidney Biopsy

In children, almost all cases of NS are due to MCD; therefore, they are empirically treated and perform a renal biopsy only if the patient is unresponsive to treatment. In adults, MCD is relatively uncommon; NS is more etiologically heterogenous compared to children and patients usually require a renal biopsy for definitive diagnosis as history, physical examination and laboratory evaluation are often not useful for differentiating the underlying cause. It also establishes the pathologic subtype of glomerular disease, helps to assess disease activity and to guide treatment decisions.

Kidney biopsy may be deferred in certain patients of adult NS like:

- Obvious underlying etiology (e.g., longstanding diabetes with progressive proteinuria).
- Less invasive, non-renal tissue biopsy establishes diagnosis (e.g., fat pad biopsy in amyloidosis).
- Positive anti-PLA2R antibody (indicates primary MGN).
- Clinically diagnosed thrombotic microangiopathy.
- Positive ANCA, anti-GBM.

However, renal biopsy may still provide important clues to disease activity and chronicity in most of these situations.

Renal Biopsy Features of Few Important Diseases

MCD: LM shows either normal glomeruli or reveals only mild mesangial cell proliferation. IF typically shows no evidence of immune complex deposition. EM characteristically shows diffuse effacement of podocyte foot processes.

FSGS: It is characterized by the presence in some but not all glomeruli, segmental areas of mesangial collapse and sclerosis. Sampling error can easily lead to misclassification of a patient with FSGS as having MCD. Perihilar variant of FSGS is characteristic of hyperfiltration injury (secondary FSGS), but does not rule out idiopathic FSGS. Degree of podocyte foot process effacement on EM is a sensitive and specific test to differentiate idiopathic from secondary FSGS.

MGN: It is characterised by basement membrane thickening with little or no cellular proliferation or infiltration, and the presence of electron dense deposits across the GBM.

Complications

The complications of NS include protein malnutrition, hypovolemia, acute kidney injury, thromboembolism [deep vein thrombosis (DVT), renal vein thrombosis (RVT), pulmonary embolism (PE)], increased susceptibility to infections, hyperlipidemia and accelerated atherosclerosis.

Suggested Reading

1. Canetta PA, Radhakrishnan J. The Evidence-Based Approach to Adult-Onset Idiopathic Nephrotic Syndrome. Front Pediatr 2015;3:78.
2. Kodner C. Nephrotic syndrome in adults: Diagnosis and management. Am Fam Physician 2009;80:1129-34.
3. Hull RP, Goldsmith DJ. Nephrotic syndrome in adults. BMJ 2008;336:1185-89.

CHAPTER

4 A Child with Nephrotic Syndrome

Aditi Sinha

Associate Professor, Division of Nephrology, Department of Pediatrics
All India Institute of Medical Sciences, New Delhi

CASE 1

A 3-year-old boy is brought to the outpatient clinic with puffiness over eyes for the last ten days and swelling over feet and abdomen associated with decrease in urine output for three days. Blood investigations are as follows: Urea: 44 mg/dl, creatinine 0.3 mg/dl, sodium 140 mEq/l, potassium 3.8 mEq/l, albumin 1.4 g/dl, total cholesterol 190 mg/dl, hemoglobin 11 g/dl, total leukocyte count 8900/mm^3 and platelet count 315 × 10^3/mm^3. Urinalysis suggests 3+ proteinuria and no sediment.

This chapter describes briefly the current view on the pathogenesis, evaluation and principles of management of idiopathic nephrotic syndrome of childhood, including both steroid sensitive and steroid resistant forms of the disease.

What is Definition of Nephrotic Syndrome?

Nephrotic syndrome is characterized by heavy proteinuria, hypoalbuminemia (serum albumin <2.5 g/dl), hyperlipidemia (serum cholesterol >200 mg/dl) and edema. Most cases (>90%) are idiopathic; a secondary cause, *e.g.*, amyloidosis, systemic lupus, Henoch-Schönlein purpura, IgA nephropathy, and infection with human immunodeficiency virus, hepatitis B and C is rare. The condition is rare, with an incidence of 1·15 to 16·9 per 100000 children.

Most (>80-85%) children with idiopathic nephrotic syndrome have disease that is 'sensitive' to therapy with oral corticosteroids. While some children have no relapses (15-20%) or 1-2 relapses a year (20-25%), about 40-50% patients show frequent relapses, while 5-10% each shows resistance at onset (initial steroid resistance) or during a relapse after initial steroid responsiveness (late steroid resistance) (Table 4.1). The prognosis in steroid sensitive disease is overall favorable, in contrast to patients with steroid resistance, of whom a significant proportion progress to end stage renal disease.

Table 4.1: Important definitions to clarify course of nephrotic syndrome
Remission: Urine albumin nil or trace (or proteinuria <4 mg/m^2/hr or Spot urine protein/creatinine ratio <0.2 mg/mg) for 3 consecutive in morning urine
Relapse: Urine albumin 3+ or 4+ (or proteinuria >40 mg/m^2/hr or spot protein: Creatinine ratio >2 mg/mg) for 3 consecutive morning specimens, having been in remission previously
Frequent relapses: Two or more relapses in initial six months or more than three relapses in any twelve months
Steroid dependence: Two consecutive relapses when on alternate day steroids or within 14 days of its discontinuation
Steroid resistance: Absence of remission despite therapy with daily prednisolone at a dose of 2 mg/kg or 60 mg/m^2 for ≥ 4 weeks

How to Evaluate a Child with Nephrotic Syndrome?

Patients typically present at 2-5 years of age with progressive edema, initially periorbital and noticed in the morning. There may be an antecedent infection. Urine appears frothy or foamy; output may be reduced. Abdominal pain is usually attributed to mesenteric ischemia but may be secondary to bacterial peritonitis.

Evaluation of a patient with suspected nephrotic syndrome includes history and physical examination, with particular attention to secondary etiology, prior therapies, edema, blood pressure, anthropometry and evidence of infections. Heavy (nephrotic range) proteinuria is presence of 3-4+ (300-1000 mg/dl) urine protein by dipstick on early morning urine for 3 consecutive days, a spot urine protein/creatinine ratio more than 2 mg/mg, or protein excretion more than 40 mg/m^2 per hour on a timed sample. A precise quantitative assessment of proteinuria is not necessary.

Urinalysis may occasionally show some red cells; persistent microscopic hematuria and/or presence of casts raises suspicion of proliferative glomerulonephritis.

Decreased serum albumin and elevated levels of cholesterol are expected. Complete blood counts and blood levels of urea and creatinine are within range.

Any Additional Evaluation Required?

Further testing is usually not necessary unless an alternative diagnosis is suspected based on history or examination. Patients with gross or persistent microscopic hematuria require testing for levels of complement C3, antistreptolysin O to rule out acute glomerulonephritis; additional testing with antinuclear antibodies may be warranted if systemic lupus erythematosus is suspected. Tuberculin test is used to rule out tuberculosis exposure before initiating corticosteroids. Universal screening for hepatitis B (surface antigen) and or urinary tract (urine culture) infection is not essential.

What are Indications for Kidney Biopsy?

Most children with idiopathic nephrotic syndrome do not require kidney biopsy. Renal biopsy is required at the onset of nephrotic syndrome in situations where a cause other than minimal change disease is suspected, such as:

1. Age at onset <9 months or >16 years.
2. Gross hematuria.
3. Persistent microscopic hematuria or low serum C3.
4. Renal failure not attributable to hypovolemia.
5. Suspected secondary cause.
6. Sustained severe hypertension.
7. A renal biopsy is considered later if the diagnosis of steroid resistance is made, or therapy with calcineurin inhibitors is planned.

What are the Common Underlying Histopathology?

Most (>80%) patients with childhood onset nephrotic syndrome show insignificant glomerular abnormalities on light microscopy, termed minimal change disease (MCD; Fig. 4.1a). Immunofluorescence examination does not show glomerular deposits of immunoglobulins or complement. Electron microscopy reveals effacement of podocytes foot processes with disruption and disorganization of actin filaments. Histology shows minimal change disease (MCD) and focal segmental glomerulosclerosis (FSGS; Fig. 4.1b) in 30-40% patients each with steroid resistance, and mesangioproliferative glomerulonephritis (MesPGN, characterized by the presence of >3 cells per mesangial lobule) in a small group. Based on location of sclerosis, subtypes of FSGS include tip, cellular or perihilar lesions and alterations not otherwise specified. Some syndromic forms of steroid resistance, such as Denys Drash syndrome, are associated with diffuse mesangial sclerosis. About 15% patients, chiefly older children, show membranoproliferative glomerulonephritis, membranous nephropathy, IgA nephropathy or amyloidosis.

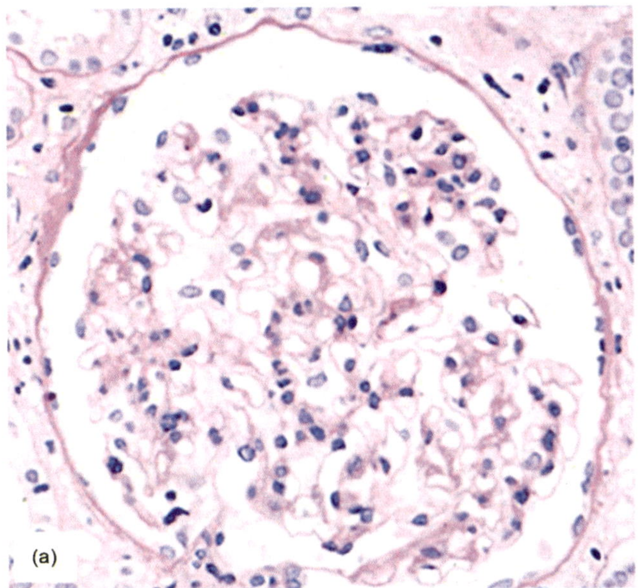

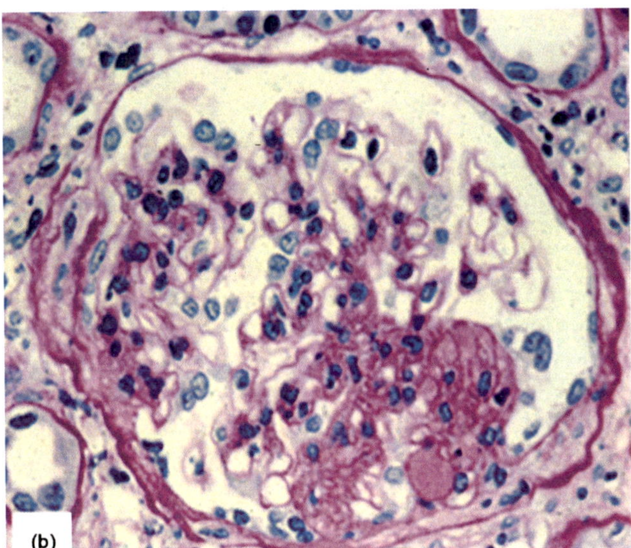

Figure 4.1: (a) Light microscopy (hematoxylin and eosin staining) in a 4-year-old girl with initial steroid resistance shows no abnormality, typical of minimal change disease (b) Light microscopy (hematoxylin and eosin staining) in a 12-year-old boy with initial steroid resistant nephrotic syndrome shows segmental sclerosis and enlarged glomerulus, indicating focal segmental glomerulosclerosis

What is Pathogenesis of Nephrotic Syndrome?

Nephrotic syndrome is considered a T cell disorder, where these cells release cytokine(s) that act on the glomeruli to induce an increase in permeability to plasma proteins. While initial evidence supported an imbalance of T helper responses, recent studies suggest alterations in both innate and adaptive immune responses. It has been speculated that immune dysfunction might result in production of an, as yet uncharacterized, circulating factor that affects the slit diaphragm, resulting in selective proteinuria. A number of proteins, including interleukin 13, soluble urokinase plasminogen activator receptor, urinary CD 80 and vascular endothelial growth factor, have been proposed to play critical role in pathogenesis. An imbalance of Th17 and T regulatory responses is suggested to allow CD 80 activation on podocytes, and/or promote T helper responses. Cross talk between B cells and T helper cells is indicated by a response to rituximab, an anti-B cell agent. An important role of the podocyte in causing proteinuria is suggested by the observation of mutations in key podocyte proteins in steroid resistant nephrotic syndrome and experimental evidence of altered podocyte signaling and cytoskeletal organization. However, there is no unifying hypothesis that combines the immunological perturbations with abnormal function at the level of the slit diaphragm.

STEROID SENSITIVE NEPHROTIC SYNDROME

How Should one Manage the Initial Episode?

Available evidence suggests that adequacy of treatment of the initial episode, both in terms of dose and duration of corticosteroids, is an important determinant of the long term course. Only prednisolone and prednisone are of proven benefit in the treatment of proteinuria in nephrotic syndrome. Other agents such as deflazacort, methylprednisolone, dexamethasone, betamethasone, triamcinolone or hydrocortisone should not be used for this purpose. Prednisolone is administered after meals to reduce its gastrointestinal side effects; concomitant administration of antacids is not required, unless there is gastrointestinal intolerance.

Prednisolone is given at a dose of 2 mg/kg or 60 mg/m^2 per day (maximum 60 mg) in single or divided doses for 6 weeks, followed by 1.5 mg/kg or 40 mg/m^2 (maximum 40 mg) as a single morning dose on alternate days for the next 6 weeks. Therapy with corticosteroids is then stopped. Evidence from controlled studies suggests that initial steroid therapy (for 8-12 weeks or longer) is associated with reduced risk for relapses than shorter regimens. Recent studies indicate that further prolongation of initial therapy may not be useful in ameliorating disease course; they also carry risk of steroid adverse effects. Based on available evidence and opinion from recent prospective studies, initial therapy with oral steroids is recommended for 12 weeks.

Most children with the initial episode enter remission within 7-10 days. Failure to achieve remission of proteinuria despite treatment with prednisolone in adequate doses for 4-8 weeks is labeled as steroid resistant nephrotic syndrome.

What is the Therapy for Relapse?

Relapses are often triggered by minor infections. Symptomatic therapy of infectious illness often results in remission of 1+/2+ proteinuria. However, persistence of 3+/4+ proteinuria with infections requires the aforementioned therapy for relapse. Prednisolone is given at a dose of 2 mg/kg/day (single or divided doses) until urine protein is trace or nil for three consecutive days *(remission)*, and subsequently as a single morning dose of 1.5 mg/kg on alternate days for 4 weeks, and then discontinued. Treatment for a relapse usually lasts for 5 to 6 weeks. In case the patient is not in remission despite two weeks treatment with daily prednisolone, the treatment is extended for 2 more weeks. Patients showing no remission despite 4 weeks' treatment with daily prednisolone should be switched to alternate day therapy and referred for evaluation for steroid resistance.

The subsequent management of a patient with steroid sensitive nephrotic syndrome depends on the course of the illness, as is described below.

Infrequent Relapses

Patients suffering from three or fewer relapses a year should receive treatment for each disease relapse as described above, i.e., prednisolone at 2 mg/kg/day (single or divided doses) until remission, followed by the same agent given in a single morning dose of 1.5 mg/kg on alternate days for 4 weeks. Therapy is then discontinued.

CASE 2

A 10-year-old girl with steroid dependent nephrotic syndrome has had three relapses on therapy with prednisolone at 0.5 mg/kg on alternate days for the past 12 months. The girl is stunted, cushingoid and hypertensive, and has bilateral subcapsular cataract. Which of the following options would be the most appropriate therapeutic strategy?

- Levamisole on alternate days.
- Oral cyclophosphamide.
- Mycophenolate mofetil.

Frequent Relapses and Steroid Dependence

Patients with frequent relapses require prolonged treatment in order to maintain disease remission. The strategies used to maintain remission in such patients are summarized below and in Table 4.2.

Table 4.2: Corticosteroid-sparing agents in frequently relapsing and steroid dependent nephrotic syndrome

Drug	Levamisole	Cyclophosphamide	MMF	Cyclosporine	Tacrolimus	Rituximab
Dose	2-2.5 mg/kg on alternate days	2-2.5 mg/kg daily	600-1200 mg/m^2 or 20-23 mg/kg daily	4-5 mg/kg day	0.1-0.2 mg/kg/day	375 mg/m^2
Duration	12-36 months	8-12 weeks (cumulative dose to not exceed 168 mg/kg)	12-36 months	12-30 months	12-30 months	2 doses a week apart
Concomitant prednisolone dose	0.25-0.5 mg/kg on alternate days; may be discontinued	1 mg/kg alternate days during therapy; rapidly taper and discontinued after therapy	0.25-0.5 mg/kg on alternate days; may be discontinued	Tapered and discontinued	Tapered and discontinued	Tapered and discontinued
Adverse effects	*Rare:* Flu-like symptoms, neutropenia, hepatotoxicity, seizures; rash	*Common:* Leukopenia *Rare* (more with IV): Alopecia, vomiting, hemorrhagic cystitis *Prolonged therapy:* Gonadal toxicity, malignancy	*Uncommon:* Abdominal discomfort; diarrhea; leukopenia	*Common:* Acute and chronic nephrotoxicity; hirsutism, gum hypertrophy; hypertension; hypercholesterolemia	*Common:* Acute and chronic nephrotoxicity; hyperglycemia; headache; seizures; hypomagnesemia, diarrhea	*Uncommon:* Infusion related (chills, rigors, fever, rash, hypotension, bronchospasm, anaphylaxis); acute lung injury; leukopenia
Monitoring	TLC and DLC q 3-4 months	TLC, DLC q 2 weeks	TLC, DLC q 2 months Avoid outside meals	Serum creatinine, potassium, lipids and trough drug levels (titrate to 80-150 ng/ml); kidney biopsy if use prolonged (>2-3 years)	Serum creatinine, potassium, glucose and trough drug levels (titrate to 4-7 ng/ml); kidney biopsy if use prolonged (>2-3 years)	Infuse over 4-6 hours under close monitoring of vital signs and for reactions
Precautions	None	Increase fluid intake Avoid at night; void often	Take in two divided doses, not with meals			Premedicate with hydrocortisone, paracetamol and diphenhydramine

DLC: Differential leukocyte count; IV: Intravenous; MMF: Mycophenolate mofetil; TLC: Total leukocyte count.

Long Term, Alternate Day Steroids

Following treatment of a relapse, prednisolone is gradually tapered to maintain the patient in remission on alternate day dose of 0.5-0.7 mg/kg, which is given for 9-18 months. This strategy is effective in maintaining remission in a proportion of patients. Relapses are often triggered by upper respiratory tract or other minor infections. Recent studies suggest that the risk of relapses might be reduced if prednisolone is administered daily for 5-7 days at the onset of infection in patients receiving corticosteroids on alternate days.

Steroid Sparing Agents

The additional of an alternative agent is recommended if: (i) the prednisolone threshold required for maintaining remission is higher than 0.5-0.7 mg/kg on alternate days; or (ii) features of corticosteroid toxicity (growth failure, hypertension and cataract) appear. The agents used, usually in successive order, are summarized in Table 4.2. Relapses during therapy with alternative agents are treated with daily steroids, followed by tapering doses of prednisolone on alternate days. The occurrence of frequent relapses despite use of alternative agent is an indication for use of another agent.

Levamisole is moderately effective in reducing relapse rates and steroid requirement in some patients with frequent relapses and steroid dependence. While therapy with prednisolone may be discontinued in some patients, many patients continue to require a small dose, given on alternate days. In contrast cyclophosphamide has a strong steroid sparing potential with remission lasting 9-18 months following therapy, allowing discontinuation of steroids. However, while therapy with levamisole is overall safe, cyclophosphamide therapy requires close supervision, especially for leukopenia. The latter is preferred in patients with: (a) Significant steroid toxicity; (b) Severe relapses with episodes of hypovolemia, life threatening infections or thrombosis, and (c) Poor compliance or difficult follow-up. Children older than 7-8 years, those with frequent relapses and lower steroid threshold do better than those who are younger and have steroid dependence or high steroid threshold. Chlorambucil, an alkylating agent like cyclophosphamide, is effective in patients with frequent relapses but is no longer recommended to be used due to significant toxicity and a low margin of safety.

In the last two decades, mycophenolate mofetil (MMF) has been used effectively in managing patients with relapsing nephrotic syndrome. Prolonged therapy results in reduced relapse rates and significant steroid sparing. While MMF is overall safe, therapy requires monitoring for gastrointestinal symptoms and leukopenia.

Therapy with oral calcineurin inhibitors or intravenous rituximab is indicated in patients with frequent relapses or steroid dependence that fail to benefit with levamisole, cyclophosphamide and/or MMF or show features of steroid toxicity while relapsing on therapy with these agents. These agents have strong steroid sparing potential, with steroid discontinuation achieved in a majority of patients. However, their administration requires close supervision for toxicity (Table 4.2) and should only be administered under the supervision of a pediatric nephrologist. Therapy with one of these agents is indicated in patients with steroid dependence that fail to benefit with milder agents. In view of a significant long-term risk of nephrotoxicity, a renal biopsy is done after 2-3 years of continuous therapy with calcineurin inhibitors.

CASE 3

A 2-year-old boy appears markedly cushingoid and has periorbital puffiness. Available documents suggest that he was diagnosed with nephrotic syndrome two months back and was given on daily (2 mg/kg for 6 weeks) followed by alternate day (1.5 mg/kg for 2 weeks) steroids since diagnosis. Urine protein tested in the clinic is 3+ by dipstick. Serum albumin was 2.2 g/dl two weeks back.

- Is this steroid resistant nephrotic syndrome or a relapse on alternate days?
- What evaluation is necessary? What is the role of genetics testing?
- How is response assessed and how long does it take to achieve it?
- How is the condition managed?

What is Steroid Resistant Nephrotic Syndrome (SRNS)?

A patient is considered to have SRNS if there is lack of remission despite treatment with prednisolone, at a dose of 2 mg/kg/day (60 mg/m^2/day) for at least 4 weeks. This definition is based on knowledge that 95% patients with steroid sensitive nephrotic syndrome achieve remission within 4 weeks of steroid therapy, and that longer therapies are associated with high incidence of medication related adverse effects. However, a small proportion of patients remit on alternate days therapy with prednisolone in the subsequent 2-3 weeks. Initial resistance is defined by the lack of remission at the first episode of nephrotic syndrome and late resistance is considered in patients who are steroid sensitive initially, but show steroid resistance during a subsequent relapse. Care is taken to exclude systemic infections (e.g., peritonitis, cellulitis, respiratory tract infections), which might result in persistent proteinuria.

How to Evaluate SRNS?

Baseline assessment of renal function, blood levels of albumin and cholesterol and quantification of urinary protein loss (spot urine protein to creatinine ratio in young children; 24-hour protein excretion in older children) guides future evaluation of response to therapy. Patients should be evaluated for hepatitis B and C virus infection before further immunosuppression; particularly in patients in whom renal histology shows membranous nephropathy or membranoproliferative glomerulonephritis, or in those having deranged liver functions.

What is the Role of Kidney Biopsy?

All children diagnosed with SRNS (initial or late) should undergo renal biopsy before instituting specific treatment. While patients with minimal change disease show a satisfactory response to therapy, the presence of FSGS with chronic tubulointerstitial changes is associated with less satisfactory outcomes. The diagnosis of entities such as membranoproliferative glomerulonephritis, IgA or membranous nephropathy, and rarely, Alport syndrome or amyloidosis is important, since their management differs from idiopathic MCD and FSGS.

What Genetic Testing is Recommended?

About 10-20% patients with familial and sporadic SRNS might carry homozygous or compound heterozygous mutations in any of over 75 genes encoding various podocyte proteins, that constitute the slit diaphragm or the podocyte cytoskeleton (NPHS1, NPHS2, CD2AP, TRCP6 and ACTN4); others are expressed in the glomerular basement membrane (LAMB2) or mitochondria (COQ2), or encode transcription factors necessary for normal development (WT1, LMX1B). These patients usually do not respond to immunosuppression, progress rapidly to end stage renal disease and, unlike non-genetic FSGS (which recurs after transplantation in 30%), do not have recurrence. Patients with syndromic forms usually have onset in early childhood; e.g., Denys Drash (diffuse mesangial sclerosis, Wilms tumor), Frasier (FSGS, male pseudohermaphroditism, gonadoblastoma) and Pierson (diffuse mesangial sclerosis, microcoria, neurological abnormalities) syndromes. While mutations are present in 10-20% patients with sporadic steroid resistance, their incidence is higher in patients with initial than late steroid resistance. Patients who do not respond to standard therapy for steroid resistant nephrotic syndrome (see later) are likely to harbor mutations. Mutations are detected in a high proportion of patients with familial steroid resistant nephrotic syndrome and in 70-80% patients with congenital nephrotic syndrome (onset at <3 months of age). Hence, mutational analysis should be offered to patients with: (i) Congenital nephrotic syndrome (onset below 3 months of age); (ii) Family history of SRNS; (iii) Sporadic initial steroid resistance that does not respond to therapy with cyclophosphamide or calcineurin inhibitors; (iv) Syndromic forms; and (v) Girls with initial steroid resistance (for WT1). Given the expanding spectrum of disease causing genes, next generation sequencing focusing on known genes (currently >75) followed by Sanger validation is a practical approach to diagnostic testing. However, novel variations require careful review of pathogenicity prediction.

How to Manage SRNS?

The management of patients with SRNS is difficult, with patients showing a variable response to immunosuppression, adverse effects of prolonged therapy and risk of progressive renal damage. Patients with idiopathic SRNS secondary to minimal change disease, FSGS or mesangioproliferative glomerulonephritis are treated similarly. Patients with minimal change disease demonstrate relatively high rates of remission and better prognosis.

The chief factor predicting renal outcome is the response of proteinuria to therapy rather than the renal histology. The aim of therapy in patients is thus to induce and maintain remission of proteinuria, while avoiding medication related adverse effects. Most regimens use a combination of an immunosuppressive agent with prednisolone (given on alternate days) and an angiotensin converting enzyme inhibitor (Table 4.3). Since adverse effects are common, immunosuppressive therapy should be stopped if there is no response after 6 months.

Calcineurin Inhibitors (Cyclosporine or Tacrolimus)

Treatment with calcineurin inhibitors (CNI) is considered 'first line' for patients with steroid resistance. Cyclosporine and tacrolimus are effective in inducing complete or partial remission in 60-80% patients.

Cyclophosphamide (Oral or IV) with Oral or IV Corticosteroids

Oral cyclophosphamide, administered alone or with oral steroids, has poor efficacy in inducing remission. Intravenous (IV) cyclophosphamide has been used, with modest success, either alone or in combination with IV steroids. IV cyclophosphamide, when administered monthly for six doses with tapering doses of alternate day prednisolone, induces remission in 40-50% patients.

Pulses of IV methylprednisolone or dexamethasone in combination with oral cyclophosphamide show moderate efficacy. The risk of steroid toxicity is high, with a significant proportion of patients developing systemic infections, hypertension and electrolyte abnormalities.

Other Agents

Therapies with limited efficacy that have not been tested in large studies include rituximab (anti-CD20 monoclonal antibody), combination of cyclosporine and MMF, abatacept (CTLA-4 agonist), anti-TNF antibodies, ACTH and plasmapheresis. Very recently, LDL apheresis using Liposorber® has been approved by the FDA for patients with refractory FSGS.

Table 4.3: Agents for management of steroid resistant nephrotic syndrome

Agent	Dose	Duration	Efficacy	Adverse effects
Calcineurin inhibitors				
Cyclosporine (CsA)	4-5 mg/kg/day	12-36 months	50-80%	*Common:* Acute and chronic nephrotoxicity; hirsutism and gum hyperplasia (CsA>Tac); hypertension; high cholesterol (CsA>Tac); hyperglycemia (Tac); elevated transaminases; neurotoxicity with headache and seizures (Tac>CsA)
Tacrolimus (Tac)	0.1-0.2 mg/kg/day	12-36 months	70-85%	
Cyclophosphamide				
Intravenous	500-750 mg/m^2	6 pulses	40-50%	Leukopenia; alopecia; nausea and vomiting (IV > oral); gonadal toxicity; hemorrhagic cystitis (IV > oral)
Oral	2-2.5 mg/kg/day	12 weeks	20-25%	
High dose corticosteroids with cyclophosphamide				
Methylprednisolone or Dexamethasone	20-30 mg/kg IV 4-5 mg/kg/day IV 'Pulses' on alternate days × 6; once weekly × 8, fortnightly × 4, monthly × 8, bimonthly × 4 [abbreviated protocols also used]		30-50%	Hypertension, hypokalemia, hyperglycemia, steroid psychosis, systemic infections Side effects of cyclophosphamide therapy and prolonged steroid therapy
Prednisolone	Tapering doses × 18 months* PO			
Cyclophosphamide	2-2.5 mg/kg/day × 12 weeks** PO			

* Prednisolone 1.5 mg/kg on alternate days × 4 weeks; 1.25 mg/kg × 4 weeks; 1 mg/kg × 4 months; 0.5-0.75 mg/kg × 12-18 months
** Cyclophosphamide is administered during weeks 3-15

Adjunctive Therapies

Prednisolone

Prednisolone is a component of all regimens used in therapy of SRNS. It is administered on alternate days at 0.75-1 mg/kg day for 1-3 months, following which the dose is tapered. Prednisolone may be discontinued if there is sustained complete remission for 6-12 months.

Angiotensin Converting Enzyme (ACE) Inhibitors, Angiotensin Receptor Blockers (ARB)

Therapy with angiotensin converting enzyme (ACE) inhibitors (e.g., enalapril 0.3-0.6 mg/kg/day, ramipril 6 mg/m^2/day) is associated with decrease in proteinuria and control of hypertension. Adverse effects include dry cough, hyperkalemia and decline in renal function. The dose of the ACE inhibitor is decreased or therapy discontinued if hyperkalemia develops or the estimated GFR falls below 30 ml/minute/1.73 m^2. ARB (e.g., losartan, valsartan) may be used in case of persistent dry cough with ACE inhibitors, or as add-on therapy to achieve better antiproteinuric effect. Recent meta-analysis indicate that use of the combination is unsafe, increasing the risk of adverse events (hyperkalemia, low GFR) while providing some additional proteinuria reduction.

Monitoring Response to Therapy

Patients should be monitored every month until response to therapy is demonstrated, and then every 2-3 months. *Complete remission* is defined as presence of trace or negative proteinuria (by dipstick) or spot urine protein to creatinine ratio (Up/Uc) <0.2 mg/mg. Patients are considered to be in *partial remission* if they show 1-2+ proteinuria (or Up/Uc between 0.2-2), blood albumin >2.5 g/dl and no edema. *Non-response* is defined as 3-4+ proteinuria (Up/Uc>2), blood albumin <2.5 g/dl or edema. The aim of treatment is the achievement of complete remission, but occurrence of partial remission is also satisfactory. Patients who respond to treatment do so within 6 months; those that fail therapy with one regimen may show response to different agents.

Drug Monitoring

Most agents used in the therapy of SRNS require monitoring for adverse effects (Table 4.3). *Monitoring for drug levels* is recommended when using either cyclosporine or tacrolimus, because individual variations in bioavailability may result in occurrence of either sub-therapeutic or toxic levels. A 12-hour trough level should be estimated about 2 weeks after introduction of therapy, after any dose change, and if suspecting drug toxicity or poor compliance. Trough levels in the range of 80-120 ng/ml for cyclosporine and 4-7 ng/ml for tacrolimus are acceptable.

Examination of renal histology is advised in patients receiving prolonged therapy (2-3 years) with calcineurin inhibitors. Histological features of nephrotoxicity include nodular hyalinosis or striped interstitial fibrosis and tubular atrophy. Prolonged duration of therapy (exceeding 2-3 years) and persistent heavy proteinuria (beyond 30 days) are risk factors for nephrotoxicity. The decision to continue calcineurin inhibitors therapy should be reviewed in presence of these changes.

Duration of Therapy

Consensus is lacking on the optimal duration of treatment with calcineurin inhibitors. Therapy is continued for 2-3 years in patients that show complete or partial remission, followed by the options: (i) taper dose of the medication to the lowest effective dose, and continue for another 1-2 years; (ii) exclude medication-related nephrotoxicity on renal histology and then continue therapy; (iii) switch treatment to a less toxic agent, e.g., mycophenolate mofetil, rituximab.

Recurrence of FSGS After Renal Transplantation

FSGS recurs in 30-50% of children following renal transplantation, leading to graft loss in half of these patients. Risk factors for recurrence include: (i) non-genetic forms of FSGS, (ii) progression to ESRD within 3 years of onset of disease, (iii) mesangial proliferation on the original biopsies; and (iv) nephrectomy of native kidneys prior to transplant. Pre-transplant plasmapheresis is an important preventive strategy. While there is no consensus on optimal therapy of patients with recurrent FSGS, options include: (i) intensive plasmapheresis; (ii) intravenous immunoglobulin (500 mg/kg/dose once a week after pheresis); (iii) rituximab (375 mg/m^2/week for 4 weeks); and (iv) oral cyclophosphamide (2-2.5 mg/kg/day for 3 months) instead of MMF.

What is Congenital Nephrotic Syndrome?

Congenital nephrotic syndrome is defined as the presence of nephrotic syndrome within the first 3 months of life. While inherited defects in genes encoding key podocyte proteins underlie almost 80% cases, rare causes include intrauterine infections and maternal drugs. Genomic sequencing of NPHS1 enables diagnosis of the Finnish nephrotic syndrome. Mutations in other genes (NPHS2, WT1, PLCE and LAMB2) might be important in other cases. A correct diagnosis is important for prognosis, therapy and genetic counseling. Immunosuppression has no role in managing infants with congenital nephrotic syndrome. ACE inhibitors (enalapril 0.2-0.5 mg/kg/day) are effective in reducing proteinuria. Supportive care includes adequate nutrition, supplementation of vitamin D, thyroxine and multivitamins, judicious use of diuretics and regular administration of IV albumin. Progression of end stage renal disease is usual during the first decade of life and parents should be counselled about the need for renal replacement therapy.

SUPPORTIVE CARE AND MANAGEMENT OF COMPLICATIONS

Patients with relapsing steroid sensitive nephrotic syndrome and those with steroid resistant or congenital disease are at risk of various complications resulting from disease or its therapy.

Edema

Daily administration of corticosteroids results in diuresis within 2-4 days; specific therapy for edema is not required in most patients in relapse. Presence of significant edema or anasarca is associated with discomfort and an increased risk of infections, meriting treatment with diuretics.

Edema that does not respond to maximal doses of oral furosemide requires coadministration of a thiazide diuretic (e.g., hydrochlorthiazide, metolazone). If furosemide is used for prolonged duration (>7 days) or in high doses (3-6 mg/kg/day), additional treatment with spironolactone (2-4 mg/kg/day) prevents the occurrence of hypokalemia. Patients with refractory edema should be hospitalized and administered IV furosemide either as bolus injections (1-3 mg/kg/dose, infused over 15-20 minutes) or as continuous infusions (0.1-1 mg/kg/hr), under careful monitoring.

Infusions of albumin (20% albumin, 0.5-1 g/kg, over 2-4 hours), with an IV bolus of furosemide, administered at the end of the infusion, are useful in patients with severe hypoalbuminemia (albumin <1.5 g/dl). The effect of these infusions is transient, necessitating repeat administration in patients with severe edema. Infusion of IV albumin in patients with oliguria can worsen hypertension and may result in pulmonary edema and congestive cardiac failure. Adequacy of urine output must be ensured prior to albumin infusion, and its administration should be avoided in individuals with respiratory distress of any cause.

Abdominal paracentesis might be necessary in patients with refractory severe ascites and respiratory distress, but should be done carefully under aseptic precautions. A daily record of weight and urine output, frequent monitoring of vital signs and daily estimation of electrolytes (hypokalemia, hyponatremia and metabolic alkalosis) are essential. Parents should be instructed to discontinue diuretics if symptoms of hypovolemia (abdominal pain, dizziness) appear, or the child has diarrhea, vomiting or poor oral intake.

Hypovolemia

Hypovolemia may occur during a severe relapse or following administration of diuretics, particularly in children with poor oral intake, diarrhea and vomiting. Features include abdominal pain, lethargy, dizziness and leg cramps, tachycardia, hypotension, delayed capillary refill, low volume pulses, and cool clammy distal extremities. Elevated ratio of blood urea to creatinine, rising hematocrit and low urine sodium and its fractional excretion (<20 mEq/l and 0.2-0.4%, respectively) indicate hypovolemia. Therapy with diuretics should be discontinued. When signs of hypovolemia are absent, an increase in oral fluid intake alone may suffice. With features of hypovolemia, patients require admission and rapid infusion of normal saline (10-20 ml/kg) over 20-30 minutes. Patients who do not respond to two boluses of saline should receive infusion of 5% albumin (10-15 ml/kg) or 20% albumin (0.5-1 g/kg).

Infections

Common infections include peritonitis and cellulitis, which should be treated using appropriate antibiotics. Since varicella may be life-threatening in patients with nephrotic syndrome receiving corticosteroids or other immunosuppressive drugs, these patients should be monitored for complications, during the illness and for 7-10 days afterwards. All patients with varicella must receive oral acyclovir for 7 days; severe illness requires admission and administration of IV acyclovir. Administration of varicella zoster immunoglobulin (in a single dose within 96 hours of exposure), or intravenous immunoglobulin (400 mg/kg, single dose) prevents or lessens the severity of the disease in susceptible individuals exposed to varicella.

Hypertension

Hypertension may be noted at the onset of disease or develop secondarily as a result of high dose steroid therapy. Persistent elevation in blood pressure, refractory to control of edema and decline of corticosteroid dose, merits treatment. An angiotensin converting enzyme inhibitor, enalapril (0.3-0.6 mg/kg/day in 2 divided doses) or ramipril is the medication of choice. The dose is increased to permissible limits in patients with persistent hypertension, while monitoring renal function and levels of potassium. Some patients require additional therapy with calcium channel blockers (e.g., amlodipine) or adrenergic blockers. The target blood pressure is between the 75th and 90th percentile for age, gender and height.

Dyslipidemia

Hyperlipidemia associated with disease relapses does not merit treatment. However, patients with steroid resistant nephrotic syndrome with persistent proteinuria have continued dyslipidemia that is undesirable, and requires treatment with statins. Therapy with HMG CoA reductase inhibitors (e.g., atorvastatin 10-20 mg daily in children >5 years) is recommended in presence of biochemical abnormalities that persist for 3-6 months: total cholesterol >200 mg/dl, LDL cholesterol >130 mg/dl or triglycerides >200 mg/dl.

Thrombosis

Children with nephrotic syndrome are predisposed to venous thromboembolism during relapses, due to multiple reasons including loss of antithrombin III, protein S, and high levels of lipoprotein A, factor V, factor VIII and fibrinogen levels. In addition, low intravascular volume (particularly with aggressive diuretic use, or diarrheal dehydration), immobilization, indwelling vascular catheters and puncture of deep vessels also predispose to thrombosis. Thrombosis should be suspected in patients with hematuria or flank pain (renal vein thrombosis); venous congestion, pain, reduced mobility of limbs (deep vein thrombosis); or seizures, vomiting, altered sensorium and neurological deficits (sagittal sinus or cortical venous thrombosis). Deep vein thrombosis can lead to pulmonary embolism. Diagnosis requires confirmation with ultrasonography, Doppler studies and cranial MRI and MR venography, depending on site of symptoms. Therapy includes the use of low-molecular-weight heparin (subcutaneously) initially, followed by oral anticoagulants for 4-6 months.

Vaccination

The administration of live vaccines (oral polio, varicella) should be deferred until the child is off immunosuppressive medications for at least 4 weeks. If essential, these vaccines may be given to patients receiving alternate day prednisolone at a dose <0.5 mg/kg. The administration of pneumococcal vaccine is desirable. Children should receive the pneumococcal conjugated vaccine, 0.5 ml intramuscularly, in the schedule advised by the Indian Academy of Pediatrics. Above 2 years of age, one dose of the polysaccharide vaccine is administered, two months following one dose of the conjugate vaccine. Children who continue to have relapses of nephrotic syndrome may receive one repeat dose of polysaccharide vaccine 5 years after the primary vaccination. Two doses of varicella vaccine should be administered 4 weeks apart while the child is in remission and off immunosuppressive medications. Injectable polio vaccine should be administered to children with nephrotic syndrome and their siblings; oral polio vaccine should not be given while on immunosuppression.

Nutrition

During remission, children should eat a balanced, nutritious diet without restrictions. If relapses are associated with edema, salt restriction is advised, by curbing the intake of snacks and foods with high salt content. Undue restriction that makes food unpalatable is not required. Patients with persistent or recurrent proteinuria should increase their daily intake of proteins to 2-2.5 g/kg. Increase in physical activity can help achieve desirable body weight in those with cushingoid features or obesity. Patients receiving prolonged therapy with prednisolone (>3 months) should receive supplements of calcium carbonate (250-500 mg) and vitamin D (125-250 IU).

Stress Dose of Steroids

Patients who have received steroids at high doses for more than 2 weeks in the past year are at risk of suppression of the hypothalamo-pituitary-adrenal axis. These children require steroid supplements during surgery, anesthesia or serious infections. Corticosteroids are supplemented, as parenteral hydrocortisone at a dose of 2-4 mg/kg/day, followed by oral prednisolone at 0.3-0.6 mg/kg/day. This is given for the duration of stress and then tapered rapidly.

Parent Education

The management of nephrotic syndrome requires frequent interactions with patients' families to ensure their cooperation in disease management. Parents are explained the natural history of the disease and its outcome, and the expected adverse effects of repeated courses of high dose steroid therapy and other medications. While steroid responsiveness remains the most important prognostic feature, patients with both steroid sensitive and steroid resistant disease require frequent monitoring of clinical course and biochemical response, and timely management of disease- and therapy-related complications in order to enable satisfactory long-term outcomes.

Key Points

- In children, nephrotic syndrome is diagnosed by presence of nephrotic range proteinurea–>50 mg/kg per day and hypoalbuminemia–serum albumin < 3 gm/dl.
- The most common cause of primary idiopathic nephrotic syndrome in children is minimal change disease especially in children < 6 years of age.
- It is characterized by diffuse foot effacement, leading to injury to glomerular filtration barrier.
- Clinical features include edema, which may progress to anasarca. Hypertension and hematuria are uncommon.
- The initial therapy consists of steroids, however, in patients with steroid resistant nephrotic syndrome, renal biopsy is required for pathological diagnosis before starting immunosuppressive therapy.

Suggested Reading

1. Bagga A, Mantan M. Nephrotic syndrome in children. Indian J Med Res 2005;122:13-28.
2. Vasudevan A, Mantan M, Bagga A. Management of edema in nephrotic syndrome. Indian Pediatr 2004;41:787-95.
3. Gulati A, Bagga A. On behalf of the Indian Society of Pediatric Nephrology. Guidelines for management of children with steroid resistant nephrotic syndrome. Indian Pediatr 2009;46:35-47.

4. Indian Society of Pediatric Nephrology. Management of steroid sensitive nephrotic syndrome: Revised guidelines. Indian Pediatr 2008;45:203-14.

5. Noone DG, Iijima K, Parekh R. Idiopathic nephrotic syndrome in children. Lancet 2018;392:61-74.

6. Hodson EM, Wong SC, Willis NS, Craig JC. Interventions for idiopathic steroid-resistant nephrotic syndrome in children. Cochrane Database Syst Rev 2016;10:CD003594.

7. Hodson EM, Hahn D, Craig JC. Corticosteroids for the initial episode of steroid-sensitive nephrotic syndrome. Pediatr Nephrol 2015;30:1043-46.

8. Pravitsitthikul N, Willis NS, Hodson EM, Craig JC. Non-corticosteroid treatment for nephrotic syndrome in children. Cochrane Database Syst Rev 2013;10:CD002290.

9. Lombel R, Gipson DG, Hodson EM. Treatment of steroid-sensitive nephrotic syndrome: New guidelines from KDIGO. Pediatr Nephrol 2013;28:415-26.

CHAPTER

5

A Patient with Plasma Cell Dyscrasia with Renal Dysfunction

Ashish Nandwani[1], **Abhyuday Rana**[2]

[1] *Consultant, Nephrology, Manipal Hospital, New Delhi*

[2] *Associate Consultant, Nephrology, Medanta, The Medicity, Gurugram*

CASE

A 68-year-old male with no previous comorbidity presented to OPD with generalized fatigue, weakness, vague abdominal pain, and outside investigations, showing renal dysfunction. He was in his usual state of health until 3 months before presentation, when he started complaining low backache which was not associated with any strenuous physical work for which he took few tablets of NSAID's. Ten days before presenting to us, he developed generalized weakness, fatigue, poor appetite, and right-sided abdominal pain. He was evaluated by his family doctor and initial laboratory tests revealed a serum creatinine (Scr) level of 10.5 mg/dl (from 1.0 mg/dl 3 months earlier), hypercalcemia (calcium, 13.6 mg/dl), and normal complete blood cell count (hemoglobin, 12.3 g/dl). Urine analysis showed bland sediment and a 24-hour urine protein estimation found proteinuria of 380 mg. He was not on any calcium supplements. His Vitamin D levels were 25 ng/ml, intact PTH level of 12 pg/ml. He was managed with IV fluids with no improvement.

With high suspicion of myeloma disease, with renal dysfunction he was referred to nephrologist. Serum protein electrophoresis (SPEP) and serum immunofixation (IFE) revealed an immunoglobulin G (IgG) κ M spike of 3.6 g/dl. Serum free light chain (FLC) assay showed κ FLC of 1041 mg/dl (reference range, 3.3-19.4 mg/l), λ FLC of 1.0 mg/dl (reference range, 5.7-26.3 mg/l), and serum FLC ratio of 1041 (reference range, 0.26-1.65). A skeletal survey was positive for lytic lesions in lumbar vertebrae. Kidney biopsy was performed, which showed intraluminal fractured casts in the distal tubules. Immunofluorescence microscopy showed that tubular casts stained 3+ for κ light chain and negative for λ light chain. Bone marrow biopsy revealed 35% κ-restricted plasma cells.

He required few sessions of hemodialysis. He was started on weekly anti-plasma cell therapy with bortezomib-dexamethasone (BorD). With this treatment, after 15 days, serum light chains were improving (κ FLC, 116 mg/dl) and had evidence of renal recovery (Scr, 3.2 mg/dl). He became dialysis independent subsequently.

What is Paraproteinemia/Monoclonal Gammopathy?

It refers to the overproduction of a *monoclonal Ig (MIg)* as a result of clonal proliferation of Ig-producing plasma-cells or B lymphocytes. Broadly divided into two main categories:

- Plasma cell dyscrasia.
- B cell lymphoproliferative disorder.

What are Various Types of Plasma Cell Dyscrasia?

- Monoclonal gammopathy of unknown significance (MGUS).
- Monoclonal gammopathy of renal significance (MGRS).
- Smoldering multiple myeloma.
- Multiple myeloma.

What is Incidence and Epidemiology of Multiple Myeloma?

1 to 2% of all cancers and > 17% of hematologic malignancies in US are attributed to multiple myeloma with annual incidence of approx 4 to 5 per 100,000. African americans and blacks from Africa have two to three times more risk of having myeloma disease than that in whites. Median age at diagnosis is 66 years; only 2 percent of patients are younger than 40 years.

Which Clinical and Laboratory Clues Suggest Myeloma as the Cause of Acute Kidney injury (AKI)?

Patient usually have severe bone pain, which is very commonly low back pain with little or no relief from rest or use of analgesics. Myeloma should be ruled out when the patient has severe cytopenia (anemia, thrombocytopenia, or pancytopenia), PTH independent hypercalcemia, recurrent infection (when all Ig classes are reduced), or an increased globulin fraction (reversal of albumin-globulin ratio). Urinalysis can be misleading because the increased urinary excretion of light chains, which is not detected by testing for albumin but can only be detected with total urine protein estimation. In case of unclear cause of AKI one should rule out myeloma disease especially in elderly population.

What are Screening Test for Monoclonal Gammopathy?

The most commonly used screening technique for detection of monoclonal protein is the serum protein electrophoresis (SPEP) and urine protein electrophoresis (UPEP). PEP is quantitative but not capable of fully characterizing the type of monoclonal immunoglobulin. To determine the identity of the monoclonal immunoglobulin (MIg), protein electrophoresis must be performed in conjunction with immunofixation which identifies the monoclonal immunoglobulin. Although Serum immunofixation is not quantative, it is around 10 times more sensitive for immunoglobulins and light chain. UPEP is generally less sensitive than SPEP for immunoglobulin detection. Urine immunofixation can detect low levels of light chains but requires concentrated urine samples.

What are Specific Diagnostic Tests for Paraproteinemias?

Sensitive quantitation of total serum free (unbound) κ-light chain and λ-light chain is useful for clones synthesizing only light chain fragment. Measurement of serum free light chain (FLC) by nephelometry is rapid (hours); more sensitive (1 to 3 mg/l); and, along with an SPE (to determine the presence or a whole Ig component), will diagnose the majority of patients with myeloma, amyloidosis, and other monoclonal immunoglobulin deposition disease (MIDD) and is now the preferred diagnostic test (Table 5.1).

Free light chains are reported in the form of ratio. Normal range for free κ-light chains is 3.3-19.4 mg/l, and normal range for free λ-light chains is 5.7-26.3 mg/l. Thus, the normal free κ to λ ratio is 0.26-1.65. In impaired renal function, the ratio rises to 0.34-3.1 owing to reduced renal clearance.

What is Diagnostic Criteria for Multiple Myeloma?

Clonal bone marrow plasma cells >10% or Biopsy proven bony or extra medullary plasmacytoma

and

1 or more Myeloma defining criteria, i.e., >=1 CRAB feature(s) or >=1 SLiM feature(s).

CRAB Criteria

- Hypercalcemia (>11 mg/dl or > 1 mg/dl above the upper normal limit).
- Renal insufficiency (Creatinine clearance <40 ml/min, or S creatinine >2 mg/dl).
- Anemia (Hb < 10 gm/l or 2 gm/l < than normal).
- Bone lesion (> 1 skeletal lesion on skeletal survey, CT or PET).

In absence of CRAB criteria, SLiM criteria can be used.

S = >60% clonal bone marrow plasma cells.

L i = Serum-free light chain involvement with an involved over uninvolved ratio of greater than 100.

M=> 1 focal lesion (>5 mm each) detected by MRI study.

What are Various Clinical Presentation (Syndromic) of Monoclonal Gammopathy?

These include acute kidney injury, nephrotic range protein, nephrotic-nephritic syndrome, rapidly progressive renal failure and chronic kidney disease (Flowchart 5.1).

How Does Myeloma Cause Acute Kidney Injury?

- Cast nephropathy (Most common).
- Hypercalcemia-induced volume depletion.
- Monoclonal immunoglobulin deposition disease (MIDD).
- Amyloidosis.
- Proximal tubulopathy/Fanconi syndrome.
- Cryoglobulinemia.

Table 5.1: Sensitivity of serum paraprotein testing for multiple myeloma, smoldering myeloma and AL amyloidosis

	Multiple Myeloma	Smoldering Multiple Myeloma	AL Amyloidosis
SPEP	87.6%	94.2%	65.9%
Serum IFE	94.4%	98.4%	73.8%
Serum FLC assay	96.8%	81.2%	88.3%
SPEP and serum FLC	100%	99.5%	94.2%
SPEP, serum IFE and serum FLC assay	100%	100%	97.1%

Note: Based on information in Katzmann *et al.* (Screening panels for detection of monoclonal gammopathies. Clin Chem. 2009; 55 (8): (1517-1522).

Abbreviations: FLC: Free light chain; IFE: Immunofixation; SPEP: Serum protein electrophoresis.

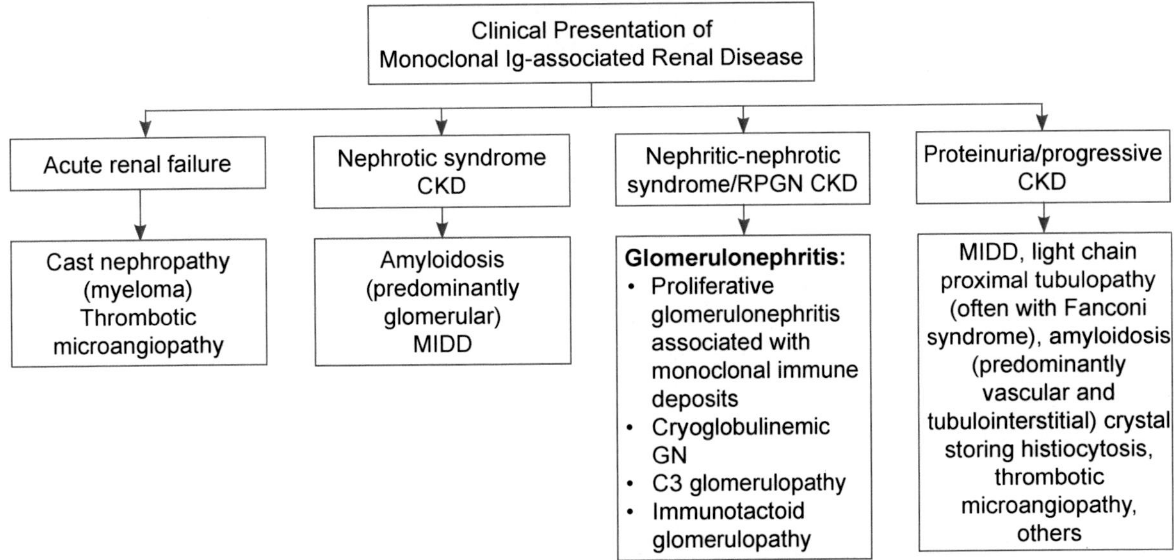

Flowchart 5.1: Various clinical presentation (syndromic) of monoclonal gammopathy
MIDD: Monoclonal immunoglobulin deposition disease; RPGN: Rapidly progressive glomerulonephritis
(Sanjeev Sethi *et al.* J Am Soc Nephrol 2018;29:1810-23)[1]

How does Cast Nephropathy Present?

Acute kidney injury is usually rapid, often occurring within days to weeks. Casts are formed when FLCs bind and precipitate with Tamm-Horsfall protein in the distal nephron. It causes tubular obstruction (typically distal) that elicits an intense immune response, resulting in a giant cell reaction around the casts and interstitial inflammation. Sometimes casts are absent but the interstitial inflammation and fibrosis are present. Kidney injury is principally related to the light chain (LC) component of monoclonal immunoglobulin. Not all LC are toxic, and some patients can excrete large quantities without AKI. Specific molecular variants of the LC molecule form specific forms of kidney injury, such as myeloma cast nephropathy or amyloidosis. It is now recognized by the International Myeloma Working Group as one of the *myeloma defining events* that makes up the CRAB criteria.

What is Role of Bone Marrow in Diagnosis?

Bone marrow is done to confirm marrow involvement by clonally expanded plasma cells and for the determination of cytogenetic abnormalities, which provide important prognostic information regarding treatment and outcome. Bone marrow shows displacement of the normal marrow by plasma cells, which ranges from complete replacement by sheets of tumor cells or as nodular aggregates. The mature plasma cells have eccentric nuclei with increased cytoplasm, and the immature forms are pleomorphic with abnormal nuclear forms. Immunoperoxidase stains show the tumor cells to stain positive with CD138 and a monoclonal LC restriction.

When Should Kidney Biopsy be Done?

In patients with laboratory analysis showing presence of monoclonal Ig and AKI who do not show a prompt response to hydration and the correction of precipitants, a diagnostic kidney biopsy to determine the cause of kidney injury is suggested because of the variability in kidney etiology and the importance of ensuring a correct histologic diagnosis. In patients with an excess of albuminuria rather than the expected LC proteinuria, a biopsy is necessary to establish the presence of amyloidosis or other glomerular disorders associated with LCs. The type and stage of disease, especially the degree of tubular atrophy and interstitial fibrosis influence the choice of chemotherapy and the consideration of adjunctive treatments such as high cut-off (HCO) dialysis. Sometimes, the diagnosis of myeloma is made by the kidney biopsy as the first investigation and subsequently confirmed with protein electrophoresis/immunofixation. Kidney biopsy is also helpful in prognostification of the renal recovery following myeloma therapy.

How do you Treat Myeloma Cast Nephropathy?

Cast nephropathy requires early diagnosis and administration of therapy to prevent permanent kidney damage.

1. First immediate management warrants removal of any precipitant.
   a. Hypercalcemia–Volume expansion.
   b. Dehydration–Volume expansion.
   c. Sepsis – Early goal directed therapy (Antibiotics).
   d. NSAID's–Discontinuation.
2. Removal of Free light chain/Cast–In patients presenting with renal dysfunction, renal recovery is improved with early reduction in serum monoclonal free light chains (FLC).

a. Increase diuresis –>3 litre a day with adequate oral fluids to prevent decrease tubular flow and eventual precipitation of free light chain.

b. Dialysis/Plasmapheresis.

3. Use of chemotherapy (Anti Myeloma Therapy)–to decrease free light chain load. Most successfully accomplished with a 3-drug regimen, of which one should be bortezomib. Cyclophosphamide, thalidomide and doxorubicin are used as second line drugs for myeloma chemotherapy. High dose steroid therapy has cytotoxic as well as anti-inflammatory effects.[2]

What is the Role of Dialysis/Plasmapheresis in Cast Nephropathy?

Plasma exchange (PLEX) was the only extracorporeal technique to remove circulating FLCs until 2005. Multiple studies have been conducted to evaluate its efficacy. Randomized and controlled clinical trials have failed to demonstrate a therapeutic effect of PLEX on renal dysfunction. In 2005, a new generation of HD membranes known as 'high cut-off membranes' (HCO) were launched. It has wide pore size, which enhanced the molecular weight cut-off to ~50-60 kDa. HCO membranes enhance FLC clearance in HD-dependent AKI secondary to cast nephropathy. The advantage of HCO-HD use upon standard of care is still controversial. It must be noted that the International Myeloma Working Group (IMWG), in their 2016 recommendations on myeloma-related renal impairment, has already stated that the current data supports the use of HCO-HD in AKI HD-dependent secondary to cast nephropathy with an evidence grade B. Plasma exchange should be used only in patients with symptoms and signs of hyperviscosity (e.g., in IgA myeloma and Waldenström macroglobulinemia [WM]) when rapid lowering of whole Igs is required to alleviate symptoms.

How does Myeloma Related Amyloidosis Present?

Amyloidosis is characterized by the abnormal deposition of fibrils in extracellular tissues derived from an abnormal protein that is bound to serum amyloid P protein. Three subtypes of Ig related amyloid exist–light chain (AL) amyloidosis–most common (95% of most cases), heavy and light chain (AHL) amyloidosis and heavy chain (AH). Approx ¾th of patients present with proteinuria, half of whom have nephrotic syndrome. Restrictive cardiomyopathy, hepatomegaly (from infiltration), and peripheral neuropathy (carpal tunnel syndrome) are also common presentations. Severe edema, often with anasarca and pleural effusions, is common, and other clinical signs include easy bruising and macroglossia. *Cardiac involvement* is as common as kidney, and the extent of cardiac involvement determines survival, whereas the extent of kidney involvement determines renal survival.

How to Diagnose Immunoglobulin Related Amyloidosis?

Finding of heavy albuminuria and bland urine sediment usually hints towards diagnosis of amyloidosis. Tissue biopsy is required to confirm diagnosis. Choice of tissue includes the rectum, abdominal fat pad, and the bone marrow, and these are biopsied in preference to the kidney. The combination of SPE and serum FLC will be abnormal in 98% of patients with primary amyloidosis. In renal biopsy, glomerular deposits are seen predominantly in the mesangium as amorphous acidophilic deposits, weakly periodic acid–Schiff positive and negative or weakly positive with Silver stain. The classical diagnostic test is the Congo red stain, which shows an orange-red color and apple-green birefringence when examined by polarized microscopy.

How to Treat Patients with Amyloidosis (AL) and What are Outcomes of Treatment Regime?

Therapy requires chemotherapy and/or autologus stem cell transplant (ASCT) to eliminate the plasma cell clone responsible for the disease. Initial treatment with melphalan and prednisone or high-dose dexamethasone had produced limited survival benefit because complete hematologic response was rarely achieved. The introduction of HDM (High dose of melphalan) followed by ASCT increased the complete hematologic response rate to 40%. Melphalan-dexamethasone, CyBorD (Cyclophosphamide + Bortezomib + Dexamethasone), bortezomib melphalan-dexamethasone and, more recently, the anti-CD 38 antibody *daratumumab have improved outcomes*. Median survival with autologous stem cell transplant (ASCT) is nearly 8 years. Achieving a minimum of a hematologic very good partial response is associated with improved overall and renal survival. Some important prognostic markers include patient's age and extent of tissue involvement particularly cardiac involvement have poor prognosis.

What are Important Aspects Associated with Renal Transplant in Patients with Monoclonal Gammopathy?

Patients with myeloma, amyloidosis, or light chain deposition disease (LCDD) are usually old and have multiple comorbidity. Disease remains incurable and has a very high chance of recurrence, hence kidney transplant is rarely considered a viable option in them. Studies have shown favourable outcomes in younger patients with myeloma, after successful induction therapy and ASCT. They may be considered suitable if prolonged disease remission (approximately 3 years) by standard criteria and if normalization of the sFLC ratio are achieved. Vigilant surveillance with regular estimation of sFLC ratio after kidney transplant for disease recurrence is usually continued life long. Few successful cases of kidney transplantation in primary amyloidosis after chemotherapy and ASCT are also reported.

What is Monoclonal Gammopathy of Undetermined Significance (MGUS)?

MGUS is defined as serum M protein (IgG or IgA) < 3 gm/dl and clonal bone marrow plasma cells < 10% and no evidence of end-organ damage (no anemia, lytic bone lesions, hypercalcemia, or kidney disease attributable to the paraprotein). Nearly 3% of individuals older than 70 years have MGUS. About 1% of patients with MGUS progress to symptomatic myeloma each year, so annual follow-up is required. The risk of progression is higher in patients with a higher level of paraprotein (>1.5 gm/dl), non-IgG paraproteins, and an abnormal sFLC ratio at diagnosis.

What is Smoldering Myeloma?

Smoldering myeloma is an intermediate clinical stage of disease between MGUS and myeloma that has a much higher risk of progression to myeloma than MGUS (10% year or more). It is defined serum M protein (IgG or IgA) ≥3 gm/dl or urinary M protein ≥ 500 mg/24 h and/or clonal bone marrow plasma cells 10%-60%, and absence of myeloma defining events or amyloidosis. These group of patients require close monitoring for any evidence of disease progression to myeloma, so that chemotherapy can be instituted at the earliest to prevent organ damage.

What is Monoclonal Gammopathy of Renal Significance (MGRS)?

MGRS is now used to define a group of B cell lymphoproliferative disorders and plasma cell disorders that do not meet criteria for myeloma, WM, or lymphoma/leukemia, yet lead to a histologically defined pattern of kidney injury directly attributable to the paraprotein or LC. The characteristics of MGRS include one or more kidney lesions that are related to the produced monoclonal immunoglobulin. The underlying B cell or plasma cell clone does not cause tumour complications or meet any current haematological criteria for specific therapy. The diagnosis of MGRS-related disease is established by kidney biopsy and immunofluorescence studies to identify the immunoglobulin deposits.

In immunotactoid glomerulonephritis, C3 glomerulopathy and proliferative glomerulonephritis with monoclonal immunoglobulin deposits (PGNMID), MGRS-associated lesions involve only the glomeruli, whereas in light-chain proximal tubulopathy (LCPT), MGRS-associated lesions involve only the proximal tubules. MGRS-associated lesions in cryoglobulinaemia, mainly involve the glomeruli but can also cause intravascular cryoglobulin thrombi or endovasculitis. Immunoglobulin-related amyloidosis and monoclonal immunoglobulin deposition disease (MIDD) usually affect glomeruli, vessels and the tubule-interstitium.[3]

What are Monoclonal Immune Deposition Disease (MIDD)?

It is histologic and clinical variant of MGRS characterized by deposition of MIg along the glomerular and tubular basement membranes. Three histologically distinct disorders:

1. Light chain deposition disease (LCDD), 80%-90% of cases.
2. Heavy chain deposition disease (HCDD).
3. Light and heavy chain deposition disease (LHCDD).
    - Light chain deposition disease (LCDD) also known as Randall's disease is associated with an underlying lymphoproliferative disorder. MIDD is almost always found in patients with LCDD, with approx 60% to 80% meeting criteria for MGRS. Overt multiple myeloma is present in 20% of patients with LCDD. Waldenstrom's macroglobulinemia associated LCDD has been rarely reported. The serum FLC assay result is abnormal in virtually all patients with LCDD. The diagnostic yield for *serum and urine IFE of 64% and 68%*, respectively. Treatment of LCDD uses clone-directed therapy with the goal of achieving hematologic response.
    - Heavy chain deposition disease (HCDD) is rare disorder. The most common involved *heavy chain is IgG* (γ), with even rarer cases showing IgA (α), IgM (μ), or IgD (δ). The pathogenic immunoglobulin in patients with HCDD is *a truncated heavy chain* that is not linked to a light chain. It is to be suspected, when initial IF is negative for MIg (Kappa, Lambda). The yield of paraprotein testing was 60% by SPEP, 80% by serum IFE, 47% by UPEP and 53% by urine IFE. Serum FLC ratio is abnormal in almost all tested patients with HCDD. Treatment of HCDD is directed at the underlying clonal cell disorder.

What are other Uncommon Renal Lesion Associated with Monoclonal Gammopathy? What is Immunotactoid Glomerulopathy?

The other lesion associated with monoclonal gammopathy which usually presents as MGRS include Proliferative Glomerulonephritis with Monoclonal Immunoglobulin deposits, Type I Cryoglobulinemic Glomerulonephritis, Light Chain Proximal Tubulopathy, Monoclonal Gammopathy–Associated C3 Glomerulopathy and Immunotactoid Glomerulopathy.

Immunotactoid Glomerulopathy accounts for <1% of kidney biopsy results. Historically grouped with *fibrillary glomerulonephritis* based on the organized substructure of deposits noted on electron microscopy, the majority of these cases stain for monoclonal immunoglobulin on immunofluorescence microscopy and are associated with underlying clonal disorders. It is characterized by proliferative lesion on LM, IgG deposits on IF, and capillary wall deposits with a microtubular substructure on EM. LM typically shows a membrano-proliferative pattern of injury with variable membranous features. It presents with renal dysfunction, microscopic hematuria, and proteinuria, with the majority of cases having full nephrotic syndrome.[4]

What is POEMS Syndrome?

The POEMS refers to:

- Polyneuropathy.
- Organomegaly.
- Endocrinopathy.
- Monoclonal protein.
- Skin involvement.

It is a paraneoplastic syndrome due to an underlying plasma cell neoplasm. The major criteria for the syndrome are polyradiculoneuropathy, clonal plasma cell disorder, sclerotic bone lesions, elevated vascular endothelial growth factor, and the presence of Castleman disease. Minor features include organomegaly, endocrinopathy, characteristic skin changes, papilledema, extravascular volume overload and thrombocytosis.

What is Waldenstrom Macroglobulinemia (WM) and What are Its Renal Manifestations?

WM is an IgM monoclonal-protein-secreting lymphoid and plasma cell malignancy. It commonly manifests with anemia and fatigue, but it also may cause constitutional symptoms (fever, weight loss), hepatosplenomegaly and lymphadenopathy; and features of hyperviscosity and cryoglobulinemia (rash). The diagnosis requires monoclonal IgM protein and a bone marrow with ≥ 10% lymphoplasmacytic cell infiltration. Usually, the FLC component is kappa only, and urinary kappa LCs can be found in around 70% of cases.

Kidney involvement with WM is uncommon and classic myeloma cast nephropathy is rare. Kidney involvement is glomerular and presents with hematuria/proteinuria, impaired kidney function, and rarely nephrotic syndrome. Histologically it takes the form of an immune-mediated glomerulonephritis with IgM deposition and/or features of cryoglobulinemia with intraglomerular thrombi. Treatment is delayed until patients develop significant end-organ damage or symptoms. Plasma exchange, rituximab, alkylating agents (chlorambucil), and the purine nucleoside analogues (fludarabine, cladribine) alone or in combination can be used.

References

1. The Complexity and Heterogeneity of Monoclonal Immunoglobulin–Associated Renal Diseases, Sanjeev Sethi S. Vincent Rajkumar, Vivette D, D'Agati JASN Jul 2018;29(7)1810-23.
2. Treatment of multiple myeloma with renal involvement: The nephrologist's view Alexandre Fava Clinical Kidney Journal 2018;1-9.
3. The evaluation of monoclonal gammopathy of renal significance: A consensus report of the International Kidney and Monoclonal Gammopathy Research Group, Nelson Leung *et al.* 2019 Nature reviews.
4. Rosner *et al.* American Society of Nephrology Onco-Nephrology Forum. Paraprotein-related kidney disease: Diagnosing and treating monoclonal gbgammopathy of renal signficance. Clin J Am Soc Nephrol 2016;11(12),2280-87. doi:10.2215/CJN.02920316.

CHAPTER

6 A Child with Acute Nephritic Syndrome

Gurinder Kumar[1], Arpana Iyengar[2]

[1] *Pediatric Nephrologist, Sheikh Khalifa Medical City, Abu Dhabi, UAE*

[2] *Professor, Department of Pediatric Nephrology, St John's Medical College Hospital, Bangalore, India*

In this chapter, we will take the examples of three case scenarios to describe and understand the clinical presentations, approach to evaluation and management of acute nephritic syndrome. We would focus on post streptococcal glomerulonephritis which is the most common cause for acute nephritic syndrome in children.

CASE 1

A 7-year-old boy presented with malaise, headache, vomiting and gross hematuria for past 2 days. Parents also noted facial edema and reduced urine output. There was history of fever 3 weeks back and antibiotics were prescribed for 5 days following which fever subsided. Examination revealed an unwell, lethargic child with periorbital edema. BP was 126/90 mm Hg (>95th centile). There was tachycardia, mild tachypnea, no crepitations, no gallop, normal JVP with mild hepatomegaly. Urine analysis revealed protein 2+ and plenty of RBCs. In addition, hemoglobin was 12 gm/dl, platelets 3.25 lakhs/cu mm, sodium 138 mEq/l, potassium 6.2 mEq/l, chloride 108 mEq/l, urea 40 mg/dl, creatinine 0.5 mg/dl and albumin of 2.8 gm/dl.

What are the Key Findings that Helps to Make Diagnosis in this Child?

Firstly, the child has four important renal symptoms of gross hematuria, edema, decreased urine output and hypertension. At this point, it is important to differentiate the clinical manifestations of acute nephritic syndrome from nephrotic syndrome (Table 6.1, Figs. 6.1 to 6.4).

Secondly, it is critical to recognize two life threatening complications namely hypertension (secondary to fluid retention) and hyperkalemia in this child. Thirdly, there is evidence of an infection preceding this illness.

These features suggest that the child is likely to have an acute nephritic syndrome following an infection. It is important to note that the absence of certain clinical

Table 6.1: Nephritic versus Nephrotic syndrome

Nephritic Syndrome	Nephrotic Syndrome
Common age 5-12 years	Common age 1-12 years
Gross hematuria with cola colored urine (Fig. 6.1)	Gross hematuria is unusual. Frothy appearance of urine is common (Fig. 6.2)
Edema is mild and limited to periorbital and pedal edema	Edema is gross and involves ascites and scrotal/labial edema
Hypertension is common	Hypertension is unusual
Proteinuria of variable degree but < 1g/m^2/day	Proteinuria >1 g/m^2/day
Hypoalbuminemia not common	Hypoalbuminemia present
Lipid profile normal	Altered lipid profile
Hyperkalemia common	Hyperkalemia uncommon
Urine microscopy RBC abundant and typically dysmorphic (Fig. 6.3) RBC casts (Fig. 6.4) Lipid elements usually absent	Microscopic hematuria may be seen in 10% of children Absence of cellular casts Free lipid droplets.

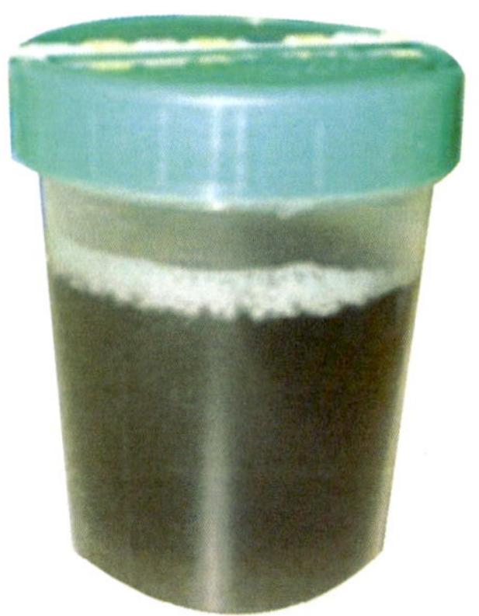
Figure 6.1: Cola colored urine with frothy appearance

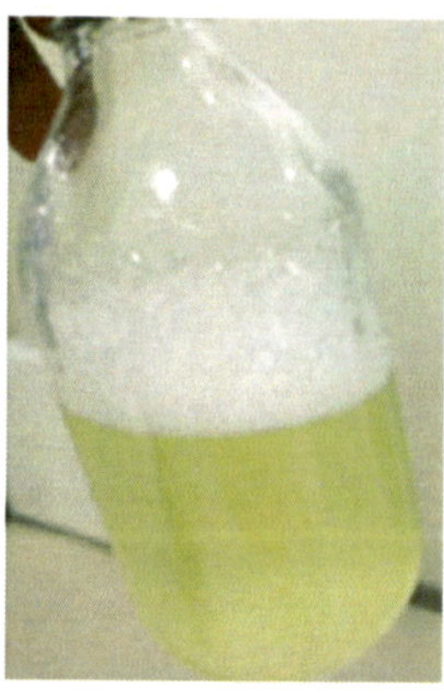
Figure 6.2: Frothy appearance of urine

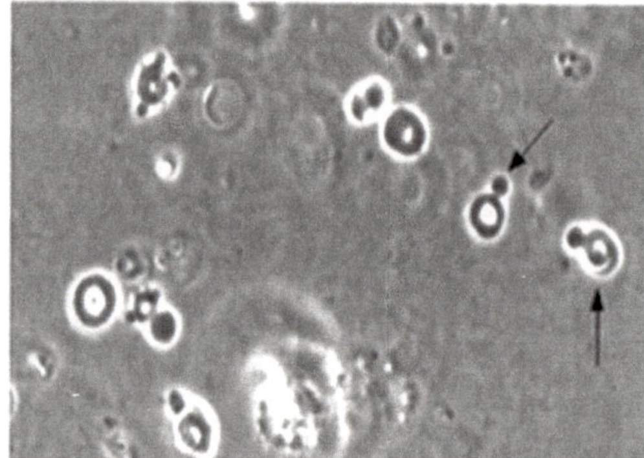
Figure 6.3: Dysmorphic red blood cells

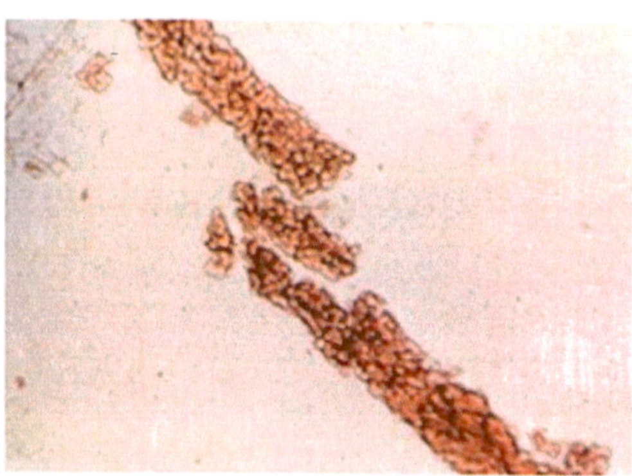
Figure 6.4: Red blood cell cast

features like pallor, rash, joint involvement help us to exclude the possibilities of immune mediated acute nephritic syndrome like lupus nephritis and Henoch-Schönlein purpura (HSP) nephritis. A diagnosis of atypical nephrotic syndrome may be considered (Membranoproliferative glomerulonephritis and IgA nephropathy) in situations where there is significant proteinuria, anasarca in addition to other features of nephritic syndrome. Occasionally, hemolytic uremic syndrome could mimic acute nephritic syndrome with a preceding infection and signs of hypertension, hematuria, edema and decreased urine output. However, the absence of pallor, thrombocytopenia and acute kidney injury can help us rule out this disorder.

What are the Common Infections that Can Cause Acute Nephritic Syndrome?

Acute nephritic syndrome usually follows an infection and hence it may be referred to as post infectious glomerulonephritis or Infection-related glomerulonephritis.

Post infectious glomerulonephritis (PIGN) is an immunologically mediated glomerular injury triggered by bacterial, viral or protozoal infections. The classical example is post streptococcal glomerulonephritis (PSGN) which often manifests a few days to weeks after streptococcal infection. Several infectious agents including non-streptococcal bacteria, viruses, fungi, and parasites can also result in immune mediated glomerular changes that fall within the broad category of infection-related glomerulonephritis. The etiology of acute nephritic syndrome is summarized in Table 6.2.

What is the Underlying Pathogenesis of PSGN?

Post streptococcal glomerulonephritis (PSGN) is the most common cause for acute nephritic syndrome especially in developing countries. The nephritogenic strains of streptococci associated with a respiratory infection are types 1, 3, 4, 12, 25, 49 and the other types 2, 49, 55, 57,

Table 6.2: Infection related etiology of acute nephritic syndrome

Post infection related:

Bacterial: Streptococci (Group A, Streptococcus viridans), Staphylococci (aureus, epidermidis), Pneumococci, Meningococci, Treponema pallidum, Salmonella (typhi and paratyphi), Leptospira, Escherichia coli, Listeria monocytogenes, Mycobacterium leprae, Yersinia enterocolitica, Coxiella burnetti, Brucella abortis, Neisseria spp.

Protozoal: Plasmodium (malariae, falciparum, vivax and ovale), Toxoplasma.

Viral: Hepatitis A, B and C, Cytomegalovirus, Parvovirus, Epstein Barr virus, Coxsackie virus, Echovirus Varicella, Parvovirus B_{19}, Human immunodeficiency virus, Mumps, Influenza and enteric cytopathic human orphan (ECHO) virus.

Fungus: Candida, Histoplasma capsulatum.

Helminthic: Filaria, Schistosoma, Trichinella spiralis, Wuchereria bancrofti.

Active infection related:

Bacterial: Pneumonia, Cellulitis, Abscess, Osteomyelitis, Endocarditis.

Viral: Hepatitis B, Cytomegalovirus, Parvovirus.

60 cause pyoderma. Antibodies bind to the streptococcal antigens planted in the glomerular basement membrane leading to alternative complement pathway activation. Glyceraldehyde phosphate dehydrogenase (also known as nephritis-associated plasmin receptor) and cationic proteinase exotoxin B (SPEB) with its zymogen precursor, have been identified in the basement membrane of PSGN patients.

NAPlr is a glyceraldehyde-3-phosphate dehydrogenase with plasmin-binding capacity, a nephritogenic property that aids circulating immune complex deposition. SPeB is a cationic protease with plasmin-binding properties which is secreted as an exotoxin and localizes to glomeruli in PSGN. Both NAPlr and SPeB activate the alternative complement pathway, resulting in low serum complement levels, and have affinity to plasmin and glomerular proteins. NAPlr and SPeB promote formation of circulating immune complexes which are deposited in sub-endothelium. These nephritogenic antigens can induce glomerular inflammation and local antibody production as depicted in Figure 6.5.

What is the Typical Clinical Course of PSGN?

PSGN affects children between 5 and 12 years of age and is rare below 3 years. Male preponderance (M : F of 2) has been reported. The classical triad includes gross hematuria, hypertension and oliguria. These symptoms can follow a sore throat or pyoderma infection. The latent period is 2 to 4 weeks for pyoderma and 7 to 14 days for sore throat. Subclinical disease (more common) is characterized by microscopic hematuria and normal or mildly increased blood pressure and low C3 levels in asymptomatic patients.

Gross hematuria is typically cola colored and does not persist beyond 1 to 2 weeks. The dark urine of glomerular hematuria reflects the lysis of the RBC membrane while traversing through varying osmolarites across the nephron and conversion of hemoglobin in urine to acid hematin (brownish). Hypertension is seen due to fluid and salt retention following a decrease in GFR and can lead to congestive cardiac failure or hypertensive encephalopathy/crisis. Variable degrees of edema and proteinuria are common. Typically all these features of edema, hypertension, gross hematuria and proteinuria resolve within 2-4 weeks of onset of nephritic syndrome (Fig. 6.6). The biochemical tests namely ASLO titer peaks at 1-4 weeks and complement C3 levels that are reduced resolves to normal levels (80-150 mg/dl) within 6 weeks of illness.

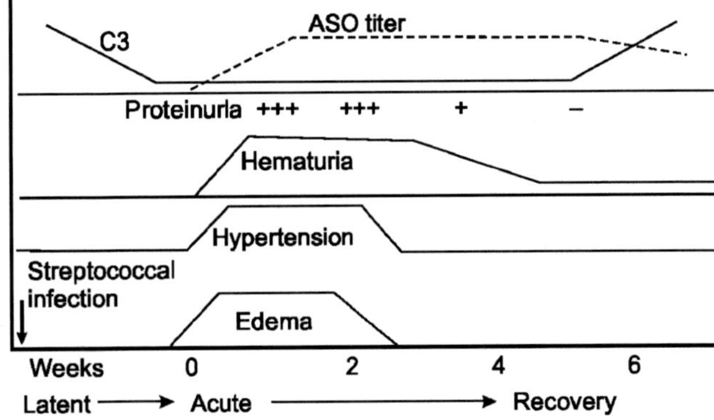

Figure 6.6: Clinical and laboratory manifestations of acute nephritic syndrome over time

What are the Initial Investigations Carried Out in a Child with Suspected Acute Nephritic Syndrome?

The approach to evaluating a child with acute nephritic syndrome is summarized in an algorithm (Fig. 6.7).

- **Complete blood count:** Dilutional anemia may be seen. Low platelets suggest hemolytic uremic syndrome or systemic lupus erythematosus.

Nephritogenic Streptococcus GAPDH (NAPlr)	Nephritogenic Streptococcus GAPDH (SpeB)
↓	↓
Mesangial and GBM binding	Anti SpeB antibodies
↓	↓
Plasmin entrapment and sustained activity Inflammatory reactivity	SpeB and Anti SpeB binding
↓	↓
Immune complex penetration through damaged GBM	Circulating SpeB and anti SpeB deposition In situ SpeB-anti SpeB formation
↓	↓

IMMUNE COMPLEX MEDIATED GLOMERULONEPHRITIS

Figure 6.5: Steps in the pathogenesis of post streptococcal glomerulonephritis (PSGN)
GAPDH: Glyceraldehyde 3-phosphate dehydrogenase; GBM: Glomerular basement membrane

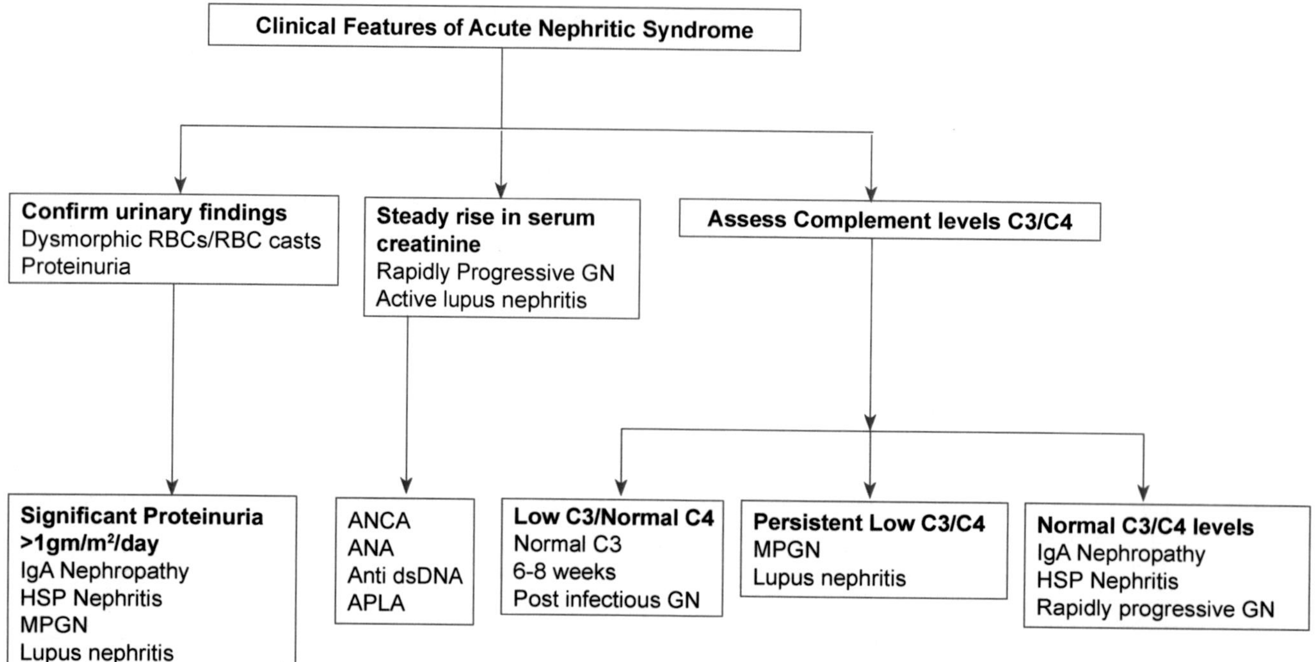

Figure 6.7: Approach to evaluation and diagnosis of acute nephritic syndrome

Abbreviations: PIGN: Post infectious glomerulonephritis; PSGN: Post streptococcal glomerulonephritis; MPGN: Membranoproliferative glomerulonephritis; APLA: Antiphospholipid antibodies; ANCA: Antineutrophilic cytoplasmic antibodies; SLE: Systemic lupus erythematosus.

- **Biochemistry:** The levels of blood urea and creatinine may be elevated to varying degrees or may be normal. Hyperkalemia is common and may be present despite normal renal function. Electrocardiogram should be done to look for changes of hyperkalemia. The initial change is peaking and narrowing of the T-wave, followed by widening of the QRS complex, loss of the P wave, and a sine wave pattern as the QRS complex merges with the T wave.
- **ASLO titer:** ASLO (antistreptolysin O) titer may be elevated (>200 IU OR >333 todd units) in 60 to 80% of the cases and indicates preceding streptococcal infection. The rise begins 1 to 3 weeks after streptococcal infection, peaks in 3 to 5 weeks and then falls in next 6 months. Given the high prevalence of streptococcal infections in general population, rising or subsiding titers are of greater diagnostic value than a single high titer. Streptolysin O is bound to lipids in the skin, preventing any demonstrable ASO elevation in nephritis following pyoderma. The height of antibody response can also be attenuated with antibiotic treatment and streptococcal skin infections frequently fail to elicit a strong ASLO antibody response. ASLO is only a marker of streptococcal infection (current or past) and does not imply or predict the presence of nephritogenic strain infection or PSGN.
- **Anti-DNAse B:** The titers are elevated in pyoderma associated PSGN.
- **Complement levels:** C3 levels are reduced in 90% of the patients. C4 is usually normal. The levels of C3 normalize by 6 to 8 weeks. However persistently low C3 for more than 12 weeks is rare in PSGN and suggests an alternative diagnosis such as lupus nephritis or membranoproliferative glomerulonephritis. CH50 (50% hemolyzing dose of complement), which is a measure of overall complement activity, may be low due to complement consumption. Measurement of complements levels is helpful to limit the differential diagnosis as C3 consumption occurs in PIGN, SLE , MPGN resulting in low levels while C3 levels are normal in IgA nephropathy.
- **Chest X-ray:** Chest X-ray may show cardiomegaly and pulmonary congestion.
- **Renal Biopsy:** The specific indications for renal biopsy in PSGN are depicted in Table 6.3.

Table 6.3: Indications for renal biopsy

- If kidney function fails to recover beyond 7 to 10 days or decline rapidly (rapidly progressive GN) requiring dialysis.
- Low C3 beyond 12 weeks.
- Nephrotic range proteinuria beyond 2 weeks or persistent proteinuria beyond 6 months.
- Systemic features of fever, rash, joint pains etc. suggesting alternate diagnosis such as SLE, MPGN etc.
- Normal levels of C3 suggestive of IgA nephropathy.
- Absence of serologic evidence of streptococcal infection.
- Gross hematuria persisting beyond 3 to 4 weeks.
- Persistent microscopic hematuria beyond 12 to 18 months.

What are the Pathological Findings in PSGN?

There is no correlation between the degree of proteinuria or hematuria and severity of glomerular changes. Renal manifestations may be minimal in the setting of biopsy proven full blown PSGN and prominent hematuria has been noted with essentially normal kidney biopsy. This clinic-pathologic disconnect could be related to the variability in time interval between the onset of symptoms and biopsy. Light microscopy (Fig. 6.8) in acute phase shows diffuse, exudative proliferative glomerulonephritis, with prominent endocapillary proliferation and numerous neutrophils. Glomeruli are diffusely enlarged and lobular pattern is accentuated.

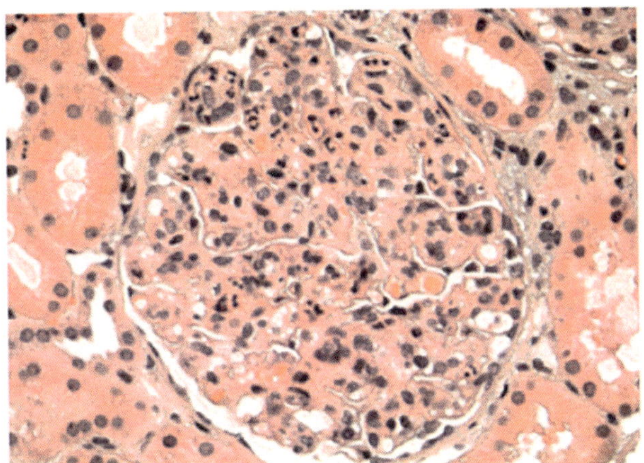

Figure 6.8: Acute post infectious glomerulonephritis. There is diffuse, global exudative proliferation with prominent endocapillary proliferation and numerous neutrophils

Hypercellularity due to proliferation of both endothelial and mesangial cells and early neutrophilic infiltration is seen with obliteration of capillary lumen resulting in glomeruli that appear bloodless.

Immunofluorescence microscopy (Fig. 6.9) shows scattered fine or large granular deposits of IgG and C3 along the glomerular basement membrane and mesangium. Three immunofluorescence patterns have been described: starry sky, garland and mesangial patterns. Starry sky refers to irregularly distributed coarse fluorescence positivity along the glomerular basement membrane while the garland pattern shows thicker and more elongated deposits along the capillary wall and has been associated with worse prognosis.

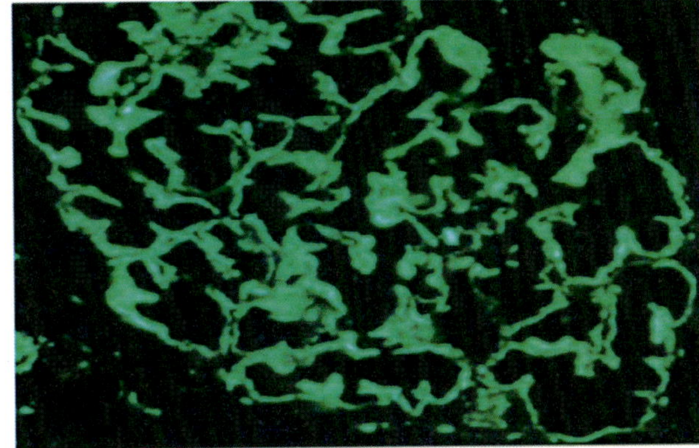

Figure 6.9: Garland pattern of immunofluorescence positivity is shown

Electron microscopy (Fig. 6.10) shows scattered subepithelial deposits or humps overlying the glomerular basement membrane without surrounding basement membrane reaction. These are more striking early and tend to disappear after 6 weeks. The histological abnormalities resolve rapidly and within 6 and 8 weeks there is considerable decrease in exudative changes (Table 6.4). Mild mesangial hypercellularity may persist for 1 to 2 years but eventually disappears.

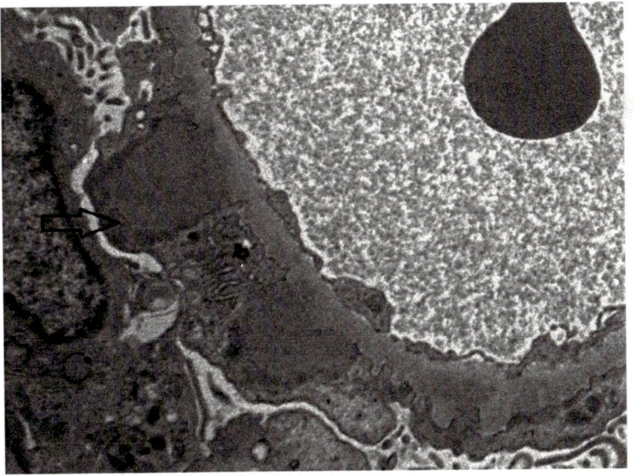

Figure 6.10: Electron microscopy showing a hump shaped sub-epithelial deposit

Table 6.4: Post streptococcal glomerulonephritis: The interval between the onset of renal symptoms and renal biopsy determines the histologic features

	Early Biopsy (<2 weeks)	Typical Features	Late Biopsy (>4-6 weeks)
Clinical Features	Mild albuminuria and hematuria	Acute nephritic syndrome	Persistent microscopic hematuria and/or proteinuria
Light Microscopy	Glomerular endocapillary proliferation: focal/diffuse	Diffuse global proliferation	Mesangial proliferation
Immunofluorescence Microscopy	C3 and IgG; Starry sky pattern	C3 and IgG; starry sky or garland pattern	C3 ± IgG; mesangial pattern
Electron Microscopy	Mesangial, subepithelial (humps), and ± subendothelial deposits	Mesangial, subepithelial (humps), and ± subendothelial deposits	Mesangial and ± rare subepithelial (humps) in the mesangial notch.

How Should one Manage a Child with PSGN?

The child would need to be admitted for close monitoring (Intake/output charts, Vital signs, JVP and BP recording) and the treatment is basically supportive.

- Fluid restriction is required as per urine output. Salt and potassium restricted diet is recommended.
- **Hypertension:** In most cases, fluid and salt restriction is sufficient to prevent edema and hypertension. Loop diuretics are indicated if there is circulatory congestion. Hypertension usually has a good response to diuretic therapy. Furosemide 1-2 mg per kg per day may be given with monitoring of urine output and weight. Particular caution is needed for patients with severe azotemia because of risk of furosemide ototoxicity. Salt intake should be limited to less than 1 g/day.

  If hypertension persists, calcium channel blockers and vasodilators are next safe options.

  Angiotensin-converting-enzyme inhibitors and angiotensin receptor antagonists should be avoided.

  In case of hypertensive emergency or urgency, oral agents like nifedipine or intravenous agents such as nitroprusside, nicardipine or labetalol may be used. There is no role for anticonvulsants in a child who has had seizures secondary to hypertensive crisis.
- **Hyperkalemia:** Hyperkalemia in acute glomerulonephritis occurs due to transient hyporeninemic hypoaldosteronism and improves spontaneously with resolution of the glomerulonephritis. It may occur in patients with normal GFR. Hence, an ECG should be done in all cases to look for tall peaked T waves which need urgent intervention. Potassium restriction along with loop diuretics as standard approach to reduce hyperkalemia is indicated.
- **Antibiotics:** Obtain throat cultures from family members and close contacts. Treat those infected to minimize spread of nephritogenic strains. Oral penicillin V for 10 days (<25 kg=250 mg bid, >25 kg=500 mg bid). Erythromycin (40 mg/kg for 10 days) or derivatives for patients allergic to penicillin.
- **Acute Kidney Injury:** Rarely, there is a rise in serum creatinine which could be due to excess use of diuretics, uncontrolled hypertension or a development of rapidly progressive glomerulonephritis. The immune mediated nephritic syndromes can present with acute kidney injury as a part of the underlying disease. Supportive therapy for AKI is indicated and specific pointers for initiation of dialysis support would be needed in the following situations:

  a. Rapidly progressive glomerulonephritis with persistent oligo anuria.

  b. Life threatening hyperkalemia not responding to medical measures.

How Long one Should Follow-up a Child with PSGN?

PSGN typically resolves within a few weeks and prognosis is excellent in children. The child should be followed up in clinic to monitor renal functions (if abnormal on presentation), blood pressure, proteinuria and microscopic hematuria. Complement C3 should normalize by 6 to 12 weeks.

Renal functions should improve within 2-4 weeks. Proteinuria may persist up to 6 months and microscopic hematuria may persist till 12 to 18 months (Fig. 6.6).

What is the Prognosis and Outcome of PSGN?

The short and long term prognosis of PSGN in children generally good. Majority (95%) of the patients recover renal function within 3 to 4 weeks. Chronic or progressive kidney disease occurs in <1% of the children. Recurrence of PSGN is extremely rare.

Key Points

- PSGN affects school going children with male preponderance and results in triad of gross hematuria, hypertension and edema.
- ASLO titer is elevated in 70 to 80% of cases of PSGN following streptococcal pharyngitis but is unreliable for streptococcal pyoderma or infection by other organisms. Complement C3 is useful in making a diagnosis of the cause for acute nephritic syndrome.
- Treatment should be focused to manage hypertension, fluid overload and hyperkalemia which may be life threatening.
- Diuretics is the mainstay of therapy to manage hypertension in PSGN.
- Hyperkalemia may occur in a child with normal renal function (mildly reduced GFR) and hence one should do a serum potassium levels and electrocardiogram in all cases to look for changes.
- Follow up of a child after a nephritic syndrome including PSGN is important to ensure complete and sustained renal recovery.

CASE 2

A 10-year-old male child presents to the emergency room with history of gross hematuria following intermittent fever, night sweats, myalgia and weight loss. Past medical history was significant for a small, muscular ventricular septal defect. On physical examination, he appears acutely ill, dyspneic and edematous. He is febrile with tachycardia. His blood pressure readings are on the 90th centile. Urine is positive for blood and protein. Lab results show a serum creatinine of 1.3 mg/dl with neutrophilia and mild anemia. ECHO done showed vegetations.

What is the Most Likely Diagnosis?

The above scenario reflects an entity where acute nephritic syndrome is associated with an active infection. Classical examples are subacute bacterial endocarditis (SBE) and ventriculoatrial (and rarely ventriculo-peritoneal) shunt nephritis. This entity is caused by immunologically mediated inflammatory process linked to the deposition of a microbial antigen, immunoglobulin and C3 in glomerular basement membranes and mesangium, induced by focal intra or extravascular infection. The most common organisms are low virulence bacterial pathogens, such as Streptococcus viridans and coagulase negative staphylococci (S epidermidis). Other organisms associated include S aureus, S pyogenes, S pneumoniae, Salmonella typhi and Brucella species.

How will you Manage a Child with Acute Nephritic Syndrome Secondary to Shunt Nephritis?

Fortunately, endocarditis-associated nephritis is quite rare in children, mainly because of effective antibiotic therapy. The diagnosis involves bacterial culture, serological or molecular antigen detection, urinalysis, and biochemical testing and evidence of complement activation. Treatment aims at treating subacute bacterial endocarditis with IV antibiotics directed by bacterial culture and sensitivity for 4 to 6 weeks. Renal outcome of glomerulonephritis associated with bacterial endocarditis, is favorable with early diagnosis and treatment.

Shunt nephritis is much more common when ventriculoatrial shunts are inserted for hydrocephalus. Approximately 30% of atrioventricular (AV) shunts become infected and of those, 0.7 to 2% are associated with glomerulonephritis. Ventriculoperitoneal shunts are rarely complicated by glomerulonephritis which results from chronic low-level bacteremia, antibody production and immune complex formation. Deposition of bacterial immune complexes in the glomeruli is associated with activation of both the classical and alternative complement pathways. Causative organisms include Staphylococcus aureus and Staphylococcus epidermidis, Propionibacterium acne, Diptheroids, Pseudomonas and Serratia species. Treatment involves appropriate antibiotic therapy and sometimes removal of the infected shunt.

Key Points

- Glomerulonephritis associated with an active infection should be differentiated from post infection related nephritis where in nephritis is seen after the cessation of infection.
- Treatment with antibiotics can treat and prevent progression of disease in contrast to post infection related nephritis wherein there is no role of antibiotics in preventing or treating the severity of nephritis.

CASE 3

A 14-year-old girl has rapid onset of periorbital edema and dark brown urine since 1 week and was admitted for the same. The child was referred to a pediatric nephrologist by a pediatrician in view of worsening hypertension, oliguria and deterioration in renal function. The patient had been in good health until 6 weeks prior to this when she developed pyoderma skin lesions accompanied by fever. Physical examination revealed an edematous child with elevated blood pressure of 150/105 mm Hg (99th centile) and facial edema. The blood tests reveal: Blood urea 80 mg/dl and serum creatinine 7 mg/dl along with RBC cast and 1+ protein on urine analysis.

What is the Most Possible Diagnosis?

The above case scenario is different from the previous cases as the patient with post infection related acute nephritic syndrome features continues to deteriorate with worsening renal functions and oliguria requiring renal replacement therapy. Hence possibility of Rapidly Progressive Glomerulonephritis (RPGN) secondary to PIGN should be considered which is a medical emergency.

Rapidly progressive glomerulonephritis (RPGN) is a clinical syndrome defined by the rapid loss of renal function (50% decline in glomerular filtration rate) within days to weeks, accompanied by features of a nephritic syndrome with proteinuria, glomerular hematuria and often oliguria. Although relatively uncommon, early recognition and prompt diagnosis and treatment are crucial to prevent irreversible loss of renal function. Histologically, RPGN is characterized by a crescentic glomerulonephritis (CGN), which is due to severe glomerular injury, resulting in rupture of the glomerular capillary loops with accumulation of leucocytes and blood constituents in Bowman's space, which in turn induces visceral epithelial cell proliferation, together forming a cellular crescent. CGN is defined pathologically (for most glomerular diseases) when >50% of glomeruli have crescents, which are identified on light microscopy by the presence of at least two layers of cells in Bowman's space (Fig. 6.11). Although uncommon in children, RPGN can result in end-stage renal failure in up to 50% of afflicted children and, if untreated, can progress to irreversible renal failure within weeks.

What are the Common Causes for RPGN?

The following are the usual causes for RPGN and majority of these disease do present initially with features of acute nephritic syndrome. Anti-glomerular basement membrane disease like Goodpasture's syndrome; systemic diseases like lupus nephritis and HSP nephritis, ANCA associated vasculitis, infection related

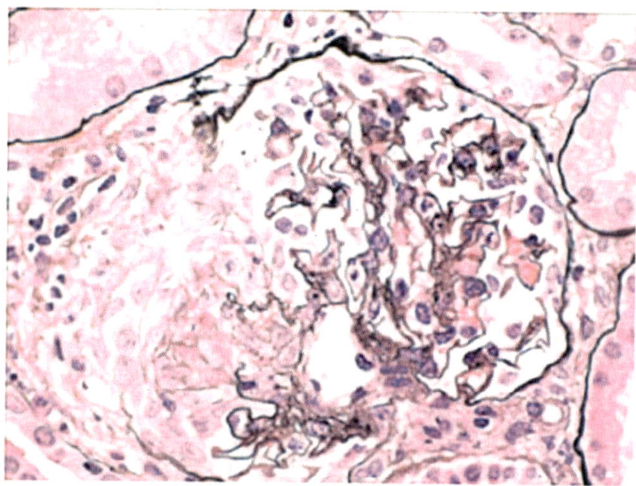

Figure 6.11: Cellular crescent (12 O'clock to 4 O'clock position) associated with endocapillary proliferation

glomerulonephritis like acute post streptococcal/post infectious glomerulonephritis, shunt nephritis, human immunodeficiency virus, Hepatitis B and C; Immune complex glomerulonephritis like IgA nephropathy and membranoproliferative glomerulonephritis.

The management of RPGN varies with the underlying cause of glomerular disease. While dialysis is the mainstay of therapy to stabilize the patient and prevent metabolic complications, certain entities would need aggressive immunosuppressive therapies.

Key Points

- RPGN is a medical emergency requiring rapid etiological diagnosis and aggressive dialysis therapy.
- Diagnosis of crescentic GN rests on the detection of crescents in >50% of glomeruli.

Conclusion

A child with acute nephritic syndrome classically presents with gross hematuria, hypertension, oliguria and edema. Occasionally, transient proteinuria and varying degrees of renal dysfunction are observed. Post-infectious glomerulonephritis remains a common cause of acute nephritic syndrome in children. Life threatening morbidities associated with acute glomerulonephritis need to be diagnosed and managed promptly. Unusual presentations, non-streptococcal glomerulonephritis, rapidly worsening renal function and systemic disease related presentations need to be managed in consultation with a pediatric nephrologist.

Acknowledgements

We thank Dr. Anila Abraham, Nephropathologist at Renopath, Chennai for providing the histopathology images.

Suggested Reading

1. Pan CG, Avner ED. Acute poststreptococcal glomerulonephritis. In Nelson Textbook of Paediatrics, 19th edn. Edited by Kliegman RM, Stanton BF, St Game JW, Schor NF, Berman RE. Elsevier Saunders. Philadelphia Pa 19103-2899,2011;1783-94.
2. Stratta P, Musetti C, Barreca A, Mazzucco G. New trends of an old disease: The acute post infectious glomerulonephritis at the beginning of the new millenium. J Nephrol 2014 Jun; 27(3):229-39.
3. Kambham N. Post-infectious glomerulonephritis. Adv Anat Pathol 2012 Sep;19(5):338-47.
4. Balasubramanian R, Marks SD. Post-infectious glomerulonephritis. Paediatr Int Child Health 2017 Nov;37(4): 240-47.
5. Bagga A, Srivastava RN, Acute and rapidly progressive glomerulonephritis in Paediatric Nephrology, 5th edn. Srivastava RN, Bagga A. Jaypee Brothers Medical Publishers (P) Ltd., New Delhi-110002, India 2011;130-50.
6. Kishore D. Phadke, Paul Goodyer, Martin Bitzan. Glomerular Diseases in Manual of Pediatric Nephrology. Springer 2014;173-84.
7. Agnes Fogo Michael Kashgarian. Acute post-infectious glomerulonephritis. Diagnostic Atlas of Renal Pathology, 3rd Edition, Elsevier 2005;1327-32.
8. Itube BR, Mezzano S. Acute post-infectious glomerulonephritis. In Paediatric Nephrology, 6th edn, edited by Avner ED, Harmon WE, Niaudet P, Yaskikawa N. Springer–Verlag Berlis Heidelberg, Germany 2009;743-55.
9. Patrick Niaudet. Nephritic Syndrome. In Denis F Geary, Franz Schaefer. Comprehensive Pediatric Nephrology, Philadelphia, PA: Mosby/Elsevier 2008;195-203.
10. Jonathan Barratt, Kevin Harris, Peter Topham. Infection-related glomerulonephritis. Oxford Desk Reference: Nephrology. Oxford University Press, New York 2008; 128-32.
11. Richard J Johnson, Jurgen Floege, John Feehally. Glomerular Diseases Associated with Infection. In Comprehensive Clinical Nephrology, 6th Edition, Philadelphia, PA: Elsevier/Saunders 2015;305-18.
12. Eison TM, Ault BH, Jones DP, Chesney RW, Wyatt RJ. Post-streptococcal acute glomerulonephritis in children: Clinical features and pathogenesis. Pediatr Nephrol 2011 Feb;26(2):165-80.
13. Gunasekaran K, Krishnamurthy S, Mahadevan S, Harish BN, Kumar AP. Clinical Characteristics and Outcome of Post-Infectious Glomerulonephritis in Children in Southern India: A Prospective Study. Indian J Pediatr 2015 Oct;82(10):896-903.

CHAPTER

7 A Patient with Rapidly Progressive Renal Failure

Ashish Nandwani[1], Prasad Dandekar[2]

[1] *Consultant, Nephrology, Manipal Hospital, Dwarka, New Delhi*

[2] *Associate Consultant, Nephrology, Fortis Hospital, Noida*

CASE

Mr X, 55-year-old male, with no past comorbidities presented with history of one spike of fever 10 days back. He went to a local practitioner where he was prescribed some antibiotics. His fever subsided but then he noticed pruritic, erythematous rash on the upper and lower limbs. He underwent evaluation after 4 days and was detected to have renal dysfunction with creatinine 2.3 mg/dl. He had no history of any decreased urine output or symptoms suggestive of volume overload. He presented to us after 1 week with creatinine 6.2 mg/dl. He was asymptomatic and had good urine output. His rash had also started to subside. IV fluids were started. His blood labs showed Hb-12.2 gm/dl, WBC count-6700/cumm, plateletes-1,56,000/cumm, creatinine-7 mg/dl, urea-113 mg/dl, sodium-142 meq/l, potassium-4.5 meq/l, normal liver function tests. Urine routine showed 1+ protein, 6-7 RBC and 5 pus cells. Urine protein creatinine ratio-0.8. Ultrasound showed bilateral normal sized kidneys, no hydronephrosis. Complements C3-92, C4-36 (normal). ANA-negative, ANCA negative. Serum protein electrophoresis showed no M band. His creatinine persisted around 7 mg/dl with IV hydration. After checking coagulation parameters, kidney biopsy was done (Fig. 7.1).

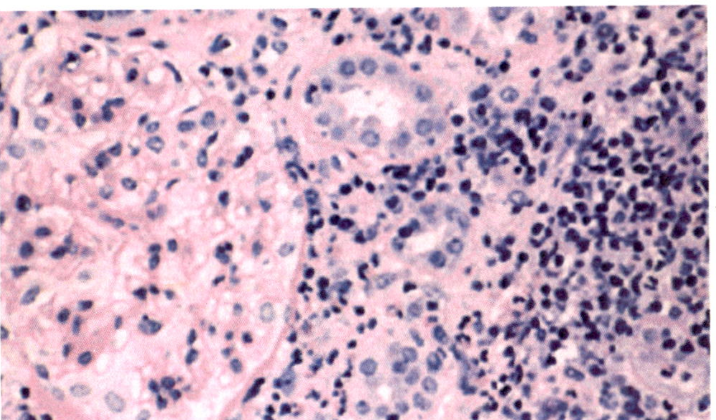

Figure 7.1: Native kidney biopsy showing acute tubulo-interstitial nephritis

He was diagnosed with rapidly progressive renal failure due to acute tubule-interstitial nephritis. He was started on prednisolone 1 mg/kg. His renal function started improving. He was subsequently discharged. On further follow-up after 1 week his serum creatinine was 1.8 mg/dl.

Discussion

The above mentioned scenario is a common presentation of rapidly progressive renal failure syndrome. *Rapidly progressive renal failure* (RPRF) is an initial clinical diagnosis in patients who present with progressive renal impairment of short duration where the timeline of onset to progression does not fit either in the definition of acute kidney injury or chronic kidney disease. It is generally defined as renal failure progressing from 2 weeks to 3 months.[1] Lately the term acute kidney disease has been coined which involve cases who present as acute kidney injury and then continue to worsen for more than 7 days.[2]

The reason why RPRF needs prompt evaluation and management is because majority of its causes are treatable and can progress to end stage renal disease if not treated on time. Renal biopsy is often required for definitive diagnosis in patients presenting with RPRF. Causes of RPRF are shown in Figure 7.2.

The most important clue for diagnosis of RPRF is the presence of active urinary sediments with normal sized kidneys. Any urinary tract infection should be ruled out before labeling. Urinary sediments can be absent in cases of acute tubulointerstitial nephritis (ATIN), atheroembolic renal failure or any obstructive causes like pelvic mass or retroperitoneal fibrosis. Ultrasound will be able to differentiate in the latter case. WBC casts can be seen in ATIN. Urinary eosinophils can be present in cases of ATIN and atheroembolic renal failure.

Thromboembolic renal disease occurs as a result of cholesterol embolism after manipulation of the aorta: angiography, angioplasty and vascular surgery.[3] Renal and systemic atheroemboli (also called cholesterol crystal emboli) usually affect older patients with diffuse atherosclerosis. Cholesterol crystal embolization occurs

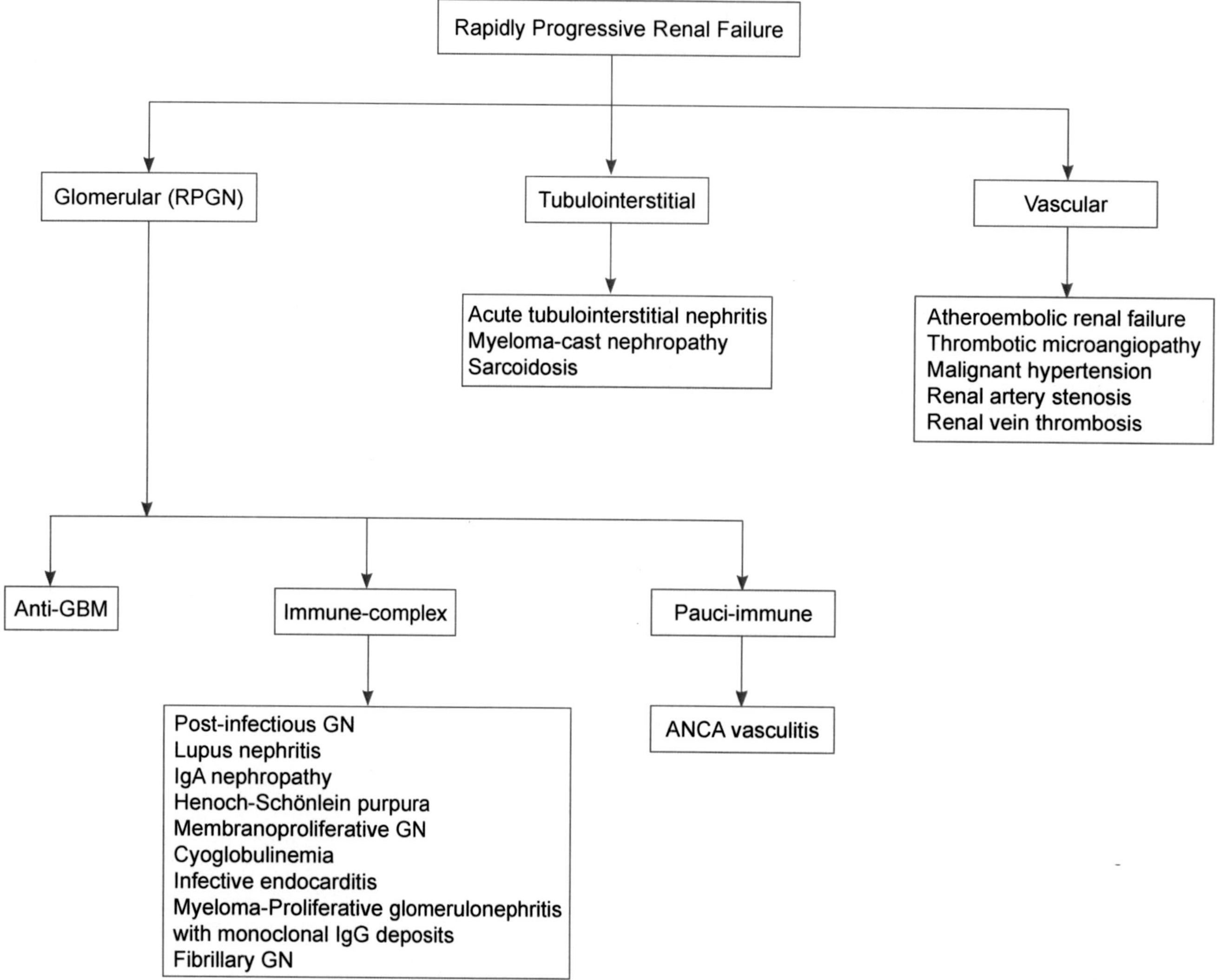

Figure 7.2: Causes of rapidly progressive renal failure

RPGN: Rapidly progressive glomerulonephritis; GBM: Glomerular basement membrane; ANCA: Antineutrophil cytoplasmic antibody; GN: Glomerulonephritis.

when portions of an atherosclerotic plaque break off and embolize distally, resulting in partial or total occlusion of small arteries (or glomerular arterioles), leading to tissue or organ ischemia. Occasionally it may occur spontaneously in patients with extensive atherosclerosis. On kidney biopsy cholesterol clefts are seen in medium sized vessels with giant cell reaction and re-canalisation.

Ultrasound doppler should be done to rule out renal artery stenosis in patients who present with accelerated hypertension and renal failure. Chronic renal vein thrombosis can have an insidious onset and present as RPRF without any acute symptoms such as flank pain.

Presence of nephritic/sub-nephrotic proteinuria with active urinary sediments usually points towards a glomerular disease. Complement levels would be able to guide towards the nature of disease. Low complement levels usually point towards immune complex disease. Low C3 or low C3+ C4 depends upon the involvement of alternative or classical pathway respectively (Table 7.1).

Table 7.1: Complement levels in immune complex glomerulonephritis

Low C3, normal C4	Low C3 + C4
Post-infectious GN	Lupus nephritis
C3 glomerulopathy	Cryoglobulinemia
	Infective endocarditis

Immune complex glomerulonephritis (GN) refers to the presence of immune deposits in the glomeruli. In most cases, the serologic and histologic findings will point to the underlying disease, such as mesangial and glomerular capillary wall immunoglobulin A (IgA) deposits in IgA nephropathy; antistreptococcal antibodies and subepithelial humps in postinfectious GN; antinuclear antibodies, a "full house" immunofluorescence staining for IgG, IgA, IgM, C3 and C1q, mesangial plus subendothelial deposits in lupus nephritis; and circulating cryoglobulins and intraluminal "thrombi" in mixed cryoglobulinemia.ANA and ENA profile support the diagnosis in autoimmune conditions.

Peripheral smear for schistocytes and LDH will be able to guide towards thrombotic microangiopathy (TMA). It is a specific pathologic lesion in which abnormalities in the vessel wall of arterioles and capillaries lead to microvascular thrombosis.[4] The primary TMA syndromes include thrombotic thrombocytopenic purpura (TTP) (hereditary or acquired), Shiga toxin-mediated hemolytic uremic syndrome (ST-HUS), drug-induced TMA (DITMA) and complement-mediated TMA (hereditary or acquired).

Paucimmune GN will have normal complements, negative IF and positive ANCA. Approximately 10% patients of pauci-immune GN are ANCA negative. Systemic complaints, and extrarenal organ involvement, are common in patients with pauci-immune crescentic GN. Most commonly affected age group is 6th-7th decade. Patients with RPGN due to Anti GBM disease present with RPRF, and may have pulmonary involvement as well. Early diagnosis with serology and renal biopsy is warranted in these patients to prevent permanent renal damage.

It is worthwhile to rule out monoclonal gammopathy in an elderly patient even without any myeloma defining history of bone pains or hypercalcemia. Myeloma can cause RPRF by glomerular involvement in the form of progressive glomerulonephritis with monoclonal immunoglobulin deposition, immuno-tactoid glomerulopathy, cryoglobulinemia or C3 glomerulopathy.[5] Tubulo-interstitial involvement by cast nephropathy can present either as acute kidney injury or as RPRF. Commonly used screening technique for detection of M protein is the serum protein electrophoresis (SPEP) and urine protein electrophoresis (UPEP). To determine the identity of the Ig, protein electrophoresis must be performed in conjunction with immunofixation.

Timely kidney biopsy is the gold standard in the diagnosis of cause of RPRF. Many patients may present in late stages wherein the role of immmunosuppression might prove doubtful and cause more harm than benefit.

Acute Tubulo-Interstitial Nephritis

Acute Tubulo-Interstitial Nephritis can present as both acute kidney injury and acute kidney disease. Suspicion for ATIN as a causative factor for RPRF arises in the light of an inciting factor–most commonly a drug and less commonly an infection. Around 1% of renal biopsies during the evaluation of hematuria or proteinuria are diagnosed as ATIN.[6]

It is an immunologically mediated hypersensitivity reaction, most commonly a delayed hypersensitivity reaction. The following factors support the hypersensitivity phenomenon as the cause of ATIN.

- Occurs only in a small percentage of individuals.
- Not dose dependent.
- Often associated with extrarenal manifestations of hypersensitivity.
- Recurs after accidental re-exposure to the same drug or to a closely related one.
- Evidence of granulomas on biopsy.

Three major categories of antigens can induce ATIN:

- Tubular basement membrane (TBM) components (such as the glycoproteins 3M-1 and TIN-Ag/TIN1).
- Secreted tubular proteins (such as Tamm-Horsfall protein).
- Extra-renal proteins (such as from immune complexes).

Majority are induced by extrarenal antigens, being produced in particular by drugs or infectious agents. Drugs/Infectious agents implicated in the etiology of ATIN are given in Tables 7.2A and 7.2B.

Table 7.2A: Drugs implicated in the etiology of ATIN

Antibiotics	Cephalosporins, Penicillins, Vancomycin, Tetracycline, Sulfonamides, Rifampicin, Macrolides, Isoniazid, Ethambutol
Diuretics	Furosemide, Thiazides, Triamterene
NSAIDs	Almost all agents
Miscellaneous	Proton Pump Inhibitors, Quinine Propylthiouracil, Phenytoin, Phenteramine, Mesalazine, Indinavir, Diltiazem, Clofibrate, Carbamazepine, Captopril, Azathioprine, Acyclovir, Allopurinol

NSAIDs: Non steroidal anti inflammatory drugs

Table 7.2B: Infectious agent implicated in the etiology of ATIN

Infectious agents	
Bacteria	Corynebacterium, Escherichia coli, Legionella, Staphylococcus, Streptococcus, Yersinia, Brucella, Campylobacter, Tuberculosis
Viruses	Cytomegalovirus, Epstein Barr Virus, Hantavirus, Hepatitis C, Herpes Simplex Virus, Human Immunodeficiency Virus, Mumps, Polyoma Virus
Others	Leptospira, Mycobacterium, Mycoplasma, Chlamydia, Rickettsia, Syphilis, Toxoplasmosis

Drug induced tubulointerstitial nephritis (D-TIN) by definition occur 48 to 72 hours after antigen exposure (delayed hypersensitivity reaction). Sterile pyuria occur at 72 hours after exposure but often goes undetected or missed. Rise in serum creatinine usually occurs 7 to 10 days after exposure to drug.

Proton pump inhibitors have recently came into light as a major cause of interstitial nephritis progressing to chronic kidney disease with prolonged exposure to the drug. Considerable higher rate of occurrence is seen in older (> 60 years) patients. In a nationwide case-control study in New Zealand by Blank ML,[7] it was found that interval between drug initiation and the onset of kidney abnormalities oscillate between 1 week and 9 months, although a timeframe of 10-11 weeks was the most common. The severity of AKI was lower than antibiotic-induced cases, but the probability of recovery by 6 months was significantly lower.

Non steroidal anti inflammatory drugs (NSAIDs) have probably a different mechanism of interstitial injury due to which response to steroids is less commonly seen as compared to other D-TIN. It has been proposed that NSAIDs cause alternative lipoxygenase pathway activation leading to production of proinflammatory leukotrienes or epoxy and hydroxy eicosanoids which cause interstitial injury. It can also present with nephrotic range proteinuria with the combination of ATIN with minimal-change glomerulopathy seen in around 0.2/1000 subjects.[8]

In cases of infection induced ATIN, tuberculosis is the most commonly implicated agent in Indian scenario. The pathogenesis involves the hypersensitive immune response against mycobacterium tuberculosis (MTB), without direct kidney invasion and injury. Ziehl-Neilsen staining and MTB PCR are typically negative in renal tissue. Biopsy shows interstitial inflammation with eosinophils and granulomas (Fig. 7.3). Anti-tuberculous therapy is followed by renal function improvement in the majority cases. Significant response to steroids is also noticed.[9]

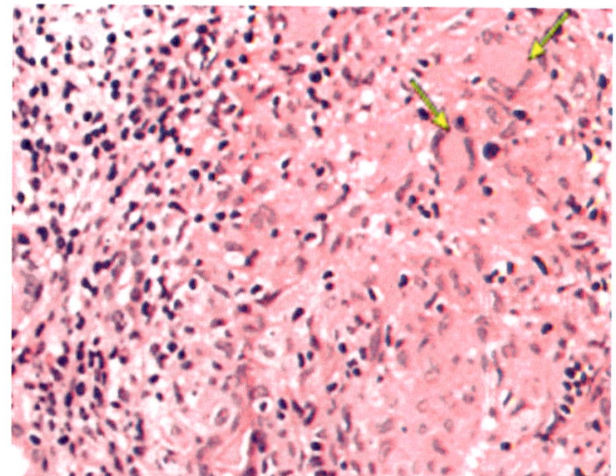

Figure 7.3: Renal biopsy showing granulomatous changes with eosinophils

Other autoimmune diseases like Sjögren syndrome, sarcoidosis, IgG4 related ATIN, Tubulointerstitial nephritis with Uveitis (TINU) and vasculitis also constitute less than 5% cases of ATIN. Lymphoproliferative disorders and paraproteinemias presenting as ATIN is not rare.

Clinical Presentation and Management of Acute Tubulointerstitial Nephritis

Patients with ATIN usually present with RPRF along with systemic features of hypersensitivity reaction, following exposure to inciting agent.

Common presentations of ATIN have been given in Table 7.3.

Table 7.3: Presentation of acute tubulointerstitial nephritis

Features	
Acute renal failure	100%
Acute renal failure requiring dialysis	40%
Arthralgias	45%
Fever	36%
Skin rash	22%
Eosinophilia (> 500 eosinophils per mm^3)	35%
Microhematuria	67%
Gross hematuria	5%
Leukocyturia	82%
Non-nephrotic proteinuria	93%
Nephrotic-range proteinuria	2.5%
Complete nephrotic syndrome	0.8%

Gonza´lez E, Kidney Int 2008[10]

Urine microscopy (Table 7.4) usually is not diagnostic. WBC casts are occasionally found (Fig. 7.4).

Table 7.4: Urinary abnormalities in acute tubulointerstitial nephritis

Urine Dipstick/Urine Microscopy	Interstitial Nephritis
Protein	0/+
Blood/RBCs	0/+
WBCs	+++
RBC casts	0
WBC casts	+++
Granular casts	+

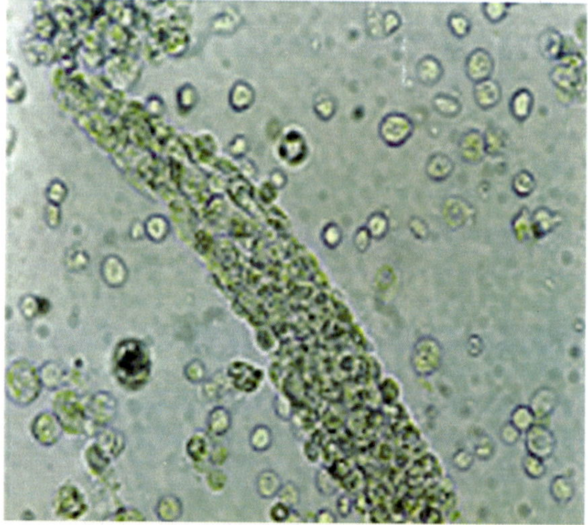

Figure 7.4: Urine microscopy showing WBC cast

There have been much speculations regarding the role of urinary eosinophils being the diagnostic factor in cases of allergic interstitial nephritis. Although recent studies have shown that they have poor sensitivity as well as specificity (Positive predictive value 38%). Urinary eosinophils should no longer be used as a biomarker for ATIN.[11]

Recently urine TNF alpha and IL9 have shown strong association with acute interstitial nephritis (AIN) and can be used as biomarkers. Further studies are required in this area.[12]

USG shows enlarged, swollen kidneys in some cases with increased echogenicity Gallium scan has been proposed to differentiate between ATN and AIN as the 67gallium binds to lactoferrin, which is expressed on inflammatory cell surfaces.

Kidney biopsy is the only confirmatory test. Lymphocyte predominant infiltration of inflammatory cells with associated edema, usually sparing glomeruli and blood vessels and tubulitis are the diagnostic features. Immunofluorescence shows linear IgG and complement on the tubular basement membrane.

It has been proposed that patients in whom kidney functions do not improve after cessation of the suspected inciting agent and with supportive measures for 3-5 days should ideally go for biopsy (Table 7.5).

Table 7.5: Supportive care measures
• Maintain adequate hydration
• Avoid volume depletion or overload
• Identify and correct electrolyte abnormalities
• Symptomatic relief for fever and systemic symptoms
• Symptomatic relief for rash
• Avoid use of drugs that impair renal blood flow
• Adjust drug dosages for existing level of renal function

The role of steroids in the treatment of ATIN is still controversial. Studies have suggested that corticosteroid therapy should be initiated early preferably in 1-2 weeks with a dose of 1 mg/kg per day of prednisone. They should be continued for approximately 1-1.5 months and should not be extended beyond it in those who fail to show any improvement in kidney function.[14] Progression to chronic interstitial nephritis in patients in whom early steroids were not started has been noted in some recent studies.

The following algorithm can guide to the management of drug-induced acute interstitial nephritis (Fig. 7.5):

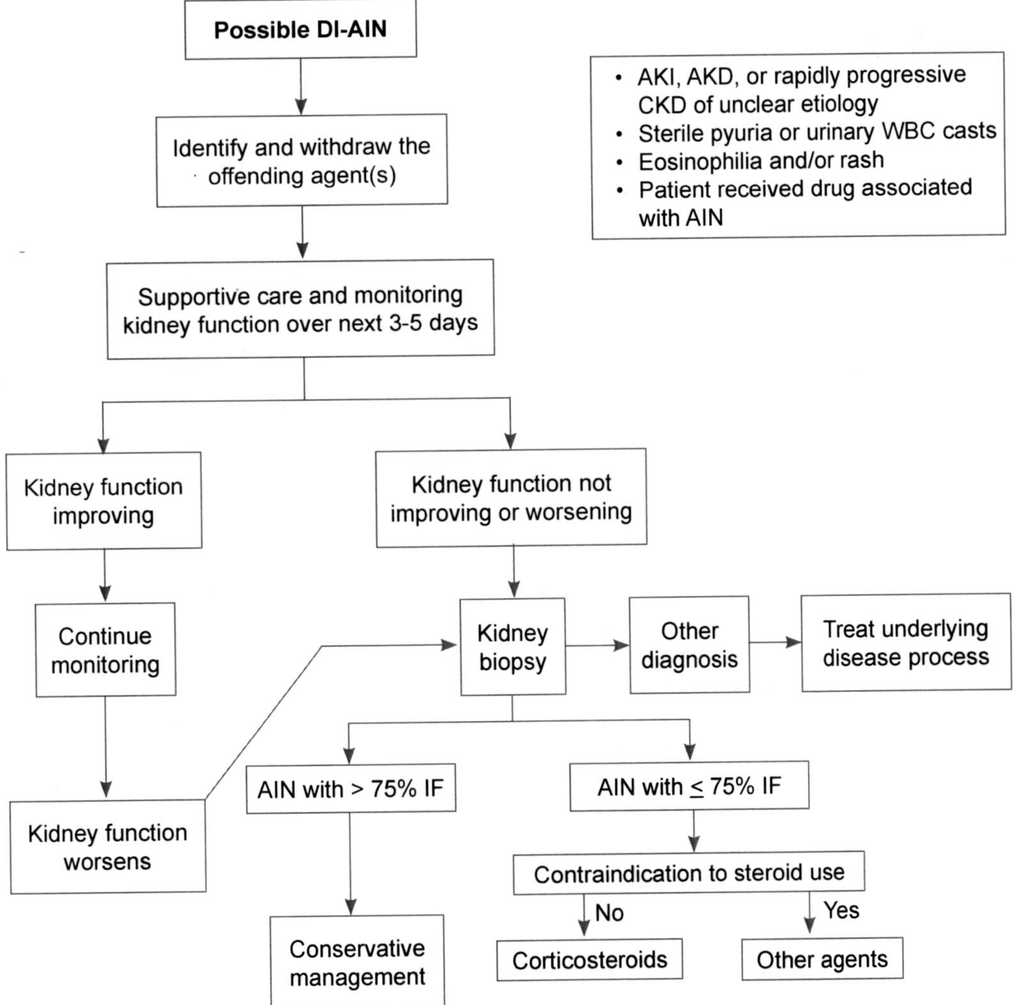

Figure 7.5: Algorithm for management of drug-induced acute interstitial nephritis[13]

AIN: Acute interstitial nephritis; AKD: Acute kidney disease; AKI: Acute kidney injury; DI-AIN: Drug-induced acute interstitial nephritis; IF: Interstitial fibrosis; WBC: White blood cell.

In patients who do not respond to corticosteroids within two to three weeks, treatment with cyclophosphamide or mycophenolate mofetil (MMF) have been used in some case studies.

The risk of progression to chronic kidney disease can be guided by the following factors[15]:

- Elderly age.
- Baseline CKD.
- Initial dialysis dependency.
- Recovery within first month.
- Degree of fibrosis on biopsy.

In conclusion ATIN is an immunologically mediated hypersensitivity reaction with drugs and infection being the major causative factors. Biopsy remains the gold standard for proving and removal of offending agent being the primary treatment. Role of steroids is controversial–early use is advised. Currently the need for better steroid sparing agents is required.

References

1. Bhowmik D, Sinha S, Agarwal SK. Clinical approach to rapidly progressive renal failure. J Assoc Physicians India 2011 Jan;59:38-41.
2. Acute kidney disease and renal recovery: Consensus report of the Acute Disease Quality Initiative (ADQI) 16 Workgroup, Nature Reviews Nephrology volume 13 (2017).
3. Tunick PA, Kronzon I. Atheroembolism. In: Vascular Medicine: A Companion to Braunwald's Heart Disease, Creager M, Dzau VJ, Loscalzo J (Eds), Elsevier, Philadelphia 2006.
4. Syndromes of thrombotic microangiopathy. George JN, Nester CM N Engl J Med 2014;371(7):654.
5. Sanjeev Sethi *et al.* J Am Soc Nephrol 2018;29:1810-23.
6. Michel DM, Kelly CJ. Acute interstitial nephritis. J Am Soc Nephrol, 1998.
7. Blank ML, Parkin L, Paul C *et al.* A nationwide nested case-control study indicates an increased risk of acute interstitial nephritis with proton pump inhibitor use. Kidney Int 2014.
8. Murray MD, Brater DC. Renal toxicity of the nonsteroidal anti-inflammatory drugs. Annu Rev Pharmacol Toxicol 1993;33:435-65.
9. Chapagain A, Dobbie H, Sheaff M *et al.* Presentation, diagnosis and treatment outcome of tuberculous-mediated tubulointerstitial nephritis. Kidney Int 2011.
10. Gonza´lez E, Kidney Int 2008;73.
11. Clinical Approach to Diagnosing Acute and Chronic Tubulointerstitial Disease Mark A. Perazella Adv Chronic Kidney Dis 2017;24(2).
12. Moledina DG, Wilson FP, Pober JS. Urine TNF-α and IL-9 for clinical diagnosis of acute interstitial nephritis. JCI Insight 2019;May 16.
13. Drug-Induced Acute Interstitial Nephritis Dennis G. Moledina and Mark A. Perazella Clin J Am Soc Nephrol 2017;12:2046-49.
14. Duration of Treatment with Corticosteroids and Recovery of Kidney Function in Acute Interstitial Nephritis CJASN December 2018.
15. Clinical characteristics, causes and outcomes of acute interstitial nephritis in the elderly Muriithi, Angela K, *et al.* Kidney International, Volume 87, Issue 2.

CHAPTER

8

A Young Female with Lupus Nephritis

Manish Rathi[1], Joyita Bharati[2]

[1] *Professor, Department of Nephrology, Postgraduate Institute of Medical Education and Research, Chandigarh*

[2] *Assistant Professor, Department of Nephrology, Postgraduate Institute of Medical Education and Research, Chandigarh*

CASE

A 24-year-old woman presented to the out-patient clinic with complaints of severe and diffuse joint pains involving small and large joints; with muscle aches and rash on her cheeks of 2 months duration. She was married for 6 months and has had normal menstrual cycles till date. Her family and personal history were non-contributory. Examination was striking for a malar rash, and multiple joint synovitis involving both small and large joints. Investigations revealed elevated erythrocyte sedimentation rate, strongly positive anti-nuclear antibody (ANA), microscopic hematuria, normal renal function and proteinuria of 0.4 gm/24 hours. A diagnosis of *systemic lupus erythematosus* (SLE) was made and a physician prescribed her prednisolone of 20 mg per day and hydroxychloroquine of 300 mg per day. There was some improvement in joint pain and myalgia. After about 3 weeks of treatment, she developed swelling of legs associated with low-grade fever. Her urine output was normal. The dose of prednisolone was increased to 60 mg per day and she was referred to a nephrologist.

On physical examination, her blood pressure was 120/80 mm Hg, heart rate was 80 per minute and respiratory rate was 20 per minute. She had a moon face with a malar "butterfly" rash and appeared pale. There was pitting pedal edema up to the ankles. The heart and chest examinations were normal. The abdomen appeared distended with reddish striae on the flanks and percussion revealed dull flanks. Analyses revealed serum creatinine of 0.6 mg/dl, blood urea 40 mg/dl, hemoglobin 8.6 g/dl, leucocytes of 4200/mm^3, platelet count of 1.0 lakh, total serum proteins 4.8 g/dl, serum albumin 2.2 g/dl, serum cholesterol 300 mg/dl, and triglycerides 169 mg/dl. Urine showed 3+ albumin by dipstick and 20-25 red blood cells per high power field. Her 24-hour urine showed proteinuria of 3.7 gm. Serology was strongly positive for ANA (3+, speckled) and anti-dsDNA titers of > 359 IU/ml with low complement levels (C3 30 mg/dl and C4 4 mg/dl). Her hemolytic work-up was normal. A working diagnosis of SLE with lupus nephritis (LN) was made.

How Common is Lupus Nephritis (LN) in Patients with SLE?

Clinically evident renal involvement occurs in 30-50% of patients with SLE at presentation and >60% patients are affected during the course of the disease.[1-3] It occurs frequently in young adults and children.

What are the Criteria for doing Renal Biopsy in a Patient with SLE?

There are six guidelines worldwide which have been published in 2012 with a mention on specific indications of renal biopsy at first clinical presentation in lupus patients. The widely used EULAR/ERA-EDTA (European League Against Rheumatism and European Renal Association–European Dialysis and Transplant Association) and ACR (American College of Rheumatology) guidelines are summarised in Table 8.1. The other 4 guidelines

Table 8.1: Indications of renal biopsy at first clinical presentation in patients with SLE

EULAR/ERA-EDTA	ACR
• Reproducible proteinuria ≥ 0.5 g/day	• Confirmed proteinuria ≥ 1g/day
• Active urine sediments	• Abnormal renal function
• Abnormal renal function otherwise not explained	• Proteinuria: 0.5 g/24 hours plus Hematuria (> 5 RBC/HPF)
	• Proteinuria: 0.5 g/24 hours plus cellular casts

EULAR/ERA-EDTA: European League Against Rheumatism and European Renal Association–European Dialysis and Transplant Association; ACR: American College of Rheumatology.

namely, GEAS (Systemic autoimmune disease group of the Spanish Society of Internal Medicine and Spanish Society of Nephology), DWP (Dutch Working Party on Systemic Lupus Erythematosus), CARRA (Childhood Arthritis and Rheumatology Research Alliance) and KDIGO (Kidney Disease: Improving Global Outcomes Glomerulonephritis Work Group) have compatible views on the indications.

All guidelines recommend renal biopsy in patients with SLE with clinical markers consistent with renal involvement by lupus. An active urine sediment includes hematuria (>5 RBCs per HPF with or without acanthocytes), leukocyturia (>5 WBCs per HPF) in the absence of infection, and RBC and WBC casts. Most guidelines consider active urine sediment as an indication of renal biopsy, often when present with proteinuria or impaired renal function. Patients who develop active urine sediment require close follow-up for proteinuria and an increase in serum creatinine. Proteinuria of more than 0.5 g to 1 g/day, which is confirmed on repeat evaluation, is usually indicative of lupus nephritis. It is prudent to do early renal biopsy at presentation so that the opportunity for aggressive treatment of active lesion is not missed. Whereas the clinical renal and pathological parameters usually correlate well at first presentation in lupus patients with rapidly progressive renal failure or nephritic syndrome, patients with sub-nephrotic proteinuria can have either aggressive proliferative or non-proliferative lesions.[4] Although these clinical clues (Table 8.2) are helpful in predicting histological involvement, there are discrepancies observed between clinical parameters and histological involvement in some patients with LN. Some patients without active urine sediment and low-level proteinuria have been reported to have significant glomerular involvement in the form of class III/IV/V LN.[4] Moreover, not all biopsy findings such as crescents and/or necrotizing lesions, which have therapeutic implication, correlate well with clinical parameters. Clinical severity does not correlate well with histological severity.[5] Therefore, renal biopsy remains indispensable and the "gold standard" to confirm the diagnosis of lupus nephritis and decide therapy.[6] Additionally, other entities specific to SLE such as lupus podocytopathy, collapsing glomerulopathy and thrombotic microangiopathy (TMA) can be revealed only on renal biopsy. Moreover, activity and chronicity indices have been reported to predict outcome in patients with LN.

How to Classify Lupus Nephritis?

Various classification schemas have been used since 1960s to describe and categorize the glomerular pathology of lupus nephritis. The first such description was by Pollack and Pirani in 1974, who, divided lupus nephritis into classes of normal glomeruli (class I), pure mesangial disease (class II), focal proliferative glomerulonephritis (class III), diffuse proliferative glomerulonephritis (class IV), and membranous glomerulonephritis (class V). The classification was modified by the International Study of Kidney Disease in Children (ISKDC), World Health Organization (WHO) and International Society of Nephrology/Renal Pathology Society (ISN/RPS) in 1982, 1995 and 2003, respectively. Too many subdivisions, inadequate clarity on separation of class III and class IV lesion, and lack of strict criteria on proportion of involved glomeruli in class VI LN in the ISKDC 1982 and WHO 1995 classification schemas made the way for a better ISN/RPS classification system in 2003.

The ISN/RPS 2003 (Table 8.3) classification stated clear definition of each class of lupus nephritis and a uniform approach to report renal biopsy. This brought in standardized and reproducible reporting of lupus nephritis pathology across the world. The classification included the following recommendations:

1. The renal biopsy should include minimum 10 glomeruli to exclude the existence of focal lesions.
2. The renal biopsy should be studied by immunofluorescence including IgG, IgA, IgM isotypes,

Table 8.2: Clinicopathological correlation in lupus nephritis

Lupus nephritis class (ISN/RPS)	Proteinuria	Active urine sediment	Increased serum creatinine	Active lupus serology	Hypertension
Class I	-*	-	-	+/-	-
Class II	+/- *	-	-	+/-	-
Class III	++ (NS: 30%)	+	+/-	+/-	+/-
Class IV	+++ (NS: 50%)	++	+/-	++/-	++/-
Class V	+++ (NS: 60%)	-	+/-	+/--	+/-
Class VI	++	+/-	+	+/--	+

(+) Represents frequent occurrence of symptom/sign; (-) Represents infrequent occurrence of symptom/sign; NS: Nephrotic syndrome; * NS is seen in class I/II LN in presence of podocytopathy.

Kappa and Lambda light chains, and C3 and C1q complement components.

3. The lack of EM should not prevent the pathologist from making LN diagnosis.

There is a recent revision of the ISN-RPS 2003 classification[7] with focus on clarifying definitions of certain histological parameters such as endocapillary hypercellularity, mesangial hypercellularity, and crescents along with modification of the NIH activity and chronicity indices as shown in Table 8.4.

Hence, renal biopsy is definitely indicated at this time in our patient. Renal biopsy was done which revealed endocapillary hypercellularity in 8 out of 12 glomeruli, presence of subendothelial deposits in 6 glomeruli and occasional fibrinoid necrosis on light microscopy. There was mild interstitial infiltration of mononuclear cells and patchy acute tubular necrosis without interstitial fibrosis or tubular atrophy. Immunofluorescence studies demonstrated immune deposits of all classes of immunoglobulins, C3 and C1q along mesangium and glomerular capillary wall.

Table 8.3: ISN/RPS 2003 classification of lupus nephritis

Class I Normal glomeruli by light microscopy (LM), but mesangial immune deposits by immunofluorescence (IF)	Minimal mesangial LN
Class II Class I + Mesangial hypercellularity with or without mesangial expansion by LM	Mesangial proliferative LN
Class III Active or inactive focal (<50% of all glomeruli) endo- or extracapillary glomerulonephritis, typically with focal subendothelial immune deposits, with or without mesangial alterations	**Focal LN** III (A): Active lesions III (A/C): Active and chronic lesions III (C): Chronic lesions
Class IV Active or inactive diffuse (≥50% of all glomeruli), segmental or global endo- or extracapillary glomerulonephritis, typically with diffuse subendothelial immune deposits, with or without mesangial alterations. This class includes cases with diffuse wire loop deposits but with little or no glomerular proliferation	Diffuse LN (≥ 50% of glomeruli) IV (S): Segmental (<50% of one glomerular tuft) IV (G): Global (>50% of one glomerular tuft) IV (A): Active lesions IV (A/C): Active and chronic lesions IV (C): Chronic lesions
Class V Subepithelial immune deposits and their morphological sequelae in light microscopy occupying at least 50% of GCL with or without mesangial alterations. It may occur in combination with class III or IV, in which case both will be diagnosed	Membranous LN
Class VI ≥ 90% globally sclerosed glomeruli without residual activity	Advanced sclerosing LN

Table 8.4: Salient differences in ISN-RPS 2003 and ISN-RPS revision 2018

ISN-RPS 2003	ISN-RPS revision 2018
Mesangial cellularity: ≥3 cells in one mesangial area	Mesangial hypercellularity redefined: 4 or more cells in one mesangial area
Endocapillary "proliferation"	Endocapillary "proliferation" changed to "hypercullarity"
Class IV-G and IV-S subdivision	No subdivision of IV-G and IV-S
Crescents occupying >25% of circumference of Bowman capsule	Cellular crescents: >10% of circumference of Bowman's capsule
NIH-AI: Endocapillary proliferation, fibrinoid necrosis or karyorrhexis, leucocyte infiltration, hyaline deposits, interstitial inflammation, cellular crescents	Interstitial inflammation is defined in the presence or absence of fibrosis Change in NIH-AI: Fibrinoid necrosis and karyorrhexis separated, no leucocyte infiltration

So, a final diagnosis of class IV G (A) LN was made and decision was made to treat the patient with induction therapy.

What are the Induction Therapies used in Proliferative Lupus Nephritis?

Once confirmed on histopathology, therapy has to be rationalized, largely based on the pathology, with due consideration of clinical characteristics. Management of active lupus nephritis usually consists of 2 phases, namely, initial or induction phase followed by maintenance phase (Fig. 8.1). Maintenance phase is to control remnant activity and to avoid relapse of disease activity so as to prevent chronic irreversible disease. Nevertheless, concerns of side-effects related to potentially toxic therapies need to be individually assessed. Till date, there are mainly two forms of induction therapies: Injection Cyclophosphamide (CYC, low or high dose) or oral Mycophenolate Mofetil (MMF) along with corticosteroids (oral or injections or both).

1. ***IV Cyclophosphamide ("NIH" Trials)***

   Randomised, controlled trials at the National Institutes of Health (NIH) paved the way to

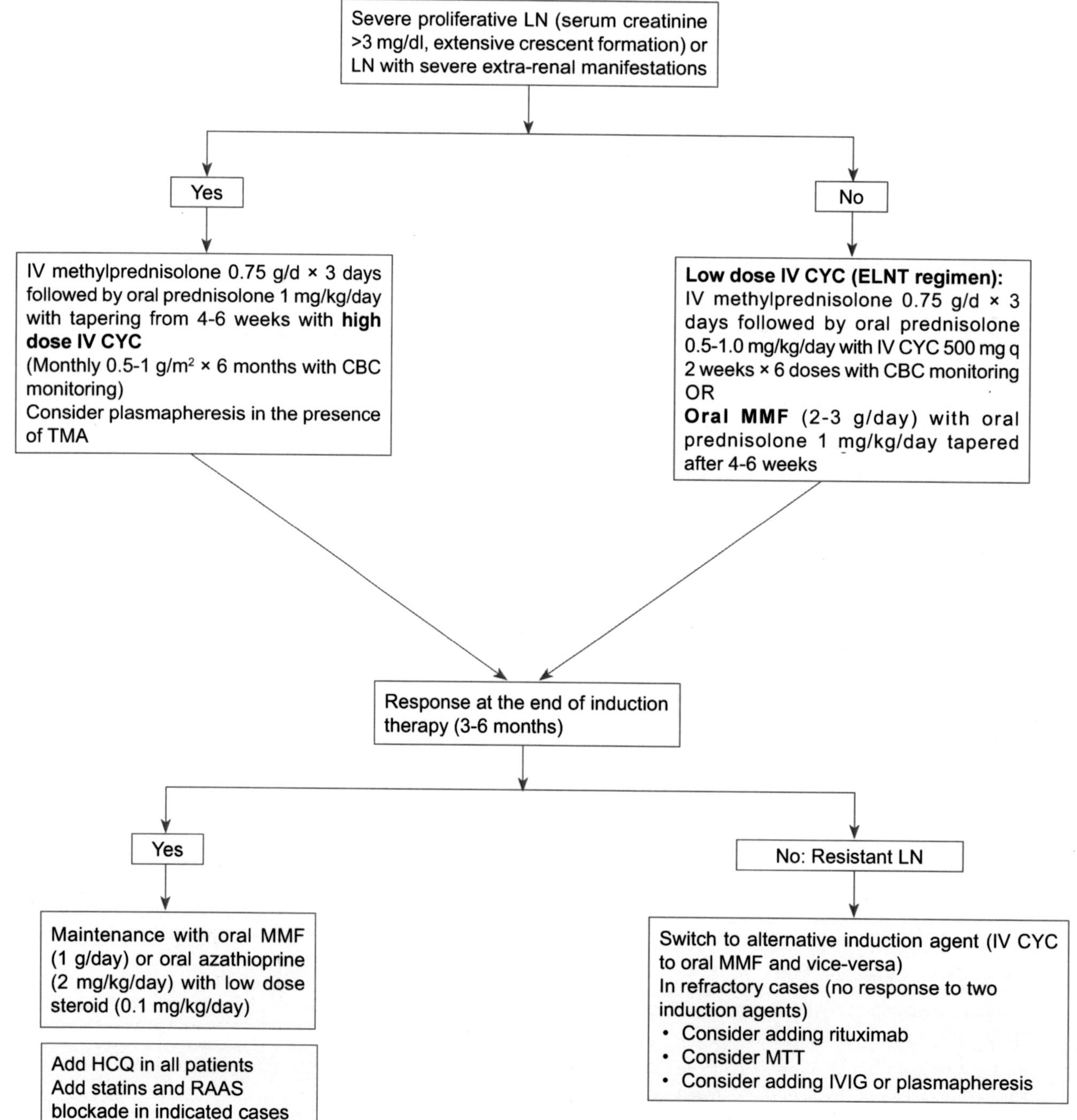

Figure 8.1: Algorithm for management of proliferative LN
CYC: Cyclophosphamide; MMF: Mycophenolate mofetil; HCQ: Hydroxy chloroquin; MTT: Multi-target therapy.

study immunosuppressive agents in addition to corticosteroids in treating proliferative lupus nephritis. The *"first NIH trial"* conducted by Austin *et al.*,[8] in 1986, compared five different immunosuppressive regimens including IV CYC, oral CYC and azathioprine with oral prednisolone to oral prednisolone alone. Addition of intravenous (IV) CYC (0.5-1 g/m^2) to oral prednisolone was found to be superior to high-dose oral prednisolone alone in preventing end-stage renal disease (ESRD) in long-term follow-up. There was no significant difference seen between IV CYC and other regimens of oral immunosuppressive agents including oral CYC with prednisolone. Since then, high dose IV CYC became the standard treatment for lupus nephritis as it involves a lower cumulative exposure to CYC than oral CYC and thus, less frequent cytopenias, hemorrhagic cystitis, and avoids problems of nonadherence. Few years later, in 1992, the *"second NIH"* trial by Boumpas *et al.*[9] described that long-term (36 months) IV CYC therapy is better than IV methylprednisolone pulses alone (monthly for 6 months) at preserving renal function and avoiding renal relapses. Gourley *et al.*[10] in the *"third NIH trial"* further established that IV CYC (0.5-1 g/m^2) every monthly pulse followed by every third monthly pulses in combination with monthly IV methylprednisolone (1 g/m^2) pulses was more effective in inducing remission than IV methylprednisolone alone. A significant finding, which became apparent, was the rate of adverse events in those on CYC. Amenorrhea was seen in about 40% of the patients on CYC. Boumpas *et al.*[11] reported rates of sustained amenorrhea of 12%, 27% and 62% patients aged ≤ 25 years, 26 to 30 years and ≥ 31 years of age, respectively (P = 0.04). Increased risk for sustained amenorrhea was also noted in those on long-term CYC (15 pulses) compared to short-term CYC (7 pulses), which was most evident in patients older than 25 years. Similarly, infections, particularly herpes zoster, were seen in 20-30% of the patients on combination therapy of CYC and steroid.

2. ***IV Cyclophosphamide (Euro Lupus Nephritis Trial)***

With the above serious concerns, Houssiau *et al.*[12] *in the Euro Lupus Nephritis Trial (ELNT),* tried lower doses of IV CYC to induce remission and simultaneously decrease side effects of high dose IV CYC. This randomized study compared standard six monthly pulse of IV CYC (0.5 to 1 g/m^2) followed by 2 every third monthly infusions to a shorter treatment course consisting of 500 mg of IV CYC every 2 weeks for six doses (total dose, 3 g), with azathioprine as the maintenance therapy (2 mg/kg per day) in proliferative lupus nephritis. Both regimens were equally effective in inducing remission with less toxicity (less severe and total infections) in the shorter regimen. The caveat was that predominantly Caucasian population with milder form of proliferative lupus nephritis were included in this trial. This may not be generalizable to world-wide populations with proliferative LN.

3. ***Mycophenolate Mofetil***

The availability of MMF brought in new options for treating lupus nephritis with a safer toxicity profile. Studies reporting efficacy of MMF as induction therapy in proliferative LN started appearing from 2000 onwards. The first report came from China,[13] where, 42 patients with proliferative lupus nephritis were randomized to either 12 months of oral MMF (2 g/d for 6 months followed by 1 g/d for 6 months) or 6 months of oral CYC (2.5 mg/kg per day), followed by oral azathioprine (1.5 mg/kg per day) for 6 months. While the rate of complete remission (81 *versus* 76%), partial remission (14 *versus* 14%), and relapses (15 *versus* 11%) were similar between the regimens, infections were less common in the MMF arm. Long-term follow-up of this cohort proved similar efficacy of MMF over CYC. Five years later, Ginzler *et al.*[14] reported superior efficacy of MMF (up to 3 g/day) over monthly IV CYC with a better side effect profile in 140 predominantly African American patients. The largest international trial *(ALMS)*[15] of induction therapy of lupus nephritis including 370 patients showed MMF (3 g/day) to be equally effective as monthly IV CYC (response rate of 56.2% in MMF group *versus* 53.0% in IV CYC, *P*=0.58). Majority of these patients had less severe LN with only 32 patients having advanced renal failure (defined as GFR 30 ml/min).

Furthermore, in a recent trial[16] done at our centre, we compared low dose IV CYC with oral MMF in patients with less severe proliferative LN. We noted that the complete remission rates and treatment response were similar in the two groups. The preference of one over the other induction agent is summarized in Table 8.5.

4. ***Others***

In addition to MMF and IV CYC, other agents used in induction therapy of LN are azathioprine, rituximab and multi-target therapy (MTT). However, the upfront use of rituximab as the only agent alongside steroid in induction therapy of lupus nephritis is not tested. Its use as additional agent alongside MMF and steroid to induce remission is not supported by evidence.[17]

A recent addition in the armamentarium of induction therapy of LN is the multi-targeted immunosuppressant regimen similar to that used in kidney transplant recipients, reported from China primarily. Combination of MMF, tacrolimus, and steroids (multi-target therapy/MTT) in patients with

Table 8.5: Indications of specific induction therapy in LN in a nutshell

Therapy	Indications
High dose IV CYC (Monthly 0.5-1.0 g/m^2 IV CYC for 6 months)	• Severe LN (S. Creatinine > 3.0 mg/dl) • Crescentic LN (> 50% crescents) • LN with TMA • LN with severe extra-renal manifestations like Neuropsychiatric SLE, pulmonary haemorrhage, etc.
Low dose IV CYC (ELNT regimen)	All other cases of proliferative LN
MMF (2-3 g/day for 6 months)	All other cases of proliferative LN Pediatric LN Women contemplating pregnancy (Seven times more expensive than ELNT regimen)

ISN class IV+V LN was shown to achieve higher rates of remission compared to IV CYC plus steroids at 6 months (50% vs. 5%).[18] This was proven in a larger trial, which included 362 patients, showing complete remission rates of 45.9% in MTT vs. 25.6% in IV CYC group in patients with LN at 6 months.[19]

To summarize, corticosteroids given along with one of the above induction agents form the backbone of treating patients with proliferative LN. In a resource-limited setting, considering the cost of therapy while choosing one induction agent over the other is important.[20] Intravenous pulse methylprednisolone (0.5-1.0 g/m^2) for 3 consecutive days is usually indicated in severe proliferative LN presenting with rapidly progressive renal failure or renal biopsy showing extensive crescentic lesions, fibrinoid necrosis or thrombotic microangiopathy involving the glomerular capillaries. Oral corticosteroids (prednisolone) at a dose between 0.5-1.0 mg/kg/day for at least 4 weeks followed by gradual tapering till 5 mg per day is the standard of care for treating proliferative LN. We, at our centre, compared two doses of oral prednisolone (0.5 mg/kg/day versus 1 mg/kg/day) given along with oral MMF as induction therapy in patients with less severe proliferative LN and found low dose (0.5 mg/kg/day) prednisolone to be inferior to standard dose (1 mg/kg/day) prednisolone in inducing remission (unpublished data). In light of the side-effects associated with high dose steroids and the inefficacy of low dose steroids, it seems prudent to use oral prednisolone at a dose more than 0.5 mg/kg/day, but, less than 1 mg/kg/day.

In addition to the induction therapies, all patients should be treated with hydroxychloroquine (HCQ) (4-6 mg/kg/day), RAAS blockade for proteinuria (>1 g/day) and if hypertensive, aggressive anti-hypertensive agents with target blood pressure of ≤ 130/80 mm Hg. Statins should be used to treat hyperlipidemia. Cotrimoxazole is added for Pneumocystis pneumoniae prophylaxis during induction therapy.

What Would be the Appropriate Choice in Our Patient?

With the background of normal renal functions, light microscopy not showing any cellular crescents and consideration of fertility preservation, MMF was proposed in this young female. She was discharged with prednisolone 40 mg per day, MMF 2 g per day, enalapril 10 mg per day, atorvastatin 20 mg per day, HCQ 300 mg per day, torsemide 50 mg per day with an advice on high protein and low salt diet. After 2 months, she presented again with generalized swelling of the body with decreased urine output and malaise. On physical examination, she was noted to have anasarca, pallor without any signs of hypercortisolism. Her blood pressure was 110/70 mm Hg, heart rate was 90 per minute and respiratory rate was 20 per minute. Analyses now revealed serum creatinine of 4.2 mg/dl, blood urea 86 mg/dl, hemoglobin 7.8 g/dl, leucocytes of 4200/mm^3, platelet count of 1.2 lakh, total serum proteins 4.2 g/dl, serum albumin 1.8 g/dl, microscopic hematuria and proteinuria of 3 gm/24 h. Serology was positive for anti-dsDNA titers of > 359 IU/ml with low complement levels (C3 46 mg/dl and C4 6 mg/dl). On questioning, patient admitted having stopped steroids and MMF for 1 month prior to admission, owing to esthetic changes caused by therapy. This could explain the progressive deterioration of disease course and probable persistent disease activity. A repeat renal biopsy was done to confirm the same and it showed persistent diffuse proliferative LN with extensive crescent formation (8 of 14 glomeruli) and fibrinoid necrosis. There was presence of moderate interstitial mononuclear cell infiltration with interstitial fibrosis/tubular atrophy in 10% of the cortical area. She was given three methylprednisolone pulses at 0.75 g/d for 3 days, followed by prednisolone 60 mg per day with tapering after 4 weeks and IV CYC 0.5 g per m^2 after repeat counseling about risks versus benefits. She was also given HCQ 300 mg per day, enalapril 10 mg per day and atorvastatin 20 mg per day. Renal function slowly improved and she was discharged with a serum creatinine of 3.2 mg/dl and hemoglobin of 8.6 g/dl. After 6 monthly pulses of cyclophosphamide, she was started on azathioprine 100 mg per day with continuation of low dose (5 mg per day) prednisolone. She followed up regularly thereafter and her serum creatinine improved to 1.6 mg/dl after completion of 8 months of therapy.

What is the Role of Repeat Renal Biopsy in Managing Lupus Nephritis?

Although there is no clinical trial that has tested the role of repeat biopsy against clinical data alone to decide therapy, repeat biopsy is frequently done to assess disease activity, class transformation, decide therapy and to prognosticate patients. Repeat renal biopsy is usually done at relapse or resistant/refractory disease and as a protocol in some centres at the end of induction and/or maintenance therapy of LN. KDIGO (2012) recommends repeat biopsy during relapse if there is suspicion that the histologic class of LN has changed, or there is uncertainty between activity or chronicity.

What are the Poor Prognostic Factors in a Patient with Lupus Nephritis?

There are various factors which predict poor outcomes in LN patients (Table 8.6). Amongst histological parameters, while increased chronicity index was found to be a poor prognostic factor in some studies,[21,22] others did not find any histological parameters to predict outcome.[23,24]

Table 8.6: Main poor prognostic factors in lupus nephritis

Demographic	Clinical
1. Age (young)	1. Class of LN (Class IV: diffuse proliferative)
2. Male Gender	2. Elevated serum creatinine
3. Black race	3. Response to treatment
	4. Anemia
	5. Thrombocytopenia

What are the Specific Issues in a Young Female?

Contraception

An effective contraceptive method in a patient with SLE should translate into an uncomplicated pregnancy during inactive phase of the disease while the patient is on non-teratogenic drugs. It should be safe in terms of side effects such as osteoporosis due to inhibition of ovulation, propensity to trigger lupus activity and thromboembolism. Progesterone intrauterine device (levonorgestrel IUD) or subdermal implant are preferable for most patients. Estrogen-containing oral contraceptives are contraindicated in patients with active disease or positive antiphospholipid antibodies (aPL).[25] Nevertheless, they were not found to add risk of causing flares in patients with mild-moderate stable disease activity in the SELENA trial.[26] Depot medroxyprogesterone acetate (DMPA) should be avoided in corticosteroid-treated patients at risk for osteoporosis.[27] Although barrier methods are less effective, they are relied on during acute illness when other methods are still not applied.

Fertility

Fertility is affected in SLE due to the following reasons:

1. Anti-corpus luteum antibodies has been shown to be associated with amenorrhea in lupus patients suggesting an autoimmune, SLE-related menstrual dysfunction.[28] Patients with high disease activity (SLEDAI ≥ 8) were more likely to have menstrual disturbance accounting for 71% of total patients.[29]
2. Ovarian failure is a frequent side effect of CYC therapy used to treat severe proliferative LN. Gonadotoxicity is dose-dependent in male patients and has an age- and dose-dependent effect on female patients. The incidence of ovarian failure in those receiving longer CYC (≥ 15 pulses) ranges from 10-100%[11,20] with rates >40% in patients between 20-30 years and 100% in those >30 years. While a cumulative dose up to 7.5 g/m^2 is the limit in males, doses up to 10-15 g/m^2 is tolerated without gonadotoxicity in young females with LN. Gonadotoxicity is considered irreversible in females (as opposed to males) owing to fixed number of oocytes throughout life and the risk of permanent infertility is unpredictable in some patients. Therefore, discussion of fertility preservation methods should be done on a case-by-case basis.
3. SLE itself can cause disorders of affect and loss of sexual function in women. These psychological factors may be responsible for a higher probability of apparent infertility.
4. Renal failure due to progressive lupus nephritis can alter the hypothalamic-pituitary-gonadal axis and result in infertility.

Measures to Prevent Infertility Due to Cyclophosphamide

1. Use of alternative immunosuppressive agents (MMF), if possible.
2. Use of lower and shorter CYC (IV administration having lower cumulative dose than oral).
3. Avoiding administration of IV CYC during ovulation period of menstrual cycle.
4. Protective agents such as concomitant monthly GnRH agonist (leuprolide) to inhibit ovulation in females (comes with risk of menopausal symptoms and exaggerated osteoporosis) and biweekly intramuscular injections of testosterone in males.
5. Oocyte cryopreservation in females (comes with the risk of flaring lupus as hormonal stimulation is required for oocyte collection)/sperm banking in males.

Referral to a fertility specialist is recommended on a case-by-case basis.

Pregnancy in a Patient with Lupus Nephritis

Multidisciplinary approach with frequent medical,

obstetric and neonatal monitoring is prudent for a successful pregnancy in patients with LN as the risks with pregnancy are high unlike patients with other glomerular diseases (Table 8.7). A stepwise approach to manage pregnancy in a patient with lupus nephritis is described as follows:

Table 8.7: Risks associated with pregnancy in patients with SLE

Disease activity during pregnancy	Ranges between 25 and 65% More commonly renal and hematological flares Active disease during the prior 6 months, history of LN and discontinuation of HCQ increases risk of flare
Pregnancy complications	Preeclampsia (3-5 times higher risk than normal population) History of LN, presence of aPL, hypocomplementemia, and thrombocytopenia are added risk factors
Fetal outcome	Fetal loss (10-20%) Pre-term birth (up to 50%) Small for gestational age babies (10-30%) Hypertension, aPL, thrombocytopenia, and LN are added risk factors

1. Ensure optimal disease control (complete remission of LN) for at least 6 months prior to conception, with pregnancy-compatible medications (including HCQ).

   Drugs, which can be safely used during pregnancy, are low-dose steroid, azathioprine (maximum dose 2 mg/kg/day), calcineurin inhibitors (cyclosporine and tacrolimus), HCQ, low dose aspirin and calcium supplements. MMF and CYC are contraindicated and should be discontinued at least 3 months before conception. Biologics (rituximab) should also be discontinued short of safety data.
2. Pre-conception counselling.
3. Maternal and fetal risk assessment with evaluation of disease activity (complement levels, anti-dsDNA titre, SLEDAI score) and set of autoantibodies (aPL and anti-Ro antibodies).

   Presence of aPL entails low dose aspirin with or without heparin depending on previous history of systemic thrombosis and fetal loss. In case of disease flare during pregnancy, higher doses of steroid (methylprednisolone) can be used with IVIG and plasmapheresis (in very severe disease).

What is Refractory Lupus Nephritis and How is it Managed?

Refractory or resistant LN is used to indicate cases that do not respond within 3-6 months of starting standard induction therapy, although, there is no formal definition of refractory LN. Refractory LN may present clinically as persistent nephrotic syndrome, renal dysfunction or asymptomatic urinary abnormalities. Early detection of refractory LN is important to prevent irreversible renal damage. KDIGO (2012) recommends switch from mycophenolate mofetil (MMF) to CYC or vice versa for patients who did not respond to either of these drugs.

In patients who do not respond to both the first line induction agents (MMF and CYC), rituximab, as add-on or monotherapy, was found to be effective in cases with persistent renal dysfunction.[30] Combination of calcineurin inhibitors, MMF and steroids (multi-target therapy) has been used successfully to treat refractory LN with persistent proteinuria.[31]

What are the Renal Replacement Therapy (RRT) Options in Lupus Nephritis Patients?

Despite the success of newer induction therapies in treating LN, 10-20% of these patients still progress to end-stage renal disease (ESRD). The choices of various modalities of RRT, as in any other patient with ESRD, are hemodialysis, peritoneal dialysis (PD), living donor renal transplant or cadaveric renal transplant. Data on long-term survival is similar in both hemodialysis and peritoneal dialysis. PD was associated with more episodes of peritonitis, other infections and technique failure in LN patients as compared to patients with non-lupus glomerulonephritis.[32] This may be related to ongoing immunosuppressive therapy in LN patients. Living donor transplantation is associated with better survival outcomes than cadaveric renal transplant as in any other patient with ESRD. It is prudent to assess for anti-phospholipid antibodies (APLA) prior to transplant to decide on peri-operative anti-coagulation as vessel thrombosis is a dreaded complication of APLA. The disease activity should also be quiescent around the time of transplant, which is usually so in LN patients with ESRD. The recurrence rate after transplant is low (about 10%) and rarely leads to graft loss, probably owing to continuous immunosuppressive therapy.

References

1. Contreras G, Roth D, Pardo V, Striker LG, Schultz DR. Lupus nephritis: A clinical review for practicing nephrologists. Clin Nephrol 2002;57(2):95-107.
2. Hogan J, Appel GB. Update on the treatment of lupus nephritis. Curr Opin Nephrol Hypertens 2013;22(2):224-30.
3. Mittal T, Rathi M. Rheumatological diseases and kidneys: A nephrologist's perspective. Int J Rheum Dis 2014; 17(8): 834-44.
4. Hsieh YP, Wen YK, Chen ML. The value of early renal biopsy in systemic lupus erythematosus patients

presenting with renal involvement. Clin Nephrol 2012; 77(1):18-24.

5. Mahmood SN, Mukhtar KN, Deen S, Khan FN. Renal Biopsy: A much needed tool in patients with Systemic Lupus Erythematosis (SLE). Pak J Med Sci 2016;32(1):70-74.
6. Rathi M, Sharma A, Nada R. Renal biopsy in lupus nephritis: To do or not to do. Indian J Rheumatol 2017;12 (1), 2.
7. Bajema IM, Wilhelmus S, Alpers CE, Bruijn JA, Colvin RB, Cook HT, *et al.* Revision of the International Society of Nephrology/Renal Pathology Society classification for lupus nephritis: Clarification of definitions, and modified National Institutes of Health activity and chronicity indices. Kidney Int 2018;93(4):789-96.
8. Austin HA, Klippel JH, Balow JE, le Riche NG, Steinberg AD, Plotz PH, *et al.* Therapy of lupus nephritis. Controlled trial of prednisone and cytotoxic drugs. N Engl J Med 1986; 314(10):614-19.
9. Boumpas DT, Austin HA, Vaughan EM, Klippel JH, Steinberg AD, Yarboro CH, *et al.* Controlled trial of pulse methylprednisolone versus two regimens of pulse cyclophosphamide in severe lupus nephritis. Lancet 1992; 340(8822):741-45.
10. Gourley MF, Austin HA, Scott D, Yarboro CH, Vaughan EM, Muir J, *et al.* Methylprednisolone and cyclophosphamide, alone or in combination, in patients with lupus nephritis. A randomized, controlled trial. Ann Intern Med 1996; 125(7):549-57.
11. Boumpas DT, Austin HA, Vaughan EM, Yarboro CH, Klippel JH, Balow JE. Risk for sustained amenorrhea in patients with systemic lupus erythematosus receiving intermittent pulse cyclophosphamide therapy. Ann Intern Med 1993;119(5):366-69.
12. Houssiau FA, Vasconcelos C, D'Cruz D, Sebastiani GD, Garrido Ed E de R, Danieli MG, *et al.* Immunosuppressive therapy in lupus nephritis: The Euro-Lupus Nephritis Trial, a randomized trial of low-dose versus high-dose intravenous cyclophosphamide. Arthritis Rheum 2002; 46(8):2121-31.
13. Chan TM, Li FK, Tang CS, Wong RW, Fang GX, Ji YL, *et al.* Efficacy of mycophenolate mofetil in patients with diffuse proliferative lupus nephritis. Hong Kong-Guangzhou Nephrology Study Group. N Engl J Med 2000;343(16): 1156-62.
14. Ginzler EM, Dooley MA, Aranow C, Kim MY, Buyon J, Merrill JT, *et al.* Mycophenolate mofetil or intravenous cyclophosphamide for lupus nephritis. N Engl J Med 2005; 353(21):2219-28.
15. Appel GB, Contreras G, Dooley MA, Ginzler EM, Isenberg D, Jayne D, *et al.* Mycophenolate mofetil versus cyclophosphamide for induction treatment of lupus nephritis. J Am Soc Nephrol 2009;20(5):1103-12.
16. Rathi M, Goyal A, Jaryal A, Sharma A, Gupta PK, Ramachandran R, *et al.* Comparison of low-dose intravenous cyclophosphamide with oral mycophenolate mofetil in the treatment of lupus nephritis. Kidney Int 2016;89(1):235-42.
17. Rovin BH, Furie R, Latinis K, Looney RJ, Fervenza FC, Sanchez-Guerrero J, *et al.* Efficacy and safety of rituximab in patients with active proliferative lupus nephritis: The Lupus Nephritis Assessment with Rituximab study. Arthritis Rheum 2012;64(4):1215-26.
18. Bao H, Liu Z-H, Xie H-L, Hu W-X, Zhang H-T, Li L-S. Successful treatment of class V+IV lupus nephritis with multitarget therapy. J Am Soc Nephrol 2008;19(10): 2001-10.
19. Liu Z, Zhang H, Liu Z, Xing C, Fu P, Ni Z, *et al.* Multitarget therapy for induction treatment of lupus nephritis: A randomized trial. Ann Intern Med 2015;162(1):18-26.
20. Rathi M, Sharma A. Mycophenolate or Cyclophosphamide in Lupus Nephritis: Which One to Use in Indian Patients? Indian J Nephrol 2018;28(2):99-100.
21. Arce-Salinas CA, Villa AR, Martínez-Rueda JO, Muñoz L, Cardiel MH, Alcocer-Varela J, *et al.* Factors associated with chronic renal failure in 121 patients with diffuse proliferative lupus nephritis: A case-control study. Lupus 1995;4(3):197-203.
22. Rijnink EC, Teng YKO, Wilhelmus S, Almekinders M, Wolterbeek R, Cransberg K, *et al.* Clinical and Histopathologic Characteristics Associated with Renal Outcomes in Lupus Nephritis. Clin J Am Soc Nephrol 2017; 12(5):734-43.
23. Schwartz MM, Bernstein J, Hill GS, Holley K, Phillips EA. Predictive value of renal pathology in diffuse proliferative lupus glomerulonephritis. Lupus Nephritis Collaborative Study Group. Kidney Int 1989;36(5):891-96.
24. Rathi M, Gupta KL, Joshi K, Gupta PK, Sharma A, Kohli HS, *et al.* Histopathological indicators of disease outcome in class IV lupus nephritis: A revisit of various indices. Rheumatol Int 2015;35(9):1511-17.
25. Culwell KR, Curtis KM. Contraception for women with systemic lupus erythematosus. J Fam Plann Reprod Health Care 2013;39(1):9-11.
26. Petri M, Kim MY, Kalunian KC, Grossman J, Hahn BH, Sammaritano LR, *et al.* Combined oral contraceptives in women with systemic lupus erythematosus. N Engl J Med 2005;353(24):2550-58.
27. Sammaritano LR. Contraception in patients with systemic lupus erythematosus and antiphospholipid syndrome. Lupus 2014;23(12):1242-45.
28. Pasoto SG, Viana VS, Mendonca BB, Yoshinari NH, Bonfa E. Anti-corpus luteum antibody: A novel serological marker for ovarian dysfunction in systemic lupus erythematosus? J Rheumatol 1999;26(5):1087-93.
29. Mok CC, Lau CS, Wong RW. Risk factors for ovarian failure in patients with systemic lupus erythematosus receiving cyclophosphamide therapy. Arthritis Rheum 1998;41(5):831-37.
30. Weidenbusch M, Römmele C, Schröttle A, Anders H-J. Beyond the LUNAR trial. Efficacy of rituximab in refractory lupus nephritis. Nephrol Dial Transplant 2013; 28(1):106-11.
31. Cortés-Hernández J, Torres-Salido MT, Medrano AS, Tarrés MV, Ordi-Ros J. Long-term outcomes–mycophenolate mofetil treatment for lupus nephritis with addition of tacrolimus for resistant cases. Nephrol Dial Transplant 2010;25(12):3939-48.
32. Siu YP, Leung KT, Tong MKH, Kwan TH, Mok CC. Clinical outcomes of systemic lupus erythematosus patients undergoing continuous ambulatory peritoneal dialysis. Nephrol Dial Transplant 2005;20(12):2797-802.

CHAPTER 9

A Patient with Rapidly Progressive Renal Failure with Skin Manifestations and Vascular Thrombosis

Shailendra Singh[1], Salil Jain[2], Abhijeet Kumar[3]

[1] *Consultant, Nephrology, Manipal Hospital, Dwarka, Delhi*

[2] *Director, Nephrology, Fortis Memorial Research Institute, Gurugram*

[3] *Consultant, Nephrology, Medanta, The Medicity, Lucknow*

In this chapter, we aim to present different clinical scenarios with history of renal failure with skin involvement and thrombotic manifestations. We will discuss few case scenarios associated with these symptoms.

CASE 1

60-year-old female with no comorbidities like diabetes or hypertension was admitted with history of generalized weakness, arthralgias, symptoms of cold intolerance and progressively increasing edema with oliguria since past 3 weeks. Lower limb examination revealed bilateral lower limb palpable purpura, peripheral sensorimotor neuropathy and left foot painful digit ulceration. Investigations revealed deranged renal function (BUN-104 mg/dl, Creatinine-4 mg/dl) along with active urinary sediments (Protein-2+, RBC-20-30 RBC/hpf, WBC-8-10 hpf), transaminitis (SGOT-300 IU/L, SGPT-200 IU/L) and anemia. Work up for RPGN revealed C3 and C4 decreased with negative ANA, ANCA, Anti GBM. Further work up revealed Anti HCV positive with negative HbsAg and HIV. Rheumatoid Factor was also positive. She had past history of multiple blood transfusions few years back for trauma. Kidney biopsy light microscopy revealed membranoproliferative pattern (MPGN) with crescents and microthrombi. IF revealed IgM and IgG deposits in capillary loop. Further electron microscopy revealed fingerprint appearance of subendothelial deposits. Serum cryoglobulins were positive and the provisional diagnosis of mixed cryoglobulinemia secondary to hepatitis C virus (HCV) was made. In view of RPGN presentation, patient was started on pulse steroids along with IV cyclophosphamide and also required 4 sessions of plasmapheresis along with intermittent dialysis. Patient started on Sofosbuvir-velpatasvir combination after HCV RNA and genotype. After a month of therapy her renal functions settled at serum creatinine 3 mg/dl along with improvement in extrarenal features. Patient has been kept on maintenance therapy with steroids.

What is Cryoglobulinemia and What is the Classification?

Cryoglobulins are immunoglobulins that precipitate at temperature <37°C and redissolve on warming in vitro. Cryoglobulinemia vasculitis refers to the presence of cryoglobulin containing immune complexes which usually involves small to medium vessels. It is classified into 3 groups based on immunoglobulin (Ig) composition. In the absence of an identifiable etiological factor (< 5% of all mixed cryoglobulinemia) it is defined as essential or idiopathic cryoglobulinemia. The classification is mentioned below (Table 9.1).[1,2]

Table 9.1: Brouet cryoglobulin classification

Cryoglobulin type	Component	Diseases associated
Type 1 (simple)	Monoclonal immunoglobulins (IgG, IgM or IgA)/monoclonal free light chains	Waldenström macroglobulinemia, Multiple myeloma, Lymphoproliferative disorder, Light chain disease
Type 2 (mixed)	Monoclonal immunoglobulins (IgG, IgM or IgA)/polyclonal free light chains (IgG)	Hepatitis C, Essential cryoglobulinemia, Sjögren syndrome, Rheumatoid arthritis, Chronic lymphocytic leukemia
Type 3 (mixed)	Polyclonal immunoglobulins of all isotypes	Essential cryoglobulinemia, Sjögren syndrome, Hepatitis B and C, Cytomegalovirus, Endocarditis

What are the Clinical Features and How is it Diagnosed?

The diagnosis of cryoglobulinemia is based on the clinical and laboratory features as shown in the Table 9.2.

Our patient had generalized weakness, arthralgia and purpura referred to as Meltzer's triad which is seen in cryoglobulinemia. Patient also had digital ulceration, rapidly progressive glomerulonephritis and peripheral neuropathy along with history of HCV. Thus, our patient fits into clinical diagnosis of mixed cryoglobulinemia as per Brouet classification.

Diagnostic Evaluation

Lab investigations: Complements (especially C4) are decreased in mixed cryoglobulinemia. Rheumatoid factor is generally raised. Multiorgan involvement can be assessed by deranged renal (raised creatinine) or liver functions (transaminits).

Viral serology including Hepatitis B, C and HIV along with screening for autoimmune diseases (SLE, Sjögren) should be done for mixed cryoglobulinemia.

Type 1 cryoglobulinemia is predominantly caused by monoclonal gammopathy (MGUS, Multiple myeloma, Waldenstrom macroglobulinemia) or lymphoproliferative disorders which cause hyperviscosity syndrome, *therefore mainly assosciated with thrombosis.*Thus screening should include protein electrophoresis, immunofixation, free light chain assays, bone marrow or CT imaging of abdomen or thorax to rule out lymphoma.

Diagnosis of serum cryoglobulins are reported as percentage of immunoglobulins precipitated at 4°C of total volume which is referred as cryocrit. > 1% cryocrit are considered as abnormal and further subtyping of immunoglobulins can be done by electrophoresis or immunofixation.

Tissue biopsy: Although biopsy is generally not required for diagnosis, it gives histopathological evidence of cryoglobulinemia. Type 1 cryoglobulinemia predominantly affects skin (leukocytoclastic vasculitis), bone marrow (plasma cells/lymphoid cells), kidney and is predominantly assosciated with thrombosis.

Mixed cryoglobulinemia: Affect skin, kidney and peripheral nerve and features are mainly suggestive of immune complex vasculitis.

Kidney Biopsy

Light microscopy and Immunofluorecence – mostly suggestive of membranoproliferative pattern (MPGN) with subendothelial deposits of cryoglobulin or immunoglobulin and hyaline intraglomerular thrombi with fibrinoid necrosis can also be seen. Electron microscopy reveals electron dense granular deposits in the subendothelial region referred to as fingerprint appearance (Fig. 9.1 a,b).

Table 9.2: Clinical and lab patterns of cryoglobulinemia

Clinical manifestation	Type 1	Type 2	Type 3
Arthralgia	+	++	+++
Purpura	+, usually unpalpable	+++ palpable	+++ palpable
Gangrene	+++	+	±
Hyperviscosity	+++	±	-
*Hematologic	++	±	±
**Renal	+	++	+
***Neurological	+	++	++
****Liver	±	++	+++
Lung	-	+	+
Cryocrit	>5%	<5% (1-2)	<5% (1-2)
C3, C4, CH 50	Normal	Decreased	Decreased
Rheumatoid factor	Normal	Decreased	Decreased
Autoantibodies (ANA, ENA, AMA)	-	++	++
Hepatitis B	-	+	+
Hepatitis C	-	+++	+++

*Hematological: Thrombosis/bleeding/thrombocytosis

**Renal: Nephrotic syndrome, Rapidly progressive glomerulonephritis

***Neurological: Peripheral neuropathy

****Liver: Transaminitis, Non alcoholic steatohepatitis

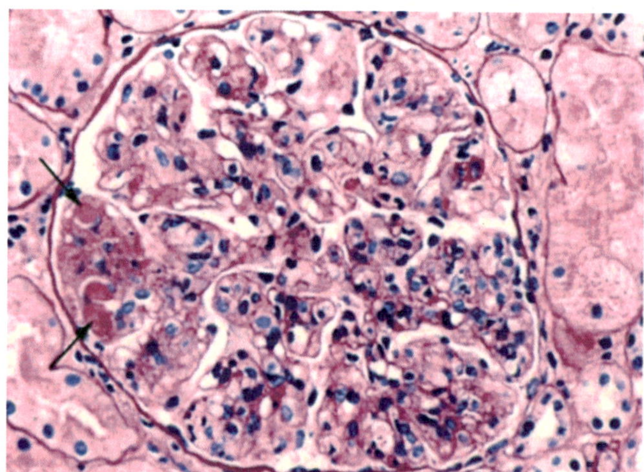

Figure 9.1a: Light microscopy revealing GBM thickening with cellular proliferation suggestive of MPGN. Hyaline microthrombi composed of cryoglobulins seen occluding capillaries in one of glomerulus (arrows)

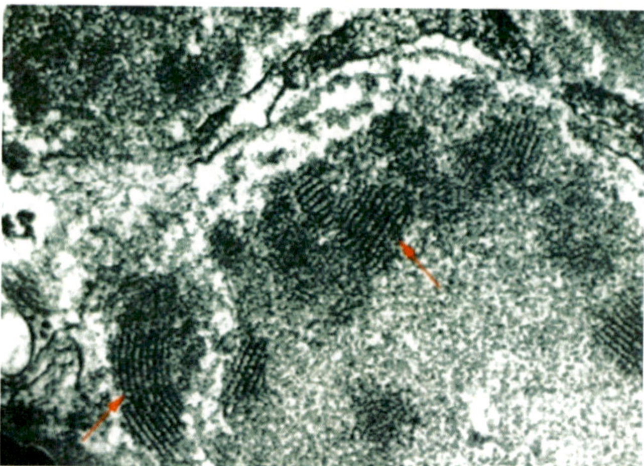

Figure 9.1b: Electron microscopy in subendothelial region showing cryoglobulins as **fingerprint appearance** (arrows)

Important point to remember is type 1 cryoglobulinemia presents predominantly with nephrotic syndrome or subnephrotic proteinuria with hematuria and may be associated with minimal cellular proliferation and predominantly foot process effacement. In contrast, mixed cryoglobulinemia presents with nephritic syndrome and has generally MPGN pattren on histopathology.

What is the Treatment and Differential Diagnosis?

The treatment of cryoglobulinemia depends on treating the underlying etiology like malignancy, autoimmune disease or viral infections.

The patient had HCV assosciated cryoglobulinemia and was treated as per underlying RPGN with steroids and cyclophosphamide and plasmapheresis. Cyclophosphamide and Rituximab improves kidney disease by reducing stimulation of B lymphocytes and cryoglobulin synthesis; steroid pulses are given to treat glomerular inflammation and plasma exchange has been employed to remove circulating cryoglobulins from the plasma and consequently reduce the deposition of immune complexes to the kidneys.

The differential diagnosis of condition like cryoglobulinemia is mentioned in Flowchart 9.1.

After the introduction of interferon (IFN) free Directly Acting Agent (DAA) regimens for treatment of HCV, there has been improvement in remission rates. Similarly, Rituximab has shown superiority as compared to old immunosuppressives (cyclophosphamide, steroids) in cryoglobulinemic vasculitis. The treatment of HCV assosciated cryoglobulinemia is given in Flowchart 9.2.

Rituximab dose is 375 mg/m^2 for 4 weeks but risk of relapse, opportunistic infection (reactivation of HCV and HBV) and most importantly cost of therapy should be kept into consideration while choosing immunosuppression.

Prior to introduction of DAA regimen, pegylated interferon along with ribavirin was used to treat HCV but was associated with side effects and low remission rates. DAA regimen has attained sustained virological response in > 90% of cases and with good tolerability.

Small vessel vasculitis can be associated with skin manifestations like purpura. The increased risk of thrombosis predominantly venous is due to either increased coagulability secondary to inflammation or immune mediated mechanism. Even middle or large vessel vasculitis is associated with thrombosis but glomerulonephritis is predominant feature of small vessel vasculitis.

The prevalence of venous thrombosis in ANCA associated vasculitis can range from 6-30%.

Among the causes for immune complex GN apart from cryoglobulinemia, the predominant causes of renal involvement with skin and thrombotic manifestations are autoimmune diseases, Infective endocarditis and shunt nephritis. Rare presentation of thrombosis is seen in Henoch-Schönlein Purpura (HSP) and post infectious GN. ANCA vasculitis has been explained in detail in chapter of RPGN.

Autoimmune Diseases

Systemic lupus erythematosus (SLE): Prevalence of arterial or venous thrombosis is a well-known clinical entity in 10-50% of cases. The most important risk factor is the presence of Antiphospholipid antibodies (APLA), however 40% of adults with SLE with thrombosis (including pulmonary embolism) are negative for APLA. Possible causes in such cases include high level of disease activity and circulating immune complexes or a higher inflammatory state. Skin manifestations in the form of photosensitivity, oral ulcers, malar or discoid lupus rash and renal involvement in form of immune complex glomerulonephritis is well-known.

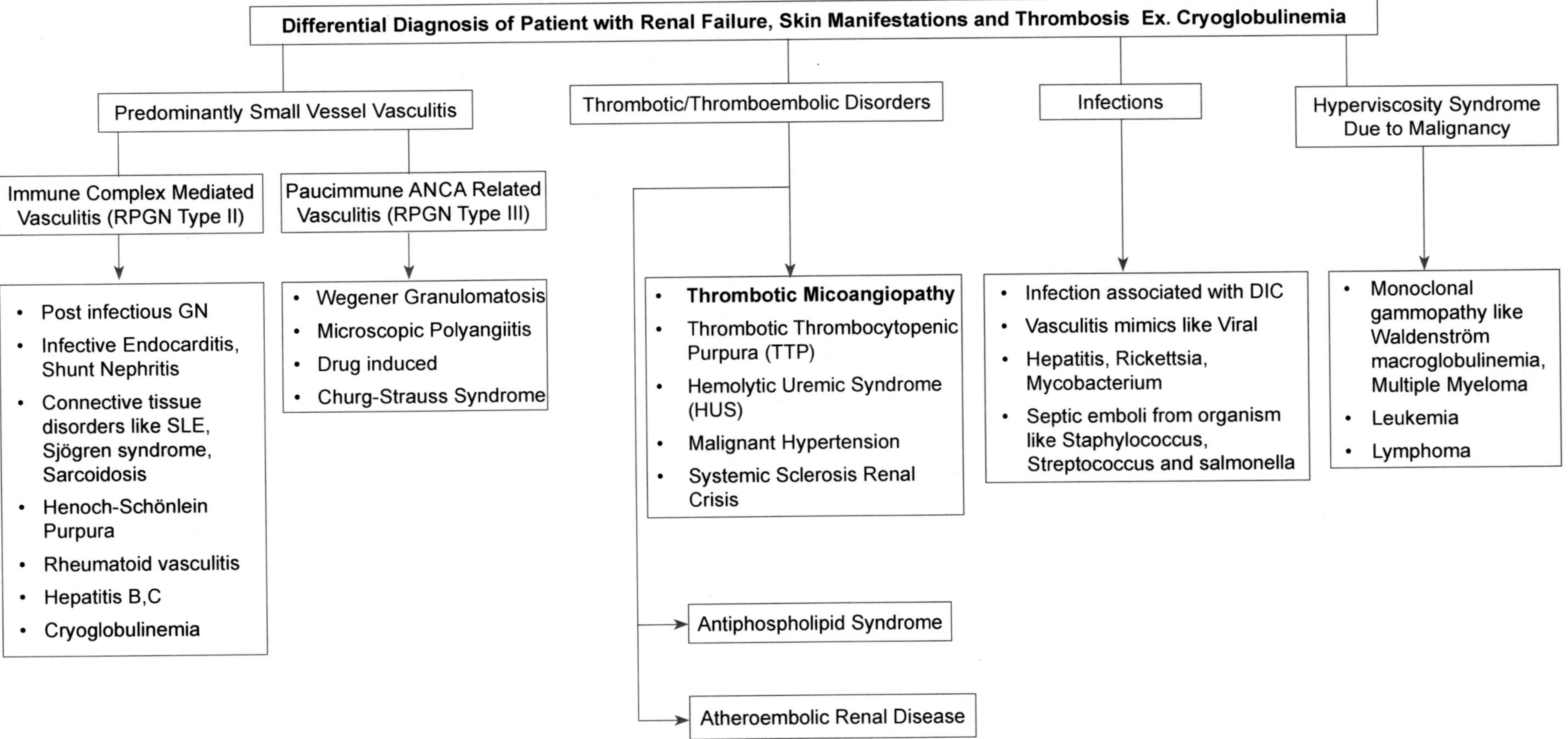

Flowchart 9.1: The differential diagnosis of conditions like cryoglobulinemia

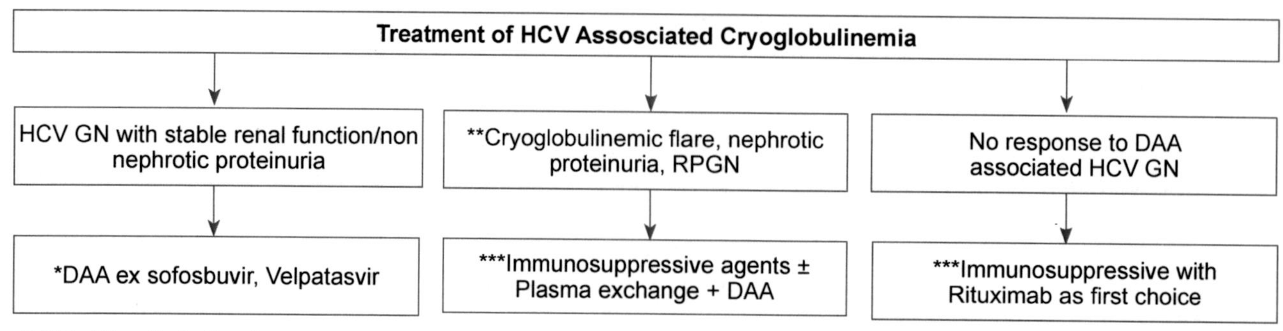

*DAA: Directly Acting Agent.

**Cryoglobulinemic flare–Multiorgan involvement like skin ulcers, peripheral neuropathy, renal involvement.

***Immunosuppressive–Steroids, cyclophosphamide, Azathioprine, Rituximab.

Flowchart 9.2: Treatment of HCV assosciated cryoglobulinemia

Sjögren Syndrome: Patients present with skin findings like xerosis, purpura, annular erythema, sclerodactyly and raynaud phenomenon. There is increased incidence of venous thrombosis and pulmonary embolism in such patients along with presence of glomerulonephritis.

Infective Endocarditis

It refers to infection of endocardial surface of heart valves or an intracardiac device by organisms like Staphylococcus aureus and Streptococcus. Patients present with high grade fever with skin manifestations include janeway lesions and osler nodes. Thromboembolic lesions include septic emboli in upto 25% of patients which can be seen in kidney, spleen, brain (embolic stroke) and other organs. Renal manifestations include immune complex glomerulonephritis, renal infarction/cortical necrosis from septic emboli.

Shunt Nephritis

Shunt nephritis is an immune complex mediated GN associated with chronically infected ventriculoatrial shunts inserted for treatment of hydrocephalus. The predominant organism is Staphylococcus. Renal manifestations include hematuria, proteinuria or RPGN presentation (endocapillary GN, MPGN). Skin manifestations include rash and thrombotic complications include clotted AV shunt, embolic stroke and pulmonary embolism.

Henoch-Schönlein Purpura (IgA Vasculitis)

The criteria for HSP is palpable purpura or petechia predominantly in lower limbs with abdominal pain, arthralgias and renal involvement (glomerulonephritis). But an important point to remember, thrombosis is a rare manifestation in HSP as there is no coagulopathy.

Post Infectious GN

This is the most common cause of nephritis predominantly seen in developing world in children. This is caused by beta hemolytic streptococcus which either causes pharyngitis (strain 12) or skin manifestation (strain 49). Renal involvement in the form of diffuse proliferative glomerulonephritis after few weeks of skin or throat infection can be seen. Risk of thrombosis is rare, seen only in case of associated vasculitis or nephrotic syndrome.

Thrombotic Disorders Associated with Renal Failure and Skin Changes

The most important cause is Thrombotic microangiopathy which is characterized by microangiopathic hemolytic anemia, renal failure and thrombocytopenia. This is divided into Thrombotic thrombocytopenic purpura and hemolytic uremic syndrome. Skin manifestations like rash or purpura are commonly present in this syndrome. As this topic has been covered in other chapters , we will not go into the details of this disorder and focus on other causes as explained below.

CASE 2

40-year-old female with no comorbidities was admitted with abdominal pain associated with constipation. Patient was provisionally diagnosed as subacute intestinal obstruction. Stool for occult blood was positive. Ultrasound abdomen followed by Upper GI endoscopy and colonoscopy were inconclusive. She was managed with conservative management and discharged. Patient was readmitted after few days with fever, severe abdominal pain, nausea and malena. Patient also had oliguria and bilateral lower limb bluish discolouration with edema. Patient gave previous history of spontaneous abortion twice followed by preterm delivery.

CT abdomen without contrast was done in view of rapid worsening renal dysfunction (creatinine 4 mg/dl) which was inconclusive. Patient had abdominal guarding and tenderness. Investigations revealed leukocytosis with worsening lactic acidosis. Patient with a high index of suspicion of bowel ischemia, underwent laparotomy and histopathological diagnosis later on confirmed the suspicion of mesenteric vein thrombosis. She developed stroke 2 days post op, was on ventilatory support and CT venography revealed cerebral venous sinus thrombosis. Work up for coagulation abnormality revealed prolonged APTT along with lupus anticoagulant positive by dilute russel viper antibody, positive antibeta 2 glycoprotein I IgG and negative anticardiolipin antibody. ANA and rest of work up for RPGN was negative. Patient had worsening renal functions (creatinine 6 mg/dl) with active urinary sediments along with RBC casts. She was initiated on low molecular weight heparin along with steroids, plasmapheresis and intermittent dialysis. Her condition improved but there was no renal recovery and patient became dialysis dependent. Lupus anticoagulant was positive repeated after 6 months. Patient has been advised lifelong warfarin therapy.

What is the Diagnosis and Clinical Features of the Syndrome?

The diagnosis is Antiphospholipid antibody syndrome (APS). APS is defined as an autoimmune multisystem disorder characterised by vascular thrombosis or pregnancy morbidity in the presence of antiphospholipid antibodies. APS can be classified as primary, i.e., idiopathic cause (almost 50%) and secondary APS with underlying autoimmune disorder, most common being SLE. The major difference between primary and secondary APS is that of thrombotic events, pregnancy associated features and clinical manifestations like arthralgias, livedo reticularis were more evident in APS secondary to SLE rather than primary.

Diagnostic Criteria of APS (Sydney Criteria)

Atleast 1 Clinical + 1 Lab Criteria.[3]

Clinical Criteria

- **Vascular thrombosis** involving vein, artery or any small vessel in any organ proven by imaging or histology, but superficial venous thrombus does not fit the criteria.
- **Pregnancy morbidity:**
  - ≥ 1 unexplained death of morphologically normal fetus at ≥ 10 weeks gestation; or
  - ≥ 1 premature births of neonate < 34 weeks due to eclampsia/placenta insufficiency; or
  - ≥ 3 consecutive pregnancy loss <10 weeks unexplained by chromosomal, anatomical or hormonal cause.

Lab Criteria

Presence of ≥1 antiphospholipid antibodies on ≥ 2 occasions 12 weeks apart

- IgG and/IgM anticardiolipin antibodies in moderate to high titres (> 40 units) by ELISA.
- IgG and/IgM anti beta 2 glycoprotein in moderate to high titres (> 40 units) by ELISA.
- Lupus anticoagulant.

Important Tips About Lupus Anticoagulant

- These are antibodies that block phospholipid surfaces important for coagulation, thus leading to hypercoagulability.
- Increase APTT which does not correct after mixing with normal plasma.
- Correction of phospholipids after addition of excess phospholipids confirms the presence of lupus anticoagulant.
- Guidelines recommend screening for Lupus anticoagulant with ≥ 2 phospholipid dependent coagulation assays like APTT, dilute Russell's viper venom time, kaolin/silica clotting time.

Clinical Presentation of APS

- With thrombotic manifestations.
- With obstetric complications/recurrent pregnancy loss.
- With simultaneous multiorgan dysfunction secondary to thrombosis.

The above said patient fits in the third category which is referred to as *Catastrophic APS.*

Diagnostic Criteria for Catastrophic APS

- Involvement of ≥ 3 organs/tissues.
- Histological evidence of intravascular thrombosis.
- Development of manifestation < 1 week.
- Presence of antiphospholipid antibodies.

Our patient had old history of recurrent pregnancy loss with preterm birth, cause of which was not evaluated. Patient was diagnosed with bowel infarction with histopathological evidence of mesenteric vein thrombosis. Patient also simultaneously presented with history of cerebral venous sinus thrombosis and renal failure, most likely due to acute thrombotic microangiopathy (TMA) within a short span of time. Skin manifestations were suggestive of livedo reticularis/racaemosa which is referred to as violaceous net like pattern on skin. Coagulopathy work up revealed positive lupus anticoagulant on 2 occasions more than 3 months apart with negative ANA.

Thus, the final diagnosis of patient is *Primary Catastrophic Antiphospholipid Syndrome (CAPS).*

Renal involvement in Primary APS can present as acute/chronic TMA. Other glomerular lesions include membranous nephropathy, minimal change disease or pauci immune glomerulonephritis, whereas APS secondary to SLE has predominantly picture of lupus nephritis with less prevalence of microthrombi.

What is the Treatment and Prognosis of APS?

For acute venous/arterial thromboembolic episode in patient with APS, the therapy of choice is heparin. Low molecular weight heparin (LMWH) is preferred over conventional heparin and treatment also includes managing complications related to thrombosis and infarction. Warfarin is the drug of choice for long term anticoagulation for ongoing event or to prevent secondary recurrence with target INR of 2-3. Aspirin (low dose) is added generally in arterial thrombosis with risk of cardiovascular complications.

In pregnancy, treatment is usually heparin as it does not cross placenta along with low dose aspirin.

If warfarin is being given, patient should discontinue warfarin and switch to heparin 6 weeks prior to gestation.

Therapy in CAPS can include pulse dose of steroids along with plasmapheresis with the aim to remove antibodies and IVIG. Therapy with rituximab and eculizumab has shown beneficial results in resistant CAPS.

Duration of therapy in APS is usually lifelong on warfarin with monitoring of INR in unprovoked thrombus. If there is a clear history of provoked thrombus or very low antiphospholipid titres, then anticoagulant can be stopped after explaining the risk of thrombosis to the patients.

The prognosis depends on the clinical manifestation. For example in CAPS, like in our patient there is high chance of morbidity and mortality. This patient developed ESRD despite immunosuppressive therapy.

CASE 3

65-year-old male diagnosed case of diabetes, hypertension was admitted with complaints of chest pain and was diagnosed to have myocardial infarction. Patient was managed with thrombolytic therapy and afterwards angioplasty was done. Patient was discharged but after 3 weeks started having progressive decreasing urine output with bluish discolouration of veins over lower limbs.

Investigations revealed deranged renal functions (BUN 128 mg/dl, creatinine 8 mg/dl) with active urinary sediments (Protein-2+, RBC-15-20/hpf, WBC-10-15/hpf) on urine analysis with baseline creatinine of 1.5 mg/dl. Work up for RPGN revealed decreased complement factors with negative ANA, Anti GBM and ANCA serology. Kidney biopsy was suggestive of features of acute tubular necrosis with evidence of thrombus present in renal artery with perivascular eosinophilia. The patient was on intermittent dialysis and managed conservatively and continued on cardioprotective medications. His renal functions gradually stabilised and settled at creatinine of 3 mg/dl.

What is the Diagnosis and What are the Clinical Features?

The diagnosis is Atheroembolic renal disease with acute tubular necrosis.

Atheroembolic renal disease usually occurs in older people with diffuse atherosclerotic disease where cholesterol crystal embolization occurs when portions of an atherosclerotic plaque break off and embolise distally, resulting in partial or total occlusion of multiple small renal vessels including glomerular arterioles leading to ischemic damage. Risk factors are similar to atherosclerosis including diabetes, hypertension, old age, hyperlipidemia, male sex and cigarette smoking.

The major inciting events for cholesterol embolization are predominantly iatrogenic like angiography, cardiovascular surgery, thrombolytic therapy or anticoagulation. Rarely, spontaneous embolization secondary to hemodynamic stress can also occur.[4]

Clinical Presentation

Kidney: Subacute renal failure progressing over several weeks is the predominant picture, although acute presentation can also occur in cases of massive embolization. Rarely, chronic renal failure secondary to ischemic nephropathy can also occur. Urine analysis can have bland sediments, microscopic hematuria, eosinophilluria or even red cell casts. There is frequent worsening of underlying hypertension along with 40% of patients developing advanced renal failure and may require dialysis. However, one must remember kidney involvement is not the most common presentation of atheroembolic disease (Flowchart 9.3).

Lab features like peripheral blood eosinophilia with hypocomplementemia and elevated inflammatory markers like ESR and CRP makes it a vasculitis mimicker and should be distinguished from true vasculitis by clinical presentation and renal histology.

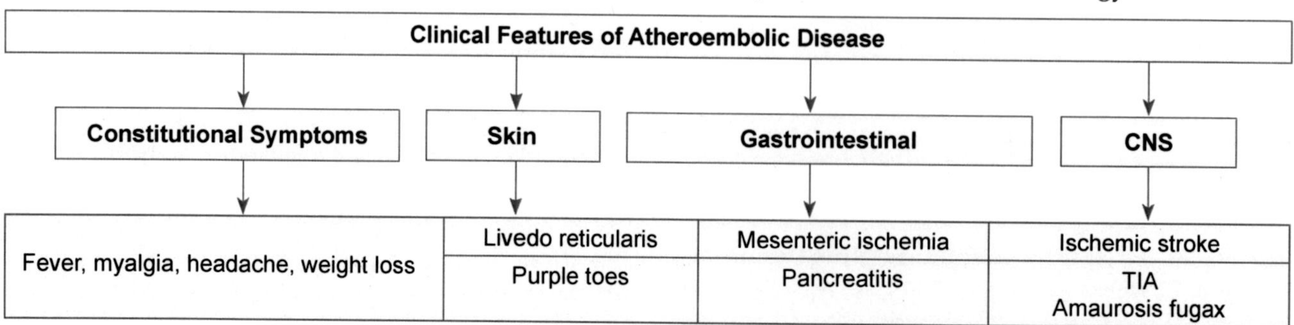

Flowchart 9.3: Clinical features of atheroembolic disease

What are Diagnostic Features on Kidney Biopsy?

Renal biopsy seems to be diagnostic in patients with atheroembolic renal disease. However, the drawback is that the typical lesions, i.e., occlusion of small renal vessel and glomerular capillaries may be focal and can be missed on biopsy. The diagnostic sensitivity of single renal biopsy is 75%. The diagnosis is established by demonstration of cholesterol emboli. The cholesterol emboli are dissolved during tissue fixation, thus pathognomonic biconvex, needle shaped clefts/ghosts are left behind within the occluded vessel. The intraluminal lesions are accompanied by a perivascular inflammatory reaction that may contain eosinophils (Fig. 9.2).

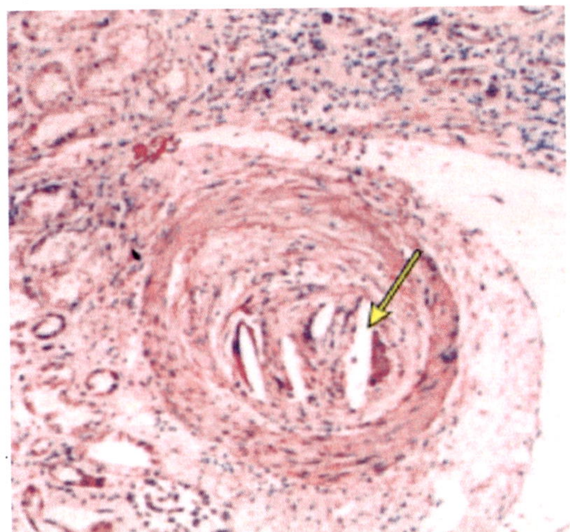

Figure 9.2: Light microscopy reveals atheroembolus in renal artery with cleft like spaces due to washout of cholesterol crystals during tissue fixation

Similarly, effect of cholesterol embolization can be demonstrated in other tissues or organs. For example on fundoscopy, retinal artery occlusion is demonstrated as Hollenhorst plaques.

What is the Treatment and Prognosis?

There is no proven effective medical therapy for atheroembolic renal disease. Therapeutic modalities are usually for secondary prevention of cardiovascular diseases. These include statin, aspirin, blood pressure and glycemic control along with cessation of smoking. In patients with diagnosed atheroembolic disease consideration should be given to withdrawal of anticoagulation, avoidance or postponement of new radiological/vascular procedures.

Prognosis is usually considered poor with high mortality, but this is also secondary to selection bias as most of biopsy proven disease have been postmortem. Similarly, our patient also presented with rapidly progressive renal failure. The most likely reason of renal recovery in our patient is that he had associated acute tubular necrosis.

Infections with Renal Failure, Thrombosis and Skin Changes

Any infection including bacterial, viral, fungal or parasitic which leads to consumptive coagulopathy, i.e., disseminated intravascular coagulation and severe systemic inflammation may predispose to thrombosis. The thrombosis can occur due to endothelial injury followed by platelet deposition leading to thrombus formation. Septic emboli like in infective endocarditis can also lead to skin involvement with renal involvement in form of thrombotic microangiopathy. Main organism include bacteria like staphylococcus, streptococcus, salmonella and fungal infections. Renal failure in underlying infections can occur because of prerenal (ex septic shock) or renal involvement. Renal involvement can occur due to glomerular or tubulointerstitial involvement as shown in Flowchart 9.4.

Skin involvement in infections can range from rash, purpura to ulcerative lesions and gangrene. In cases with underlying predominant hemolysis or liver failure jaundice is usually evident like leptospirosis, complicated malaria.

Hyperviscosity Syndromes

Hyperviscosity syndrome is an emergency that presents with elevated blood viscosity that results due

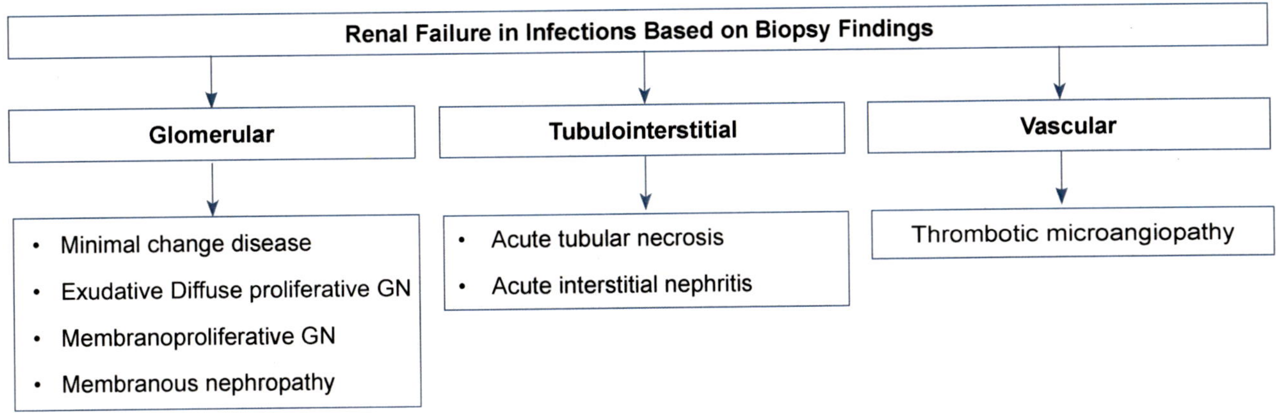

Flowchart 9.4: Renal involvement in infections

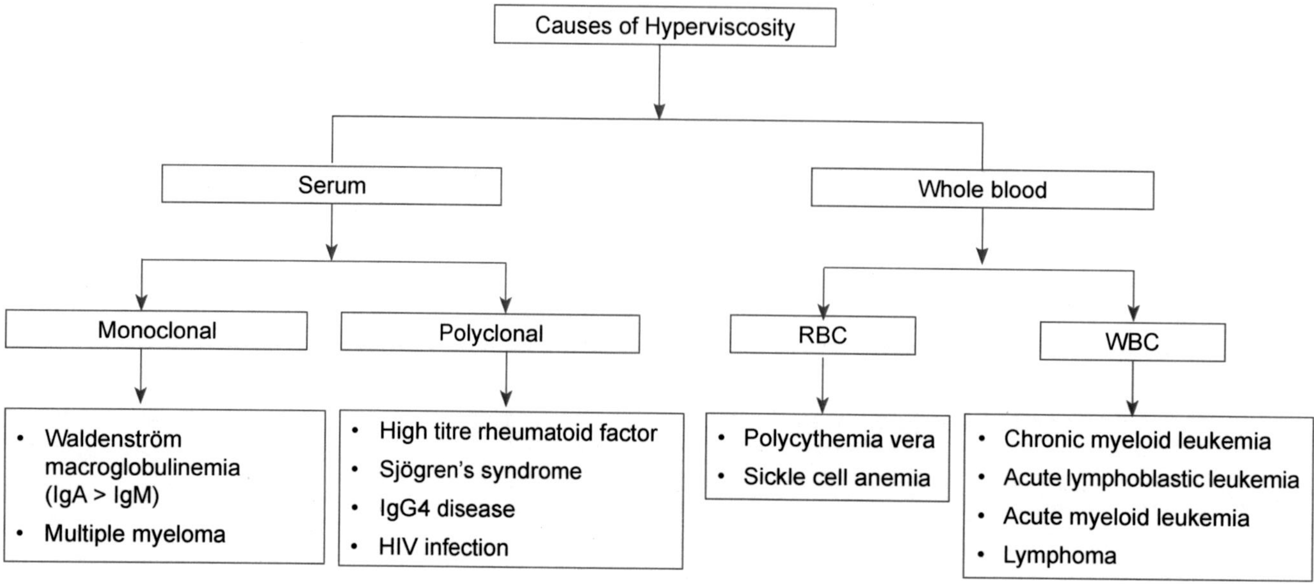

Flowchart 9.5: Renal involvement in hyperviscosity syndromes

to RBC deformity or pathological increase in serum proteins, RBC, WBC or platelets. The most common cause of hyperviscosity syndrome is Waldenström macroglobulinemia (WM) (Flowchart 9.5).[5]

The clinical manifestations present with triad of neurological manifestations, visual changes and mucosal bleeding. Multiple myeloma commonly presents with renal failure like cast nephropathy whereas WM, leukemia and lymphoma have infiltrations but clinical disease is less common.

Skin manifestations in malignancies can range from maculopapular rash, urticaria, purpura, livedo reticularis, Raynaud phenomenon and ulcers.

Sickle cell disease is an inherited disorder leading to polymerisation of deoxygenated RBC leading to microvascular occlusion with thrombosis, hemolytic crisis and end organ manifestations like sickle cell nephropathy. Renal medullary hypoxia with vasocclusion leading to predominantly tubular and later on glomerular damage is seen. Renal failure in form of chronic renal failure and recurrent AKI at times of sickle cell crisis can occur. FSGS is predominant glomerular lesion seen. Hemolytic crisis may present with rashes and jaundice.

Management of hyperviscosity syndrome includes supportive care with IV fluids, plasmapheresis and treatment of underlying hematological conditions.

References

1. Motyckova G and Murali M, Laboratory testing for cryoglobulins. Am. J Hematol 2011;86:500-02. doi:10.1002/ajh.22023.
2. Ramos-Casals M, Trejo O, García-Carrasco M, Cervera R, Font J. Mixed cryoglobulinemia: New concepts. Lupus. 2000;9(2):83-91. doi:10.1191/096120300678828127.
3. Miyakis S, Lockshin MD, Atsumi T, *et al.* International consensus statement on an update of the classification criteria for definite antiphospholipid syndrome (APS). J Thromb Haemost 2006;4(2):295-306. doi:10.1111/j.1538-7836.2006.01753.x.
4. Modi KS, Rao VK. Atheroembolic renal disease. Journal of the American Society of Nephrology 2001 Aug 1;12(8): 1781-87.
5. Rogers AP, Estes M. Hyperviscosity Syndrome. InStatPearls [Internet] 2019 Feb 18. StatPearls Publishing.

CHAPTER 10

A Patient with Rapidly Progressive Glomerulonephritis

Shailendra Singh[1], Saurabh Pokhariyal[2], Davinder Kundra[3]

[1] *Consultant, Nephrology, Manipal Hospital, Delhi*
[2] *Head of Department, Nephrology, Manipal Hospital, Delhi*
[3] *Consultant, Pulmonology, Manipal Hospital, Delhi*

Introduction

The World Health Organization defines rapidly progressive glomerulonephritis (RPGN) as an abrupt or insidious onset of macroscopic hematuria, proteinuria, anemia and rapidly progressing renal failure. Clinically, RPGN has less incidence of hypertension and edema as compared to acute glomerulonephritis. The exact timeline of this entity is undefined varying from few weeks to < 3 months, thus falling in the category between Acute Kidney Injury (AKI) and Chronic Kidney Disease (CKD). On ultrasonography, patients with RPGN have normal sized kidneys while presence of small, contracted kidneys points in favour of CKD. Kidney biopsy along with serology is mostly required for establishing the diagnosis of RPGN. In most cases, the histopathological diagnosis is necrotizing crescentic glomerulonephritis (NCGN). Crescentic glomerulonephritis, a term synonymously used for RPGN refers to extensive glomerular crescent formation (i.e., >50% of sampled glomeruli contain crescents). NCGN is classified into three types–linear, granular and pauci immune pattern–based on immunofluorescence (IF) microscopic findings. A linear pattern indicates anti-glomerular basement disease (Anti-GBM) whereas granular staining is seen in circulating immune complex diseases such as systemic lupus erythematosus (SLE) and IgA vasculitis. Most cases with the pauci immune pattern are glomerulonephritis induced by anti-neutrophil cytoplasmic autoantibody (ANCA)-associated vasculitis (Table 10.1).

Treatment usually involves pulse methylprednisolone followed by daily oral prednisolone, oral/IV cyclophosphamide or rituximab (in certain cases) and plasmapheresis. Plasmapheresis removes circulating antibodies, whereas immunosuppressive agents like steroids, cyclophosphamide minimize new antibody formation.

Time is of the essence in the management of RPGN, otherwise most of the patients will develop end stage renal failure. Thus, in fact, RPGN should be considered as "Renal Emergency"and timely biopsy followed by immunosuppressive therapy is required to prevent irreversible renal failure.

CASE 1

47-year-old male, smoker presented with complaints of fever lasting for around 20 days followed by generalized swelling of body along with decreased urine output. On evaluation, he was found to have renal dysfunction with serum creatinine 7.1 mg/dl and active urinary sediments (protein 2+, RBC-40-50/hpf, WBC-20-30/hpf) with anemia (HB-8.5 gm/dl). USG abdomen revealed normal sized kidneys. Patient had persistent breathlessness, for which HRCT chest was done which was suggestive of pulmonary hemorrhage. In view of possibility of RPGN serology work up was done which revealed normal C3 and C4. cANCA and pANCA serology was negative but Anti-GBM titres were positive (76.8 AU/ml). Biopsy revealed (14/16) glomeruli having cellular crescents on light microscopy with linear IgG deposits on immunofluorescence. The patient was managed with plasmapheresis with immunosuppressive therapy, along with dialysis. Patient also developed sepsis for which IV antibiotics were escalated. Patient condition improved, became dialysis independent but eventually developed chronic kidney disease with eGFR 30 ml/min.

What is the Diagnosis and Underlying Etiopathogenesis?

The diagnosis is Goodpasture Syndrome, as the patient has RPGN (Anti-GBM disease) with features of lung hemorrhage. It comes under the category of pulmonary renal syndrome which has both immune and non-immune causes. The most common etiologies are autoimmune conditions like ANCA vasculitis, SLE and Goodpasture disease. Non-immune conditions include infections with Hantavirus, Legionella and paraquat poisoning.

The patient was a smoker which is the risk factor for precipitation of lung hemorrhage in such a patient. Other precipitating factors include infections, fluid overload and hydrocarbon exposure.

Table 10.1: Classification of RPGN based on etiopathogenesis and histology

Types of RPGN	Percentage of RPGN cases	Causes
Type 1 RPGN Anti-GBM Disease	≤ 10%	Anti-GBM disease (without lung hemorrhage) Goodpasture syndrome (with lung hemorrhage)
Type 2 RPGN Immune Complex Mediated	≤ 40%	**Post Infectious Causes** Antistreptolysin O (ASLO) and subepthelial humps–Streptococcus (predominant) Infective endocarditis, Vascular prosthetic nephritis, Viral hepatitis B infection, Visceral abscess/sepsis **Connective tissue disorders** Lupus Nephritis–ANA, Anti dsDNA positive "full house" IF staining for IgG, IgA, IgM, C3 and C1 q, mesangial plus subendothelial deposits IgA vasculitis–Henoch-Schölein Purpura Cryoglobulinemia–Mixed IgM/IgG **Other glomerulopathies** IgA Nephropathy–IgA deposits Membranous nephropathy–Subepithelial deposits MPGN 1–Mesangiocapillary proliferation MPGN 2–Dense deposit disease Idiopathic crescentic GN (rare)
Type 3 RPGN Pauci Immune (IF negative)	≤ 50%	Wegener Granulomatosis/Granulomatosis with Polyangiitis (GPA) (Predominant cANCA) Churg-Strauss Syndrome/Eosinophilic Granulomatosis with Polyangiitis (EGPA) (Predominant pANCA) Microscopic Polyangiitis (Both cANCA and pANCA) Renal limited Vasculitis (Predominant pANCA) Drug induced-levamisole, adulterated cocaine, hydralazine, propylthiouracil, minocycline (Predominant pANCA)
Type 4 RPGN Double Antibody Positive (Anti-GBM + ANCA)	Rare	Same as for Anti-GBM and ANCA
Type 5 RPGN Pauci Immune ANCA negative	5-10%	Cause not known, Idiopathic cresentic GN

Anti-GBM disease is a rare disorder in which circulating antibodies are directed against an antigen intrinsic to the glomerular basement membrane (GBM). The principal antigen target is noncollagenous (NC1) domain of a type IV collagen chain, α3 (IV) NC1 which is highly expressed in kidney and alveoli.

What are Crescents and What is Its Significance?

Cellular crescents are defined as 2 or more layers of proliferating cells in bowman space. Crescents are formed due to rupture of glomerular capillaries, which allows cytokines and growth factors cross the GBM to initiate proliferation of the parietal epithelial cells. The proliferation of parietal epithelial cells and macrophages is associated with fibrin deposition, slowly choking the glomerular tuft until filtration becomes impossible. This leads to oligoanuria and rapid renal failure.

This pathology was initially referred to as 'subacute nephritis' or 'extracapillary nephritis'. Later on this crescentic glomerulonephritis was termed as RPGN.

The best predictor of outcome for RPGN is severity of renal failure at the time of presentation. The crescents evolve from cellular (early stage < 1 week)– fibrocellular (middle stage with fibrin deposition) – fibrous crecscents (late stage with irreversible glomerular damage).

Thus, crescentic glomerulonephritis should be promptly diagnosed and early therapy initiated, i.e., at cellular crescent stage for better prognosis. If there is predominant fibrosis, i.e., chronic damage then aggressive immunosupression should only be initiated if benefits outweigh the risk assosciated, i.e., infections.

What are the Diagnostic Features of Anti-GBM Disease and the Atypical Variants?

The diagnosis is based on clinical symptoms, serology and kidney biopsy.

Clinical Scenario: Oligoanuria with modest proteinuria, with hematuria and dysmorphic red blood cells on urine analysis is seen. Pulmonary symptoms like cough and hemoptysis signifies lung hemorrhage which can be present in 40-60% of patients. The higher risk of kidney disease as compared with lung hemorrhage is because alveolar capillary endothelial cells more effectively block circulating immunoglobulin from the underlying basement membrane. Although diffusion capacity of lungs for carbonmonoxide (DLCO) is most sensitive indicator for lung hemorrhage, usually HRCT is done which also helps in diagnosing any underlying lung consolidation/ground glass opacities apart from alveolar hemorrhage. In case of significant lung hemorrhage, iron deficiency anemia can be seen and on bronchoalveolar lavage hemosideren laden macrophages are observed.

Serology

Raised anti-GBM titres are usually detected by direct ELISA and the specificity confirmed by Western Blot assays.

Kidney Biopsy

Unless the patient requires urgent treatment for any underlying pulmonary hemorrhage or sepsis, kidney biopsy should be done as early as possible to corroborate the diagnosis. Light microscopy reveals crescentic glomerulonephritis whereas, IF demonstrates linear IgG along the GBM which is pathognomonic of anti-GBM disease. Diffferential diagnosis of diseases with IgG bound to GBM include diabetes, SLE, light chain deposition disease, Alport syndrome after renal transplant. Characteristically, the *crescents appear to be of similar age and cellularity,* similar to the patient whose biopsy revealed all cellular crescents. Anti-GBM glomerulonephritis is the most aggressive form of RPGN with the highest frequency of crescents at the time of diagnosis (approximately 85% patients have 50% or more of glomeruli with crescents). It is important to note that therapy should not be delayed, if kidney biopsy is not possible.

Variants of Anti-GBM

Double Positive Anti-GBM and ANCA Associated Disease

ANCA titres (usually pANCA) may be present at low levels prior to onset of clinical symptoms and increased anti-GBM titres in up to 25% of patients. Anti-GBM titers tend to be lower in ANCA-positive anti-GBM antibody-positive patients than in patients with anti-GBM antibodies alone. Such "double-positive" patients have a better clinical course and response to treatment which is more typical of vasculitis than of Goodpasture disease.

Anti-GBM Disease Associated with Membranous Nephropathy

Usually the course of membranous nephropathy is benign, progressive in nature, but if there is any rapid loss of renal function, associated anti-GBM disease should always be suspected.

Anti-GBM Disease Without Detectable Circulating Antibodies

A rare variant referred to as 'Atypical anti-GBM nephritis'. Here, patient has mild renal course with no pulmonary hemorrhage. Kidney biopsy reveals no crescents but diffuse linear IgG deposits on IF are seen.

Anti-GBM Disease Post Renal Transplant

Upto 5% of kidney transplant patients with underlying Alport syndrome can develop anti-GBM disease which occurs usually early post transplant.

What are Factors Determining Treatment Modality and Prognosis?

Oliguria and dialysis dependency on presentation are factors against any aggressive immunosuppressive treatment. As per the KDIGO 2020 draft guidelines, conservative approach has been adviced for 85-100% crescents on kidney biopsy without alveolar haemorrhage.

Although the patient had above criteria, patient also had lung hemorrhage along with cellular crescents on biopsy which favour therapy. Cellular crescents signify recent rapid progression and early therapy can help in salvaging kidney function.

Other factors for therapy include "double positivity" as ANCA positive patients have less severe disease.

Aggressive treatment includes pulse with methyl-prednisolone (usually 3 doses of 500 mg-1000 mg) followed by daily steroids, along with oral cyclophosphamide (2 mg/kg) usually upto 3 months. Plasmapheresis can be initiated if there is probability of renal recovery (creatinine < 5.5 mg/dl) or the patient has pulmonary hemorrhage. Plasmapheresis sessions are done until anti-GBM titres are not detectable, usually the duration is of 2 weeks. Replacement volume is 40-50 ml/kg bodyweight with 5% albumin. Fresh frozen plasma can be given at end of plasma exchange in case of pulmonary hemorrhage or kidney biopsy. Anti-GBM titres are measured to assess prognosis. In refractory cases, Rituximab has been tried and even mycophenolate has been used in cases of cyclophosphamide intoleance or toxicity. Practically, we need to be cautious to avoid overt immunosuppression as infection is one of the common cause of mortality in anti-GBM disease apart from lung hemorrhage. Therefore, in cases in which the use of immunosuppressive agents is not desirable because of adverse effects, initial therapy with corticosteroids alone is recommended, usually combined with plasmapheresis. Important thing to remember is that in contrast to advanced renal failure, in which plasmapheresis is unlikely to lead to recovery of renal function, even severe lung hemorrhage is likely to respond to treatment with plasmapheresis. Clinical relapses are rare and if they occur, there is high likelihood of double positive disease or patients who are heavy smokers. Patients with double positive disease require long-term maintenance therapy similar to ANCA vasculitis as compared to Anti-GBM disease.

Newer Therapies in trial phase for anti-GBM disease are: *Imlifidase*–this is an IgG degrading endopeptidase derived from streptococcus pyogens, which cleaves the human IgG mmunoglobulin and can clear anti-GBM antibodies from the circulation. It has been tried for desensitization in high risk patients getting kidney transplant.

Immunoadsorption–which specifically binds and removes the anti-GBM antibodies.

Finally, anti-GBM disease has worst prognosis amongst RPGN as it has maximum number of crescents on presentation. Like in our patient, with aggressive immunosuppression, although patient became dialysis independent but he eventually developed chronic kidney disease.

Recurrence can occur post transplant if circulating anti-GBM antibodies are present. Thus , it is recommended that transplant should be deferred until circulating anti-GBM antibodies are undetectable for 6 months.

CASE 2

A 16-year-old female presented with a 6 months history of malar rash, arthralgias and arthritis in her hand joints and recent pedal edema. Her evaluation revealed positive ANA and anti-DNA Ab with low complement levels. Urine analysis showed 3 + proteinuria and 2 + hematuria and a creatinine of 2.0 mg/dl. Kidney biopsy light microscopy showed diffuse proliferative glomerulonephritis (DPGN) suggestive of class IV lupus nephritis with (3/10) glomeruli with cellular crescents and (2/10) fibrocellular crescents and IF was suggestive of "full house" immune deposits. Patient was initiated on IV pulse cyclophosphamide and steroids. She responded to treatment and later on switched to maintenance treatment with mycophenolate mofetil (MMF) along with low dose steroids.

What is the Diagnosis and Associated Etiologies?

The patient has RPGN secondary to immune complex crescentic glomerulonephritis (ICCGN)–Class IV lupus nephritis with crescents. Although ANCA assosciated vasculitis is the most common cause of RPGN, in children and adolescents like our 16-year-old patient, immune complex glomerulonephritis is the most common cause.

ICCGN refers to immune deposits in the glomeruli. In most cases, serology and histolologic findings will point to underlying diagnosis (Table 10.1).

In contrast, to Anti-GBM disease/ANCA vasculitis, ICCGN, similar to our patient, has lower frequency of crescents, rarely affecting > 50% of glomeruli. Another important point, is that ICCGN has low frequency of systemic vasculitis, apart from conditions like Henoch-Schönlein purpura (HSP).

What is the Treatment and Prognosis?

The treatment for the patient is similar to Diffuse proliferative glomerulonephritis (DPGN) (class IV lupus nephritis), i.e., either NIH or Eurolupus regimen which includes pulse of cyclophosphamide and methylprednisolone. Mycophenolate mofetil (MMF) can also be used for induction remission in lupus nephritis with crescents, although cyclophosphamide is usually preferred. This is followed by tapering doses of steroids along with MMF as maintenance therapy for the underlying lupus and extrarenal manifestations. Plasmapheresis is usually not advocated unless patient is refractory to initial therapy.

The prognosis as already explained before depends on the frequency of crescents. Among the etiologies for ICCGN patients with postinfectious glomerulonephritis, IgA nephropathy, MPGN Type 1 have better prognosis than patients having lupus nephritis, HSP and MPGN Type 2 as overall they present with lesser frequency of crescents (Table 10.2).

Table 10.2: Frequency of crescentic glomerulonephritis

Causes	Proportion of conditions with > 50% crescents (in %)
Anti-GBM Disease	85
ANCA GN	50
Lupus Nephritis	13
Henoch-Schönlein Purpura	10
IgA Nephropathy	4
Post-infectious GN	3
Type 1 MPGN	5
Type 2 MPGN	19
Fibrillary GN	5

CASE 3

A 65-year-old male with history of hypertension and recurrent sinusitis started having migratory polyarthralgia for around 6 months for which he was on NSAIDs. Work up for Rheumatoid arthritis was negative. Patient started having low grade fever, along with cough, breathlessness and intermittent hemoptysis. Patient was empirically treated for tuberculosis based on chest X-ray findings (sputum AFB –ve). Patient also started having oliguria with generalized swelling with worsening chest symptoms. CT chest revealed bilateral pulmonary infiltrates and nodules. Blood investigations revealed Hb-8 gm/dl, serum creatinine-5.0 mg/dl. Urine analysis revealed protein 2+, RBC-20-30 RBC/hpf, WBC-

10-20/hpf. Work up for RPGN revelaed normal C3, C4, ANA, Anti-GBM. pANCA was negative with positive cANCA titres. Kidney biopsy–light microscopy revealed 16 glomeruli with features of fibrinoid necrosis and crescents (4 cellular, 4 fibrocellular and 2 fibrous) whereas IF was negative for any immune deposits. Patient was initiated on immunosuppression along with plasmapheresis and intermittent hemodialysis. Patient renal functions did not improve despite therapy and he became dialysis dependent.

What is the Diagnosis? What are Types of ANCA Vasculitis and Clinical Features Assosciated?

The diagnosis is Wegener's granulomatosis – cANCA associated pauciimmune crescentic glomerulonephritis.

As per Chapel Hill Classification, ANCA vasculitis is divided as Wegener's granulomatosis (Granulomatosis with Polyangiitis), Microscopic Polyangiitis and Churg-Strauss Syndrome (Eosinophilia with Granulomatous Polyangiitis). Flowchart 10.1.

Shared Features of ANCA-Associated Vasculitis: They can be considered together in view of a number of shared pathologic, clinical and laboratory features.

- Preferentially cause *small vessels* vasculitis.
- Age > 50 years.

Similar glomerular lesions (crescents, focal necrosis, pauci-immune).

- Propensity to present as *pulmonary renal syndromes.*

Varying Prevalence of ANCA Positivity

The patient mentioned has been diagnosed as Granulomatosis with Polyangiitis (GPA)/Wegener's granulomatosis based on clinical, histopathological and serology findings. Wegener's granulomatosis presents as a triad of symptoms involving:

Upper Respiratory Tract

Chronic sinusitis*, otitis media, saddle nose, laryngeal stridor and eye manifestations.

Lower Respiratory Tract

Cough, hemoptysis,* and pleuritis are the most common pulmonary symptoms.

CT chest findings include fleeting pulmonary infiltrates and nodular cavities.*

Most commonly in India, such patients with history of low grade fever and above chest findings are misdiagnosed as tuberculosis, similar to our patient. So a high index of clinical suspicion should be kept and serology for ANCA should be sent.

Kidney Involvement: It occurs in the form of RPGN presentation and biopsy having necrotizing crescentic glomerulonephritis*. Granulomas are usually present in upper and lower respiratory tract and may be absent on kidney biopsy.

Important difference from Anti-GBM disease is that the crescents are comparatively less frequent and may be of different age and cellularity on kidney biopsy as seen in our patient. Other extrarenal features include constitutional symptoms like fever, polyarthralgia, palpable purpura, peripheral neuropathy.

Serology–cANCA positive*.

* Manifestations present in the abovesaid patient.

Important Clinical Features of other ANCA Vasculitis

Microscopic Polyangiitis: Kidney involvement is highest among ANCA vasculitis (>90%) and can present as RPGN and renal lesion is similar to Wegener's granulomatosis. Diffuse alveolar hemorrhage on imaging can be seen and pulmonary capillaritis is a characteristic lung histopathology. Constitutional symptoms and extrarenal features similar to GPA can be seen.

Serology: Variable geographical distribution and almost equal distribution of pANCA and cANCA has been seen in the overall population.

Churg-Strauss Syndrome

Eosinophilic granulomatosis with polyangiitis (EGPA)—or, as it was traditionally termed, Churg-Strauss syndrome—is a rare systemic necrotizing vasculitis that affects small-to-medium-sized vessels and is associated with severe asthma and blood and tissue eosinophilia. Predominantly pANCA vasculitis with less frequent kidney involvement (20%) and RPGN presentation.

Syndrome is characterized by history of allergic rhinitis or asthma preceding vasculitis. Peripheral neuropathy in the form of mononeuritis multiplex predominates and cardiac disease is the most common cause of mortality.

What are Different Types of ANCA and What is Their Prognostic Implications?

ANCA are a group of autoantibodies, mainly of IgG type against antigens MPO/PR 3 which are colocalized in azurophillic granules in cytoplasm of neutrophils. ANCAs were originally described based on their IF patterns:

Cytoplasmic (c-ANCA) against antigen MPO (myeloperoxidase).

Perinuclear (p-ANCA) against antigen PR3 (proteinase 3).

ANCA can be positive in other connective tissue disorders like lupus, rheumatoid arthritis, endocarditis, inflammatory bowel diseases and drugs.

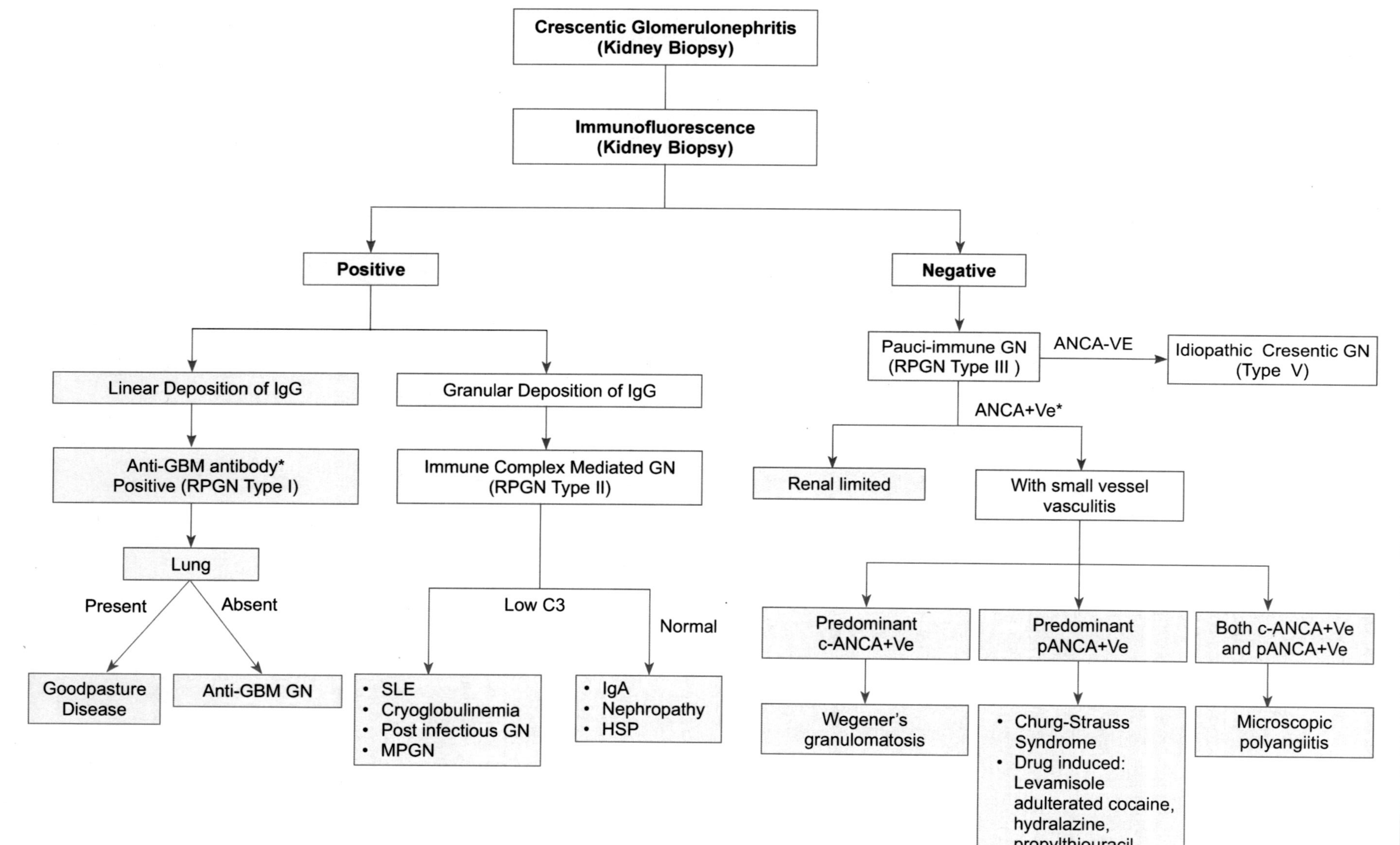

Variations:
* Double positivity including Anti-GBM + ANCA+Ve (RPGN TYPE IV)

Flowchart 10.1: Algorithm for rapidly progresssive glomerulonephritis

As per 1999 consensus statement, all sera should be screened for ANCA by indirect IF and then confirmed by direct ELISA. However, as per 2017 revised ANCA guidelines, high quality immunoassays like ELISA can be used for primary screening, without categorical need for indirect IF.

10-20% pauci-immune vasculitis can be ANCA negative and clinicopathologic and outcome characteristics are similar to ANCA positive vasculitis.

Prognosis: pANCA vs cANCA

pANCA has better renal prognosis although they have more renal impairment and chronic renal pathological changes at presentation. cANCA patients have more extrarenal involvement (especially respiratory tract), higher chances of relapse and mortality. Regardless of category of ANCA, best clinical predictor is GFR at presentation.

Double positive disease (ANCA+Anti-GBM) has worse prognosis than ANCA alone in view of presence of more frequency of crescents. So, thus in terms of prognosis - ANCA > ANCA + Anti-GBM > Anti-GBM disease. Changes in ANCA titers over time may correlate with disease activity. In general, titers decrease with treatment and increase before or at disease recurrence. However, results should be interpreted with caution and treatment decision should be based on clinical features and biopsy findings rather than ANCA titres alone.

What is the Treatment of ANCA Related RPGN and Overall Prognosis?

ANCA assosciated RPGN is treated with pulse cyclophosphamide (IV preferred over oral) along with methylprednisolone as induction followed by maintenance therapy with azathioprine or MMF and low dose steroids.

Remission Induction

1. *Pulse IV Cyclophosphamide (CYC) Regimen*

   The standard dose is 15 mg/kg, reduced for age and renal function.

   Pre-hydration (considering fluid status) and mesna administration should be encouraged to prevent bladder toxicity (hemorrhagic cystitis and malignancy).

   The first three pulses are usually given at intervals of 2 weeks and thereafter at 3-week intervals, upto maximum dose of 10 pulses and the duration of pulse therapy should be either 3 months or maximum upto 6 months.

   Patient should be monitored for leucopenia (TLC<4,000) and thrombocytopenia (platelet count <1 lakh) after 10-14 days of giving pulse cyclophosphamide to avoid chances of infection. If leucopenia or thrombocytopenia is present, next dose should be delayed and dose reduction for further doses advised.

   Table 10.3 shows comparison between IV and oral cyclophosphamide therapy.

Table 10.3: IV CYC vs Oral CYC

IV Pulse (CYCLOPS)	Oral
Remission rate similar	
Less cumulative dose	More cumulative dose
Less adverse effects	More adverse effects
More relapse	Less relapse

2. *Rituximab (RTX)*

   B cell targeted therapy has been recently introduced for ANCA assosciated vasculitis considering B cells are predominantly involved in the production of ANCA.

   RTX is a chimeric monoclonal antibody against anti CD 20 which is primarily found on the surface of B cells. RTX is as effective as CYC for remission induction of previously untreated patients and is preferable when CYC avoidance is desirable or in relapse or refractory cases.

Dose: The licensed and recommended RTX dosing protocol for the treatment of ANCA disease is 375 mg/m^2/week, i.e., 500 mg for 4 weeks. The alternative regimen can be 1 gram 2 doses after a gap of 15 days. Ideally IgG levels should be measured at baseline and every 6 months for patients treated with RTX. Thus, level of hypogammaglobulinemia may predict dosing interval and associated adverse effects, e.g., IgG levels <3 gm/l at baseline may predict a greater risk of secondary immunodeficiency and can be a deterrent in using RTX for induction.

Which Drug to use for Induction?

As per 2020 KDIGO draft guidelines in RPGN, either cyclophosphamide or rituximab can be used for remission induction along with steroids. Since the framework of RAVE trial did not include patients with serum creatinine > 4 mg/dl and pulmonary hemorrhage, limited data for RTX is available and cyclophosphamide is the preferred induction agent. In contrast RITUXIVAS trial included dialysis dependent patients along with pulmonary hemorrhage, whose outcome including rate of remission and adverse effects were comparable to cyclophosphamide. This included a hybrid therapy comprising 2 doses of CYC along with 4 doses of RTX. Thus as per the findings of this trial RTX can be considered as an alternative agent to CYC for remission induction in patients with RPGN (Table 10.4).

Table 10.4: Induction Therapy-Cyclophosphamide vs Rituximab

Cyclophosphamide	Rituximab
Cheap	Costly
Infertility	No infertility
Higher rates of infection	Low infection rate
More relapse (Primary induction)	Less relapse (Secondary induction) (RAVE Trial)
	Intolerant to or Contraindication of CYC

Glucocorticoids: IV pulse of methyl prednisolone 500 mg-1000 mg /day for 3 consecutive doses, followed by 1 mg/kg oral prednisolone, tapered to 5 mg/day by 6 months. However, following RTX induction, prednisolone can be with drawn by 6 months.

Plasmapheresis: As per the MEPEX trial, patients with ANCA vasculitis, presenting with severe renal failure (creatinine > 5.6 mg/dl) or pulmonary hemorrhage should be treated with plasmapheresis. However, the recently concluded PEXIVAS trial failed to show any benefit in prevention of ESRD or death in ANCA vasculitis patients, with eGFR < 50 ml/min. Thus, in conclusion, if there is history of recent oliguria with creatinine > 5.6 mg/dl and pulmonary hemorrhage is present, trial of plasmapheresis should be given.

Plasma Exchange – Dosing and Frequency

1. ANCA with RPGN presentation-7 treatments on alternate days, usually for duration of 2 weeks with 60 ml/kg of replacement volume with albumin as substitution fluid.
2. ANCA vasculitis with alveolar hemorrhage–More aggressive daily plasmapheresis until bleeding stops and fresh frozen plasma is the preferred substitution fluid.
3. ANCA + Anti-GBM–Similar to Anti-GBM plasmapheresis protocol as mentioned above.

IVIg: This can be used as an alternative option for patients with refractory ANCA-associated vasculitis or those with concurrent complications such as severe infections when it is advisable to avoid the standard therapy with high-dose steroids and immunosuppressant. Various trials for remission induction are shown in Table 10.5.

Maintenance Therapy

Maintenance Therapy of ANCA Vasculitis

Patients require long-term maintenance therapy as approximately 25-50% of ANCA patients relapse (Tables 10.6 and 10.7). Factors that increase the risk of relapse include, PR3 ANCA subgroup, low renal with high extra renal manifestations including extensive lung or cardiovascular disease. Other factors include, history of relapse, level of ANCA titre and withdrawl of immunosuppression.

Initially, azathioprin (AZA) was considered as the standard therapy for remission maintenance. However, with new evidence gathered from MAINRITSAN and RITAZERAM trials, RTX can be considered as first line therapy for maintenance.

Table 10.5: Summary of trials for remission induction

Trial	Therapy	Conclusion
CYCLOPS	IV CYC vs oral CYC	IV CYC is non-inferior to oral CYC and is assosciated with reduced cumulative exposure and leukopenia, but relapse rates are higher with IV regimen
RITUXIVAS	RTX + 2 IV CYC pulse vs IV CYC	RTX non-inferior to IV CYC for remission induction
RAVE	RTX vs oral CYC	RTX non-inferior to oral CYC for remission induction and no significant difference in renal outcomes
MEPEX	PLEX vs methylpredni-solone + oral CYC	Plasma exchange superior to high dose methylprednisolone+ CYC for preventing dialysis dependence at 3 and 12 months but not survival
PEXIVAS	2 × 2 factorial design where PLEX vs no PLEX as adjunct to standard dose vs low dose steroid has been studied	No significant difference in renal recovery or death comparing PLEX vs no PLEX and standard vs low dose steroid
NORAM	Oral MTX vs oral CYC in non severe disease	MTX was non-inferior to CYC in inducing remission
MYCYC	Oral MMF vs oral CYC in patients with non-severe renal disease	MMF was non inferior to CYC for remission induction

Abbreviations: CYC: Cyclophosphamide; RTX: Rituximab; PLEX: Plasmapheresis; MTX: Methotrexate; MMF: Mycophenolate mofetil.

Table 10.6: Maintenance immunosuppression in ANCA vasculitis		
RTX	**AZA**	**MMF**
500 mg infusion at remission and at 6, 12 and 18 months (Modified Mainritsan Scheme)	1.5 - 2 mg/kg/day upto 1 year followed by decrease 25 mg every 3 months	1 gm twice daily
OR	PLUS	
1 gm infusion at 4, 8, 12 and 16 months after remission (Ritazeram Scheme)	Steroids–5-7.5 mg/day	
No oral steroids if maintenance on RTX		
	Duration of Maintenance Therapy	
1.5 years (As per Mainritsan)	Duration of therapy–1.5-4 years	Duration–2 years

Table 10.7: Summary of trials for maintenance remission		
Trial	**Therapy**	**Conclusion**
CYCAZERAM	AZA VS oral CYC both in combination with prednisolone after achieving remission	AZA and CYC both associated with similar rates of relapse at 18 months whereas toxicity of CYC is avoided if AZA is preferred
IMPROVE	AZA vs MMF after achieving remission	AZA superior to MMF in maintaining remission with similar adverse effects
WEGENT	AZA VS MTX	AZA and MTX associated with similar adverse effects and relapse
MAINRITSAN	RTX VS AZA	RTX superior to AZA in maintaining remission and adverse effects
RITAZERAM	RTX VS AZA after achieving remission with RTX and steroids	RTX was superior to AZA for preventing disease relapse in patients with a prior history of relapse

Abbreviations: RTX: Rituximab; AZA: Azathioprine; CYC: Cyclophosphamide; MTX: Methotrexate; MMF: Mycophenolate mofetil.

Rituximab is preferred in relapsing disease, PR3 ANCA subgroup, azathioprin allergy or where steroid sparing is required. Azathioprin is more cost effective and is a preferred drug in patients with hypogammaglobulinemia (IgG < 300) and HbsAg positive patients. Regarding the patient mentioned, the patient had severe renal insufficiency with predominating fibrocellular and fibrous crescents, thus the patient did not respond to immunosuppression and became dialysis dependent.

Transplant in ANCA Disease

Recurrence can occur in upto 20% of patients and graft loss in upto 10%.

As per KDIGO, patient should be in extrarenal remission upto 1 year prior to transplant and there should be no delay based on ANCA titres alone.

Key Points

RPGN is rapid onset renal failure within few weeks characterized by crescents involving a > 50% of sampled glomeruli.

Prognosis in RPGN predominantly depends on frequency of crescents and GFR at presentation. Thus, Anti-GBM disease has worst prognosis amongst RPGN.

Treatment for RPGN usually includes pulse of methylprednisolone along with pulse/oral cyclophosphamide for remission induction.

Plasmapheresis is preferred in early renal insufficiency (creatinine < 5.6 mg/dl) in Anti-GBM and severe renal insufficiency (creatinine > 5.6 mg/dl) in ANCA.

Maintenance therapy usually includes tapering steroids along with other immunosuppresants (MMF, AZA).

With the availability of newer data, rituximab is being increasingly used especially in resistant/refractory cases.

Cotrimoxazole should be given to all patients of RPGN as it reduces overall mortality related to Pneumocystis carini pneumonia which can occur in these patients due to exposure to high dose immunosuppressants.

Finally, RPGN is a renal emergency where patients should undergo timely biopsy and receive immunosuppressive therapy to avoid irreversible renal damage.

Suggested Reading

1. Bhowmik D, Sinha S, Gupt A, Tiwari SC, Agarwal SK. Clinical approach to rapidly progressive renal failure. J Assoc Physicians India 2011 Jan;59(2):38-41.
2. Jennette JC. Rapidly progressive crescentic glomerulonephritis. Kidney international 2003 Mar 1;63(3):1164-77.

3. Arimura Y, Muso E, Fujimoto S, Hasegawa M, Kaname S, Usui J, Ihara T, Kobayashi M, Itabashi M, Kitagawa K, Hirahashi J. Evidence-based clinical practice guidelines for rapidly progressive glomerulonephritis 2014. Clinical and experimental nephrology 2016 Jun 1;20(3):322-41.
4. Parmar MS, Bashir K. Crescentic Glomerulonephritis. [Updated 2020 Jun 4]. In: StatPearls [Internet]. Treasure Island (FL): StatPearls Publishing; 2020 Jan. Available from: https://www.ncbi.nlm.nih.gov/books/NBK430727/.
5. Couser WG. Rapidly progressive glomerulonephritis: Classification, pathogenetic mechanisms and therapy. Am J Kidney Dis 1988;11:449.

CHAPTER 11

A Patient with Acute Kidney Injury in Pregnancy

Pulkit Nandwani[1], Abhyuday Rana[2], Ashish Nandwani[3]

[1] *Consultant, Obstetrics and Gynecology, Saroj Medical Institute, Delhi*
[2] *Associate Consultant, Nephrology, Medanta, The Medicity, Gurugram*
[3] *Consultant, Nephrology, Manipal Hospital, Dwarka, Delhi*

CASE

A 32-year-old gravida 2 para 1, female was admitted at 29th week of gestation with severe abdominal pain, emesis, and diarrhea of 1 day duration. She had mild hypertension during this pregnancy. Her preceding pregnancy was complicated by eclampsia, but she delivered a viable male infant at 35-week gestation. Her mother also had history of pregnancy-induced hypertension. The patient was found to be hypertensive (BP 180/108 mm Hg) and was treated with intravenous labetalol and hydralazine. An ultrasound Doppler revealed partial placental abruption. A stillborn fetus was delivered after spontaneous rupture of membranes. The placenta appeared intact, and no retained products of conception were identified on postpartum ultrasound.

The clinical course was further complicated by a generalized tonic-clonic seizure and oligoanuria. Laboratory evaluation revealed anemia (hemoglobin dropped from 14.8 to 6.9 g/dl), schistocytes on peripheral blood film, and thrombocytopenia (platelet count declined from 183,000 to 62,000/cmm). Over the next 4 days, her serum creatinine rose from 1.9 to 6.7 mg/dl (baseline prior to pregnancy 0.8 mg/dl). Persistent anuria and hyperkalemia (serum potassium 6.4 mEq/l) prompted initiation of hemodialysis on day 3. The patient had elevated lactate dehydrogenase (5641 IU/l) and worsening liver functions (serum aspartate transaminase rose from 71 to 692 IU/l, and alanine transaminase from 36 to 292 IU/l).

Patient was diagnosed to have acute kidney injury (AKI) requiring dialytic support. The approach to such case will be discussed.

What is Incidence of Acute Kidney Injury (AKI) in Pregnancy?

AKI is a rare complication of pregnancy in the developed countries. There are huge differences in the epidemiological characteristic of pregnancy related AKI with respect to incidence, causes, and outcome between developing and developed countries. Differences are due to environmental, socioeconomic and different health delivery systems. The incidence has decreased to 1/15,000–1/20,000 in the recent years from 1/3000 in 1960, with respect to the total number of pregnancies in developed countries. The current incidence of pregnancy related AKI in developing countries has a declining trend owning to better health facilities. It still accounts for 5%–20% of total AKI population.

What are Anatomical and Physiological Changes Occurring in Kidney During Pregnancy?

1. **Kidney size:** The kidney length increases by 1-1.5 cm and kidney volume increases by up to 30%.
2. **Hydronephrosis:** Physiological dilation of the urinary collecting system with hydronephrosis in up to 80% of women (right > left).
3. **Renal blood flow:** Increased by 80% above baseline.
4. **Glomerular filtration rate (GFR):** 150-200 ml/min (rise 40-50% above baseline).
5. **Serum creatinine:** Falls to 0.4-0.5 mg/dl.
6. **Uric acid:** Falls to 2.0-3.0 mg/dl.
7. **BUN:** Falls to 8-10 mg/dl.
8. **Sodium:** Mild hyponatremia (fall of 4-5 mmol/l).
9. **Osmolality:** Falls to about 270 mosm/kg.
10. **Bicarbonate:** Drops to 18 to 20 mEq/l (respiratory alkalosis with a compensatory drop in bicarbonate).

What are Various Causes of Acute Kidney Injury in Pregnancy? (Flowchart 11.1)

Obstetrical Complications:

- Septic abortion.
- Abruptio placentae.
- Placenta previa.
- Uterine hemorrhage.
- Intrauterine fetal death.
- Puerperal sepsis.

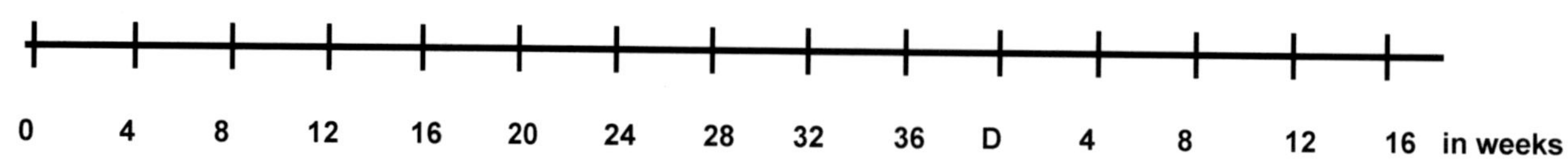

Septic abortion

Abruptio placentae

Severe hemorrhage/DIC

Sepsis

Pre-eclampsia/Eclampsia

HELLP syndrome

Acute fatty liver

ADAMTS13 deficiency–TMA

CAP dysregulation–TMA

TMA of unknown mechanism

Flowchart 11.1: Time line of various causes of AKI in pregnancy
TMA: Thrombotic microangiopathy; D: Delivery; Indian J Nephrol 2017;27(4):258-270

Pregnancy Specific Disorders:

- Pre-eclampsia/eclampsia.
- HELLP syndrome.
- Acute Fatty Liver of Pregnancy (AFLP).
- Thrombotic Microangiopathy (TMA).
- Atypical Hemolytic Uremic Syndrome (aHUS).
- Thrombotic Thrombocytopenic Purpura (TTP).
- Hyperemesis gravidarum.

Miscellaneous (cause not related to pregnancy):

- Acute postinfectious glomerulonephritis.
- Lupus nephritis.
- Acute pyelonephritis.
- Dehydration.
- Calculus of urinary tract.

What is Pre-eclampsia, Definition, Risk Factors?

The International Society for the Study of Hypertension in Pregnancy (ISSHP) defines pre-eclampsia (PE) as *de novo* hypertension (blood pressure >140/90 mm Hg) manifesting after 20 weeks of gestation combined with one or more of the following:

1. Proteinuria (spot urine protein/creatinine >30 mg/mmol [0.3 mg/mg] or >300 mg/day or [2+] on dipstick testing).
2. **Other maternal organ dysfunction:**
   - Renal impairment (serum creatinine ≥1 mg/dl.
   - Liver involvement (elevated transaminases—at least twice the upper limit of normal) right upper quadrant or epigastric abdominal pain.
   - Neurologic complications—altered mental status, blindness, stroke, or, more commonly, hyperreflexia with clonus, severe headaches with hyperreflexia, persistent visual scotomata.
   - Hematologic complications (thrombocytopenia–platelet count below $150 \times 10^9/l$, DIC, hemolysis).
3. **Uteroplacental Dysfunction:** Fetal growth restriction.

It is the most common hypertensive disorders of pregnancy, incidence ranging between 5% and 7% of pregnancies. It remains a major contributor to maternal, fetal and neonatal mortality worldwide. Over the last decade, long-term follow-up of large populations of women with pre-eclampsia has shown a subsequent increased risk of cardiovascular disease, kidney disease leading to end-stage kidney disease. Pre-eclampsia/Eclampsia were responsible for AKI in 43.9% and 35.3% of cases in pregnant women from India.

Risk Factors

Paternal Obstetric Factors

- Father born from pre-eclamptic pregnancy.
- Family history of pre-eclampsia (Fetal HLA-G variants).

Maternal Obstetric Factors

- Nulliparity.
- Multiple-gestation pregnancy.
- History of previous preeclampsia.
- Prior intrauterine growth restriction.
- Prior placental abruption.
- Artificial reproductive technology.
- Molar pregnancy.
- Trisomy 13 or fetal hydrops.
- Gestational diabetes.

Maternal Comorbid Conditions

- Chronic hypertension.
- Chronic kidney disease.
- Pregestational diabetes.
- Obesity (body mass index >30 kg/m^2).
- Antiphospholipid antibody.
- Systemic lupus erythematosus.
- Polycystic ovarian syndrome.

Maternal Genetic Factor

- Thrombophilia.
- Preeclampsia in pregnancy of first-degree relative.

Other Maternal Factors

- Age older than 40 years.
- Having been born small for gestational age.
- Pregnancy interval greater than 10 years.

What is Pathogenesis of Renal Disease in Pre-Eclampsia, Its Complications and How Do You Manage It?

The pathogenesis of PE is not fully understood but involves defects in placentation and systemic endothelial activation. The initiating factor in pre-eclampsia is incomplete remodeling of uterine spiral arteries, which results in placental ischemia which produces high levels of the antiangiogenic factors, soluble Fms-like tyrosine kinase (sFlt1) and soluble endoglin which are released into the circulation. Levels of placental growth factor (PlGF) and vascular endothelial growth factor (VEGF) are low. sFlt1 antagonizes the angiogenic activity of VEGF and PlGF, causing diffuse vasoconstriction and glomerular endothelial damage. Regardless of cause, preeclampsia is characterized by vasoconstriction, platelet activation with intravascular coagulation (usually local but occasionally disseminated), and maternal plasma volume contraction associated with capillary leak.

PE is associated with altered hemodynamic abnormalities such as decreased renal plasma flow, reduction in GFR by 30%–40%, and renal vasoconstriction. Thus, kidney in preeclamptic women is highly susceptible to ischemic injury. Renal tubular secretion of uric acid is impaired in PE, resulting in elevated concentration of uric acid in the blood. The urine sediment is usually bland. AKI occurs in approximately 1% of women with severe PE. On renal biopsy, "Glomerular endotheliosis" is characterized by glomerular endothelial swelling with loss of endothelial fenestrae and occlusion of the capillary lumens. Associated thrombosis is unusual.

The most common maternal complications of PE include:

- Disseminated coagulopathy (10%–20%).
- HELLP syndrome (20%).
- Pulmonary edema (2%–5%).
- AKI (1%–5%).
- Placental abruption (1%–2%).

AKI usually occurs in the setting of PE complicated by placental abruption, disseminated intravascular coagulation, sepsis, postpartum bleeding, or intrauterine fetal death.

The treatment of severe PE/HELLP syndrome depends on illness severity, gestational age, and fetal well being. Before 24 weeks of gestation, pregnancy discontinuance is recommended since studies show no fetal survival benefit and only increase the risk of severe maternal complications. Between 24 and 32 weeks of gestation, expectant management is a reasonable approach. The first-line treatment options in pregnant women with hypertension are methyldopa and labetalol. The dihydropyridine calcium-channel blockers can also be used safely in pregnancy. Delivery is the treatment of choice for pregnancy ≥32 weeks. There is no specific treatment of PE yet available. Removal of sFlt1 from circulation using therapeutic apheresis is associated with proteinuria reduction and prolongation of pregnancy,further controlled study is needed to confirm the beneficial effect of apheresis in patients with PE.

What are Various Thrombotic Microangiopathies of Pregnancy?

Pregnancy related thrombotic microangiopathy (TMA) accounts for 8%–18% of all cases of TMA, and it is a secondary form of TMA. Pregnancy related TMA can be classified into three groups based on underlying pathogenic mechanism:

(1) ADAMTS13 deficiency related-TTP.

(2) Complement alternative pathway (CAP) dysregulation related-Atypical HUS.

(3) Unknown mechanism.

Thrombotic Thrombocytopenic Purpura (TTP)

The combination of fever, severe thrombocytopenia, microangiopathic hemolytic anemia (MAHA), and predominant neurologic symptoms (disorientation, ataxia, headache, focal deficits, seizures, or aphasia) are the presenting features of TTP. It is often diagnosed before delivery, especially in the second and third trimester, because the ADAMTS 13 level physiologically tends to be decreased during the last trimester. The highest risk of TTP during the late second and third trimester seems to be due to progressive decrease in ADAMTS 13 activity and simultaneous steady increase in plasma concentration of von Willebrand factor during normal gestation.

Atypical Hemolytic Uremic Syndrome

Pregnancy related TMA associated with complement activation pathway (CAP) dysregulation clinically presents as atypical hemolytic uremic syndrome (aHUS). Clinical features of aHUS are similar to TTP, but renal involvement is more severe and the neurological manifestation is rare. aHUS occurs mainly in the first 6 months postpartum. TMA caused by CAP dysregulation occurred mainly (80% of cases) during the postpartum period. Infections and bleeding, which frequently complicate the postpartum period, may trigger complement activation leading to TMA (aHUS). Eighty percent of pregnancy associated Hemolytic uremic syndrome had CAP dysregulation with factor H (FH) and factor I (FI) encoding gene (CFH and CFI, respectively) mutation, and 80% of patients reached end stage renal disease during the first aHUS episode.

The treatment of TMA occurring during pregnancy should be tailored to the underlying pathogenic mechanisms. The treatment of TTP includes fresh frozen plasma infusion and plasmapheresis to correct ADAMTS-13 deficiency and remove the ADAMTS-13 circulating antibodies. In suspected case of autoimmune ADAMTS-13 deficiency, steroids are recommended as initial immunosuppressive therapy.

The B-cell depleting antibody rituximab is probably the optimal second-line therapy for cases resistant to plasma exchange or fresh frozen plasma infusion. However, potential fetal toxicity associated with rituximab is of concern. Platelet transfusions should be avoided if possible because of risk of increased microvascular thrombosis. The maternal mortality in TMA has declined in recent years and is now between 10% and 20%.

What is Acute Fatty Liver of Pregnancy, Presentation and Its Outcomes?

Acute fatty liver of pregnancy (AFLP) is obstetric emergency that progresses to fulminant liver failure if left untreated. It is characterized by sudden onset of acute liver failure with coagulopathy. Incidence of AFLP is 1/7000–1/20,000 pregnancies. It is an autosomal recessive genetic disorder which causes defective function of long chain 3 hydroxyacyl CoA dehydrogenase. The presence of lipid microvesicles infiltration of the hepatocytes, without inflammation, or necrosis are the typical histological findings in patients with AFLP.

The early presenting symptoms of AFLP are nonspecific with malaise, fever, nausea, vomiting, and abdominal pain. With progression of disease (jaundice and hepatic encephalopathy), other physical signs evolve. The low fibrinogen level, prolonged prothrombin time, depressed antithrombin III levels, and thrombocytopenia are the main features of disease which lead to coagulopathy. Hyperbilirubinemia, increased hepatic transaminases, hypoglycemia, and leukocytosis are the other laboratory abnormalities in patients with AFLP. The absence of hypertension supports viral hepatitis rather than AFLP.

AKI is seen in 20%–100% of cases and etiology of AKI is multifactorial. Renal insufficiency in AFLP is usually nonoliguric although oliguria and ATN can occur in the setting of hemorrhage induced hypovolemia. The urgent and immediate delivery of fetus is associated with favorable maternal and fetal prognosis. The prompt and urgent delivery with supportive care is the essential component in the management of women with AFLP.

What is HELLP Syndrome, Clinical Manifestation, Diagnosis?

HELLP syndrome is widely considered a variant of pre-eclampsia and occurs only in pregnant women. It resolves with delivery and is frequently but not always associated with hypertension and proteinuria. The pathogenesis of HELLP syndrome is not fully known. However, increased level of antiangiogenic factors (sFlt 1 and sEng) and decrease concentration of proangiogenic mediators (PIGF) have been proposed in the pathogenesis of HELLP syndrome similar to PE.

HELLP syndrome seems to be a TMA like disorder because of several clinical similarities between these two disorders: mechanical hemolysis, thrombocytopenia, and AKI. The link between HELLP syndrome and complement dysregulation has been suspected in various study.

It occurs typically in the third trimester but may be diagnosed in the second trimester or in the postpartum period.The clinical features are variable. The most common symptoms are epigastric/right upper quadrant pain, nausea, vomiting and headache, but it may manifest by its complications such as DIC, placental abruption, AKI, pulmonary edema, hepatic capsular hematoma and retinal detachment.

The diagnosis of HELLP syndrome is based on the following laboratory criteria: (a) microangiopathic hemolytic anemia (MAHA): Schistocytes in blood smear, serum bilirubin $\geq$1.2 mg/dl, lactate dehydrogenase (LDH) >600 U/L; (b) increased liver transaminases (alanine aminotransferase >70 U/L); and (c) platelet count <100 × 10^3 cells/mm^3.

AKI is reported in 3%–15% cases of HELLP syndrome, and overall, it may account for 40% of all cases of pregnancy related AKI and may increase up to 60% of cases in severe form of disease. The progression to CKD is reported to occur in <10% of patients who developed AKI on preexisting renal disease and/or hypertension.

What are Indications and Special Care Taken During Hemodialysis in Pregnancy Associated AKI?

Indications for dialysis in pregnancy related AKI are similar to the non-pregnant cases and they include uremic symptoms (encephalopathy, pericarditis, or neuropathy), volume overload, hyperkalemia, and/or metabolic acidosis unresponsive to initial medical treatment. However, early start of dialysis is recommended when GFR falls to below 20 ml/min/1.73 m^2.

It is essential to keep certain aspects in mind when dialysis is prescribed in pregnant women with AKI.

- Increased dialysis dose (daily dialysis with duration of more than 20 hours/week). This will improve the uremic environment, a high risk factor for prematurity and poor fetal outcome.
- The hemodialysis related hemodynamic fluctuation and volume depletion can cause diminished uteroplacental perfusion and increased placental oxidative state.
- It is advised to maintain certain dialysis parameters in narrow range in pregnant women, such as bicarbonate to 25 mEq/l and sodium to 135 mEq/l.

Both conventional and low molecular weight heparin are safe to use in pregnancy during hemodialysis treatment because they do not cross the placental barrier.

Indications of Renal Biopsy During Pregnancy

- Newly diagnosed lupus nephritis.
- Unexplained AKI.
- Nephrotic syndrome severe enough to require treatment.
- Graft dysfunction in transplant patient with suspicion of rejection.

In view of increased renal blood flow during pregnancy, the risk of bleeding is increased, hence biopsy should be postponed until after delivery unless management is determined by biopsy results.

Suggested Reading

1. Prakash J. The kidney in pregnancy: A journey of three decades. Indian J Nephrol 2012;22:159-67.
2. Maynard SE, Karumanchi SA, Thadhani R. Hypertension and kidney disease in pregnancy. In: Brenner BM, Rector B, editors. The Kidney, 11th ed. Philadelphia: Saunders, Elsevier 2019;1567-95.
3. Pregnancies complicated by HELLP syndrome (hemolysis, elevated liver enzymes and low platelets): Subsequent pregnancy outcome and long-term prognosis. American Journal of Obstetrics and Gynecology 172;125-29.
4. Phipps *et al.* Preeclampsia: Updates in pathogenesis, definitions and guideline. Clinical Journal of the American Society of Nephrology 11;1102-13.
5. Chaiworapongsa T, Chaemsaithong P, Yeo L, Romero R. Pre-eclampsia part 1: Current understanding of its pathophysiology. Nat Rev Nephrol 2014;10:466-80.
6. American College of Obstetricians and Gynecologists; Task Force on Hypertension in Pregnancy. Hypertension in Pregnancy. Report of the American College of Obstetricians and Gynecologists' Task Force on Hypertension in Pregnancy. Obstet Gynecol 2013;122:1122-31.
7. Prakash J, Ganiger VC. Acute kidney injury in pregnancy-specific disorders. Indian J Nephrol 2017;27:258-70.

CHAPTER

A Pregnant Female with Chronic Kidney Disease

Pulkit Nandwani[1], Ashish Nandwani[2], Shalu Gupta[3]

[1] *Consultant, Obstetrics and Gynecology, Saroj Medical Institute, Delhi*

[2] *Consultant, Nephrology, Manipal Hospital, Delhi*

[3] *Consultant, Obstetrics and Gynecology, Cloudnine Hospital, Gurugram*

CASE

26 years old female, known case of chronic kidney disease (CKD) stage 3 secondary to biopsy proven class IV lupus nephritis, hypertension, presented with 8 weeks of pregnancy. She had no urinary complaints with normal appetite and mild nausea. On evaluation her HR 70/min, BP was 140/80 mm Hg, pallor present, no edema, systemic exam was normal. Labs revealed normocytic hypochromic anemia with Hb 10 gm/dl. Urine analysis revealed protein + with no active sediments. Spot urine protein/creatinine ratio was 0.50. Serum creatinine 1.5 mg/dl with normal electrolytes.USG abdomen showed normal size kidneys with increased cortical echogenicity. Her drugs included amlodipin, metoprolol, hydroxy chloroquin (HCQS), azathioprin and oral iron tablets. Her ANA was negative and complement levels were within range. 2D Echo was normal. There were no other extra renal manifestation of lupus. She had received steroids and rituximab in past for lupus nephritis and had been in remission for last 1 year with well controlled hypertension on drugs.

This is a patient with CKD due to lupus nephritis in remission, who became pregnant, the approach to such patient will be discussed.

CKD is estimated to affect 3% of pregnant women. The prevalence of CKD in pregnancy is rising due to increasing maternal age, obesity, hypertension and diabetes mellitus.

Women with CKD are at an increased risk of adverse pregnancy outcomes including pre-eclampsia, fetal growth retardation, preterm delivery and deterioration in maternal renal function. Such patients should be managed by a team of obstetrician, nephrologist and physician.

Effect of Pregnancy on Kidney Disease

There are anatomic and physiologic changes in kidney during pregnancy. There is an increase in size by 1-1.5 cm and collecting system dilatation. Glomerular filtration rate increases by 50% during first trimester leading to decrease in serum creatinine to 0.5-0.7 mg/dl. Also there is respiratory alkalosis compensated by drop in serum bicarbonate level. Pregnancy can hasten the progression of CKD. The risk is dependent upon the baseline glomerular filtration rate, proteinuria, and hypertension. In pregnant patient with CKD, there is:

- Increase in proteinuria.
- Worsening of hypertension.
- Increased risk of pre-eclampsia.
- Worsening of renal function-temporary or permanent.
- Worsening of anemia.

Effect of Kidney Disease on Pregnancy

- Degree of renal dysfunction determines outcome rather than underlying etiology of disease.
- Absence of hypertension significantly decreases chance of poor outcomes.
- Inability to use ACE inhibitors (angiotensin converting enzyme inhibitors) and ARBs (angiotensin-receptor blockers) in pregnancy.
- Both the presence of GFR <40 ml/min and proteinuria > 1gm predicts poor maternal and fetal outcomes.

What Pre-Pregnancy Care/Counselling is Required?

Contraception

CKD patients of reproductive age group should be offered safe and effective contraception. Patients who are taking teratogenic/cytotoxic medication, patients with active lupus nephritis, and during first year after transplantation should be offered contraception.

Progesterone only-pill, a progesterone subdermal implant, and the progesterone intrauterine device are safe and effective for women with CKD. All oestrogen-containing contraceptives are associated with risk of hypertension, venous and arterial thrombosis and cervical cancer. These risks are important in women with CKD and hypertension, so are best avoided.

Pre-Pregnancy Counselling

Pregnant women with CKD are at an increased risk of complications like pre-eclampsia, preterm birth and fetal growth restriction. Neonatal outcomes in women with CKD are poor. These include premature births, small for gestational age, neonatal mortality, and stillbirths. The likelihood of adverse outcomes are predominantly dependent on baseline renal function (eGFR <60 ml/min/1.73 m^2), hypertension (>140/90 mm Hg), and proteinuria (nephrotic range proteinuria), women with active renal disease, women with lupus nephritis, women with renal transplants and all women with previous adverse obstetric history.

How to Optimize Maternal and Neonatal Outcomes in Women with CKD?

- Renal disease activity should be stabilized in advance of pregnancy on minimal doses of pregnancy safe medications.
- Blood pressure control (< 140/90 mm Hg) on pregnancy-appropriate medications.
- Glycemic control in women with diabetes mellitus.
- Minimize exposure to teratogenic medications.
- Treatment plan in the event of disease activity exacerbation/relapse/graft rejection during pregnancy.
- Access to regular antenatal checkups.

Pregnancy Care in CKD Patient

Renal function monitoring in pregnancy is based on serum creatinine as estimated GFR (eGFR) is not valid for use in pregnancy. There is increased plasma flow and dynamic changes in filtration fraction during pregnancy, leading to increase in glomerular filtration up to 50% with a consequent fall in serum creatinine concentrations. The dynamic nature of gestational and immediate post-partum change in renal function means that steady state cannot be presumed, prohibiting the use of eGFR equation in this setting.

Quantification of Proteinuria in Pregnancy

As there is increase in renal blood flow with a corresponding increase in glomerular filtration, and altered tubular reabsorption, the proteinuria increases in pregnancy. Abnormal proteinuria is defined as proteinuria levels of > 300 mg/24 hours, twice the normal limit in non-pregnant women.

Quantification of proteinuria is undertaken by urine protein : creatinine ratio (uPCR) or albumin : creatinine ratio (uACR). 24 hours urine collection is time-consuming and subject to inadequacies in collection. In women without pre-existing proteinuria, diagnostic performance equivalent to 30 mg/mmol of uPCR is achieved with a uACR cut-off of 8 mg/mmol.

Quantification of proteinuria particularly after 20 weeks' gestation is required when pre-eclampsia may develop and in conditions where an increase in proteinuria may represent disease flare or progression. Proteinuria in early pregnancy predicts adverse fetal and maternal outcomes in women with CKD. Women with albuminuria ≥300 mg/24 hours or proteinuria ≥500 mg/24 hours had an increased risk of pre-eclampsia and preterm birth.

Antenatal Care in CKD Patient

Pregnant women with CKD should receive routine antenatal care.

- Pregnant women with CKD should have access to usual trisomy screening.
- Women with CKD exposed to teratogenic drugs in the first trimester are referred to a specialist fetal medicine unit for fetal abnormalities.
- Pregnant women with CKD should undergo scans to assess fetal growth and well-being in the third trimester.
- Pregnant women taking prednisolone and/or calcineurin inhibitors should be screened for gestational diabetes. Fasting plasma glucose and glycated hemoglobin in patients with pre-gestational diabetes mellitus.
- Assessment of disease activity in patients with SLE should be done.
- Renal transplant recipients should be monitored more frequently to detect graft dysfunction and dosage adjustment of immunosuppressive medications.
- Vaccinations – Patients should receive standard vaccinations included in obstetric care.

Pre-Eclampsia Prophylaxis

Women with CKD are offered low dose aspirin (75-150 mg) in pregnancy to reduce the risk of pre-eclampsia. Kidney donors are also offered low dose aspirin (75-150 mg) to reduce the risk of pre-eclampsia.

Low dose aspirin is associated with a reduced incidence of pre-eclampsia, although there is limited definitive evidence as to the optimal dose for women with CKD. Current guidelines recommend 75-150 mg of aspirin from 12 weeks' gestation onwards but future research may elucidate optimization of prophylaxis in women with CKD.

Blood Pressure Management

Target blood pressure during pregnancy for women with CKD is 135/85 mm Hg or less, which should be recorded in the woman's antenatal health care record. Anti-hypertensive treatment in women with CKD is continued in pregnancy unless systolic blood pressure is consistently <110 mm Hg systolic, or diastolic blood is pressure consistently <70 mm Hg, or there is symptomatic hypotension. Labetalol, nifedipine and methyldopa can be used to treat hypertension in pregnancy. Angiotensin converting enzyme inhibitors, angiotensin receptor anatgonists and diuretics are not used to treat hypertension in pregnancy.

Diagnosis of Pre-Eclampsia

In patients with CKD, diagnosis of superimposed pre-eclampsia is considered:

- In a woman with non-proteinuric CKD, if she develops new hypertension (BP >140/>90 mm Hg) and proteinuria (uPCR >30 mg/mmol or uACR >8 mg/mmol) or maternal organ dysfunction after 20 weeks of gestation.
- In a woman with proteinuric CKD if she develops new hypertension (BP >140/90 mm Hg) or maternal organ dysfunction after 20 weeks of gestation
- In a woman with chronic hypertension and proteinuria, if she develops maternal organ dysfunction after 20 weeks of gestation.

In women with chronic hypertension and proteinuria, development of sustained severe hypertension '(BP >160/110 mm Hg or doubling of anti-hypertensive agents) and/or a substantial rise in proteinuria (doubling of uPCR or uACR compared to early pregnancy) should prompt clinical assessment for superimposed pre-eclampsia. Angiogenic markers soluble fms-like tyrosine kinase 1 (sFlt-1) and placental growth factor (PlGF) may be considered as an adjunct to diagnose of pre-eclampsia.

Venous Thromboembolism

Women with nephrotic-range proteinuria (uPCR >300 mg/mmol or ACR >250 mg/mmol) should be given thromboprophylaxis with low molecular weight heparin (LMWH) in pregnancy and the postpartum period unless there is a specific contraindication including risk of labour or active bleeding.

Anemia

Pregnant women with CKD are given parenteral iron and erythropoietin stimulating agents if indicated.

The most common cause of anemia in pregnancy is iron deficiency. Iron deficiency anemia can be diagnosed with ferritin (<100 µg/l), transferrin saturation (<20%), hypochromic red cells (>6%) and reticulocyte hemoglobin content (<25 pg). Oral iron is cheap and accessible, however, the intravenous route offer better bioavailability and tolerability in pregnancy. Erythropoietin (EPO) concentrations increase approximately two-fold during pregnancy. In women with CKD, the supplementation with synthetic EPO may be required, even in the context of mild or moderate renal impairment. As EPO is a large molecule that does not cross the placental barrier, hence, its use is considered safe in pregnancy however, a theoretical risk of exacerbating pre-existing or new-onset hypertension exists.

Bone Health

Women with CKD, who are vitamin D deficient, should be given vitamin D supplementation in pregnancy. Vitamin D deficiency is associated with increased risk of pre-eclampsia and gestational diabetes. For women with CKD, a maintenance daily dose of vitamin D 400-1000 IU can be given in pregnancy. Calcimimetics (cinecalcet, etelcalcetide) and non-calcium phosphate binders (sevelamer hydrochloride, lanthanum carbonate) have insufficient safety data in pregnancy and should therefore be discontinued in advance of pregnancy.

Timing of Delivery

Timing of birth for women with CKD is determined by obstetric indications, with consideration of maternal renal factors including deteriorating renal function, symptomatic hypoalbuminemia, pulmonary oedema, pre-eclampsia and refractory hypertension. If maternal complications develop before 34 weeks of gestation, attempt should be made to continue the pregnancy under strict supervision to attain sufficient fetal maturity to reduce adverse neonatal and developmental outcomes, although this decision will depend upon maternal condition. There is no evidence that mode of delivery affects maternal renal function. Mode of delivery should therefore be based on obstetric indications and maternal preference according to guidance in women without CKD.

Pregnancy in Renal Transplant Recipient

The Risk of Pregnancy on Kidney Allograft Function

Women with renal transplants should wait until their kidney function is stable on immunosuppressive medications that are safe in pregnancy before conceiving, which is usually more than one year after transplantation. In women with renal transplant, maternal and neonatal complications remain higher compared to the general population. There is an increased risk of pre-eclampsia, induction of labour, cesarean delivery, preterm delivery <37 weeks, and small for gestational age babies.

The Effect of Immunosuppression on Fetus

Standard immunosuppression regimens routinely include mycophenolate mofetil in the first year after transplantation. Due to the teratogenicity of mycophenolate mofetil, switching to alternative agents is recommended before pregnancy, thus at least a year after transplantation is advised before attempting to conceive. Calcineurin inhibitors can be used safely in pregnancy with regular monitoring of levels as trough level falls during pregnancy.

The Risk of Opportunistic Infections

There is increased risk of urinary tract infections along with viral infections like CMV and herpes during pregnancy. CMV infection may lead to developmental delay and sensorineural hearing loss.

Other important factor include any recent episodes of rejection, stability and level of graft function, maternal age, diabetes and blood pressure control, but direct evidence regarding impact of these factors on pregnancy and graft outcomes is limited.

Mode and timing of delivery in women with renal transplants is based on obstetric indications and maternal preference.

Pregnancy in Dialysis Patient

Women on dialysis prior to pregnancy should receive pre-pregnancy counselling for use of contraception to avoid pregnancy.

Women established on hemodialysis prior to pregnancy should receive long, frequent hemodialysis either in centre or at home to improve pregnancy outcomes. Women receiving hemodialysis during pregnancy have dialysis dose, aiming for a pre-dialysis urea <75 mg/dl. Women on peritoneal dialysis prior to pregnancy should convert to hemodialysis during pregnancy.

Studies show an association between increased dialysis dose and improved fertility and pregnancy outcomes. A cohort of women who received 48 ± 5 hours of dialysis per week had a conception rate of 32 pregnancies per 1000 women/year compared with 5 per 1000 women/year in a separate cohort receiving fewer than 20 hours of dialysis per week. Dialysis in pregnancy for 37–56 hours/week compared to fewer than 20 hours/week also resulted in a higher live birth rate (85% versus 48%), higher median gestational age at delivery (38 weeks versus 28 weeks) and a greater median birth weight (2600 g versus 1800 g).

Long, frequent hemodialysis has implications for electrolyte and nutritional provision. Dialysate concentrations of potassium, calcium and phosphate may need to be increased. Dialysate losses of water-soluble vitamins and folic acid need to be considered, with increased supplementation as required, including high-dose folic acid pre-pregnancy and in the first trimester.

Initiating Dialysis During Pregnancy

Hemodialysis should be initiated in pregnancy when the maternal urea concentration is 100-120 mg/dl and eGFR declines to below 20 ml/min/1.73 m^2. Renal function, fluid balance, biochemical parameters, blood pressure and uremic symptoms should be considered in addition to maternal urea concentration. However, this decision must be individualized.

Pregnancy in Lupus Nephritis

Women with lupus nephritis should be advised to wait until their disease is quiescent for at least 6 months before conceiving. Active lupus nephritis is associated with adverse pregnancy outcomes. The presence of antiphospholipid antibodies is also a major risk factor in pregnancy. Presently, treatment for active lupus nephritis involves the use of cyclophosphamide as induction agent, and mycophenolate mofetil is used for maintenance therapy. Women in remission, should discontinue these teratogenic medications three months prior to conception and need to be maintained on azathioprine. All women with lupus should be advised to take hydroxy chloroquine in pregnancy unless it is contraindicated as it is associated with a lower risk of lupus flare.

Women with lupus should be monitored for disease activity during pregnancy. Women who are positive for anti-Ro (SSA) or anti-La (SSB) antibodies should get fetal echocardiography in the second trimester.

Women with antiphospholipid syndrome and a history of a confirmed thromboembolic event or previous adverse obstetric outcome (excluding recurrent early fetal loss) should receive low molecular weight heparin in pregnancy and for six weeks postpartum. Steroids, azathioprine, calcineurin inhibitors, intravenous immunoglobulin and plasma exchange can be used to treat lupus in pregnancy.

Pregnancy in Diabetic Nephropathy

Women with diabetic nephropathy should have optimal control of blood glucose, blood pressure and proteinuria prior to conception. Women with diabetic nephropathy continue angiotensin converting enzyme inhibitors until conception, with regular pregnancy testing during attempts to conceive.

Most women with diabetic nephropathy have successful pregnancy outcomes. However, diabetic nephropathy in pregnancy is associated with an increased risk of adverse outcomes including pregnancy loss, congenital malformation, pre-eclampsia, preterm delivery, growth restriction and neonatal unit admission.

Proteinuria increases in pregnancy in the majority of women with diabetic nephropathy, including progression to the nephrotic range. Low molecular weight heparin may be indicated for the prevention of venous thromboembolism, although the level of proteinuria at which the risk of venous thromboembolism becomes clinically significant is unknown.

Which Medications can be Taken Safely in Pregnancy?

Medication should be prescribed in pregnancy if the benefit to the woman outweighs the potential risk to the fetus.

- Low dose aspirin, low molecular weight heparin, labetalol, nifedipine, methyldopa, hydralazine, prednisolone, azathioprine, cyclosporine, tacrolimus, and hydroxychloroquin are safe for use in pregnancy.
- Trough levels of calcineurin inhibitors need to be checked throughout pregnancy and immediately postpartum, as blood concentrations change with volume status changes during pregnancy.
- Mycophenolate mofetil (MMF), methotrexate and cyclophosphamide are teratogenic drugs and thus are contraindicated in pregnancy. MMF is associated with an increased risk of spontaneous abortion and fetal abnormality. A 3-month interval is advised before conception to allow conversion to a safe alternative and ensure stable renal function.
- mTOR inhibitors, *e.g.*, Sirolimus and everolimus are avoided in pregnancy due to insufficient safety data in pregnancy.
- Metformin can be used in pregnancy for women with a pre-pregnancy eGFR > 30 ml/min/1.73 m^2 and stable renal function during pregnancy.
- Angiotensin converting enzyme inhibitor (ACEi) and receptor antagonists (ARB) are fetotoxic in the second and third trimesters and are associated with major birth defects including renal agenesis, oligohydroamnios. These agents should be stopped prior to pregnancy, or as soon as pregnancy is confirmed.

Suggested Reading

1. Kate Wiles, Lucy Chappell, Katherine Clark, Louise Elman, Matt Hall, Liz Lightstone, Germin Mohamed, Durba Mukherjee, Catherine Nelson-Piercy, Philip Webster, Rebecca Whybrow and Kate Bramham. Clinical practice guideline on pregnancy and renal disease. BMC Nephrology 2019; 20:401 https://doi.org/10.1186/s12882-019-1560-2.
2. Gill JS, Zalunardo N, Rose C, Tonelli M. The pregnancy rate and live birth rate in kidney transplant recipients. Am J Transplant 2009; 9:1541.
3. Zhang JJ, Ma XX, Hao L, *et al.* A Systematic Review and Meta-Analysis of Outcomes of Pregnancy in CKD and CKD Outcomes in Pregnancy. Clin J Am Soc Nephrol 2015; 10:1964.
4. Nevis IF, Reitsma A, Dominic A, *et al.* Pregnancy outcomes in women with chronic kidney disease: A systematic review. Clin J Am Soc Nephrol 2011;6:2587.
5. Piccoli GB, Cabiddu G, Attini R, *et al.* Risk of Adverse Pregnancy Outcomes in Women with CKD. J Am Soc Nephrol 2015;26:2011.

CHAPTER 13

A Child with Thrombotic Microangiopathy

Suprita Kalra[1], Sidharth Kumar Sethi[2]

[1]Associate Professor, Pediatric Nephrology, Army Hospital R&R, Delhi Cantt
[2]Senior Consultant, Pediatric Nephrology, Medanta, The Medicity, Gurugram, Haryana

What is Thrombotic Microangiopathy?

Thrombotic microangiopathy (TMA) is defined as a pathology of vessel wall (mainly arterioles or capillaries), intraluminal platelet thrombosis and partial or complete obstruction of the vessel lumina. TMA may develop secondary to various diverse etiologies as seen in Figure 13.1 but the two most commonly described entities are: hemolytic uremic syndrome (HUS) with predominantly renal manifestations and thrombotic thrombocytopenic purpura (TTP) which has mainly neurological involvement. Injury to the endothelial cell is the chief inciting factor leading to TMA.

In children HUS is the most common etiology of TMA. HUS is a clinical triad of microangiopathic hemolysis with thrombocytopenia and deranged renal function. Broadly it has two forms. The first one is shiga toxin-associated HUS (earlier known as D+ HUS or typical HUS) which is seen mostly in young children. This is associated with shiga toxin producing enteropathogens, typically enterohemorrhagic Escherichia coli or Shigella dysenteriae. In the second form, known as the atypical HUS (aHUS), shiga toxin has no role and includes HUS caused by diverse etiologies in dysregulation of the complement cascade, cobalamin pathway etc. The HUS may also be seen following infections, drugs, transplantation, pregnancy and autoimmune conditions and is then termed secondary aHUS.

Based on the above background let us consider a few case scenarios:

CASE 1

8-year-old boy, previously healthy was brought to the ER with vomiting since last 2 days with history of reduced urine output and bluish-purple rash on the extremities

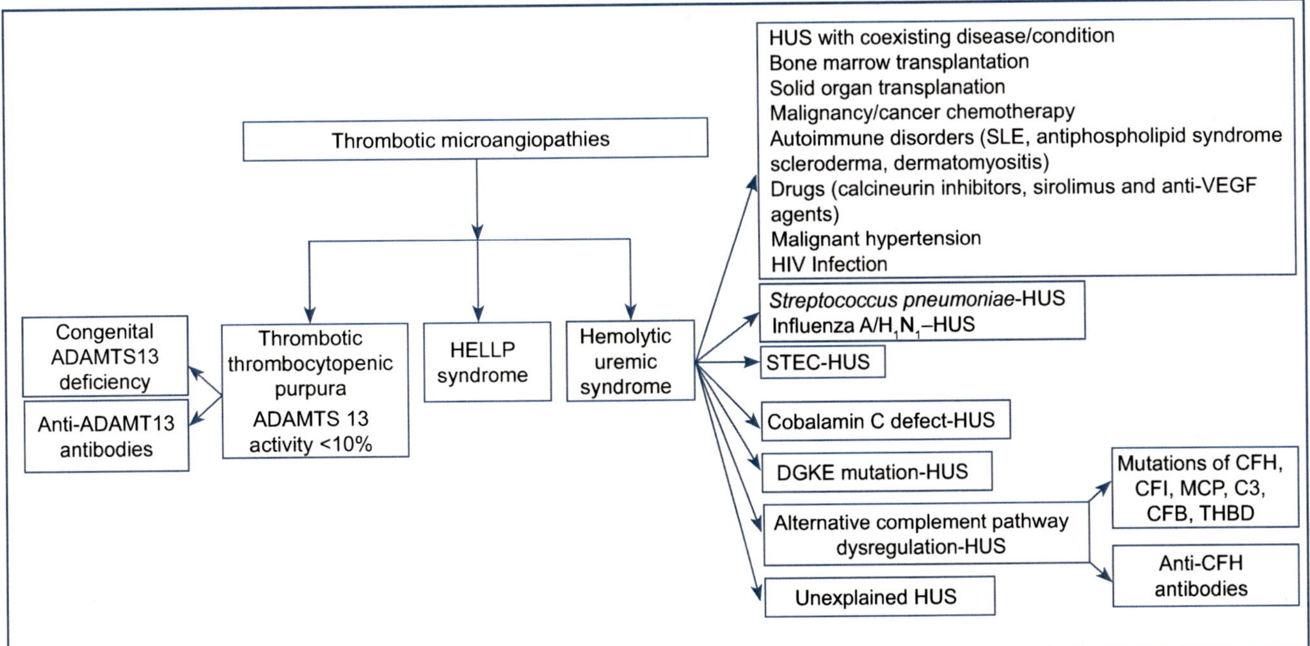

Figure 13.1: Etiologies and presentations of thrombotic microangiopathy
DGKE: Diacylglycerol kinase ε; STEC: Shiga toxin E coli; CFH: Complement factor H; CFI: Complement factor I; MCP: Membrane cofactor protein; CFB: Complement factor B; THBD: Thrombomodulin.

and trunk since yesterday. Clinical examination revealed severe pallor with petechiae on all 4 limbs and stage II hypertension with essentially normal systemic examination.

What is the Diagnosis? How will You Evaluate this Child?

Table 13.1 gives the investigations needed to confirm the diagnosis of HUS, its etiology and relevant investigations to rule out common conditions which may have similar presentation.

In the absence of history of dysentery, step by step evaluation for atypical HUS should be done as summarizes in Figure 13.2.

60% to 70% of all aHUS patients have one or more known mutations in complement genes or anti-CFH antibodies. Complement factor H (CFH) is the main fluid phase regulator of the complement alternative. The

Table 13.1: Evaluation in patients with hemolytic uremic syndrome

To confirm presence of HUS	Renal function tests, Complete blood counts with peripheral smear to look for schistocytes; reticulocyte count, Lactate dehydrogenase (LDH), haptoglobulin
To rule out other differential diagnoses with similar presentations	Direct Coombs test, antinuclear antibodies (ANA), antiphospholipid antibodies (APLA), antineutrophil cytoplasmic antibodies (ANCA) Antibodies to human immunodeficiency virus, Leptospira Polymerase chain reaction (PCR) for Cytomegalovirus, Epstein-Barr virus: If strongly suspected clinically
For underlying etiology	**For Shiga toxin mediated HUS** Stool or rectal swab culture, PCR for shiga toxin in stool **For Genetic Disorders of complement pathway regulation** Serum C3 levels Complement factors H, I by ELISA Membrane cofactor protein (CD46) by flow cytometry Antifactor H antibodies by ELISA Sequencing for genes encoding factor H, I, B, C3, CD46 and diacyglycerol kinase ε Multiplex ligation based probe amplification for complement factor H related proteins 1-5 **For S pneumoniae associated TMA** DCT, blood culture, positive T-antigen (peanut agglutination) **In suspected defective cobalamin metabolism** Serum homocysteine and methionine levels by high performance liquid chromatography (HPLC) and Urine methylmalonic acid by tandem mass spectrometry (TMS) **In suspected TTP** ADAMTS13 activity, ADAMTS13 antigen, anti-ADAMTS13 antibodies

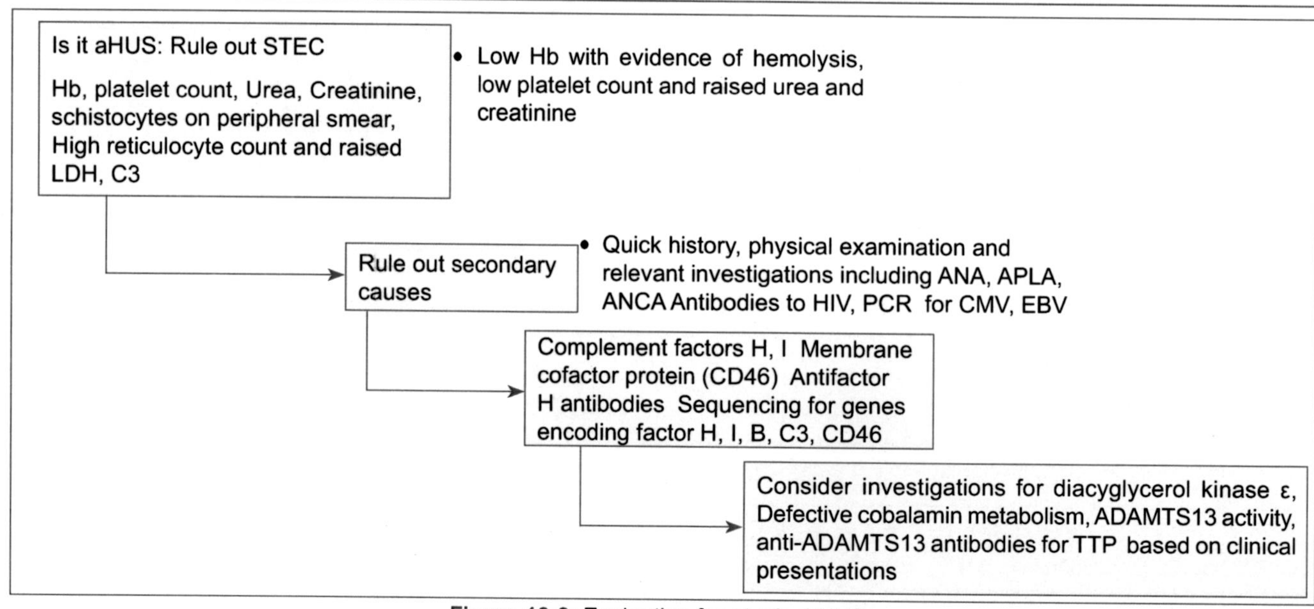

Figure 13.2: Evaluation for atypical HUS

inherited defects and autoantibody formation to CFH are the two main pathogenic mechanisms that cause aHUS. From the time it was first reported by Dragon-Durey *et al.* in 2005, Anti factor H antibody disease has been seen increasingly worldwide and remains the most common cause of aHUS in the Indian subcontinent. 90-95% of patients with anti-CFH antibodies have a complete deficiency of CFH-related proteins 1 (CFHR1) and 3 (CFHR3), due to a homozygous deletion of CFHR1-R3 which may also be seen in a small percentage of the healthy population. CFH autoantibody IgG titers by ELISA using the Paris protocol has been used widely though some other research laboratories may have a slightly different protocol for the same. The antibody assay results are usually available in a few days and may be used to guide treatment decisions in conjunction with the clinical condition of the patient.

Mutations in 6 genes have been associated with increased susceptibility for aHUS (CFH, CFI, MCP, C3, CFB and thrombomodulin). They should be analyzed by direct sequencing. Multiplex ligation dependent probe amplification (MLPA) is required to detect hybrid CFH genes and copy number variations in the genes encoding CFH and CFH-related (CFHRs) proteins. Screening for DGKE mutation should be performed in infants and young children aHUS.

Renal biopsy is not mandatory for establishing the diagnosis and cannot be performed in the acute stage due to thrombocytopenia. It is indicated if the diagnosis is in doubt, or in recurrent or severe disease. The pathognomic finding of TMA is seen in all types. In aHUS, the thrombi made up of fibrin, platelet and VWF clumps are seen in renal and interlobular arterioles along with glomerular capillary wall thickening and narrowing of capillary lumens. Mesangial expansion and mesangiolysis may also occur. Cortical necrosis is present in severe cases and indicates a poor outcome (Fig. 13.3).

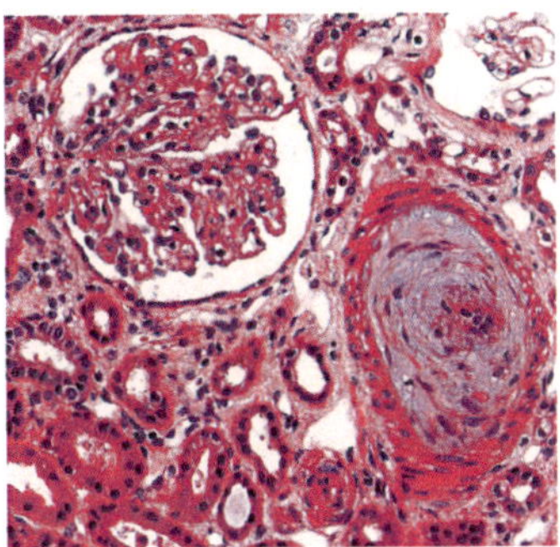

Figure 13.3: Kidney biopsy with TMA. Kidney biopsy image showing intimal hyperplasia with occlusion of the lumen in the arteriole and shrunken capillary tuft in the glomerulus in chronic TMA

How will You Treat this Patient?

For children with a clinical diagnosis of aHUS, eculizumab is now recommended as first-line treatment and should be started within 24-48 hours of onset as it has implications on renal recovery and risk of progression to end stage renal disease (ESRD). The guidelines also recommend therapeutic plasma exchange (TPE) as primary treatment option if eculizumab is not (or not immediately) available.

Due to non-availability eculizumab in India we have to continue to follow protocols with plasma exchange as primary treatment option. Plasma exchange may be by plasma filtration or centrifugal separator, according to availability of resources and expertise. Figure 13.4 gives the line diagram for plasma exchange by filtration method. The first plasma exchange with fresh frozen

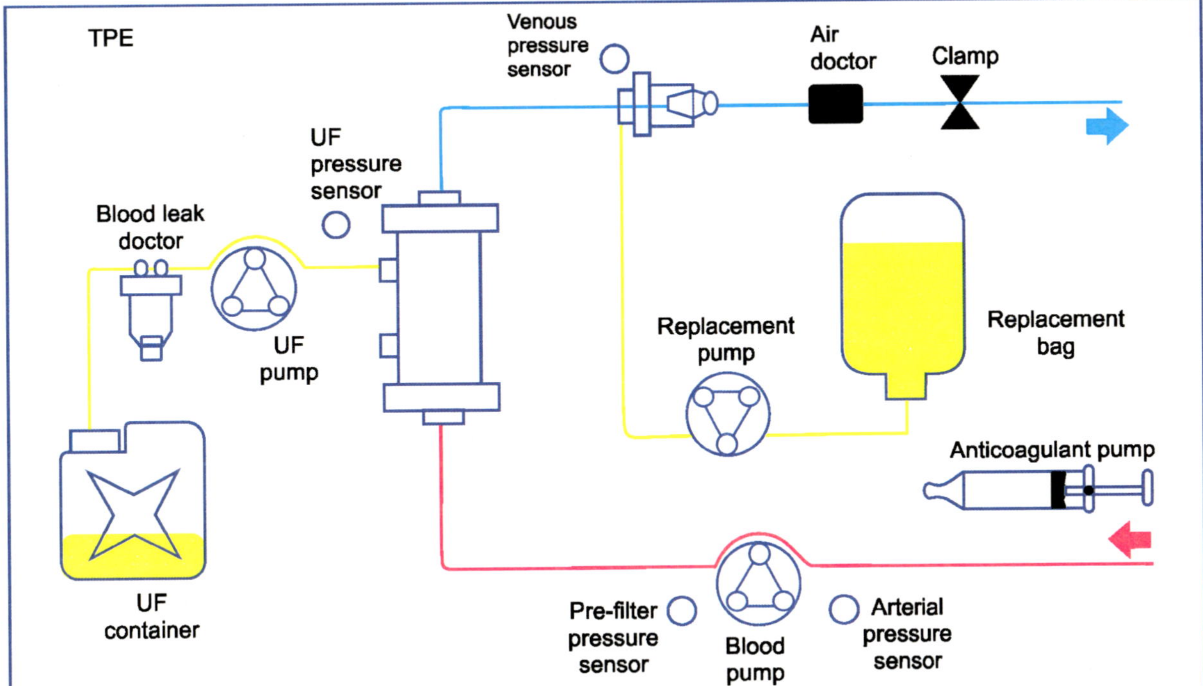

Figure 13.4: Line diagram for plasma exchange by filtration method

plasma should be initiated under close monitoring as soon as feasible and the child is hemodynamically stable.

Further Treatment Plan Would be:

Daily double volume plasma exchanges (75 ml/kg body weight) till hematological remission

Alternate day 1.5 times volume plasma exchanges (60 ml/kg body weight) for 4 sessions

Twice weekly 1.5 times volume plasma exchanges (60 ml/kg body weight) for 6 sessions

The plasma exchanges are stopped at this point in case of anti Factor H antibody disease. The exchanges may however need to be continued for prolonged periods once or twice a week to maintain hematological remission in children with aHUS due to other genetic abnormalities in the complement pathway.

Eculizumab is recommended for children managed with plasma exchange in case of: (i) Lack of remission despite 5-7 plasma exchanges; (ii) Life-threatening manifestations like seizures, myocardial dysfunction etc.; (iii) Complications associated with plasma exchange or vascular access; and (iv) Disease due to a genetic mutation known to respond to complement blockade.

The hematological remission has been defined as a platelet count >150 × 10^9/l for 2 weeks and no signs of hemolysis (absence of schistocytes, normal LDH levels). This is independent of renal function. A hematological relapse is defined as presence of microangiopathic hemolytic anemia and thrombocytopenia after being documented as normal for at least 2 weeks.

Baseline serum LDH, reticulocyte count and liver function tests should be done and repeated at day 3, 7 and thereafter weekly while the plasma exchanges are being carried on. The child's haemoglobin, platelet counts and renal function tests need to be checked daily to decide the number of daily exchanges required.

Most children require 7-10 sessions of hemodialysis in view of grossly elevated urea and creatinine, oliguria and fluid overload but renal recovery starts after first few sessions of plasma exchange.

Anti factor H antibody disease: In patients with anti factor H antibody disease plasmapheresis along with immunosuppression to prevent further antibody production has been shown to have best results. Oral prednisolone (1 mg/kg/d; for 4 weeks followed by 1 mg/kg alternate day tapered slowly over next 12-18 months) and either intravenous cyclophosphamide (500 mg/m^2 3-weekly for 6 doses) or intravenous rituximab (375 mg/m^2 weekly for 2 doses) followed by mycophenolate mofetil 750-1000 mg/kg/day for 18-24 months is the recommended protocol.

CASE 2

5-year-old girl admitted with history of oligo-anuria 3 days and history of epistaxis since morning. Examination revealed marked pallor with petechial rash on her neck and trunk. There is similar history one year back when she underwent 12 plasma exchanges and 4 sessions of hemodialysis after which the child improved and was discharged on oral amlodipine 0.3 mg/kg/day. She was advised some investigations but the patient did not come for the follow up visit.

What are the Causes of Relapsing aHUS?

While most causes of aHUS can have clinical relapses, the risk for relapse depends on the underlying condition. For instance mutations in C3 and CFH have almost 50% risk for relapse, whereas in mutations in Membrane Cofactor Protein the same increases to 100%. As mentioned earlier, genetic workup for the 6 most commonly implicated genes namely CFH, CFI, MCP, C3, CFB and thrombomodulin should be carried out in all children especially if they relapse.

CASE 3

9-month male infant brought with history of excessive irritability and vomiting of two days duration. Clinical evaluation revealed stage II hypertension. His initial investigations showed the triad of aHUS, i.e., presence of hemolytic anemia, thrombocytopenia and deranged renal function test (RFT). There was no history of diarrhea or history suggestive of pneumonia before the onset of the illness.

What are the Causes of aHUS in Infants?

Infants presenting with aHUS are likely to have a diacyglycerol kinase ε mutation or defective cobalamin metabolism or inherited deficiency of ADAMTS13 (Upshaw-Schulman syndrome) though it may be an early presentation of the other complement and coagulation pathway defects as mentioned earlier. They should undergo sequencing for genes encoding factor H, I, B, C3, CD 46 and diacyglycerol kinase ε along with ADAMTS13 activity. For defective cobalamin metabolism serum homocysteine and methionine can be measured by high performance liquid chromatography and tandem mass spectrometry can be done to estimate the urine methylmalonic acid levels.

Monitoring and follow-up: Patients should be monitored closely for hematological remission, renal dysfunction, proteinuria and hypertension at follow-up. Twenty to thirty percent of all cases with aHUS have residual defects including deranged renal function tests,

Table 13.2: Clinical course and outcomes in children with aHUS due to common genetic conditions

Abnormal/deficient factor	Cause of HUS in %	% progressing to ESRD	% experiencing clinical relapses	% with recurrence post transplant
C3	2-10%	60%	50%	40-70%
Complement factor H	20-30%	50-70%	50%	75-90%
Complement factor I	4-10%	50%	10-30%	60-80%
Membrane cofactor protein B (CD46)	5-15%	0-10%	70-90%	<20%
Complement factor B	1-4%	50%	Common	100%
Anti factor H antibody	6-50%	30-40%	20-50%	Low
Thrombomodulin	3-5%	50%	30%	Not known

ESRD: End stage renal disease

proteinuria and hypertension and depends upon the underlying etiology as well as the severity of disease at presentation. The long-term disease course and outcomes as well as risk for post transplant recurrence is as summarised in Table 13.2. Combined liver and kidney transplant may be required in children with aHUS due to mutations of complement factors synthesized in the liver including those in CFH, CFB and C3.

Suggested Reading

1. Ariceta G, Besbas N, Johnson S. European Pediatric Study Group for HUS: Guideline for the investigation and initial therapy of diarrhea negative hemolytic uremic syndrome. Pediatr Nephrol 2009;24:687-96.
2. Loirat C, Fakhouri F, Ariceta G, *et al.* for HUS International. An international consensus approach to the management of atypical hemolytic uremic syndrome in children. Pediatr Nephrol 2015;31(1):15-39.
3. Nelson W, Kliegman R, Stanton B, St Geme J, Schor N, Behrman R. Nelson textbook of pediatrics. International: Elsevier; 2016.
4. Sinha A, Gulati A, Saini S, Blanc C, Gupta A, Gurjar B *et al.* Prompt plasma exchanges and immunosuppressive treatment improves the outcomes of anti-factor H autoantibody-associated hemolytic uremic syndrome in children. Kidney International 2014;85(5):1151-60.

CHAPTER

A Patient with Acute Kidney Injury Due to Contrast Induced Nephropathy

Ashish Nandwani[1], Prasad Dandekar[2]

[1] *Consultant, Nephrology, Manipal Hospital, Dwarka, New Delhi*

[2] *Associate Consultant, Nephrology, Fortis Hospital, Noida*

CASE

65 years old male with Type 2 diabetes mellitus and hypertension presented with complaints of chest pain and breathlessness of one day duration. On exam, BP 180/100 mm Hg, pedal edema +, chest revealed bilateral basal crepts. He had no past history of any renal disease.

Lab evaluation revealed urea 65 mg/dl, serum creatinine 1.5 mg/dl with normal electrolytes. Urine exam showed 3+ protein with no active sediments. Spot urine protein/creatinine ratio was 3.2. USG revealed bilateral normal size kidneys with increased echogenicity and poor cortico-medullary differentiation. 2D Echocardiography was suggestive of hypo kinetic left ventricular wall with LV EF 30%. Patient was diagnosed to have acute myocardial infarction and underwent primary angioplasty.

Post procedure, on day 1, his serum creatinine started rising reaching upto 4.6 mg/dl on day 4. Patient remained non oliguric during the episode. He was managed conservatively with hydration and supportive care. Serum creatinine started decreasing from day 6 onwards and patient was discharged with serum creatinine of 1.7 mg/dl.

What is Contrast Induced Nephropathy?

Contrast induced nephropathy (CIN) is characterized by a decrease in kidney function that occurs within days after the intravascular administration of iodinated contrast material. In past, case reports of contrast nephropathy in patients with preexisting kidney disease who were undergoing intravenous pyelography were published. Since then the quality and content of contrast materials for procedure, has improved significantly leading to reduction in the nephropathy. In addition recognition of risk factors and implementation of preventive care resulted in lower rates of acute kidney injury after the administration of contrast material. The over looming risk of acute kidney injury leading to underutilization of lifesaving procedures like coronary angiography is a matter of concern. Recent studies have suggested that the risk is somewhat overestimated.

The Kidney Disease Improving Global Outcomes (KDIGO) working group proposed the term "contrast induced acute kidney injury" in 2012 . It was defined as rise in plasma creatinine by a factor of 1.5 times or more over the baseline value within 7 days after exposure to contrast medium or > 0.3 mg/dl increase over the baseline value within 48 hours after exposure to contrast medium or a urinary volume of less than 0.5 ml/kg of body weight per hour that persists for at least 6 hours after exposure.

How Contrast Causes Acute Kidney Injury?

Contrast can affect a nephron in either direct or indirect ways or both.

Direct Mechanisms

These effects are related to the biochemical properties of the particular contrast medium causing injury to tubular epithelium which leads to loss of function, apoptosis, and eventually, necrosis.

a. Early tubular epithelial injury is characterized by the loss of cell polarity due to the redistribution of Na^+/K^+-ATPase from the baso lateral to the luminal surface of the tubular cells, resulting in abnormal ion transport across the cells and increased sodium delivery to the distal tubules. This phenomenon leads to further renal vasoconstriction through tubuloglomerular feedback.
b. As the injury progresses the epithelial cells detach from the basement membranes and cause luminal obstruction, increased intratubular pressure, and finally, a decrease in the glomerular filtration rate.

Indirect Mechanisms

a. Contrast agents lead to release of local vasoactive substances such as endothelin, nitric oxide and prostaglandin resulting in vasoconstriction. This causes decrease in glomerular blood flow and reduced oxygen delivery to the metabolically active parts of the nephron.

b. Contrast agents increase blood viscosity leading to further reduction of the microcirculatory flow and changes in blood osmolality, which in turn impair the plasticity of erythrocytes and may increase the risk of microvascular thrombosis.

What are the Risk Factors for Contrast Induced Nephropathy?

Many risk factors have been proposed to accentuate the effect of contrast on the kidneys. Combination of risk factors as compared to a presence of a single risk factor worsens the outcome.

a. **Type of contrast material:** The high osmolarity contrast materials were initially used and had the most number of cases of contrast induced nephropathy. But over the time the design of contrast material has evolved making it iso osmolar leading to less chances of causing hyperviscosity related indirect effects on the tubules. Low osmolality and iso-osmolality agents are associated with a lower risk of kidney injury and their use is recommended (class I recommendation, level of evidence A) by the European Society of Cardiology and the American Heart Association–American College of Cardiology (Table 14.1).

b. **Amount of contrast material:** High volume (>350 ml or >4 ml per kilogram) or repeated administration within 72 hours after initial administration has been shown to be associated with an increased risk.

c. **Preexisting chronic kidney disease:** It is the strongest well established patient-related risk factor for CIN. An analysis of 985,737 patients from the NCDR Cath-PCI registry undergoing percutaneous coronary intervention showed that lower levels of kidney function associated with higher degrees of nephropathy.

d. **Indication for contrast use:** The risk of acute kidney injury varies with the clinical presentation. In patients who have myocardial infarction and are undergoing PCI have a particularly high risk of contrast-associated kidney injury. Likewise patients who are in shock or who are posted for surgeries associated with hemodynamic instability like coronary artery bypass grafting/valve replacement are more prone for CIN.

e. **Type of imaging procedure:** Arteriography is associated with a higher risk than computed tomography (CT), owing to delivery of more concentrated contrast material to the kidneys with arteriographic procedures and the higher overall risk profile of patients requiring such procedures.

f. Old age (> 75 years), diabetic nephropathy, heart failure, acute myocardial infarction, hypotension, use of intra aortic balloon pump, renal transplant recipient are some of other important risk factors for CIN.

Most of the risk stratification models designed to estimate the risk of CIN were developed in studies involving patients undergoing PCI, which limits their generalizability. However the strength of these models is that they are derived from data based on large numbers of patients.

The most common model that is used is developed by Mehran *et al.* in patients undergoing PCI. 5,571 patients were studied with a validation cohort of 2,786 subjects. CIN was defined as >0.5 mg/dl of absolute or 25% relative increase in pre-PCI serum creatinine at 48 hours after PCI.

Mehran Contrast Induced Nephropathy Risk Scoring System

The Mehran Risk Score (MRS) has been demonstrated to be clinically useful for prediction of contrast-induced nephropathy (CIN) (Tables 14.2 and 14.3).

Implications of Contrast Induced Nephropathy

Mild increments in plasma creatinine levels are common in patients who have undergone contrast enhanced

Table 14.1: Type of contrast material

Type	High osmolality	Low osmolality	ISO osmolality
Generic Name (mg contrast/ml)	Diatrizoate meglumine and Diatrizoate sodium (760)	Ioxaglate meglumine and Ioxaglate sodium (589) Iopamidol (408) Iopamidol (510) Iopamidol (612) Iopamidol (755)	Iodixanol (550) Iodixanol (652)
Iodine concentration (mg/ml)	370	200-370	270-320
Osmolality (mOsm/kg H_2O)	1551	413-796	290
Viscosity (mPa. sec at 37°C)	10.5	2.0-9.4	6.3-11.8

Table 14.2: Mehran contrast induced nephropathy risk scoring system

Risk factor	Score
Hypotension	5
Advanced congestive heart failure	5
Impaired renal function	
-Serum creatinine >1.5 mg/dl	4
or	
-eGFR:	
40-60 ml/min/1.73 m^2	2
20-40 ml/min/1.73 m^2	4
<20 ml/min/1.73 m^2	6
Age >75 years	4
Anemia	3
Diabetes	3
Contrast media volume/100 ml	1
Elective use of intra-aortic balloon pump	5

Table 14.3: Risk of contrast-associated acute kidney injury according to score stratification

Scores	Risk
Scores: 0 to 5	→7.5%
Scores: 6 to 10	→14.0%
Scores: 11 to 16	→26.1%
Scores: >16	→57.3%

procedures. Studies have shown that contrast-associated acute kidney injury is associated with increased mortality. But such increases are not uncommon among hospitalized patients in general. However, the incidence of severe acute kidney injury characterized by substantial decrements in kidney function or the need for renal replacement therapy is quite low.

Deteriorating kidney function after angiography or angioplasty has been characterized as a major procedural complication in the National Cardiovascular Data Registry. Although there have been no adequately powered clinical trials showing that prevention of contrast-associated acute kidney injury results in a survival benefit.

Acute kidney injury following coronary angiography is associated with a long-term decline in kidney function.

Contrast-associated acute kidney injury is also correlated with accelerated progression of underlying chronic kidney disease. The risk of a sustained reduction in kidney function at 90 days is greater for patients who had acute kidney injury after contrast exposure than for those who did not have acute kidney injury.

Prevention of Contrast Induced Nephropathy

Preventive strategies for CIN have been a debatable question since a long time. Benefits of prophylactic renal replacement therapy and of most pharmaceutical agents have not been proved.

a. **Volume Expansion:** It is the only preventive strategy that has stood the test of time. Several observational studies have shown a protective effect of intravenous fluids, evidence from randomized clinical trials is relatively sparse. Marked lower incidence of contrast-related acute kidney injury with saline (3.7% vs. 34.6%, P = 0.005) was showen in a study by Trivedi *et al.* American College of Radiology guidelines on the administration of contrast material recommend the use of intravenous isotonic saline at an infusion rate of 100 ml per hour for 6 to 12 hours before and 4 to 12 hours after angiography. Alternatively an intravenous infusion of isotonic saline for 1 to 3 hours before and 6 hours after the procedure also suffices (3-6 ml/kg/hr). AMACING (A Maastricht Contrast-Induced Nephropathy Guideline) trial showed no significant difference in the incidence of acute kidney injury between the hydration group and the no-hydration group (2.7% and 2.6%, respectively). Although the evidence in favour of volume expansion is far greater to conclude the futility of this measure.

   It was hypothesized that intravenous isotonic sodium bicarbonate with isotonic sodium chloride causing urinary alkalinization would reduce contrast-induced generation of injurious oxygen free radicals. The theory was tested in Prevention of Serious Adverse Events Following Angiography (PRESERVE) study which showed no significant difference in the incidence of contrast associated acute kidney injury (9.5% with bicarbonate and 8.3% with saline).

b. **Avoid Nephrotoxic Drugs:** Potentially nephrotoxic agents, including NSAIDs and aminoglycosides should be stopped or avoided before the use of contrast. Data is insufficient to support discontinuation of diuretics, angiotensin-converting–enzyme inhibitors, or angiotensin-receptor blockers.

c. **Low Dose of Contrast:** It is advisable to use the lowest necessary total dose of low osmolality or iso osmolality contrast medium. It has been suggested that the total volume to less than double the patient's baseline glomerular filtration rate.

d. **Acetylcysteine:** Routine administration of acetylcysteine is not recommended for the prevention of acute kidney injury or longer-term adverse events after angiographic procedures. Still it has been widely used in clinical practice because of its low cost, ease of use, and limited toxic effects. The efficacy of acetylcysteine was tested in the PRESERVE trial where oral acetylcysteine was administered at a dose of 1200 mg twice daily for 5 days, beginning on the day of angiography. No benefit in reducing the incidence of CIN was seen over a placebo (4.6% with acetylcysteine and 4.5% with placebo).

e. **Statins:** PRATO-ACS (Protective Effect of Rosuvastatin and Antiplatelet Therapy on Contrast-Induced Acute Kidney Injury and Myocardial Damage in Patients with Acute Coronary Syndrome) trial showed a significant benefit in reducing acute kidney injury after PCI in patients treated with high-dose rosuvastatin as compared with patients who did not receive statin treatment. The hypothesis that statins reduce the risk of contrast-associated acute kidney injury is based on their anti-inflammatory and antioxidant properties. Although other trials have failed to show any benefit.

Contrast induced nephropathy is an important and potentially preventable complication of IV contrast administration. Patients should be adequately hydrated and all nephrotoxic drugs should be discontinued before contrast administration to decrease this complication.

Suggested Reading

1. Rudnick MR, Berns JS, Cohen RM, Goldfarb S. Nephrotoxic risks of renal angiography: Contrast media-associated nephropathy and atheroembolism–A critical review. Am J Kidney Dis 1994;24:713-27.
2. Lasser EC, Lyon SG, Berry CC. Reports on contrast media reactions: Analysis of data from reports to the U.S. Food and Drug Administration. Radiology 1997;203:605-10.
3. Weisbord SD, Mor MK, Resnick AL, *et al.* Prevention, incidence and outcomes of contrast-induced acute kidney injury. Arch Intern Med 2008;168:1325-32.
4. Kidney Disease Improving Global Outcomes (KDIGO). Clinical practice guideline for acute kidney injury. Kidney Int Suppl 2012;2:1-138.
5. Heyman SN, Clark BA, Kaiser N, *et al.* Radiocontrast agents induce endothelin release in vivo and in vitro. J Am Soc Nephrol 1992;3:58-65.
6. Heyman SN, Rosen S, Brezis M. Radiocontrast nephropathy: A paradigm for the synergism between toxic and hypoxic insults in the kidney. Exp Nephrol 1994;2:153-57.
7. Mehran R *et al.* N Engl J Med 2019;380:2146-55.
8. Rudnick MR, Goldfarb S, Wexler L, *et al.* Nephropathy of ionic and nonionic contrast media in 1196 patients: A randomized trial: The Iohexol Cooperative Study. Kidney Int 1995;47:254-61.
9. Goldfarb S, Spinler S, Berns JS, Rudnick MR. Low-osmolality contrast media and the risk of contrast-associated nephrotoxicity. Invest Radiol 1993;28:Suppl 5:S7-10.
10. Amsterdam EA, Wenger NK, Brindis RG, *et al.* 2014 AHA/ACC Guideline for the Management of Patients with Non-STElevation Acute Coronary Syndromes: A report of the American College of Cardiology/American Heart Association Task Force on Practice Guidelines. J Am Coll Cardiol 2014;64(24):e139-e228.
11. Mehran R, Aymong ED, Nikolsky E, *et al.* A simple risk score for prediction of contrast-induced nephropathy after percutaneous coronary intervention: Development and initial validation. J Am Coll Cardiol 2004;44:1393-99.

CHAPTER

An End Stage Renal Disease Patient with Metabolic Bone Disease

Santosh Varughese[1], Suceena Alexander[2]

[1]*Professor and Head, Department of Nephrology, Christian Medical College, Vellore*
[2]*Professor, Department of Nephrology, Christian Medical College, Vellore*

Metabolic bone disease is a common complication of chronic kidney disease (CKD) and is part of a broad spectrum of disorders of mineral metabolism that occur in this clinical setting and result in both skeletal and extraskeletal consequences.

CASE

55-year-old Ms G presents with symptoms of fatigue for 2 months; pain in her hips and lower back for the past 6 months and nausea and vomiting for a week. There was no significant past medical history. For these symptoms, she was evaluated and told to have advanced chronic kidney disease and she was started on medications, the names of which she was unable to recall. She was also told that she would need dialysis. A tunnelled jugular venous catheter was inserted into the right side of the neck a day ago and she was started on hemodialysis yesterday.

Clinical examination showed pallor. There was no edema. Blood pressure 110/70 mm Hg; pulse 68/min, normal. There was a tunnelled dialysis catheter below her right collar bone with the tunnel entering the lower neck. The rest of the examination was unremarkable including absence of additional heart sounds.

Clinical Diagnosis

Chronic Kidney Disease G5 D.

Possible etiology: Chronic Interstitial Nephritis.

Current symptoms/complications: Anemia; possible chronic kidney disease (CKD) – mineral and bone disorder (MBD).

Discussion on CKD-MBD

CKD-MBD is known as the "silent crippler" of the disease. Metabolic abnormalities onset in patients with CKD is associated with progressive fall in glomerular filtration rate (GFR) (Table 15.1).

Table 15.1: Relationship between metabolic abnormalities onset and eGFR

	Abnormality	**eGFR at onset**
1	↑ plasma phosphate	~ 20 ml/min
2	↓ plasma calcium	~ 20 ml/min
3	↓ calcitriol	< 60 ml/min (occ. 80 ml/min)
4	↑ PTH	< 60 ml/min
5	Onset of bone disease	eGFR 60 to 89 ml/min
6	↑ FGF 23	eGFR <70 ml/min
7	↓ Klotho	eGFR <70 ml/min

Definition

Systemic disorder of mineral and bone metabolism, with ≥ 1 manifestation:

- Abnormalities of calcium, phosphorus, parathyroid hormone (PTH), fibroblast growth factor 23 (FGF23) and vitamin D metabolism.
- Abnormalities in bone turnover, mineralization, volume linear growth, or strength.
- Extraskeletal calcification.

"Renal osteodystrophy" is used exclusively for diagnosis made by bone biopsy.

Etiopathogenesis of Secondary Hyperparathyroidism

- Phosphate retention.
- Decreased free ionized calcium concentration.
- Decreased 1, 25-dihydroxyvitamin D (calcitriol) concentration (Fig. 15.1).
- Increased fibroblast growth factor 23 (FGF23) concentration.
- Changes in the parathyroid glands – ↓ vitamin D receptors (VDRs), ↓ calcium-sensing receptors (CaSRs), ↓ fibroblast growth factor receptors, ↓ klotho in the parathyroid glands.

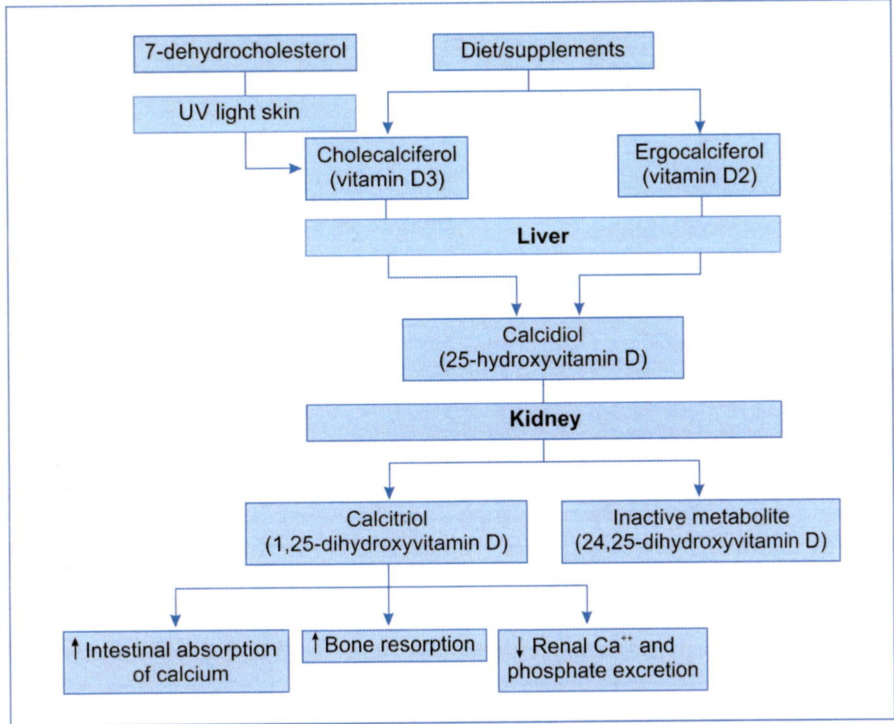

Figure 15.1: Metabolism of vitamin D *[Ref: Uptodate.com]*

Etiology of Phosphate Retention

- Decreased formation or activity of calcitriol.
- Increased PTH gene expression.
- Hypocalcemia.

Serum phosphate levels are not elevated in early stages of CKD due to a reduced renal tubular phosphate resorption mediated by increased levels of PTH and FGF23. Klotho deficiency that occurs early in CKD may blunt the effect of FGF23 on phosphate excretion. Then, PTH may be the primary factor in maintaining serum phosphate level. Normal proximal tubule phosphate reabsorption is about 80-95% of filtered phosphate.

Pathogenetic Mechanism of Hyperphosphatemia Induced Hyperparathyroidism:

- Decreased formation or activity of calcitriol.
- Decreased plasma calcium.
- Direct effect–through reduction of PTH messenger RNA (mRNA) concentrations via increasing post-transcriptional PTH mRNA message stability.
- Opposite effect by stimulating FGF23 secretion that suppresses PTH.

Hyperparathyroidism in CKD is initially appropriate to cause phosphaturia and lower the plasma phosphate concentration toward normal. When glomerular filtration rate (GFR) is severely reduced, PTH inhibits proximal tubule phosphate reabsorption to 15% but the compensatory increase in the levels of PTH and FGF23 becomes inadequate resulting in hyperphosphatemia. Also, continued PTH-induced release of phosphate from bone exacerbates hyperphosphatemia.

Hyperphosphatemia causes osteoblastic transformation of the vascular smooth muscle cell in the vasculature and directly contributes to cardiovascular calcification and arterial stiffness.

Hyperparathyroidism corrects hypocalcemia by increasing bone resorption. Hyperparathyroidism corrects calcitriol deficiency by stimulating the 1-hydroxylation of calcidiol [25-hydroxyvitamin D] in the proximal tubule.

Causes of Low Calcitriol in CKD

- Initially, due to the increase in FGF23 concentration.
- Reduced renal mass.
- Hyperphosphatemia.
- Phosphate retention leads to suppression of 1-alpha hydroxylase.
- Increased FGF23 leads to suppression of 1-alpha hydroxylase.

FGF23 secretion from bone osteocytes is stimulated by dietary phosphate load and increased calcitriol. FGF23 secretion increases soon after initial renal injury and increases with worsening of renal function.

How Decrease in Calcitriol Concentrations Leads to Increase in PTH?

- **Indirect effects:** Decrease in intestinal absorption of calcium and calcium release from bone leading to hypocalcemia and stimulates PTH secretion.

- **Direct effects:**
  - Calcitriol normally acts on vitamin D receptor (VDR) in the parathyroid gland to suppress PTH transcription but not PTH secretion. Removal of inhibitory effect of calcitriol on PTH.
  - Decrease in calcitriol lowers the number of VDRs in parathyroid. Worsened with retained uremic toxins which additionally blocks binding to VDRs.

  [Both of these cause parathyroid chief cell hyperplasia].
- **Decreased Responsiveness to Calcitriol:** Administration of calcitriol/vitamin D analogs can partially reverse the hyperparathyroidism both in early and advanced disease by blocking the increase in transforming growth factor-alpha (TGF-alpha). Supraphysiological doses are needed as there is decreased responsiveness to calcitriol due to a reduction in the number of VDRs in the parathyroid gland.

  Both hypocalcemia and hypercalcemia are associated with increased mortality in CKD patients. Hypocalcemia is more common.

Etiology of Hypocalcemia in CKD

- Phosphate retention.
- Decreased calcitriol concentration.
- Resistance to the calcemic actions of PTH on bone (PTH secretion varies inversely with serum calcium concentration).

Hypocalcemia is associated with increased PTH secretion and abnormal bone remodelling. Hypercalcemia has been implicated in pathogenesis of extraskeletal calcification. Positive calcium balance in the absence of hypercalcemia may cause aorta, heart, and aortic valve calcification.

Calcium-Sensing Receptor (CaSR) in CKD

- It is a specific membrane receptor on the surface of the chief cells of the parathyroid glands, senses minute changes in serum ionized calcium to tight regulation of PTH transcription, secretion and parathyroid gland hyperplasia secretion.
- Number of CaSRs are reduced in hypertrophied parathyroid glands, particularly in areas of nodular hypertrophy and can lead to inadequate suppression of PTH secretion by calcium, resulting in inappropriately high PTH concentrations in the setting of normal or even high calcium concentrations.

  Calcimimetic agents in CKD reduce PTH by > 50%.

Mechanisms of Action

- Increases sensitivity of CaSR to extracellular calcium and decrease PTH secretion.
- Directly reduce PTH gene expression.
- Increase VDR expression in parathyroid glands.

FGF23 in CKD

- FGF23 is secreted by bone osteocytes and osteoblasts in response to calcitriol, increased dietary phosphate load, PTH and calcium.
- Another cause of increased FGF23 concentrations is due to decreased clearance (prolonged half life).
- FGF23 levels are associated with increased risk of cardiovascular disease and mortality in patients with CKD. There is a direct pathogenic effect causing left ventricular hypertrophy.
- FGF23 increases apical membrane expression of the sodium-chloride cotransporter and epithelial calcium channel, through klotho-dependent activation of WNK4. This leads to sodium and calcium reabsorption in the distal tubule and can lead to sodium retention, volume overload, hypertension and cardiac hypertrophy.
- Primary function of FGF23 is to maintain normal serum phosphate concentration:
  - In renal proximal tubular cells, FGF23 binds to FGF receptor (FGFR) and klotho causing downregulation of the luminal membrane sodium phosphate cotransporters Na/Pi IIa and Na/Pi IIc causing reduced phosphate reabsorption from urine and increased urinary phosphate excretion.
  - FGF23 inhibits proximal tubular 1-alpha-hydroxylase expression leading to decreased calcitriol synthesis.
  - FGF23 reduces intestinal phosphate absorption through decreased calcitriol production.

Klotho in CKD

- Klotho is a transmembrane protein produced by osteocytes and is required for FGF23 receptor activation. Klotho does not directly bind to FGF23 but enhances FGF23 binding to its receptor complex with an increased affinity than to the FGFR alone.
- Decline in Klotho may be partially responsible for the progressive rise in FGF23 concentration and decreased expression on hyperplastic parathyroid glands may contribute to the resistance and impaired parathyroid suppression by FGF23.

Mechanisms of Resistance of Bone to PTH in CKD

- Downregulation of PTH receptors induced by the high circulating PTH concentrations, calcitriol deficiency and hyperphosphatemia.

- Presence of inactive 7-84 PTH fragments in addition to the whole 1-84 hormone that inhibit the effects of 1-84 PTH, reducing biologic activity.
- PTH's target cell in bone is the osteoblast and acts via the PTH/PTHrP receptor (PTH1R). Binding of PTH to this receptor leads to osteoblast activation, bone anabolism, and indirect activation of the osteoclasts through the RANK-RANKL system. Decreased density of PTH1R mRNA seen in bone biopsies of uremic patients. It is more severe in patients with adynamic bone disease.
- RANK-RANKL interaction triggers osteoclast differentiation and activity. Osteoprotegerin (OPG) is secreted by osteoblasts to block the osteoclastogenesis induced by RANKL. Normally, PTH inhibits OPG production and stimulates RANKL production and therefore enhancing bone resorption. Serum OPG concentrations increase progressively with serum creatinine in predialysis patients and are markedly elevated in dialysis patients. Elevated levels of OPG reduces the bone resorptive effect of PTH in uremia.

Tertiary Hyperparathyroidism

Tertiary hyperparathyroidism is markedly elevated PTH concentrations, often associated with hypercalcemia. This is due to severe parathyroid hyperplasia, with autonomous secretion of PTH that does not adequately respond to plasma calcium concentration. This results from the increase in parathyroid gland mass rather than an alteration in the set point of PTH release unlike what is seen in familial hypocalciuric hypercalcemia (in which it is the primary defect) and primary hyperparathyroidism (in which there is both a set-point error and increased gland mass). There is decreased expression of CaSR and VDRs and results in a lack of suppression of PTH by increasing calcium or vitamin D analogs.

Nodular hyperplasia results from prolonged stimulation of parathyroid cell growth due to high phosphate, low calcitriol and hypocalcemia. These glands do not undergo involution, despite resolution of some of the triggering mechanisms and may explain high PTH concentrations and hypercalcemia that may persist after renal transplantation. Another important pathogenetic factor is neoplastic transformation–monoclonal parathyroid adenoma.

Bone turnover is the ratio between bone formation and bone resorption. PTH level, used either alone or in combination with bone-specific alkaline phosphatase, is used as a marker of bone turnover. Plain radiographs may show osteomalacia (Looser-Milkman zones) and quantified computerized tomography is superior but expensive and dual-energy X-ray absorptiometry is unreliable.

Gold standard for the diagnosis and classification of bone disease in CKD is bone biopsy obtained from the iliac crest after two tetracycline markers are administered separated by 21 days. The second labeling period is two days before biopsy. The specimen is stained with Goldner Masson trichrome for differentiation of mineralized lamellar bone and nonmineralized osteoid and Villanueva stain for tetracycline fluorescence. Three parameters are used to assess bone pathology – bone turnover, mineralization and volume (TMV). The specimen consists of osteoid, stained red brown with the Goldner-Masson (trichrome) stain, and mineralized bone, stained blue under light microscopy. The osteoid appears orange, and the mineralized bone is green under fluorescent light. The luminescent tetracycline bands within bone represent active mineralized bone formation beneath the osteoid surface. The osteoid appears lamellar occupying < 25% of bone, covered with mature osteoblasts (~ 40%). Bone resorption is minimal (<7%) and osteoclasts are < 2% on the bone surface. Various pathological lesion found on bone biopsy are:

- **Osteitis fibrosa cystica:** Characterized by high bone turnover due to secondary hyperparathyroidism. Histologically, there is marrow fibrosis, woven osteoid, increased number and activity of osteoblasts, expansion of osteoid surfaces, and numerous osteoclasts and resorptive surfaces. The woven osteoid indicates disordered collagen contrasting with the parallel collagen strands of normal bone. Distinct tetracycline labels cover most of the bone surfaces, indicating accelerated bone formation and the absence of a mineralization defect.
- **Adynamic bone disease:** Characterized by low bone turnover. Results from excessive suppression of the parathyroid glands and is the most common bone lesion in ESRD patients. This is the most common type and possibly is the earliest to occur. More common in diabetics and peritoneal dialysis. Other risk factors are use of calcium containing phosphate binders, high dialysate calcium, use of active vitamin D analogs and increased age. The most common symptom is bone pain. On biopsy, there is reduced osteoblast and osteoclast number and activity resulting in low bone formation and resorption, manifesting histologically by thin osteoid seams that display no active mineralization, inactive appearing osteoblasts, and decreases in osteoclast number and bone resorptive surfaces. Adynamic bone disease is treated by decreasing/stopping calcium-based phosphate binders and vitamin D/analogues and use of low calcium dialysate allowing the PTH level to rise. Use of non-calcium based phosphate binders may increase bone formation rate. Teriparatide (recombinant human PTH) has been tried with resolution of bone pain and increased bone formation.
- **Osteomalacia:** Characterized by low bone turnover in combination with abnormal mineralization.

The mineralization lag time is more than 100 days comparison to less than 35 days in normal subjects and those with pure osteitis fibrosa. Histologically, there is marked increase in the fraction of bone exhibiting wide osteoid seams and by the absence of osteoblasts or erosive surfaces. Fluorescent microscopy reveals little or no tetracycline deposition. Historically, osteomalacia used to be related to aluminum exposure from aluminum-containing antacids that were used as phosphate binders and water contamination. Combination with citrate increases intestinal absorption. The action is by formation of soluble aluminum citrate and by chelating calcium in the intestinal wall. There is no safe dosage of aluminum that is permitted in ESRD. Serum aluminum > 20 mcg/l are abnormal. Aluminum levels rise (6 to 7 mcg/l) in those treated with ferric citrate as phosphate binder, long-term consequences of which are unknown. Screening aluminum levels is restricted to those receiving aluminum containing phosphate binders, in areas where water purification is inadequate and perhaps prior to parathyroidectomy. Bone biopsy shows osteomalacia with extensive aluminum deposition on bone surfaces. Aluminum is detected histologically with a Villanueva-prestained section stained with aurintricarboxylic acid where osteoid is light blue, and the mineralized bone is white. Aluminum stains as a red band at the osteoid-bone interface.

- **Mixed uremic osteodystrophy:** Characterized by either high or low bone turnover and by abnormal mineralization. On biopsy, it resembles osteitis fibrosa with greater degree of osteoid accumulation. Fluorescent microscopy shows impaired mineralization, evidenced by diffuse tetracycline deposition and absence of tetracycline in some bone-forming surfaces. There is also a decreased mineralization lag time.

Indications for Bone Biopsy

The indications for bone biopsy are controversial and is usually done only when the exact histological diagnosis is likely to make a difference to management. Currently acceptable indications are:

- Confirmation of presence of PTH-mediated high-turnover bone disease in patients with ESRD undergoing parathyroidectomy with persistent symptoms of hyperparathyroidism having lower PTH level (< 450 pg/ml).
- Unexplained bone pain or fractures with minimal or no trauma.
- Suspected osteomalacia due to aluminum toxicity.
- Confirmation of adynamic bone disease in patients with bone pain and persistent serum PTH levels <100 pg/ml, despite withdrawal of calcitriol or vitamin D analogues.

Vascular Calcification

Vascular calcification is common in ESRD patients. All large and medium-sized muscular arteries and arterioles can calcify. Differences in the mechanical forces and histologic structure between arteries and veins lead to veins usually not calcifying, unless injured or arterialized. Two types of vascular calcification are seen in CKD – medial and intimal calcification. *Medial* calcification is a result of a phenotype switch of vascular smooth muscle cells to osteoblast-like cells and local inflammation. These changes are caused by hyperphosphatemia, hypercalcemia, and high PTH levels. Hyperphosphatemia increases activity of the sodium-dependent cotransporters, PiT-1 and PiT-2 which upregulates genes associated with matrix mineralization. Hypercalcemia and hyperphosphatemia both increase the release of matrix vesicles, resulting in the deposition of hydroxyapatite. Systemic and local inflammation contribute to vascular calcification. Infiltrating macrophages release proinflammatory cytokines and cause influx of lymphocytes and smooth muscle cells. The cellular microvesicles released from macrophages or apoptotic macrophages form a nidus for calcification, and macrophage-derived inflammatory regulators, such as matrix metalloproteinases (MMPs) and cathepsin S, contribute to the disintegration of elastic fibers and matrix components in the vessel wall, all which may promote calcification. *Intimal* calcification is a result of ongoing atherosclerosis, similar to the general population. Mechanisms that contribute to intimal calcification, e.g., shear stress, local inflammation, calcification of macrophage- and vascular smooth muscle cell-derived microvesicles, are amplified in CKD patients. Also, the factors causing medial calcification may worsen intimal calcification and the resultant arterial stiffness may directly contribute to the shear stress, atherosclerosis, and calcification of the intima.

Risk Factors for Vascular Calcification are:

- Increased age.
- Dialysis vintage.
- Persistent hyperphosphatemia.
- Hypercalcemia.
- Increased calcium-phosphate product.
- Increased oral calcium intake.
- Secondary hyperparathyroidism.
- Adynamic bone disease.
- Vitamin D deficiency.
- High dialysate calcium (3.5 mEq/l worse than 2.5 mEq/l).
- Hypomagnesemia.
- Diabetes mellitus.
- Dyslipidemia.

- Warfarin.

The risk is reduced in those using non-calcium phosphate binders and calcimimetics.

Vascular calcification is inhibited by multiple circulating regulatory proteins called calciprotein particles made up of calcium-phosphate crystals and chaperone-binding proteins inhibit the crystallization of calcium/phosphate in blood. Fetuin A is the major chaperone protein, low levels of which leads to precipitation of calcium-phosphate and thus to vascular calcification. Both inflammation and malnutrition in patients with CKD are associated with low levels of fetuin A. Other inhibitory proteins in the calciprotein particles are matrix Gla-protein (MGP) and gamma-carboxylated Gla-rich protein (GRP), both of which are vitamin K dependent. (The inhibition of GRP and MGP may contribute to vascular calcification in patients on warfarin). Other inhibitors of vascular calcification are klotho and pyrophosphate, the latter is produced by vascular smooth muscle cells and inhibits formation of hydroxyapatite. Pyrophosphate is reduced in CKD patients, especially in those on dialysis. Osteoprotegerin competes with the receptor activator of NF-kB ligand (RANKL) and its receptor, RANK, on osteoclast precursor cell membranes. RANKL promotes against vascular calcification and osteoprotegerin is protective.

Refractory Hyperparathyroidism

Refractory hyperparathyroidism is severe, persistent and progressive PTH elevation that cannot be lowered to acceptable levels by medical therapy (including both vitamin D analogs and cinacalcet) without causing significant hyperphosphatemia or hypercalcemia. The level at which parathyroidectomy may be considered is varied. Some have suggested 800 pg/ml or 585 pg/ml, the latter being derived from nine times above the upper limit the normal range. The most common clinical manifestations are hypercalcemia, hyperphosphatemia, bone and joint pain and/or fractures, proximal muscle weakness, extraskeletal calcification, calciphylaxis and pruritus. Osteitis fibrosa cystica is the main cause of bone and joint pain and is primarily in weightbearing joints. The pain is relieved by rest. The common indications for parathyroidectomy are those with refractory hyperparathyroidism and significant associated clinical manifestations despite optimal management with phosphate binders, active vitamin D analogues, and calcimimetics. Extremely elevated PTH (as discussed above) with hypercalcemia, refractory hyperphosphatemia, bone pain, myopathy and pruritis may possibly benefit from parathyroidectomy. Parathyroidectomy in those with PTH greater than 1000 pg/ml without symptoms may also benefit as parathyroidectomy may confer reduced risk of mortality, cardiovascular disease and fractures, decreased erythropoietin resistance and improved nutrition. Parathyroidectomy in patients on dialysis may result in "hungry bone syndrome". Parathyroidectomy leads to functional or relative hypoparathyroidism leading to transient but often severe hypocalcemia. The relative hypoparathyroidism leads to reduced bone reabsorption and increased bone formation, leading to an increased influx of calcium into bone. Another less important factor is acute calcitonin release. Hypocalcemia is generally transient (usually lasts less than a week). When the postoperative hypocalcemia is severe and prolonged, despite normal or even elevated levels of PTH, the condition is called "hungry bone syndrome" and is seen in patients who have bone disease preoperatively due to a chronic bone resorption due to prolonged high levels of PTH (osteitis fibrosa cystica). Sudden decrease in PTH leads to an imbalance between osteoblast-mediated bone formation and osteoclast-mediated bone resorption leading to a marked net increase in bone uptake of calcium, phosphate and magnesium. Hypophosphatemia, hypomagnesemia and hyperkalemia may be seen. Typically two to four days after surgery, the serum calcium is at its lowest point. Tetany and seizures can occur. Overt heart failure may be seen in patients with cardiac dysfunction. The hypocalcemia may take up to three months to normalize. Treatment involves correction of metabolic abnormalities.

Thus, patients with CKD require evaluation and management of MBD to prevent complications. The suggested frequency of monitoring is given in Table 15.2.

Table 15.2: Suggested frequency of monitoring

eGFR (ml/min/1.73m^2)	Ca	PO_4	PTH	Vitamin D
30 – 50	6 to 12 monthly	6 to 12 monthly	12 monthly (or 6 monthly if baseline is elevated or being treated)	12 monthly (or 6 monthly if being treated)
15 – 29	3 to 6 monthly	3 to 6 monthly	6 to 12 monthly (or 6 monthly if baseline is elevated or being treated)	
< 15	1 to 3 monthly	1 to 3 monthly	3 to 6 monthly	

Suggested Reading

1. Kidney Disease: Improving Global Outcomes (KDIGO) CKD-MBD Update Work Group. KDIGO 2017 Clinical Practice Guideline Update for the Diagnosis, Evaluation, Prevention and Treatment of Chronic Kidney Disease–Mineral and Bone Disorder (CKD-MBD). Kidney Int Suppl 2017;7:1-59.
2. Block GA, Klassen PS, Lazarus JM, *et al.* Mineral metabolism, mortality and morbidity in maintenance hemodialysis. J Am Soc Nephrol 2004;15:2208-18.
3. Young EW, Albert JM, Satayathum S, *et al.* Predictors and consequences of altered mineral metabolism: The Dialysis Outcomes and Practice Patterns Study. Kidney Int 2005;67:1179-87.
4. Noordzij M, Korevaar JC, Boeschoten EW, *et al.* The Kidney Disease Outcomes Quality Initiative (K/DOQI) Guideline for Bone Metabolism and Disease in CKD: Association with mortality in dialysis patients. Am J Kidney Dis 2005;46: 925-32.
5. Slinin Y, Foley RN, Collins AJ. Calcium, phosphorus, parathyroid hormone and cardiovascular disease in hemodialysis patients: The USRDS waves 1, 3 and 4 study. J Am Soc Nephrol 2005;16:1788-93.

CHAPTER

16 An End Stage Renal Disease Patient with Multiple Vascular Access Failures

Gaurav Sagar[1], Sanjiv Jasuja[2]

[1] *Senior Consultant, Interventional Nephrologist, Indraprastha Apollo Hospital, New Delhi*

[2] *Senior Consultant, Nephrologist, Indraprastha Apollo Hospital, New Delhi*

Hemodialysis (HD) remains the most common modality of dialysis therapy for end stage renal disease (ESRD) treatment worldwide.[1] The advances in technology and improved process of care have led to longer survival of patients on dialysis. Longevity on dialysis is dependent on multiple factors, of which a good functional vascular access (VA) remains in the forefront. Increasing dialysis patient longevity, repeated punctures of dialysis access, multiple comorbidities, suboptimal blood vessel anatomy, procoagulant states, changing blood rheology, persistently activated endothelial architecture and exhausted conventional access sites often poses difficulties in creating a suitable upper extremity arteriovenous access. VA is the lifeline of a dialysis patient. In dialysis patients, VA dysfunction contributes to 25-30% annual admissions, contributing significantly to mortality and morbidity as shown in multiple studies.[2]

How to Define Multiple Vascular Access Failure?

Despite increasing prevalence of HD, for the patients with complex access issue, there remains no consensus on the definition of vascular access (VA) failure or end stage VA or end of road for conventional VA. In this chapter we have considered VA failure or end stage VA when standard upper limb option becomes non-viable. At any point of time in a HD unit, there would be 10-15% patients with problematic VA or multiple VA failures in serious cases.

Management of the patients with multiple VA failures can be challenging and may require a multi-disciplinary approach. These patients with multiple VA failures can't be managed with any pre-defined protocol, rather the treatment approach has to be customized and tailored based on patient's need. The author has presented few case scenarios with personal experience in the management of this difficult subset of patient.

CASE 1

A 62 years old female with Type 2 diabetes mellitus, diabetic kidney disease (DKD), ESRD was initiated on maintenance HD through an Internal Jugular (IJ) dialysis catheter. She was obese with very thin and deep venous vasculature on duplex mapping. An attempted brachiocephalic arteriovenous fistula (AVF) in the left upper limb stopped flowing a day after it was made. A forearm loop graft was created in the right upper limb which became dysfunctional due to thrombosis after 4 weeks. Work up for hypercoagulable state was non-contributory, which is often the case in most of such patients. These patients generally have stiff atherosclerotic arteries with poor inflows. The patient was continued on HD through an IJ dialysis catheter and was switched to Continuous Ambulatory Peritoneal Dialysis (CAPD). CAPD is therefore an appropriate choice of renal replacement therapy (RRT) modality in patients with multiple vascular access failures.

CASE 2

A 38 years old male patient on CAPD since last 3 years presented to the hospital with high grade fever, pain abdomen and purulent peritoneal effluent. He had history of multiple VA failures and on examination features of central venous stenosis, prominent collaterals on the anterior chest wall and suffused face were recorded. Because of fungal peritonitis, CAPD catheter was removed and HD was initiated. Doppler evaluation revealed bilateral obliterated internal jugular, subclavian and left femoral vein. He was dialyzed through the right femoral vein but this had to be preserved for future kidney transplant. The peripheral angiogram and central CT angiography showed obliteration of the Superior Vena Cava (SVC) with prominent mediastinal collaterals draining from head and neck region into Inferior Vena Cava (IVC). This collateral was used for placement of tunneled HD catheter through which he received dialysis for next 3 months before receiving kidney.

CASE 3

A 42 years old female patient known case of ADPKD and on maintenance HD presented with a thrombosed AV

Graft. On examination she had features of central venous stenosis and history of multiple VA failures in both upper limbs. CT-Angiography confirmed total occlusion of the SVC, bilateral brachiocephalic, subclavian and internal jugular veins with prominent collateralization. The patient was not willing for CAPD because of bulky polycystic kidneys. Option of an AV access in the lower limb was discussed which she denied.

A prosthetic axillary subclavian arterial loop graft was created around breast. There was a risk of distal ischemia but fortunately there was no such occurrence. She received dialysis through this access for 9 months before she succumbed due to a cardiac event. Thus, Necklace grafts are saviors in such patients with multiple access failures.

CASE 4

A 58 years old female patient was being worked up for kidney transplant; she had a history of multiple VA failures. Presently she was getting HD through a right IJ tunneled dialysis catheter. She presented to the hospital with poor flow in the catheter. She had received intracatheter r-TPA instillations multiple times in previous sessions of HD. The peripheral angiogram (PAG) revealed obliteration of the Superior Vena Cava (SVC) and the catheter's tip in the Azygos vein.The Azygos vein had good diameter, we decided to "push in" a longer cuffed tunnel catheter over a stiff guidewire into the Azygos vein and good flows were achieved. She could get HD through this tunneled dialysis catheter for next two months before she got a kidney transplant.

CASE 5

A 48 years old male patient, known case of Diabetes Mellitus since 15 years presented with multiple VA failures. A loop mid-thigh lower extremity AV Graft was done by anastomosing the PTFE loop to the mid-superficial femoral artery and vein. The patient received HD for 6 months at our facility before moving out and then turned lost to follow-up. Lower extremity permanent dialysis VA is also an option in patients with exhausted multiple accesses in the upper limb.[3] Similar to upper extremity VA options, lower extremity arteriovenous fistula remains a preferred access over arteriovenous synthetic grafts. Lack of surgical skills, fear of complications particularly distal steal/ischemia and limited involvement of the treating nephrologist in the decision making process are some of the reasons why lower extremity permanent dialysis remains an infrequently used access option (Table 16.1).

Table 16.1: Lower extremity permanent dialysis vascular access options

1.	Autogenous lower extremity AVF	a.	Femoral (superficial femoral artery)–great saphenous vein looped transposition
		b.	Femoral artery–femoral vein transposition
		c.	Posterior tibial artery Great Saphenous Vein
2.	Synthetic lower extremity AVG	a.	Upper thigh synthetic graft
		b.	Mid-thigh synthetic graft
3.	Lower extremity central venous catheter		

CASE 6

Central venous stenosis (CVS) is reason for VA failure in many cases. History of central venous catheters is the most important cause of CVS.[4] Patients with CVS presents with upper limb and facial edema, pleural effusions, inability to tolerate ultrafiltration during HD along with prominent collaterals on the anterior chest wall. Pleural effusion, subarachnoid hemorrhage with myoclonic seizures, unilateral high pressure glaucoma, unilateral conduction hearing loss, cerebral infarct and bleeding oesophageal varices could be additional complication.

A 70 years old female patient on maintenance HD for last 12 years presented to the hospital with poor flows in the right IJ dialysis catheter and possible central venous stenosis. All options of VA were exhausted in bilateral upper limbs. Peripheral angiogram was performed for further investigations, which revealed a long segment stenosis of the Superior Vena Cava. To manage the same, the tunneled dialysis catheter was dissected out and subsequently angioplasty and stenting of the stenotic lesion was performed. A fresh catheter was inserted through the stent to continue the HD.Thus the management of CVS many a times provides an opportunity to create a vascular access in these patients.

CASE 7

A 24 years old female patient with 7 years of kidney transplant presented to the hospital with ESRD, severe paraparesis and inability to walk. She was initiated on HD through a left radiocephalic AVF a month ago. The patient also had left pleural effusion, uncontrolled blood pressure and breathlessness on minimal exertion. Neurological workup towards diagnosis of paraparesis was non-contributory, while CT angiography of upper limb veins revealed complete obliteration of left brachiocephalic vein with prominent collaterals. CT findings were confirmed by conventional angiography. The attempt for left brachiocephalic vein angioplasty got failed as the wire could not be crossed across the lesion. Since right brachiocephalic vein also had smaller caliber, it was decided to do plasty and stenting of right subclavian vein. The left radio-cephalic AVF was surgically closed and a right brachiocephalic AVF was constructed. Meanwhile HD was continued through a right femoral sheath. Her chest X-ray was found normal after four days of procedure and she secured independent walking over next 2 weeks. Reason for paraparesis could probably have been due to central venous stenosis in prominent vertebral venous channels. This case is discussed to demonstrate the varied clinical presentations of central venous stenosis.

Innovative Technique–HeRO Graft

In patients with CVS Hemodialysis Reliable Outflow (HeRO) graft is an innovative option.[5] The HeRO Graft is a fully subcutaneous vascular access system that bypasses the central venous system to provide reliable, continuous blood flow directly from a target artery to the heart. HeRO Graft is classified by the FDA as a graft but differs from a conventional AV graft since it has no venous anastomosis. The HeRO Graft Arterial Graft Component has a 6 mm inner diameter (ID), 7.4 mm outer diameter (OD), and is 53 cm long, inclusive of the connector. It consists of an ePTFE hemodialysis graft with PTFE beading to provide kink resistance near the proprietary titanium connector. The titanium connector attaches the Arterial Graft Component to the Venous Outflow Component.The Arterial Graft Component is cannulated using standard technique according to KDOQI guidelines.

Translumbar and Transhepatic tunneled hemodialysis catheter are other access options for patients with multiple VA failures.[6]

To conclude, managing a patient with multiple VA failures is a challenging clinical situation. It involves a multi-disciplinary approach with active participation of the treating nephrologist and surgical skills. Managing such complex situation is always an expensive affair adding to the cost of treatment.

References

1. US Renal Data System: USRDS 2013 Annual Data Report: Atlas of End Stage Renal Disease in the United States, National Institutes of Health, National Institute of Diabetes and Digestive and Kidney Diseases, Bethesda, MD, 2013.
2. Mortality and hospitalization in hemodialysis patients in 52 European countries: Results from the Dialysis Outcomes and Practice Patterns Study (DOPPS), Nephrol Dial Transplant 2004;19:108-20.
3. Vishal B Parekh, Vandana D Niyyar and Tushar J. Vachharajani Lower Extremity Permanent Dialysis Vascular Access CJASN September 07,2016;11:(9) 1693-702.
4. Agarwal AK, Patel BM, Haddad NJ. Central vein stenosis: A nephrologist's perspective. Semin Dial 2007;20:53.
5. Modified use of the Hemodialysis Reliable Outflow (HeRO) graft for salvage of threatened dialysis access, Bassan J Allan, Angela T Prescott, Marwan Tabbara, Arash Bornak, Lee J Goldstein, Journal of Vascular Surgery,Volume 56, Issue 4, October 2012;1127-29.
6. Mohamed El Gharib, Gamal Niazi, Waleed Hetta, Yahya Makkeyah. Transhepatic venous catheters for hemodialysis, The Egyptian Journal of Radiology and Nuclear Medicine, Volume 45, Issue 2, 2014;431-38.

CHAPTER 17

An Adult End Stage Renal Disease Patient with Peritoneal Dialysis (PD) Peritonitis

Manish Jain[1], Dhawal Khetia[2]

[1] *Director, Nephrology, Medanta, The Medicity, Gurugram*

[2] *Consultant, Nephrology, Bankers Heart Hospital, Vadodara*

CASE

Mr XYZ is a 48-year-old patient with Type 2 diabetes mellitus, hypertension since 10 years and chronic kidney disease stage 5 since 2 years on continuous ambulatory peritoneal dialysis (CAPD). He is using a 7.5% icodextrin solution 2 liters for his night dwell (10-12 hours) and three 1.5% dextrose solutions during day time (dwell time 4 hours each). With this prescription he had ultrafiltration of around 1.5 liters/24 hours. His urine output is around 500 ml in 24 hours. There was no history of peritonitis or exit site or tunnel infection till date.

Patient presented with following complaints – turbid effluent fluid and abdominal pain since 3 days and fever since 2 days.

Considering the above clinical picture of possible peritoneal dialysis (PD) related peritonitis, his peritoneal fluid examination was done – fluid was turbid. PD fluid cytology revealed cell count of 550 cells/micro liter with 70% polymorphonuclear (PMN) cells. Culture of PD fluid was sent and he was started on intra peritoneal Injection Vancomycin 1 gram in 6 hours day time dwell every 5th day and Injection Ceftazidime 2 grams in 6 hours day time dwell daily.

His symptoms improved within 2 days, PD fluid cleared and repeat cytology on day 3 was suggestive of 30 cells/hpf with 50% PMNs.

This patient on CAPD developed peritonitis. Approach to such a patient will be discussed.

What are the Measures to Prevent PD Peritonitis?

Hand hygiene while performing PD exchanges is extremely important. Keeping the exit site clean and applying Mupirocin or gentamycin ointment reduces exit site infection rates. Prompt treatment of episodes of exit site infection reduces peritonitis rates.

What are the Risk Factors for PD Peritonitis?

The following are risk factors for developing PD peritonitis:

- Social–Smoking, Living distantly from PD unit, Pets.
- Medical–Obesity, Depression, Hypokalemia, Hypoalbuminemia.
- Invasive interventions–Colonoscopy or gynecological intervention.
- Dialysis related–Prior hemodialysis, PD against patient's choice, Contamination of PD fluid.
- Infection related–Previous exit site infection, Nasal staphylococcal carrier state.

What are the Symptoms of PD Peritonitis?

PD peritonitis commonly presents with abdominal pain, turbid PD effluent fluid and fever. Patient may have associated exit site infection (discharge or redness at exit site). Ultrafiltration volume reduces as more fluid get reabsorbed due to inflamed peritoneal surfaces. Patient with severe peritonitis may present with features of septic shock.

On examination, patient have generalized abdominal tenderness, and occasionally rebound tenderness may be present. On gross examination, PD fluid appears turbid, and a newspaper kept under PD bag cannot be read clearly – a bedside test for turbidity of PD fluid.

As Per ISPD Guidelines, How Peritonitis is Diagnosed?

Peritonitis is diagnosed when at least two of the following are present:

1. Clinical features consistent with peritonitis–abdominal pain and/or cloudy dialysis effluent.
2. Dialysis effluent WBC count >100/micro liter with more than 50% PMNs.
3. Positive dialysate effluent culture.

How a PD Fluid Sample Should be Cultured for Diagnosis of PD Peritonitis?

- Bedside inoculation of 5-10 ml of PD fluid in 2 blood culture bottles (aerobic and anerobic) has good sensitivity with culture negative rate of around 10-20%.

- Yield of culture can be increased by inoculating PD fluid directly into rapid blood culture bottle kits, centrifuging PD fluid and culturing the pellet.
- Specimen should arrive at laboratory within 6 hours of collection.
- When culture remains negative after 3-5 days of incubation, PD effluent should be sent for repeat cell count, differential count, fungal and mycobacterial culture.

What are the Differential Diagnosis of Cloudy Effluent?

- Culture positive infectious peritonitis.
- Culture negative infectious peritonitis.
- Specimen taken from dry abdomen.
- Chemical peritonitis.
- Eosinophilia of effluent.
- Calcium channel blockers.
- Hemoperitoneum.
- Malignancy.
- Chylous effluent.

What are Common Empirical Antibiotic Regimen for PD Peritonitis?

- Empirical antibiotic rēgimen should be center specific and should cover both gram positive and gram negative organisms.
- It is recommended that for gram positive organism Vancomycin or a first generation cephalosporin and for gram negative organism, third generation cephalosporin or an aminoglycoside (if anuric) should be used.
- Intraperitoneal (IP) route is preferred unless patient has features of systemic sepsis. IP vancomycin is administered intermittently once in 3 to 5 days and serum vancomycin level is kept above 15 micro gram/ml. IP aminoglycoside should be administered as daily intermittent dosing.
- In intermittent dosing, the antibiotic containing dialysis solution should dwell for at least 6 hours for adequate absorption.
- There is under dosing in APD patients as rapid exchanges in APD lead to inadequate time to achieve therapeutic levels. APD patients who develop peritonitis may be switched to CAPD temporarily.

How would you Subsequently Manage Peritonitis?

- Antibiotic therapy should be adjusted once culture results and sensitivities are known. Within 48 hours of initiating therapy, most patients show clinical improvement. Assess clinical improvement and repeat dialysis effluent cell count and cultures at days 3-5. Effluent should be visually inspected to see whether its clearing or not.
- For gram positive cocci continue IP antibiotics based on sensitivities for 2-3 weeks depending on organism, e.g., coagulase negative staphylococci for 2 weeks, S. aureus, enterococci – treat for 3 weeks.
- Gram negative bacilli treat minimum for 3 weeks. For pseudomonas or stenotrophomonas species give 2 effective antibiotics based on sensitivities for 3 to 4 weeks.

What is the Role of Heparin in Treatment of Peritonitis?

Heparin 500 units/l intra peritoneal prevents occlusion of catheter by fibrin.

Definitions of Peritonitis

Recurrent: An episode that occurs within 4 weeks of completion of therapy of a prior episode but with a different organism.

Relapsing: An episode that occurs within 4 weeks of completion of therapy of a prior episode with the same organism or one sterile episode.

Repeat: An episode that occurs more than 4 weeks after completion of therapy of a prior episode with the same organism.

Refractory: Failure of the effluent to clear after 5 days of appropriate antibiotics.

Catheter-related peritonitis: Peritonitis in conjunc-tion with an exit site or tunnel infection.

Exit-site infection(ESI): Presence of purulent discharge, with or without erythema of the skin at the catheter-epidermal interface.

Tunnel infection: Presence of clinical inflammation or ultrasonographic evidence of collection along the catheter tunnel.

What are Indications for Catheter Removal?

- Fungal peritonitis.
- Refractory peritonitis.
- Relapsing peritonitis.
- Refractory exit and tunnel site infection.
- Catheter removal also considered for:
  - Repeat peritonitis.

- Mycobacterial peritonitis.
- Multiple enteric organisms.

When can Catheter be Reinserted?

Reinsertion should be performed at least 2 to 3 weeks after catheter removal and complete resolution of peritoneal symptoms. Reinsertion of new catheter should be done by laparoscopic or mini laparotomy approach so that adhesions can be directly visualized.

Is There Any Recommendation on Catheter Design for Prevention of Peritonitis?

There is no specific recommendation on catheter design for prevention of peritonitis.

Which Connection Method is Associated with Lower Peritonitis Rate?

It is recommended to use Y connection system with flush before fill design for CAPD as this results in lower peritonitis rate than traditional spike systems.

Is There Any Recommendation on Dialysis Solutions for Prevention of Peritonitis?

There is no specific recommendation on choice of dialysis solutions for prevention of peritonitis.

Suggested Reading

1. ISPD Guidelines/Recommendations: 2016. PDI. Vol 36, 481-508.

CHAPTER 18

A Chronic Kidney Disease Stage 5D Patient on Peritoneal Dialysis with Ultrafiltration Failure

Amit Gupta[1], **Manas Ranjan Patel**[2]

[1] *Senior Consultant, Apollomedics Super Specialty Hospitals, Lucknow*

[2] *Assistant Professor, Nephrology, Sanjay Gandhi Postgraduate Institute of Medical Sciences, Lucknow*

CASE

A 45-year-male patient with diabetes and CKD stage 5 on peritoneal dialysis for past 5 years presents with progressive swelling of legs, decreasing ultrafiltration and has gained 8 kgs of weight in last 1 month. He is on 2 day exchanges with 1.5% 2L and one night exchange with 2.5% 2L bag with an ultrafiltration of 800 to 1100 ml/day with a urine output of 200 ml/day. On investigation his laboratory parameters were Hb-10.2 gm/dl, serum creatinine-5.6 mg/dl, BUN-43 mg/dl, FBS-123 mg/dl, PP-210 mg/dl, HbA1C-7.3, Na-132 meq/l, K-3.8 meq/l, Ca-8.9 mg/dl, PO 4-4.1 mg/dl. Chest X-ray PA view was normal.

Some of the important questions in such a patient are:

a. Adequate history about compliance to fluid/diet and dialysis prescription along with blood sugar control is essential before diagnosing ultrafiltration failure (UFF).

b. Exclusion of mechanical causes of catheter dysfunction and fluid leaks are prerequisites before performing a peritoneal equilibration test (PET).

c. A standard PET is more informative and is preferable than a modified PET for characterization of membrane dysfunction.

d. Poor ultrafiltration along with poor small solute clearance is the most common type of abnormality found in PET.

e. Icodextrin containing dialysate and automated peritoneal dialysis (PD) are the mainstay of treatment of most cases of UFF.

Answer: A. True, B. True, C. False, D. False, E. True.

Discussion

Fluid overload is an important clinical issue in patients on peritoneal dialysis (PD). It may be caused by high fluid intake, noncompliance, or by a low drained volume. The latter can be due to inappropriate selection of dialysate, mechanical problems of catheter or obscured leaks, or per se due to peritoneal membrane failure, i.e., ultrafiltration failure (UFF). UFF is one of a major cause of decreased ultrafiltration and/or drain volume but both are not necessarily synonymous. Ultrafiltration failure is defined as clinical evidence of fluid overload with an ultrafiltration volume <400 ml in a modified peritoneal equilibration test (PET). The modified PET using a 4.25% 2L dialysate dwell is preferable to 2.5% 2L bag used in the standard PET as it exerts maximal osmotic drive required for ultrafiltration and allows determination of sodium sieving along with small solute clearance profiles. UFF is one of a major cause of decreased ultrafiltration/drain volume but both are not necessarily synonymous. UFF should not be diagnosed unless catheter malfunction and leaks have been excluded.

Once UFF has been confirmed, the next step is to review the patient's solute transport characteristics (Fig. 18.1). There are four types of ultrafiltration failure each characterized by a different etiology and pathophysiology.

Type I Ultrafiltration Failure

High transporter with poor ultrafiltration is the most common cause and is often called Type I UFF. Dialysate dextrose concentration falls rapidly (D/P Creatinine >0.8) resulting in loss of the concentration gradient but small solute remains unaffected. It is caused by increase in the effective peritoneal surface area due to increased membrane vascularity, can also occur transiently during and after peritonitis. This can be either late acquired or early inherent. Late phenotype usually develops after a long duration of PD, typically 3 years or more and is due to increase in the effective surface area secondary to an increased vascularity. They have high mass transfer area of coefficients and normal lymphatic flow rates. Uremia, high glucose load, exposure to Glucose degradation products (GDPs), Advanced Glycosylated End Products (AGEs) and low pH of dialysate fluid; and recurrent peritonitis result in the production of various proinflammatory and angiogenic mediators

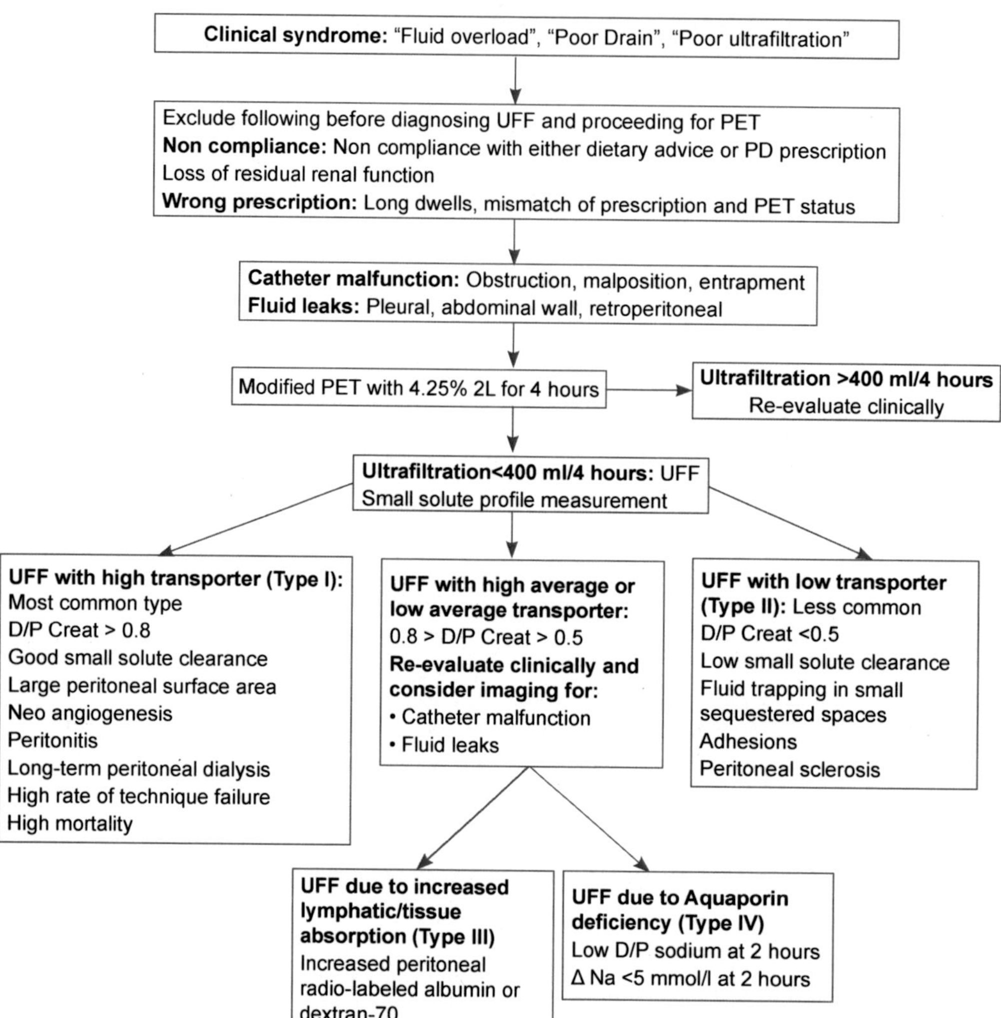

Figure 18.1: Diagnostic approach of volume overload and ultrafiltration failure
UFF: Ultrafiltration failure; PET: Peritoneal equilibration test.

including various cytokines, endothelial nitric oxide synthase (eNOS), and various growth factors and vascular endothelial growth factor (VEGF).Treatment of this form of ultrafiltration failure is difficult. Peritoneal resting, i.e., cessation of peritoneal dialysis for a period of 4-8 weeks has been occasionally successful in restoring ultrafiltration capacity, which remains sustained for few years thereafter. Patients using a single daily exchange of icodextrin exhibited no change in D/P creatinine and no loss of ultrafiltration capacity over two years, hence is usually recommended for treatment of this type of UFF. Recent evidence suggests use of neutral pH low GDP fluids may be beneficial but the evidence is inconclusive. Early inherent phenotype can be either due to systemic inflammation (i.e., increased CRP and IL-6 in serum and PD effluent) or increased surface area (increased CA125 in PD effluent). Early inherent type usually doesn't respond to peritoneal membrane resting and has poor prognosis.

Type II Ultrafiltration Failure

Low transporters with UFF have reduced small solute clearance with normal to reduced glucose absorption profile. This is also called Type II UFF and is less common. It reflects decreased membrane surface area and is due to adhesions and scarring after sclerosing peritonitis or other intra-abdominal complications. It is caused by TGF-β causing epithelial mesenchymal transition (EMT), sub-mesothelial fibrosis and obliterative vasculopathy. More severe phenotype is encapsulating peritoneal sclerosis (EPS), characterized by the symptoms of bowel obstruction with extensive adhesion by hypertrophied and calcified peritoneum. Though, rare is seen mostly after 8 years of peritoneal dialysis. Moderate sclerosis of peritoneum results in diminution in transport but in more severe form, this may lead to bowel obstruction caused by adhesions of a diffusely hypertrophied and often calcified peritoneum. Generally, peritoneal dialysis should be discontinued in patients with EPS and surgical enterolysis may be considered.

UFF with transport in the normal range (usually high average or low average) is usually unrelated to membrane, thus imaging to exclude obscure leaks and catheter malfunction should be considered actively.True UFF with normal transport characteristics can rarely

Table 18.1: General and cause specific management strategies of fluid overload and UFF

Cause	Possible management
Noncompliance with salt and water restriction Poor blood glucose control Noncompliance with PD prescription	Dietary counseling Hyperglycemia control Enhanced compliance-Education
Loss of residual renal function	Protection of RRF by ACEI or ARB Loop diuretics if RRF is present Avoidance of nephrotoxic drugs and contrast agents
Inappropriate PD prescription for patient PET status Long dwells with dextrose dialysate	Routine standardized monitoring and tailoring prescription to transport profile determined by PET
Catheter malfunction: Obstruction, malposition, entrapment	Identification by imaging including peritoneography Heparin for fibrin clots Omentectomy, reinsertion of catheter
Abdominal or retroperitoneal leaks	Identification by imaging including peritoneography Repair of defects Plurodesis
Peritoneal membrane dysfunction	Preservation of peritoneal membrane function Reduction in episodes of peritonitis Avoidance of high dextrose concentration PD fluid Biocompatible PD solutions
High transport status (Type I UFF)	Shorter dwells of dextrose dialysate Automated PD Icodextrin for long dwells Two icodextrin exchanges in 24 hours period Treatment of peritonitis
Loss of functional peritoneum (Type II UFF)	Loop diuretics and adjunctive hemodialysis if good residual renal function Transfer to hemodialysis if no residual renal function Peritoneography and adhesiolysis if indicated
Aquaporin deficiency (Type IV UFF)	Icodextrin for long dwells Avoid higher dextrose concentration
Exaggerated lymphatic/tissue reabsorption (Type III UFF)	Shorter dwells Avoid large dwell volumes Higher dextrose concentration

be seen in two conditions, i.e., in increased lymphatic absorption of peritoneal fluid and in aquaporin channel deficiency.

Type III Ultrafiltration Failure

Increased lymphatic absorption of peritoneal fluid called Type III UFF. It can be quantified by measuring the disappearance rate of radio-labeled albumin or dextran-70 from the peritoneal cavity. Failure to achieve desired ultrafiltration with icodextrin is the usual clinical scenario in this type of UFF, as icodextrin is reabsorbed through lymphatics. Though rare, these patients have poor prognosis and are usually managed by permanent shifting to hemodialysis or renal transplant.

Type IV Ultrafiltration Failure

The transcapillary movement of free water via aquaporin channels accounts for 40-50% of total ultrafiltration.The hallmark of this type of UFF is attenuation of sodium sieving, i.e., dampening of the decrease in dialysate sodium during the first hour of a dwell. Studies indicate this condition is probably due to a functional defect rather than a quantitative decrease in aquaporin numbers as an investigational agent has increased activity of these channels in experimental models. Aquaporin deficiency related UFF is suggested when the difference between the sodium level of the 4.25% and 1.5% dextrose dwell samples taken at 60 minutes is <5 mmol/l. Aquaporin transport water but not sodium (sodium sieving), responsible for initial fall in dialysate sodium by 5-10 mmol/l with 4.25% dextrose dwell, that doesn't occurs in aquaporin deficiency. Free water clearance is less than 26% of total ultrafiltration is consistent with AQP-1 dysfunction can be diagnosed with mini-PET.

Summary of general and cause specific management strategies are given in Table 18.1. Overall, patients with UFF on continuous ambulatory peritoneal dialysis may do well with use of icodextrin and/or by switching to automated peritoneal dialysis (APD).

Suggested Reading

1. Gokal R, Khanna R, Krediet RT and Nolph KD (Eds.). (2013). Textbook of peritoneal dialysis. Springer Science and Business Media.
2. Daugirdas JT, Blake PG and Ing TS (2012). Handbook of dialysis. Lippincott Williams and Wilkins.

CHAPTER

19

A Chronic Kidney Disease Patient Due to Diabetic Nephropathy

Mohit Madken[1], Vijay Kher[2]

[1] *Fellow, Nephrology, The Ottawa Hospital, Canada*

[2] *Chairman, Institute of Nephrlogy and Urology, Medanta, The Medicity, Gurugram*

CASE

55-year-old male Mr AB with Type 2 diabetes mellitus (DM) presented with history of easy fatigability and progressive bilateral lower limb swelling since 3 months. On examination blood pressure (BP) is 150/100 mm Hg. On physical examination there is pallor and bilateral lower limb pedal edema. Fundus examination shows evidence of proliferative diabetic retinopathy with otherwise unremarkable systemic examination. He is obese with BMI of 30 kg/m^2.

He was diagnosed to be diabetic 10 years back. Initially his renal functions were normal with serum creatinine of 0.7 mg/dl and he was told to have microalbuminuria with urine albumin-creatinine ratio (UACR) of 200 mg/gram. He was followed up by the physician annually and after 5 years he was told to have renal impairment with serum creatinine of 1.3 mg/dl with an UACR of 500 mg/gram. His blood pressure was uncontrolled at this time and was started on telmisartan 40 mg once a day.

He gives history of tingling and numbness over extremities. He also underwent laser of left eye for diabetic retinopathy 2 years back.

His renal functions deteriorated gradually and his serum creatinine was 2.5 mg/dl two years back. Telmisartan was stopped by the physician in view of hyperkalemia.

Current laboratory values include the following: Hemoglobin-10.1 gm/dl, serum creatinine 4.9 mg/dl; potassium 4.7 mEq/l, albumin-creatinine ratio 750 mg/g; and glycated hemoglobin (HbA1c), 8.1%. Urine sediment is otherwise bland.

He is presently using regular insulin for diabetes. His antihypertensives include metoprolol and amlodipine.

This case describes natural progression of chronic kidney disease (CKD) in a patient with diabetic nephropathy.

Diabetic Nephropathy

Diabetes mellitus is a growing epidemic and is the single most common cause of end stage renal disease (ESRD) worldwide with diabetic patients accounting for 25% to 45% of all patients enrolled in ESRD programs.[1]

Diabetic nephropathy (DN) develops in 15% to 35% of patients with diabetes. Early identification and management are critical to prevent development and slowing progression of diabetic nephropathy.

Classically, diabetic nephropathy, as a syndrome, has been defined as:

- Persistent albuminuria (>300 mg/d or >200 μg/min) confirmed on at least 2 occasions 3-6 months apart.
- Progressive decline in the glomerular filtration rate (GFR).
- Hypertension.

Following additional criteria required for diagnosis include–presence of diabetic retinopathy and absence of clinical or laboratory evidence of other kidney or urinary tract disease.

Natural History of Disease

Natural history of diabetic nephropathy has been classically described with Type 1 Diabetes Mellitus and is less defined in Type 2 Diabetes Mellitus as onset of the disease is not apparent. Diabetic nephropathy evolves through different phases such as phase of glomerular hyperfiltration, incipient nephropathy characterized by microalbuminuria, overt nephropathy characterized by macroalbuminuria and end stage renal disease characterized by decrease in GFR to less than 15 ml/min.

There are five stages in the development of diabetic nephropathy:

- **Stage 1** is characterized by hyperfunction and hypertrophy that are present at the time of diagnosis of diabetes. In this stage, GFR is either normal or increased. The size of the kidneys is increased by approximately 20% and renal plasma flow is increased by 10%-15%, while albuminuria and blood pressure remain within the normal range. Changes are at least partly reversible by intensive glycemic control.

- **Stage 2** develops silently over many years and is characterized by morphologic lesions without signs of clinical disease. This stage is characterized by basement membrane thickening and mesangial proliferation. There are still no clinical signs of the disease.
- **Stage 3** incipient diabetic nephropathy, is the forerunner of overt diabetic nephropathy. Patients develop microalbuminuria (albumin 30-300 mg/day) and is the first clinically detectable sign of glomerular damage. It usually occurs five to ten years after the onset of the disease. Blood pressure may be increased or normal. Approximately 40% of patients reach this stage.
- **Stage 4** is overt diabetic nephropathy, the classic entity characterized by persistent proteinuria (>0.5 g/24 h). When the associated high blood pressure is left untreated, renal function (GFR) declines, the mean fall rate being around 1 ml/min/month.
- **Stage 5** is end stage renal disease with uremia due to diabetic nephropathy (Fig. 19.1).

Risk Factors

Genetic susceptibility: Likelihood of developing diabetic nephropathy is markedly increased in patients with a diabetic sibling or parent who has diabetic nephropathy.

There is a 14% probability for a child of the parents without proteinuria to develop clinical proteinuria, 23% probability in cases where one of the parents has proteinuria, and 46% probability in case that both parents have proteinuria. This increased risk cannot be explained by the duration of DM, increased blood pressure or glycemic regulation.

Blood pressure: There is association between the development of diabetic nephropathy and higher systemic blood pressure.

Glycemic control: Diabetic nephropathy is more likely to develop in patients with poor glycemic control. The importance of tight glycemic control for protection against microvascular and cardiovascular disease in diabetes was established in the Diabetes Control and Complications Trial (DCCT) study for Type 1 diabetes and in the United Kingdom Prospective Diabetes Study (UKPDS) in Type 2 diabetes.

Race: The incidence and severity of diabetic nephropathy are increased in blacks (3- to 6-fold compared to Caucasians), Mexican-Americans and Pima Indians with Type 2 diabetes.

Obesity: High body mass index (BMI) has been associated with an increased risk of chronic kidney disease among patients with diabetes. In addition, diet and weight loss may reduce albuminuria and improve kidney function among patients with diabetes.

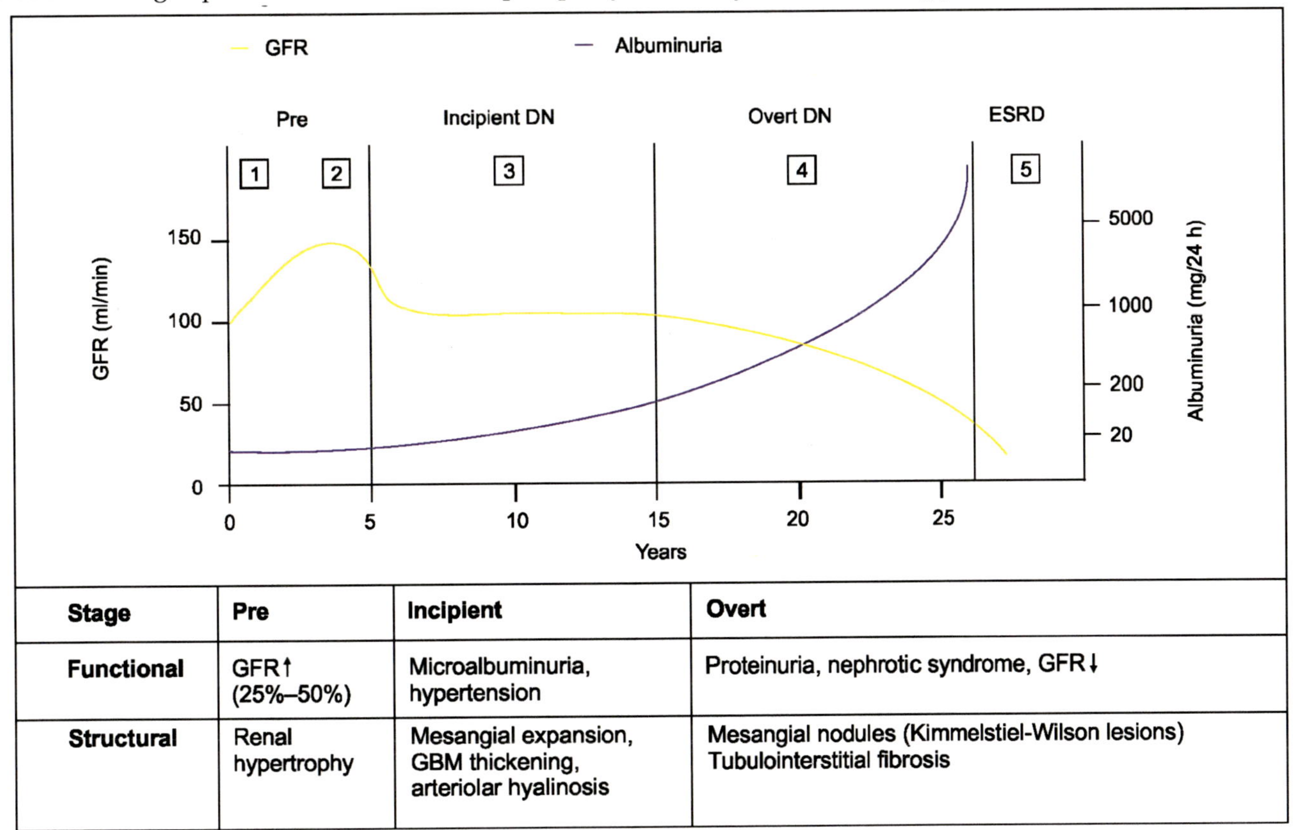

Stage	Pre	Incipient	Overt
Functional	GFR↑ (25%–50%)	Microalbuminuria, hypertension	Proteinuria, nephrotic syndrome, GFR↓
Structural	Renal hypertrophy	Mesangial expansion, GBM thickening, arteriolar hyalinosis	Mesangial nodules (Kimmelstiel-Wilson lesions) Tubulointerstitial fibrosis

Figure 19.1: Natural history of diabetic nephropathy in type 1 diabetes mellitus
ESRD: End stage renal disease; DN: Diabetic nephropathy; GFR: Glomerular filtration rate.

Smoking: Smoking is associated with a variety of adverse effects in patients with diabetes. This includes evidence of increases in albuminuria and the risk of end-stage renal disease and of decreased survival once dialysis is begun.

Relation Between Diabetic Nephropathy and Retinopathy

Patients with nephropathy and Type 1 diabetes almost always have other signs of diabetic microvascular disease, such as retinopathy and neuropathy. The retinopathy typically precedes the onset of overt nephropathy in these patients.

The relationship between diabetic nephropathy and retinopathy is less predictable in Type 2 diabetes and 50% to 60% of proteinuric Type 2 diabetic patients have retinopathy. The absence of retinopathy should prompt further investigation for non diabetic glomerulopathies.[2]

Screening and Diagnosis

- Blood glycemic profile: Fasting and Postprandial blood sugars or Glucose tolerance test (GTT) and a HbA1c.
- Urine albumin excretion annually in Type 1 Diabetes Mellitus of >5 years and in Type 2 Diabetes Mellitus from the time of diagnosis.
- Serum creatinine and estimation of GFR annually in all diabetic patients regardless of albuminuria (Table 19.1).
- Urinalysis with urine microscopy.
- Ophthalmological evaluation: Fundus for evidence of diabetic retinopathy.
- A renal USG/doppler to look for bilateral kidney size, echogenicity and patency of the renal arteries.
- Measurement of blood pressure.

Non-Diabetic Renal Disease

Proteinuria and/or hematuria in diabetes mellitus is occasionally due to a glomerular disease other than diabetic nephropathy.

Studies[3] have evaluated most common causes of non-diabetic kidney disease were focal segmental glomerulosclerosis (FSGS) (22%), hypertensive nephrosclerosis (18%), acute tubular necrosis (17%), IgA nephropathy (11%), membranous nephropathy (8%), and pauci-immune glomerulonephritis (7%).

Major clinical clues suggesting the presence of nondiabetic glomerular disease necessitating kidney biopsy are:

1. Absence of diabetic retinopathy.
2. Sudden and rapid onset of nephrotic range proteinuria.
3. Duration of diabetes mellitus (in Type 1 – less than 5 years).
4. Atypical progression, without transition through the usual stages – for e.g., development of nephrotic syndrome without previous microalbuminuria.
5. Macroscopic hematuria or active nephritic sediment – numerous RBCs, many dysmorphic red cells or red cell casts or acanthocytes.
6. Rapid decline in renal function (usual decline in diabetic nephropathy is 0.5-1.5 ml/min/1.73 sq.m./month).
7. Renal dysfunction in presence of systemic disease.

Clinical Features

- There are no specific clinical features of nephropathy in its early stages. In people with Type 1 diabetes a rise in blood pressure is a subtle sign but usually accompanies an increase in albuminuria.
- The clinical features of established nephropathy are often dictated by concomitant microvascular (retinopathy and neuropathy) or macrovascular complications (disease in the coronary, cerebral or peripheral vasculature). The majority of people entering end-stage renal disease due to diabetic nephropathy will have evidence of microvascular or macrovascular complications of diabetes.
- Blindness due to severe proliferative retinopathy or maculopathy is approximately five times more frequent in Types 1 and 2 diabetic patients with nephropathy than in normoalbuminuric patients. Peripheral neuropathy is present in almost all patients with advanced nephropathy.

Table 19.1: Urinary albumin excretion in different stages of diabetic nephropathy

	Normal	Stage of microalbuminuria (Incipient nephropathy)	Stage of macroalbuminuria (Overt nephropathy)
Albumin creatinine ratio (ACR) – Spot (mcg/mg creatinine)	<30	30-299	≥300
24 hours urinary albumin excretion (mg/day)	<30	30-299	≥300
Timed collection (mcg/min)	<20	20-199	≥200

- Foot ulcers with sepsis leading to amputation occurs frequently due to a combination of neuropathy and peripheral vascular disease in diabetic patients.
- Macrovascular complications like stroke, coronary artery disease, and peripheral vascular disease are two to five times more common in patients with diabetic nephropathy.
- Autonomic neuropathy, diabetic cystopathy and recurrent urinary tract infections (UTIs) are other complications commonly encountered in patients with diabetic nephropathy.
- Anemia due to erythropoietin deficiency is more common and occurs earlier in people with diabetic nephropathy compared with those with non-diabetic kidney disease. Symptoms of uremia such as nausea, anorexia, pruritus, tiredness and weight loss develop in advanced CKD. The occurrence of these symptoms suggest need for renal replacement therapy (RRT).
- Even the asymptomatic diabetic patient with CKD must be monitored at regular intervals for timely detection of microvascular and macrovascular complications.

Prevention of Diabetic Nephropathy

The natural history of diabetic nephropathy has prolonged course so appropriate measures can be taken to prevent development or to slow the progression of diabetic nephropathy.

Life Style Modification

All diabetic patients should undergo life style modification to lower risk of progression as well as cardiovascular disease. The measures include:

- Dietary restriction of salt and saturated fats.
- Weight reduction.
- Exercise.
- Smoking cessation.

Glycemic Control

One keystone in the prevention and management of diabetic nephropathy is tight glycemic control.

- Poor glycemic control is a risk factor for both the development of microalbuminuria and for progression to macroalbuminuria in patients with Type 2 diabetes.
- In the Diabetes Control and Complications Trial (DCCT),[4] intensive glycemic control reduced the incidence of microalbuminuria by 39% and macroalbuminuria by 56%, and the benefits persisted in the follow-up study known as the Epidemiology of Diabetes Interventions Complications trial (EDIC).[5] Comprehensive prospective data also link glycemic control to diabetic nephropathy in T2DM. In the UKPDS,[6] the intensively treated group showed a 30% risk reduction for the development of microalbuminuria.The Kumamoto study,[7] albeit a much smaller study than the UKPDS, also demonstrated that intensive glycemic control reduced the rate of microalbuminuria and macroalbuminuria.
- Based on available evidence (Table 19.2),[8] a goal HbA1c concentration of 7.0% to reduce microvascular complications and diabetic nephropathy progression is advised. Further reduction of HbA1c is of unproven benefit and would likely put the patient at risk for hypoglycemic events. This is congruent with current American Diabetes Association and KDOQI clinical practice guidelines.
- Target HbA1c should be extended above 7.0% in individuals with comorbidities or limited life expectancy and risk of hypoglycemia.
- Thirty percent to 45% of insulin is metabolized and cleared by the kidneys. Therefore, as kidney function decreases, insulin lasts longer, putting patients at risk for hypoglycemic episodes.
- Additionally, most oral hypoglycemic medications are metabolized and cleared by the kidney. Thus, doses of these agents and insulin must often be reduced as kidney function decreases. Additionally, if hypoglycemia occurs, it may last for a prolonged period that may necessitate hospitalization for observation.
- Metformin is contraindicated in patients with eGFRs< 30 ml/min/1.73 m^2 due to its association with severe lactic acidosis in these patients.
- SGLT2 inhibitors, have demonstrated cardiovascular disease benefit. Their mechanism of action is to block glucose and sodium uptake in the proximal tubule, thereby generating natriuresis and glucosuria.
- Recently, 2 studies, designed as cardiovascular safety studies, EMPA-REG Outcome (Empagliflozin, Cardiovascular Outcomes, and Mortality in Type 2 Diabetes)[9] and CANVAS (Canagliflozin Cardiovascular Assessment Study)[10] have demonstrated significant cardiovascular risk reduction when used for the treatment of diabetes. In these cardiovascular outcome trials, the SGLT2 inhibitors had positive effects on kidney outcomes, namely albuminuria reduction and a reduction in the occurrence of a composite renal outcome.
- SGLT2 inhibitors are contraindicated in patients with eGFR< 45 ml/min/1.73 m^2 and must be used at lower doses at eGFR of 45-60 ml/min/1.73 m^2.
- **Sulfonylureas:** Shorter acting drugs, especially those metabolized in the liver (glipizide and glimepiride) are relatively safe and preferred in patients with CKD.

Table 19.2: Glycemic control studies in patient with diabetes mellitus

Trial	Population	N	Intervention Target	Achieved Interven-tion	Findings in Intensive Care Group	Comments
DCCT	T1DM	1,441	Intensive therapy targeting fasting and postprandial blood glucose vs conventional therapy	HbA1c 7.3% vs 9.1%	Decreased microvascular complications (including microalbuminuria, proteinuria, retinopathy and neuropathy)	
EDIC	T1DM	1,375 patients that completed DCCT	Observational follow-up of DCCT with all getting intensive therapy	HbA1c 7.8% vs 7.9%	Reduction in microalbuminuria and proteinuria	
UKPDS	Newly Diagnosed T2DM	3,867	Intensive therapy targeting a fasting blood glucose vs conventional therapy	HbA1c 7% vs 7.9%	Reduction in any diabetes-related end point in aggregate	Reduction not seen in kidney-specific events (microabuminuria, proteinuria, or doubling of SCr)
ACCORD	T2DM and CV event history or risk	10,251	HbA1c < 6.0% vs 7%-7.9%	HbA1c 6.4% vs 7.5%	Increased CV and total mortality	No benefit on kidney end points
ADVANCE	T2DM and CV event history or risk	11,140	HbA1c < 6.5% vs routine care	HbA1c 6.3% vs 7.0%	No benefit on CV outcomes; reduction in microvascular events	Albuminuria reduced by 21%
VADT	T2DM and poor BP control	1,791	Reduction in HbA1c of 1.5% vs routine care	HbA1c 6.9% vs 8.4%	No benefit	No benefit on kidney end points

- **Thiazolidinediones:** All thiazolidinediones cause fluid retention that may lead to heart failure, a problem especially pertinent to patients with CKD. Their use also is associated with increased risk of fractures making them less preferable drug in CKD.
- **DPP-4 Inhibitors:** Sitagliptin, saxagliptin, alogliptin and linagliptin are the drugs in this class. These drugs becoming more popular in patients with CKD because of their better tolerability and low risk of hypoglycemia. Sitagliptin and saxagliptin need dose adjustment for reduced eGFR. Linagliptin can be safely given in all stages of CKD as it is not metabolized by the kidney.
- **GLP-1 Receptor Agonists:** Exenatide undergoes renal excretion and is not approved for patients with eGFRs <30 ml/min/1.73 m^2.
- **α-Glucosidase Inhibitors:** Their main limitation is frequent dosing and gastrointestinal side effects, mainly flatulence. These drugs are contraindicated in patients with serum creatinine levels >2 mg/dl due to the risk of accumulation that may cause liver failure.

Blood Pressure Control

- Blocking the Renin–Angiotensin–Aldosterone (RAS) pathway has proved to be the single most effective therapy for slowing the progression of diabetic nephropathy especially if started early in the course of the disease.
- The initial mechanism in development of diabetic nephropathy is renal hypertrophy, hyperfunction and glomerular hyperfiltration. This results from intraglomerular hypertension due to Angiotensin-II induced vasoconstriction of efferent arteriole. So the blockade of Angiotensin-II with Angiotensin receptor blockers (ARB) or Angiotensin converting enzyme (ACE) inhibitors helps in prevention of onset of microalbiminuria.
- In diabetic patients with established nephropathy, RAS blockade with ACE inhibitors or ARBs confers preferential renoprotection that is independent of BP reduction. Intraglomerular hemodynamic and nonhemodynamic renal effects of angiotensin II (Ang II) best explain the observed renoprotection.

- Data from randomized clinical trials testing an intervention in patients with T2DM, IDNT (Irbesartan Diabetic Nephropathy Trial),[11] IRMA-2 (Effect of Irbesartan in the Development of Diabetic Nephropathy in Patients with T2DM)[12] and the RENAAL[13] (Reduction in End-Points in Non-Insulin Dependent Diabetes Mellitus with the Angiotensin II Antagonist Losartan) 11 trial are known for demonstrating the benefit of angiotensin receptor blockers (ARBs) to delay the progression of kidney disease.
- The effect of achieved BPs was analyzed in detail in IDNT and suggested the presence of a J-shaped curve such that kidney benefit reached a plateau at systolic BP < 130 mm Hg, and all-cause mortality increased at systolic BP < 120 mm Hg.
- In the SPRINT[14] trial primary cardiovascular outcomes were reduced with intensive treatment with blood pressure goal of less than 120/80 mm Hg for patients with pre-existing CKD; however there was no difference in rates of 50% reduction of eGFR or ESRD rates in patients with intensive blood pressure control.
- Based on the current evidence (Table 19.3),[8] it is clear that BP reduction is important in the management of patients with diabetic nephropathy. Cardiovascular and kidney event rates are higher with increasing BP and are reduced progressively with therapy to lower BP.
- There may be a point beyond which further BP reduction may not be helpful or even be harmful despite a reduction in proteinuria. The current KDOQI guideline recommends a goal BP <130/80 mm Hg, whereas the Eighth Joint National Committee (JNC 8) guidelines recommend a goal BP < 140/90 mm Hg for most patients with T2DM and diabetic nephropathy, but with individualization.

Control of Dyslipidemia

Dyslipidemia is common in people with diabetes and CKD. Cardiovascular events are a frequent cause of morbidity and mortality in this population. Lowering low-density lipoprotein cholesterol (LDL-C) with statin-based therapies reduces risk of major atherosclerotic events, but not all-cause mortality, in patients with CKD including those with diabetes.

Goal for low-density lipoprotein (LDL) cholesterol is:

- <100 mg/dl (2.57 mmol/l) for diabetic patients in general and below.
- <70 mg/dl (1.81 mmol/l) for diabetic patients with CVD.

Table 19.3: Blood pressure control studies in patients with diabetes mellitus

Trial	Population	N	Intervention	Conclusions	Comments
ROAD MAP	T2DM without microalbuminuria	4,449	Olmesartan vs placebo	Olmesartan delayed the onset of microalbuminuria	Olmesartan group had lower BPs and more CV deaths
IRMA-2	T2DM and microalbuminuria	590	Irbesartan 150 mg vs irbesar-tan 300 mg vs placebo	Irbesartan reduced the development of overt proteinuria	Subgroup analysis suggested a dose-dependent effect
Captopril Trial	T1DM with proteinuria	409	Captopril 25 mg 3×/d vs placebo	Captopril reduced the risk for doubling of SCr as a primary outcome and death, dialysis therapy, or transplantation as a secondary outcome	
IDNT	T2DM with proteinuria and reduced kidney function	1,715	Irbesartan vs amlodipine vs placebo	Irbesartan reduced the risk for doubling of SCr, ESRD, or death	
RENAAL	T2DM with proteinuria and reduced kidney function	1,513	Losartan vs placebo	Losartan reduced the risk for doubling of SCr, ESRD, or death	

It is recommended using LDL-C lowering medicines, such as statins or statin/ezetimibe combination, to reduce risk of major atherosclerotic events in patients with diabetes and CKD, including those who have received a kidney transplant. It is not recommended initiating statin therapy in patients with diabetes who are treated by dialysis.

Dietary Changes

It is advisable to avoid protein supplements such as protein shakes or powders, but do not otherwise restrict protein from the diet. Protein intake recommended is:

- 0.8-1.0 g/kg body wt/day in individuals with diabetes and the earlier stages of CKD.
- 0.8 g/kg body wt/day in the later stages of CKD.

It is important to maintain a low-sodium diet in diabetic nephropathy. Low-sodium diet of 2.3 g or lower (5.8 g of NaCl) or 100 mEq/day in patients with diabetes and hypertension or any degree of proteinuria is recommended.

Avoidance of Nephrotoxins

- It is important to avoid nephrotoxic agents, if possible, in patients with diabetic nephropathy.
- Nonsteroidal anti-inflammatory drugs (NSAIDs) can cause a significant drop in GFR in patients with diabetic nephropathy, particularly when used with angiotensin-blocking agents.
- Radiocontrast media is particularly nephrotoxic for diabetics. Even with a normal serum creatinine level, patients with diabetes and proteinuria should be hydrated with saline 12 hours before and after exposure to contrast. Diuretics should be temporarily discontinued, and hyperglycemia should be controlled. Risk benefit assessment should be done before deciding for radio contrast study especially in patients with diabetes and kidney disease due to increased risk for contrast induced acute kidney injury (CIAKI).

Future Strategies

Various novel drugs targeted against different steps in diabetic pathophysiology are currently under research and different phases of trials such as:

- Bardoxolone–Inflammation modulator.
- Sulodexide–Glycosaminoglycan.
- Pirefenidone–TGF-B inhibitor.
- Ruboxistaurine–Protein Kinase-C inhibitor.
- Benfothiamine.
- Vitamin D Receptor Activation–Paricalcitol.
- Pentoxifylline.
- Baricitinib–JAK-STAT pathway inhibition.

End Stage Renal Disease (ESRD) in Diabetic Patients

Diabetic patient with ESRD has several options for renal replacement therapy:

1. Transplantation (kidney only, pancreas plus kidney simultaneously, pancreas after kidney).
2. Hemodialysis.
3. Peritoneal dialysis.
    - Currently, there is consensus that survival rates are best after transplantation.
    - Survival on peritoneal dialysis and hemodialysis are inferior to transplantation, but comparable between peritoneal dialysis and hemodialysis.
    - Blindness from proliferative diabetic retinopathy may limit a patient's ability to perform peritoneal dialysis.
    - Rates of recurrent peritonitis are also higher in patients with DM.
    - Patients with DM have an accelerated course to peritoneal membrane failure.
    - Systemic glucose absorption from the dialysate may lead to worsening hyperglycemia and increasing insulin requirements in patients undergoing peritoneal dialysis.
    - In patients undergoing hemodialysis, the preponderance of vascular disease in those with diabetes limits the maturity and increases the rate of complications of vascular access.
    - The increased rate of cardiac disease, left ventricular hypertrophy, and autonomic insufficiency observed in patients with diabetes can contribute to intradialytic hypotension, arrhythmias, or even sudden death on hemodialysis.

Conclusion

As diabetes becomes a global epidemic worldwide, incidence and prevalence of diabetic nephropathy is steadily increasing. Early detection of diabetic nephropathy combined with multifactorial interventional approach and use of ACE-Inhibitors and ARB's hold the key to slowing renal disease progression. For patients reaching ESRD, renal transplantation has definite survival advantage over hemodialysis and peritoneal dialysis.

References

1. Warram JH, Gearin G, Laffel L, Krolewski AS. Effect of duration of type 1 diabetes on the prevalence of stages of diabetic nephropathy defined by urinary albumin/creatinine ratio. J Am Soc Nephrol 1996;7(6):930-37.
2. Gall MA, Rossing P, Skott P, *et al.* Prevalence of micro- and macroalbuminuria, arterial hypertension, retinopathy and large vessel disease in European type 2 (non-insulin-dependent) diabetic patients. Diabetologia 1991;34:655-61.

3. Sharma SG, Bomback AS, Radhakrishnan J, Herlitz LC, Stokes MB, Markowitz GS, D'Agati VD: The modern spectrum of renal biopsy findings in patients with diabetes. Clin J Am Soc Nephrol 2013;8:1718-24.

4. The Diabetes Control and Complications (DCCT) Research Group. Effect of intensive therapy on the development and progression of diabetic nephropathy in the Diabetes Control and Complications Trial. Kidney Int 1995;47: 1703-20.

5. Writing Team for the Diabetes Control Complications Trial/ Epidemiology of Diabetes Interventions Complications Research Group. Effect of intensive therapy on the microvascular complications of type 1 diabetes mellitus. JAMA 2002;287,2563-69.

6. UK Prospective Diabetes Study (UKPDS) Group. Intensive blood-glucose control with sulphonylureas or insulin compared with conventional treatment and risk of complications in patients with type 2 diabetes (UKPDS 33). UK Prospective Diabetes Study (UKPDS) Group. Lancet 1998;352:837-53.

7. Shichiri M, Kishikawa H, Ohkubo Y and Wake N. Long-term results of the Kumamoto Study on optimal diabetes control in type 2 diabetic patients. Diabetes Care 2000;23 (Suppl. 2),B21-B29.

8. Umanath K, Lewis JB. Update on Diabetic Nephropathy: Core Curriculum 2018. Am J Kidney Dis 2018 Jun;71(6): 884-95.

9. Wanner C, Inzucchi SE, Lachin JM, *et al.* Empagliflozin and progression of kidney disease in type 2 diabetes. N Engl J Med 2016;375:323-34.

10. Neal B, Perkovic V, Mahaffey KW, *et al.* CANVAS Program Collaborative Group. Canagliflozin and cardiovascular and renal events in type 2 diabetes. N Engl J Med 2017;17;377:644-57.

11. Pohl MA, Blumenthal S, Cordonnier DJ, *et al.* Independent and additive impact of blood pressure control and angiotensin II receptor blockade on renal outcomes in the Irbesartan Diabetic Nephropathy Trial: Clinical implications and limitations. J Am Soc Nephrol 2005;16:3027-37.

12. Parving HH, Lehnert H, Brochner-Mortensen J, *et al.* The effect of irbesartan on the development of diabetic nephropathy in patients with type 2 diabetes. N Engl J Med 2001;345:870-78.

13. Eijkelkamp WB, Zhang Z, Remuzzi G, *et al.* Albuminuria is a target for renoprotective therapy independent from blood pressure in patients with type 2 diabetic nephropathy: Post hoc analysis from the Reduction of Endpoints in NIDDM with the Angiotensin II Antagonist Losartan (RENAAL) trial. J Am Soc Nephrol 2007;18:1540-46.

14. Wright JT Jr, Williamson JD, Whelton PK, *et al.* A randomized trial of intensive versus standard blood-pressure control. N Engl J Med 2015;373(22):2103-16.

CHAPTER

20 An Elderly Patient with Resistant Hypertension Due to Renal Artery Stenosis

Ashish Nandwani[1], Saurabh Shukla[2]

[1] *Consultant, Nephrologist, Manipal Hospital, New Delhi*

[2] *Consultant, Nephrologist, Arvy Hospital, Gurugram*

CASE

70 years old male known case of diabetes mellitus for last 15 years, presented with new onset hypertension, which was detected during routine evaluation. There was no history of any urinary complaints or swelling feet. His evaluation revealed BP 170/100 mm Hg and all peripheral pulses were present. CVS exam was unremarkable. Lab evaluation showed normal blood counts. Urea 50 mg/dl and creatinine 1.6 mg/dl with trace protein on urine analysis. USG revealed right kidney 7.5 cm with increased echogenicity and left kidney 8.8 cm with increased echogenicity. USG doppler revealed presence of parvus tardus pattern in bilateral renal arteries, suggestive of renal artery stenosis, which was confirmed by MR angiography. Patient was managed with antihypertensive medication with amlodipin, metoprolol and hydrochlorthiazide. However, his BP control remained poor and he presented in ER with accelerated hypertension and pulmonary edema, which was managed with IV NTG and Labetalol infusion. After optimization of antihypertensive medication, he was kept on regular follow-up with monitoring of BP control and renal functions.

What is Renovascular Hypertension (RVH)?

It is a form of secondary hypertension occurring due to decreased perfusion of kidney. This may occur even though patient may have higher than normal blood pressure, which the kidneys perceive it to be low. A fall in renal perfusion pressure sufficient to initiate renovascular hypertension only occurs when 70 to 80% of artery lumen is occluded.

What is Underlying Pathophysiology of RVH?

Reduction in renal perfusion sets into action counter regulatory pathways from the kidney, majority of which is mediated by Renin Angiotensin Aldosterone system (RAAS).

Various lesions that can lead to RVH are as follows:

- Atherosclerotic renal vascular disease (ASRVD).
- Fibromuscular dysplasia (FMD).
- Vasculitis.
- Aneurysm and fistulas.
- Systemic emboli.
- Aortic dissection.
- Renin secreting renal tumor.
- Compression–Metastatic/Neurofibromatosis/Hematoma.

What is Critical Stenosis?

Kidneys have enormous capacity to autoregulate blood flow, such that 50-60% obstruction does not cause change in parenchymal blood flows. Latex Rubber cast studies have elucidated that at least 70-80% of narrowing is required to cause measurable flow and pressure gradient changes across the lesion. Renin-Angiotensin Aldosterone system (RAAS) is the key effector counter regulatory mechanism which sets into action as renovascular hypertension develops. Pathophysiology of renovascular hypertension depends on what percentage of renal parenchyma is facing diminished perfusion.

Role of Renin-Angiotensin Aldosterone System (RAAS)

In bilateral renal artery stenosis or stenosis in single kidney all of the renal mass is ischemic, this is analogous to *Goldblatt's two kidney 1 clip model.* In this model decreased perfusion to the stenosed kidney causes activation of RAAS pathway, consequently Renin, Angiotensin II and Aldosterone increases. These cause salt and water retention which raises blood pressure. However as salt and water retention occurs, pressure natriuresis by contra lateral kidneys occurs, which is mediated by natriuretic peptides, hence the blood pressure is RAAS dependent. This has important implications in both anti-hypertensive management, its effects and diagnostic tests.

The other model of renovascular hypertension is *Goldblatt's one kidney one clip model,* entire renal mass is hypoperfused leading to RAAS activation with sodium and water retention, however, there is no contralateral or normal kidney to counteract these changes. With sodium retention and volume expansion, there is negative feedback to inhibit the RAAS activation resulting in decrease in angiotensin II levels. Thus, hypertension in this situation is not angiotensin II dependent.

The role of RAAS in tissue injury is more than just causing hypertension mediated by salt and water retention. It also has vascular and cellular effects:

- Angiotensin II causes efferent arteriolar constriction.
- Induces cellular hypertrophy and hyperplasia of extracellular matrix, vascular smooth muscles, myocytes.
- Platelet aggregation, generation of superoxide radicals oxidation of low density lipoproteins.
- Activation of adhesion molecules and macrophages.
- Induction of proto-oncogen.

Role of Vasoactive Factors

Nitric oxide level decreases in post stenotic renal artery segments due to decreased perfusion. Nitric oxide has vaso dilatory actions. *Endothelin peptides* are produced in endothelial cells and also renal epithelial cells following TGF-β, IL1 and TNF up regulation. It is a potent vasoconstrictor which further enhance in hypoperfusion. *Prostaglandins* are arachidonic acid derivatives, which are important regulators of renal blood flow and filtration. Tissue hypoperfusion causes enhanced production of prostacyclin and PGE_2 which are renoprotective. Thrombaxane A2(TXA2) is vasoconstrictor that lower GFR by lowering renal blood flow, TXA2 also modulates vascular permeability and AT–II hemodynamic properties. Interplay of above factors along with TGF-β, PDGF, br FGF cause progressive interstitial fibrosis.

Epidemiology of RVH

In all hypertensive patient cohort incidence of RVH has been estimated to be around 0.6 - 3%. However refractory hypertension cohort may have prevalence of more than 20%.

Clinical scenarios where renovascular hypertension should be suspected are:

- Atherosclerosis in other vascular territories.
- Onset of HTN <30 years or >55 years.
- Diastolic abdominal bruit.
- Worsening of previously controlled hypertension.
- History of accelerated/malignant/refractory hypertension despite 3 drug regimen.
- Unilateral small kidney; Difference of >1.5 cm.
- RAAS inhibition induced deterioration of renal functions.
- Recurrent pulmonary edema.
- High grade hypertensive retinopathy.
- Angina with normal coronaries.

Atherosclerotic Renovascular Disease (ASRVD)

- Risk factors–age > 50 years, smoking, diabetes mellitus, hyperlipidemia and hypertension.
- Atherosclerotic narrowing of the renal arteries range from focal stenosis to complete occlusion of one or both renal arteries leading to renal ischemia and subsequent renal atrophy.
- Present along with macrovascular disease in other organ systems; coronary, peripheral and cerebral arteries.
- Atherosclerotic plaques are commonly present in the first or second centimeter of renal artery and may extend into aorta. Renal artery stenosis may be bilateral in 20% to 40% cases.
- ASRVD may be detected incidentally, while doing coronary or peripheral angiography. Renovascular hypertension is most common clinical manifestation and may be associated with other target organ damage.
- Patients with RVH may have abnormal circadian rhythm with loss of nocturnal pressure fall.
- Patients may have resistant hypertension requiring three or more antihypertensive medication. RAAS inhibition with ACE inhibitor or ARB may lead to acute kidney injury in patients with ASRVD.
- Patients with advanced disease present with renal dysfunction progressing to end stage renal disease or flash pulmonary edema due to rapid volume expansion.

Fibromuscular Dysplasia (FMD)

- FMD is an idiopathic noninflammatory, nonathero-matous arteriopathy associated with proliferation of medial smooth muscle cells and fibrous tissue leading to renal artery stenosis.
- The most common age group is 15 to 50 years and 90% of cases are in females.
- The prevalence of renovascular FMD is estimated at 4 in 1000.
- FMD may be associated with disorders like Marfan syndrome, tuberous sclerosis, Ehlers-Danlos syndrome and cystic medial necrosis.
- The FMD involves mainly renal and cerebral vessels. Renal arteries are involved in 65-70% of cases and cerebrovascular involvement is seen in 25-30% of cases. It may also involve coronary, mesenteric and peripheral extremity vessels.

- Histologically, medial fibroplasia is the most common variety; other rare forms include perimedial fibroplasias and medial hyperplasia.
- On angiography, the characteristic appearance is that of string of beads, with bead diameter larger than lumen.
- Most common clinical presentation of FMD is renovascular hypertension, headaches, dizziness and pulsatile tinnitus. While hypertension is the leading manifestation of renovascular FMD, some patients may have flank pain due to renal infarction either from dissection of renal artery or embolism from the proximal aneurysm. Flank pain may also be due to rupture of a renal artery aneurysm with retroperitoneal bleed.
- FMD rarely causes ESRD unless hypertension is uncontrolled or thrombosis of renal artery results in the renal infarction.

Inflammatory Arteritis

- Takayasu arteritis (TA) is the most common inflammatory arteritis leading to renovascular hypertension.
- Other causes include polyarteritis nodosa, giant cell arteritis, kawasaki disease and idiopathic aortitis.
- Takayasu arteritis is an inflammatory granulomatous arteritis involving aorta and its first order branches.
- TA is usually presents in 25-40 years of age group.
- The common clinical presentation is fatigue and discomfort in the muscles of one or more extremities especially upper limbs.
- Decreased pulsation of one or both brachial arteries with difference in systolic blood pressure in both arms.
- Bruit may be heard on abdominal aorta or subclavian arteries.
- Hypertension due to proximal renal artery stenosis may be the sole manifestation.
- Diagnosis is usually based on angiographic findings of narrowing or occlusion of aorta and its primary branches.

Other Causes

- Coarctation of aorta.
- Middle aortic syndrome.
- Radiation induced RAS due to previous abdominal radiation.

Diagnosis of Renovascular Hypertension

The diagnosis of the renovascular hypertension depends on demonstrating both critical stenosis of renal artery and activation of renin angiotensin aldosterone system. These include both invasive and non-invasive imaging modalities. The gold standard for diagnosing renal artery stenosis is renal angiography.

Duplex Doppler Ultrasonography

- Doppler ultrasonography (USG) is used for renal vascular anatomy and functional status.
- Doppler ultrasonography is used to obtain the renal resistive index, which is calculated from the following formula:

  (Peak systolic velocity–end diastolic velocity) ÷ Peak systolic velocity.
- Lesions can also be detected by comparing the systolic flow velocity in the renal artery to that in the aorta since the velocity of flow increases as the artery narrows; end-diastolic velocity may also be increased distal to a stenotic lesion.
- Features of significant renal artery stenosis are:
  - *Elevated peak systolic velocity:* Velocities in the stenotic segment >1.8-2.0 m/s correlate well with stenosis of > 60% diameter reduction.
  - *Renal artery/aorta ratio:* An RAR >3.5 correlates with stenosis >60%.
  - *Acceleration time:* An AT >0.07s correlates with a stenosis >60%.
  - *Loss of the early systolic peak (ESP):* Proximal stenosis results in changes to the intrarenal waveform with loss of the ESP and a 'tardus parvus' appearance.
- Using these criteria, sensitivity and specificity with angiographic estimation of lesions exceeding > 60% is 90% and 96% respectively.
- Doppler USG is an inexpensive, noninvasive test and is widely available. However, limitations include that this is operator dependent and may be difficult to perform in obese patients. Also, Doppler USG will not be able to differentiate between fibromuscular dysplasia and atherosclerotic lesion.

Computed Tomographic Angiography (CTA)

- A spiral computed tomography scan with intravenous contrast injection is a highly accurate noninvasive diagnostic test, which provides excellent images of both kidneys and the vascular tree.
- Provide excellent sensitivity (96%) and specificity (97%).
- The risk of contrast induced nephrotoxicity is high especially in patients with impaired renal functions due to underlying ischemic nephropathy.
- CT imaging with 3-D reconstruction, and higher resolution with less contrast use, continue to improve the value of CT angiography as a diagnostic tool for renovascular disease.

Magnetic Resonance Angiography (MRA)

- MRA with gadolinium contrast gives excellent vascular imaging of the renal arteries.
- This technique is useful in patients who cannot be given iodinated contrast agent due to either allergic reactions or impaired renal functions due to risk of contrast induced nephrotoxicity.
- MRA has sensitivity of 83-100% and specificity of 92%-97%.
- Limitations of MRA include overestimation of luminal narrowing and limited sensitivity for middle and distal vascular lesions.
- Patients with metallic stents are not candidate for MRA.
- The use of breath-hold MRA with paramagnetic contrast material improves the ability to visualize small accessory arteries.
- Blood oxygen level dependent (BOLD) MRI is non-invasive method that detects local levels of the deoxyhemoglobin without requiring contrast.

Renal Angiography

- Renal angiography remains gold standard for defining the stenotic lesions of renal vasculature.
- It can identify whether stenosis is unilateral or bilateral, atherosclerotic or fibromuscular dysplasia and post stenotic dilatation.
- It is also useful for planning the endovascular procedure like angioplasty and stenting.
- Contrast induced nephrotoxicity and catheter related complications are main issues associated with renal angiography.
- As it is invasive procedure with potential complications, it is suitable only for those patients in whom renal vascular intervention is planned.

Captopril Renogram

- Radionuclide imaging provides a functional assessment of the kidneys allowing the comparison of blood flow and glomerular filtration rate (GFR) between two kidneys.
- DTPA and MAG3 are the commonly used radiopharmaceuticals used for radionuclide renography.
- MAG3 may be more reliable in patients with renal insufficiency. MAG3 also has clearance characteristic similar to hippuran and represents the renal blood flow.
- Change in the GFR after ACE inhibition allows inferences regarding the presence of renal artery stenosis.
- When this test is completely negative, it has a high negative predictive value.
- The predictive value can be increased by administration of oral captopril (25 to 50 mg) one hour before the isotope is injected. The interpretation of captopril renogram is based upon the ACE inhibitor-induced decline in GFR in the stenotic kidney, accompanied by an increase in GFR in the contralateral kidney due to removal of angiotensin II-mediated vasoconstriction. The net result is that the difference between the two kidneys is enhanced.
- The sensitivity and specificity range from 65% to 96% and 62% to 100% respectively. Sensitivity further decreases in the presence of the renal insufficiency with reduced GFR (serum creatinine >2.0 mg/dl).

Plasma Renin Activity (PRA)

- Peripheral venous PRA demonstrates the activation of renin angiotensin system as a marker of underlying renovascular hypertension.
- PRA is elevated in only 50 to 80% of patients with renovascular hypertension.
- Levels of PRA may be suppressed by a high dietary sodium intake, bilateral renal arterial disease, volume expansion related to intrinsic kidney disease, and various antihypertensive drugs.
- The predictive value of the PRA can be increased by measuring the rise in PRA one hour after the administration of 25 to 50 mg of captopril. Patients with renal artery stenosis have an increase in the PRA as compared with normal individuals, due to removal of the normal suppressive effect of high angiotensin II levels on renin secretion in the stenotic kidney.

Renal Vein Renin Measurements

Measurement of renal vein renin levels helps to lateralize the stenotic kidney (> 1.5:1 stenotic-nonstenotic kidney ratio). The presence of highly lateralizing renal renin values indicate the presence of physiologically significant renal artery stenosis. The accuracy of these measurements may be enhanced by administration of an ACE inhibitor and/or diuretics, which will increase renin secretion on the affected side.

These peripheral PRA, stimulated PRA, renal vein renin level and the captopril renogram are no longer considered suitable for initial testing patients with suspected renovascular disease because of their poor sensitivity and specificity and thus have no meaningful role.

Management of Renovascular Hypertension

It is important to know the likely cause of renal artery stenosis, i.e., atherosclerotic or FMD or inflammatory and whether the lesion is unilateral or bilateral. The main therapeutic options available are: (Fig. 20.1)

1. Medical therapy.
2. Percutaneous angioplasty with or without stenting.
3. Surgical revascularization or, in some cases, resection of a "pressor" kidney.

The most difficult aspect of management of RVH is whether to treat medically or with revascularization procedure. General approaches in patients with renovascular hypertension include control of hypertension by medical therapy. Revascularization is reasonable in patients who have short duration of blood pressure elevation prior to the diagnosis of renovascular disease or in patients who don't respond to optimal medical therapy or are intolerant to medical therapy. Patients with recurrent flash pulmonary edema and/or refractory heart failure may also require revascularization procedure. In addition, revascularization may be required in patients having progressive renal insufficiency due to bilateral renal artery stenosis (or unilateral stenosis to a solitary functioning kidney).

Medical Therapy

Medical therapy include the control of hypertension, dyslipidemia and life style changes including smoking cessation. Angiotensin-converting enzyme (ACE) inhibitors and angiotensin II receptor blockers (ARBs) are the mainstay of drugs to control the blood pressure in patients with renovascular disease. If blood pressure goals are not achieved with angiotensin inhibition alone, other antihypertensive drugs, such as a calcium channel blocker, diuretic, or a beta blocker, should be added as necessary. The potential concerns associated with medical treatment are progressive worsening of stenotic lesion over a period of time leading to impaired GFR due to ischemic damage. Angiotensin inhibition may lead to acute kidney injury and hyperkalemia especially in patients with bilateral renal artery stenosis. Patients with advanced age, advanced renal insufficiency (serum creatinine >3.0 mg/dl), atherosclerotic as opposed to FMD and small kidneys on imaging have poor response to antihypertensive medications.

Endovascular Treatment of Renal Artery Stenosis

For patients with renal artery stenosis with uncontrolled hypertension despite three antihypertensive medications, progressive deterioration in renal function and cardiac failure, revascularization may restore the renal blood flow and stabilize the renal function. Stent placement is superior to angioplasty alone especially in ostial stenosis. Patients with FMD are usually treated with angioplasty without stenting. The risks associated with the procedure are renal artery dissection, embolization into the kidney, rupture of renal artery and contrast induced nephrotoxicity.

Revascularization versus Medical Therapy Alone

Multiple randomized trials have compared revascularization using percutaneous transluminal renal angioplasty (PTRA) with or without stent in combination with medical therapy in patients with atherosclerotic renovascular disease.

The largest and most recent of these was the *Cardiovascular Outcomes in Renal Atherosclerotic Lesions*

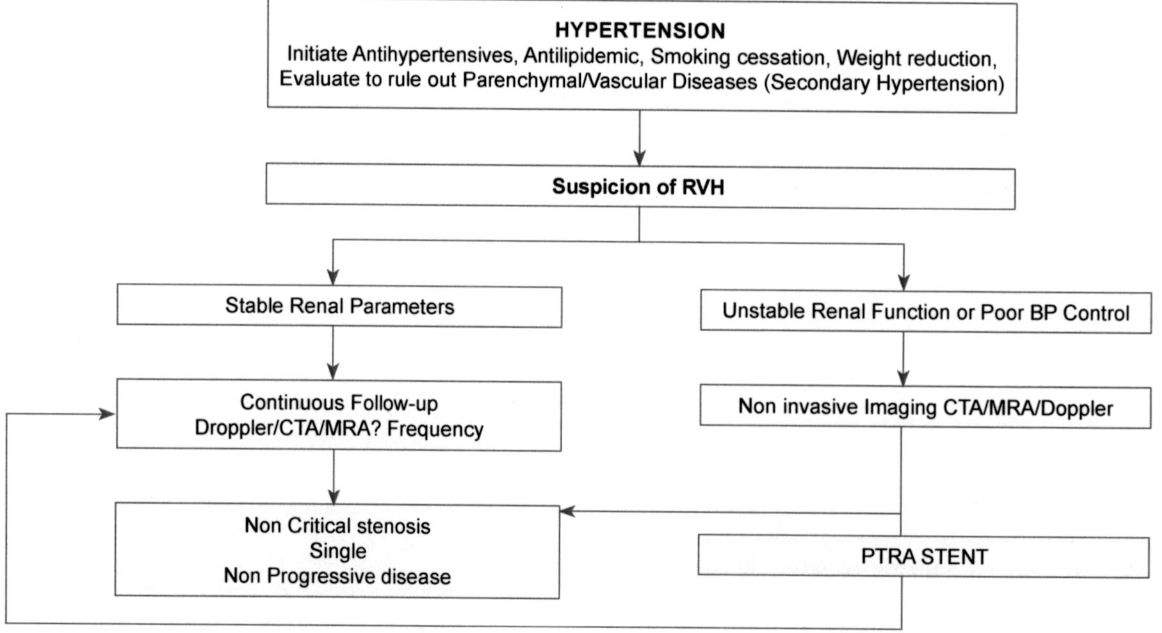

Figure 20.1: Management of patient with renovascular disease
PTRA: Percutaneous transluminal renal angioplasty; RVH: Renovascular hypertension.

(CORAL) trial, which included 947 patients, who had unilateral or bilateral atherosclerotic renal artery stenosis. These patients had systolic hypertension despite two or more antihypertensive medications and/or an eGFR <60 ml/min/1.73 m^2. All patients received antiplatelet therapy plus standardized medical treatments for diabetes, hypertension and hyperlipidemia. Candesartan was given as an angiotensin receptor blocking agent to all the patients. Patients were then randomly assigned to revascularization or to no revascularization.

The primary outcomes were a composite of cardiovascular or renal death, stroke, myocardial infarction, hospitalization for heart failure, a reduction in eGFR by more than 30 percent, or end-stage renal disease. After a median of 3.6 years, revascularization had no additional effect on the primary outcome as compared with medical therapy alone (35.1 versus 35.8%). Also, revascularization had no effect on any of the individual components of the primary outcome. The most frequent complication was renal artery dissection, occurred in 11 (2.2%) revascularized patients.

The Angioplasty and Stenting for renal Artery lesion trial (ASTRAL) and *Stent placement in patients with atherosclerotic renal artery stenosis and impaired renal function trial* (STAR) randomized patients to medical therapy or intervention. ACE inhibitors were used in two thirds of patients in STAR and 38% patients in ASTRAL trial. There were no significant differences in the blood pressure control, number of antihypertensive medications, renal functions or cardiovascular outcomes in these patients.

In a meta-analysis, including CORAL and ASTRAL patients treated with PTRA with or without stent required an average of 0.2 lesser antihypertensive medications. There was no difference with regard to change in renal function, or the incidence of heart failure, stroke, myocardial infarction, or total mortality. Periprocedural complications were–procedure-related deaths occurred in 0.4% of patients, and renal artery perforations or dissections occurred in 2.5%. Apart from slight reduction in antihypertensive medication, none of these studies demonstrated any significant clinical benefit from PTRA.

Earlier studies by Van Jaarsveld *et al.* and Plouin *et al.* evaluated blood pressure control in patients with medical therapy vs PTRA in patients who required two or more anti-hypertensive drugs for BP control and serum creatinine < 2.3 mg/dl. The study was unable to demonstrate any benefit in respect of renal function or event free survival. The main drawbacks of these studies are that high risk group patients were excluded, who may have benefited most from the procedure, e.g., patients with bilateral RAS, recurrent pulmonary edema and renal dysfunction.

The current data demonstrate that most of the patients with renovascular disease can be effectively managed with optimal medical therapy with antihypertensive therapy as compared to PTRA with or without stent therapy. No significant difference in patient survival or renal function could be identified.

Surgical Revascularization

Surgical revascularization carries a considerable cost, risk and morbidity. It is reserved for patients, who fail medical and endovascular therapies or have associated aortic disease that is not amenable to endovascular therapy. Some patients with total occlusion of renal artery resulting in non-functioning kidney may require nephrectomy for control of blood pressure.

Conclusion

Renovascular hypertension caused by renal artery stenosis especially due to atherosclerosis is an important cause of secondary hypertension especially in elderly patients. Most of the patients can be managed by medical therapy with antihypertensive medications and with statin therapy. Resistant hypertension, flash pulmonary edema and deteriorating renal functions despite medical therapy may warrant revascularization therapy. There is potential of recurrent disease or restenosis after revascularization requiring regular follow-up.

Suggested Reading

1. Derkx FH, Schalekamp MA. Renal artery stenosis and hypertension. Lancet 1994;344:237-39.
2. Ram CV. Renovascular hypertension. Curr Opin Nephrol Hypertens 1997;6:575-79.
3. Olin JW, Melia M, Young JR, Graor RA, Risius B. Prevalence of atherosclerotic renal artery stenosis in patients with atherosclerosis elsewhere. Am J Med 1990;88:46N-51N.
4. The ASTRAL Investigators: Revascularization versus medical therapy for renal-artery stenosis. N Engl J Med 2009;361:1953-62.
5. Cooper CJ, Murphy TP, Cutlip DE, *et al*. Stenting and medical therapy for atherosclerotic renal artery stenosis. N Engl J Med 2014;370:13-22.
6. Herrmann SM, Saad A, Textor SC. Management of atherosclerotic renovascular disease after Cardiovascular Outcomes in Renal Atherosclerotic Lesions (CORAL). Nephrol Dial Transplant 2015;30:366-75.
7. Textor SC, Misra S, Oderich G. Percutaneous revascularization for ischemic nephropathy: The past, present and future. Kidney Int 2013;83(1):28-40.
8. Conlon PJ, O'Riordan E, Kalra PA. Epidemiology and clinical manifestations of atherosclerotic renal artery stenosis. Am J Kidney Dis 2000;35:573-87.

CHAPTER

21 A Young Female with Renovascular Hypertension

Rahul Grover

Senior Consultant, Nephrology, Max Super Speciality Hospital, Saket, New Delhi

CASE

Mrs YN, 23-year-old female presented to OPD for uncontrolled hypertension for the past 3-4 months. She was first diagnosed hypertensive around 7 years ago. Her blood pressures remained poorly controlled. Around 1 year later, she developed hypertensive encephalopathy and required ICU admission. She was found to be having uveitis in left eye with posterior synechiae formation and secondary cataract. Investigations revealed presence of bilateral renal artery stenosis (RAS). CT imaging revealed presence of mediastinal lymphadenopathy and Mantoux test was strongly positive. She was also detected to be Treponema pallidum hemagglutination assay (TPHA) and rapid plasma reagin (RPR) reactive. She underwent left renal artery angioplasty and stenting. She also received treatment for tuberculosis and syphilis. Post angioplasty her blood pressures became well controlled on single anti-hypertensive medication.

Since last 2 years her antihypertensive medication requirement had increased. For last 3-4 months her blood pressures were uncontrolled on 3 antihypertensive medications including an angiotensin receptor blocker. She was further investigated. Her routine labs including blood counts, lipid profile, liver and renal functions were within normal limits (creatinine 0.9 mg/dl) and ESR was 13. Ultrasound revealed asymmetric kidneys (RK 7.9 cm, LK 10.2 cm). CT angiography revealed normal abdominal aorta, > 70% stenosis in right renal artery (2.6 cm segment narrowing of right renal artery with ostial diameter 1 mm and post stenotic diameter 5 mm). A normal left renal artery, with around 50% in stent restenosis and moderate to severe circumferential stenosis of osteo-proximal celiac trunk with mild narrowing of superior mesenteric artery. A dedicated renal stent (Ivnatec Hippocampus 6.0 × 15 mm) was placed in left renal artery. Blood pressure got controlled on olmesartan 40 mg once a day.

Renovascular Hypertension

Seminal work by pathologist Harry Goldblatt on experimental production of hypertension by partially constricting major renal artery in dogs was published in 1934.[1] This discovery led to the concept of renovascular hypertension as well as the further discovery of renin and renin-angiotensin-aldosterone axis, that are so important in current cardiovascular medicine. Renal artery stenosis can be associated with a spectrum of clinical states from incidental detection with no functional significance to renovascular hypertension caused by excessive activation of renin-angiotensin system to accelerated cardiovascular disease and ischemic nephropathy.[2]

What are Etiologies of Renovascular Hypertension?

A multitude of etiologies can lead to development of renal artery stenosis. The stenosis can be either unilateral of bilateral. The common etiologies include atherosclerotic renal artery stenosis (60%-90%), fibromuscular dysplasia (10-30%) and other less common entities like vasculitis (Takayasu's arteritis, Buerger's disease, polyarteritis nodosa, post radiation), Neurofibromatosis Type 1, thromboembolic disease, arterial dissection, infrarenal aortic aneurysm etc. At younger ages (<50 years) atherosclerotic disease is less likely with fibromuscular dysplasia and vasculitis being more likely etiologies.

When to Suspect Renovascular Hypertension?

The prevalence of renal artery stenosis is low in patients with mild hypertension (around 1%) but increases sharply in severe or uncontrolled hypertensive patients (up to 30%-40%). Presence of severe hypertension, young age of onset, abrupt onset, flash pulmonary edema, hypertensive urgency/emergencies, presence of hypokalemia, asymmetric kidney size, or acute and sustained deterioration of renal functions with ACE inhibitors or ARBs are some of the clinical clues suggesting presence of renovascular hypertension.

How to Diagnose Renal Artery Stenosis (RAS)?

Imaging studies like duplex ultrasonography and angiography (CT, MR or conventional) are required to achieve the diagnosis.[3] ACE inhibitor scintigraphy and intravascular ultrasound with simultaneous pressure measurement are sometimes used for assessment of functional significance of the lesion. Catheter based angiography remains the gold standard but is generally preformed if there intervention is planned.

Unlike atherosclerotic renal artery stenosis where role of renal artery interventions (percutaneous and surgical) is controversial, their role in conditions like fibromuscular dysplasia and vasculitis like Takayasu's arteritis is better defined and is sometimes curative. Regular monitoring is required as lesions tend to recur and sometimes multiple interventions are required.

While atherosclerosis is the most common cause of renovascular hypertension in the elderly while there is a spectrum of disorders that can lead to renovascular hypertension in the young. The common etiologies of renovascular hypertension in the young adults are discussed further.

Fibromuscular Dysplasia (FMD)

FMD is an idiopathic non-inflammatory, non-atherosclerotic vascular disease with a prevalence ranging from 1.1% (autopsy series) to 6.6% (angiography in renal donors). It predominantly affects young women (F:M–3:1-9:1) and is responsible for around 10% to 20% of cases of renal artery stenosis.[4] There are no large epidemiological studies from India but it is considered that the prevalence may be lower than that seen in caucasian population. In a retrospective case series of renovascular hypertension from north India that included 205 patients over a period of 16 years, chugh KS *et al.*, reported fibromuscular dysplasia as the second most common etiology [N=58 (28.3%)] with Takayasu's arteritis being the most common etiology [N=125 (61%)] of RAS.[5]

The etiology of fibromuscular dysplasia remains unknown. An association with environmental factors like smoking and renal mobility (more common in right kidney) has been reported. Genetic predispositions is suggested as it is reported to occur in twins, has association with HLA DRw6 as well as with other connective tissue disorders like Marfans, Tuberous sclerosis, Ehlers-Danlos syndrome, neurofibramatosis, Williams syndrome etc. Recently an association with phosphatase and actin regulator 1 gene (PHACTR1) has been identified further supporting genetic basis.[6]

FMD affects small and medium sized arterial walls and leads to stenosis, aneurysms and dissections. It commonly affects renal (58%) and cranio-cervical arteries (32%) but can affect any arterial bed. Depending on the arterial layer affected by dysplasia it is classified as intimal, medial or peri-advential.

Peri-adventitial FMD is the rarest of the group (~1% of all FMD). It is characterized by dense deposition of collagen leading to a smooth narrowing appearance. Intimal is the next most common (5%-10%) and is characterized by circumferential deposition of collagen in intima with fragmentation of elastic lamina. This also results in smooth narrowing/stenosis on imaging. The most common variant is that of medial FMD (85%). There are alternating ridges of collagen and loss of elastic membrane but internal elastic lamina is preserved. This gives the classical imaging findings of 'string of beads' appearance. Unlike atherosclerotic renal artery stenosis, FMD rarely affects ostia of the arteries. Medial FMD is further sub-classified into perimedial fibroplasia, medial fibroplasia and medial hyperplasia.

Resistant hypertension and stroke are common clinical presentations of FMD. Renal involvement can also occur in form of renal artery dissection, infarction, loin pain and hematuria. Diagnosis of FMD should prompt screening for its involvement in other vascular beds. Headaches, pulsatile tinnitus, cervical artery dissection, strokes can occur in cranio cervical FMD; weight loss with post-prandial epigastric/abdominal pain may suggest mesenteric FMD involvement, upper or lower limb claudication and chest pain can suggest involvement of subclavian, lower limb vessels or coronaries by FMD respectively. Young onset or resistant hypertension, strokes in young, aortic or other vascular aneurysms at age <60 or a positive family history should prompt screening for FMD.

Angiography (CT and MR) helps to diagnose and classify the disease. Angiographically FMD is classified as Multifocal (string of bead), tubular (> 1 cm), focal (<1 cm) or mixed depending on the appearance and length of stenosis.

Percutaneous transluminal angioplasty (PTA) with bailout stent placement is performed for resistant hypertension in FMD. It enjoys a good technical success rate with majority achieving good blood pressure control and 40-50% achieving a cure of hypertension. FMD with severe intimal hyperplasia, branch renal artery stenosis, associated aneurysms, failed PTA may sometimes warrant surgical correction.[7]

Takayasu's Arteritis

Takayasu's arteritis or the "pulseless disease" was first described in 1908 by a Japanese ophthalmologist Dr Mikito Takayasu with having "wreathlike" appearance of retinal vessels. Its association with absence of wrist pulses was noted at same time.

It is a large vessel vasculitis that involves aorta and its major branches and sometimes coronary and pulmonary arteries. It leads to stenosis, occlusion or aneurysmal dilatation of the involved vessels.

It is a rare disease with a worldwide incidence of 1-2/million. It is more common in Asian population (40/million in Japan vs 0.09/million in Mexico). It has a predilection for young age (<40-50) and female gender [F:M–9.4:1 (Japan) to 1.7:1 (India)].[8]

It is an inflammatory, granulomatous vasculitis that causes transmural fibrous thickening of arterial wall. Inflammation initially involves the vasa vasoram and medio-adventitial junction and subsequently inflammation leads to marked adventitial and peri-adventitial fibrosis making the arterial walls very stiff. Pathogenesis is unclear and infectious as well as immunological basis has been suggested. Heightened reactivity to mycobacterial proteins in view of high incidence of mantoux positivity has been contemplated but remains unproven.[8]

Clinical course is considered to follow three stages. The first stage is an early systemic inflammatory phase that presents with non-specific constitutional symptoms, is often subclinical and passes undiagnosed. This is followed by a vascular inflammatory phase, a protracted phase in which patient progressively develops symptoms of vascular insufficiency. Symptoms depend on the vascular bed involved. Abdominal aortic involvement with renovascular hypertension is common in India while aortic arch involvement with aortic regurgitation is most common in Japan. The third phase is when inflammation subsides and chronic arterial stenosis or aneurysms are left. There may be additional renal parenchymal involvement in form of mesangioproliferative glomerulonephritis or amyloidosis is a subset of patients.[9]

Ishikawa in 1988 proposed the initial diagnostic criteria for Takayasu's arteritis, consisting of obligatory criteria of age < 40, two major criteria (including subclavian artery involvement) and 9 minor criteria (including ESR, hypertension, angiographic demonstration of various lesions). American College of Rheumatology and subsequently Sharma BK *et al.* have proposed modifications to improve sensitivity and specificity (Table 21.1).

On angiography four patterns of arterial involvement are seen including varying degrees of narrowing, complete occlusion, aneurysm formation (fusiform/saccular) and irregularity of vessel wall. The arterial involvement is classified as follows.[11]

- Type I involves only the branches of the aortic arch.
- Type IIa involves ascending aorta, aortic arch and its branches.
- Type IIb affects ascending aorta, aortic arch and its branches, and thoracic descending aorta.

Table 21.1: Diagnostic criteria for Takayasu's arteritis[10] [Sharma BK *et al.*]*

Major criteria	
Left mid subclavian artery lesion	The most severe stenosis or occlusions present in the mid portion from the point 1 cm proximal to the vertebral artery orifice determined by angiography.
Right mid subclavian artery lesion	The most severe stenosis or occlusions present in the mid portion from the right vertebral artery to the point 3 cm distal to orifice determined by angiography.
Characteristic signs and symptoms of at least one month duration	These include limb claudication, pulselessness or pulse difference (>10 mm Hg systolic blood pressure difference in limb), fever, neck pain, transient amaurosis, blurred vision, syncope, dyspnea or palpitations.
Minor criteria	
High ESR	Unexplained persistent high ESR >20 mm/hr (Westergreen) at diagnosis or presence of the evidence in patient's history.
Carotid artery tenderness	Unilateral or bilateral tenderness of common carotid arteries on palpation. Neck muscle tenderness is unacceptable.
Hypertension	Persistent blood pressure in brachial >149 mm Hg, or popliteal >160/90 mm Hg by auscultation or Doppler echocardiography or angiography.
Aortic regurgitation or Annulo-aortic ectasia	By angiography or two-dimensional echocardiography.
Pulmonary artery lesion	Lobar or segmental arterial occlusion or equivalent determined by angiography or perfusion scintigraphy, or presence of stenosis, aneurysm, luminal irregularity or any combination on pulmonary trunk or in unilateral or bilateral pulmonary arteries determined by angiography.
Left mid common carotid lesion	Presence of the most severe stenosis or occlusion in the mid portion of 5 cm in length from the point 2 cm distal to its orifice determined by angiography.
Distal brachiocephalic trunk lesion	Presence of the most severe stenosis or occlusion in the distal third determined by angiography.
Descending thoracic aorta lesion	Narrowing, dilation or aneurysm, luminal irregularity or any combination determined by angiography: Tortuosity alone is unacceptable.
Abdominal aorta lesion	Narrowing, dilation or aneurysm, luminal irregularity or aneurysm combination.
Coronary artery lesion	Documented on angiography below the age of 30 years in the absence of risk factors like hyperlipidemia or diabetes mellitus.
*Two major, one major and two minor or 4 minor criteria have high sensitivity and specificity (92.5% and 95% respectively).	

- Type III involves the descending thoracic aorta, the abdominal aorta and/or the renal arteries. The ascending aorta, the aortic arch and its branches are not affected.
- Type IV involves only the abdominal aorta and/or renal arteries.
- Type V has combined features of Type IIb and IV.

Management

Disease activity assessment is challenging, there is no specific immunological marker. ESR and CRP are not always reliable. Radiological imaging with digital subtraction angiography has been the gold standard for diagnosis. MR angiography and FDG –PET scan imaging techniques have an advantage that they can image vessel wall in addition to the vascular lumen and can possibly delineate minor non occlusive lesions as well as assess disease activity.[12]

ITAS 2010: Indian Takayasu's Arteritis Activity Scale has been derived from earlier Disease Extent Index (DEI.Tak) and combines imagine data to capture clinical disease activity. ITAS-A uses ESR or CRP as acute phase response parameters in addition to clinical and image abnormalities for activity assessment. They have been validated for assessment of disease activity and treatment response.[13]

Corticosteroids are the mainstay of therapy for control of disease activity. Around half the patients may be resistant to steroid therapy alone. Conventional immunomodulating drugs like azathioprine, mycophenolate, methotrexate, calcineurin inhibitors (CNIs), leflunomide are often combined to achieve a remission and for their steroid sparing effects. Cyclophosphamide has been used in severe vasculitis like retinal arteritis, myocarditis etc. Corticosteroids are generally tapered gradually closely watching disease activity for any relapse of disease activity.

Refractory disease is poorly defined. Turkish TA study group defined it as prednisolone dose > 7.5 mg/day at 6 months despite adding conventional immunosuppressant medication, new surgery due to persistent disease activity, frequent attacks and death due to disease activity.[14] Biological agents like Infliximab, rituximab and tociluzimab have been used in refractory disease with promising results. There are no good comparative studies between different immunosuppressive agents and therapy needs to be individualised.[15] Revascularization of renal arteries/ other involved arteries is required to improve tissue perfusion due to stenotic vascular lesions. Both, percutaneous angioplasty and vascular grafting are employed. Generally, interventions are performed when a satisfactory control of vascular inflammation has been achieved. Long segment lesions or heavily scarred arteries are better managed with vascular grafts due to difficulty in performing angioplasty procedures and high re-stenosis rates. In view of chronic inflammatory nature and high restenosis rates after angioplasty, surgical options are gaining favor in this predominantly young population.[16]

Other Vasculitis

Polyarteritis Nodosa (PAN)

PAN was first described in 1866 by Adolph Kussmaul and Rudolph Maier. It is a necrotizing systemic vasculitis that affects medium sized arteries and typically spares small sized blood vessels like arterioles, capillaries and venules. Clinical manifestations are similar to other systemic vasculitis, difference being that there is no small vessel involvement like pulmonary capillaritis or glomerulonephritis. American College of Rheumatology in 1990 gave classification criteria for PAN, Chapel Hill International Consensus Conference distinguished it from microscopic polyangitis (1994) and specified it as not being associated with ANCA and not involving glomeruli, capillaries, venules and arterioles (2012).[17] It thus often remains a diagnosis of exclusion. It is a rare form of vasculitis with a prevalence ranging from 2-33/ million population. Its peak incidence is in 4th-6th decade with male predominance (M:F–1.5:1).[18]

PAN had been classified as idiopathic or classical PAN and PAN secondary to infections like HBV, HCV, HIV and malignancies like hairy cell leukemia.[19] There have been newer insights in pathogenesis of necrotizing vasculitis. Association with autoinflammatory diseases and genetic disorders have been found. A high incidence of PAN is seen in patients with Familial Mediterranian Fever (FMF) an autoinflammatory disorder associated with mutation in gene MEFV encoding pyrin. Similarly, childhood onset PAN like vasculitis is seen with monogenic recessive mutation in CERC 1 gene that encodes adenosine-deaminase 2 (DADA2).[20,21] Hepatitis B associated PAN is now classified separately from classical PAN. HBV infection has been the most common infection associated with PAN and its prevalence has gone down with universal use of hepatitis B vaccinations. It is considered to be precipitated by immune complex deposition in the vessels.[22]

Idiopathic/Classical PAN by far remains the most common form of PAN with secondary causes and genetic causes being less frequent. The lesions in PAN are segmental and tend to involve areas of bifurcation. They are characterized by neutrophilic infiltration, fibrinoid necrosis of vessel wall with mural and perivascular inflammation. In the late phase infiltrate is replaced by mononuclear cells but there is lack of any granulomatous inflammation. Inflammation leads to formation of aneurysms, thrombosis and rupture of vessels.

Imaging reveals presence of microaneurysms, (1-5 mm), occlusions and stenosis in medium sized arteries. Renal involvement is common (50%-70%) followed by peripheral nerves and skin (~50%), mesentery and skeletal muscles (~30%) and CNS (~10%). Renal involvement is additionally characterized by cortical infarctions.[23]

Clinical manifestations follow the vascular bed involvement with hypertension, hematuria, pain abdomen, GI bleeds, skin ulcers and mononeuritis multiplex being common manifestations in addition to constitutional symptoms.[24,25]

Guillevin *et al.* proposed the five-factor score for prognostication of disease. This score is also used to decide intensity of treatment.[26] Corticosteroids alone may be helpful for milder disease while cyclophosphamide is added in severe cases. Azathioprine and methotrexate are used for maintenance therapy. Plasma exchange and antiviral drugs in addition to corticosteroids are recommended for HBV associated PAN and colchicine and anti-TNF therapy is employed in FMF associated PAN and DADA2 vasculitis.[20]

Behcet's Disease

It is a vasculitic illness characterized by a chronic remitting and relapsing course with recurrent oral aphthous ulcers, genital ulcerations and ocular involvement including panuveitis. It is common in Far Eastern and Mediterranean countries with highest prevalence in Turkey. HLA B 51 carrier state predisposes and infections like herpes simplex virus (HSV), streptococcus, and staphylococcus often act as triggers. It is a rare form of vasculitis that involves both arterial and venous beds. Venous involvement in Behcet's disease occurs in the form of superficial thrombophlebitis or venous thrombosis (deep venous thrombosis, Budd Chiari syndrome, portal venous or cerebral venous thrombosis etc.). Venous involvement in Behcet's disease is much more common than arterial lesions. Arterial complications are seen in only 1%-7% of patients. Arterial involvement commonly affects the aortic arch causing aneurysms and aortic regurgitation. It can also involve visceral arteries like mesenteric, splenic etc. causing stenosis. Femoral artery and coronary arterial involvement is also documented.[27]

Management is similar to other forms of vasculitis with steroids and conventional or biological immunosuppressive drugs.

Secondary Vasculitis

Connective tissue disorders like SLE, rheumatoid arthritis as well as antiphospholipid syndrome can be associated with renal vascular involvement in addition to more common renal parenchymal involvement.[28]

Vascular syphilis is an infectious aortitis and a late manifestation of syphilis. It is rare in the current post antibiotic era. It predominantly affects ascending and thoracic aorta causing aneurysmal dilatation of aortic root. It can rarely cause abdominal aortic with renal artery involvement.

Middle Aortic Syndrome

It is an anatomically described entity characterized by narrowing of aorta in the perirenal segment of abdominal aorta. It is a disorder of childhood and young adults and constitutes 0.5%-2% of all cases of aortic stenosis. There is segmental or diffuse narrowing of abdominal or distal descending thoracic aorta.

Majority of the cases are idiopathic. Association with genetic disorders like Neurofibromatosis Type 1, Alagille's syndrome, Williams syndrome as well as inflammatory disorders like Takayasu's arteritis and congenital Rubella infection has been documented.

Renal artery stenosis is the initial presentation in the majority with 60% having bilateral and another 20% having unilateral renal artery involvement. Superior mesenteric artery [around 30%] and celiac artery [around~20%] involvement is common while inferior mesenteric artery is usually spared. Isolated aortic coarctation without visceral artery involvement is seen in ~30% cases. Cases associated with genetic disorders have more extensive involvement compared to those associated with inflammatory disorders.[29]

Management is based on judicious use of anti-hypertensive medications with endovascular and surgical corrective therapy.

Summary

A variety of inflammatory and non-inflammatory conditions can result in renovascular hypertension in a young female patient. Takayasu's arteritis may be the most common cause of renovascular hypertension in young females in India. A possibility of fibromuscular dysplasia must be considered in young female patients with renovascular hypertension. Secondary causes of vasculitis and connective tissue disorders and antiphospholipid syndrome must be ruled out. As the disorders involve multiple vascular beds and may have extra vascular features, a thorough clinical examination and detailed radiological examination is mandated. Rare entities like middle aortic syndrome and auto-inflammatory disorders must be kept in differential diagnosis in appropriate clinical situations.

Diagnosis of renal artery stenosis follows standard imaging and nuclear scintigraphy techniques. MRI and FDG PET imaging may help gauge vessel wall involvement in addition to lumen and help assess disease activity in cases of vasculitis.

Hypertensive urgencies and emergencies often lead to initiation of diagnostic workup for renovascular hypertension in previously undiagnosed patient.

Management rests on making the correct diagnosis. Conditions like fibromuscular dysplasia are immensely responsive to percutaneous interventions and percutaneous transluminal angioplasty is often curative. On the other hand, inflammatory vessel wall involvement as in Takayasu's vasculitis requires both a control of disease activity with steroids and conventional or biological immunomodulating agents as well as vascular interventions either surgical or percutaneous. In view of young age of these patients and a high rate of restenosis after percutaneous interventions surgical correction is gaining preference.

Regular monitoring, clinical and radiological, is required to prevent restenosis, relapse of disease activity and organ damage.

References

1. Goldblatt H. Studies on experimental hypertension: XII. The experimental production and pathogenesis of hypertension due to renal ischemia. Am J Clin Pathol 1940;10(10):40-72.
2. Stephen CT. Renal Arterial Disease and Hypertension. Med Clin North Am 2017;101(1):65-79.
3. Al-Katib S, Shetty M, Jafri SM, Jafri SZ. Radiologic Assessment of Native Renal Vasculature: A Multimodality Review. Radiographics 2017;37(1):136-56.
4. Plouin PF, Perdu J, La Batide-Alanore A *et al.* Fibromuscular dysplasia. Orphanet J Rare Dis 2007;2:28.
5. Chugh KS, Jain S, Sakhuja V, *et al.* Renovascular hypertension due to Takayasu's arteritis among Indian patients. Quart J Med 1992;85:833-43.
6. Narula N1, Kadian-Dodov D1, Olin JW2. Fibromuscular Dysplasia: Contemporary Concepts and Future Directions. Prog Cardiovasc Dis 2018 Mar-Apr;60(6):580-85.
7. Olin JW, Gornik HL, Bacharach JM *et al.* Fibromuscular Dysplasia: State of the Science and Critical Unanswered Questions. A Scientific Statement From the American Heart Association. Circulation 2014;129:1048-78.
8. Jain S, Pondaiah SK Takayasu's arteritis: Review of epidemiology and etiopathogenesis. Indian Journal of Rheumatology 2015;10(1):S22-S29.
9. Parakh R, Yadav A.Takayasu's Arteritis: An Indian Perspective, Eur J Vasc Endovasc Surg 2007;33,578-82.
10. Sharma BK, Siveski-Iliskovic N, Singal PK. Takayasu arteritis may be underdiagnosed in North America. Can I Cardiol 1995;11:311-16.
11. Hata A, Noda M, Moriwaki R, Numano F. Angiographic findings of Takayasu arteritis: New classification. Int J Cardiol 1996;54 Suppl:S155-63.
12. Alibaz-Öner F, Aydın SZ, Direskeneli H. Recent advances in Takayasu's arteritis. Eur J Rheumatol 2015;1:24-30.
13. Misra R, Danda D, Rajappa SM, Ghosh A, Gupta R, Mahendranath KM, *et al.* Indian Rheumatology Vasculitis (IRAVAS) group. Development and initial validation of the Indian Takayasu Clinical Activity Score (ITAS2010). Rheumatology (Oxford) 2013;52:1795-801.
14. Sahin Z, Bıcakcıgil M, Aksu K, Kamali S, Akar S, Onen F, *et al.* Takayasu's arteritis is associated with HLA-B*52, but not with HLA-B*51, in Turkey. Arthritis Res Ther 2012; 14: R27.
15. Pacheco RL, Latorraca COC, de Souza AWS, Pachito DV, Riera R. Clinical interventions for Takayasu arteritis: A systematic review. Int. J. Clin. Pract 2017;71(11).
16. Comarmond C, Biard L, Lambert M, *et al.* French Takayasu Network. Long-Term Outcomes and Prognostic Factors of Complications in Takayasu Arteritis: A Multicenter Study of 318 patients. Circulation 2017;136(12):1114-22.
17. Jennette JC *et al.* (2013) 2012 revised International Chapel Hill Consensus Conference Nomenclature of Vasculitides. Arthritis Rheum 65(1):1-11.
18. Watts RA *et al.* Epidemiology of systemic vasculitis: A 10-year study in the United Kingdom. Arthritis Rheum 2000;43(2):414-19.
19. Hernandez-Rodriguez J *et al.* Diagnosis and classification of polyarteritis nodosa. J Autoimmun 2014;48-49:84-89.
20. Ozen S. The changing face of polyarteritis nodosa and necrotizing vasculitis. Nat Rev Rheumatol 2017 Jun; 13(6):381-86.
21. Navon Elkan P *et al.* (2014) Mutant adenosine deaminase 2 in a polyarteritis nodosa vasculopathy. N Engl J Med 2014; 370(10):921-31.
22. Guillevin L *et al.* Polyarteritis nodosa related to hepatitis B virus. A prospective study with long-term observation of 41 patients. Medicine (Baltimore) 1995;74,238-53.
23. Travers RL *et al.* Polyarteritis nodosa: A clinical and angiographic analysis of 17 cases. Semin Arthritis Rheum 1979;8(3):184-99.
24. Pagnoux C *et al.* Clinical features and outcomes in 348 patients with polyarteritis nodosa: A systematic retrospective study of patients diagnosed between 1963 and 2005 and entered into the French Vasculitis Study Group Database. Arthritis Rheum 2010;62(2):616-26.
25. el-Reshaid K *et al.* The spectrum of renal disease associated with microscopic polyangiitis and classic polyarteritis nodosa in Kuwait. Nephrol Dial Transplant 1997;12(9):1874-82.
26. Guillevin L *et al.* The Five-Factor Score revisited: Assessment of prognoses of systemic necrotizing vasculitides based on the French Vasculitis Study Group (FVSG) cohort. Medicine (Baltimore) 2011;90(1):19-27.
27. Calamiaa KT, Schirmerb M and Melikogluc M. Major vessel involvement in Behcet's disease: An update. Current Opinion in Rheumatology 2011;23:24-31.
28. Turrent-Carriles A, Herrera-Félix JP, Amigo MC. Renal Involvement in Antiphospholipid Syndrome. Front Immunol 2018;9:1008.
29. Rumman RK, Nickel C, Matsuda-Abedini M. Disease Beyond the Arch: A Systematic Review of Middle Aortic Syndrome in Childhood. American Journal of Hypertension 2015;28:833-46.

CHAPTER

A Patient with Polycystic Kidney Disease

Vikas Makkar[1], Hemanth Kumar MK[2], Sudhir Mehta[3]

[1] *Professor, Nephrology, Dayanand Medical College, Ludhiana*

[2] *Associate Consultant, Nephrology, Paras Hospital, Gurugram*

[3] *Assistant Professor, Nephrology, Maharishi Markandeshwar Institute of Medical Sciences and Research, Mullana, Ambala, Haryana*

CASE

A 32 years old male patient presented to the clinic with history of right flank pain and gross hematuria since 3 days. There was no history of fever or dysuria. He had no previous history of hypertension and no history of any previous episodes of hematuria. Family history was positive for presence of renal failure with polycystic kidney disease in the mother and maternal grandfather.

On examination, he had tachycardia, BP- 150/90 mm Hg. Per abdomen examination revealed bilateral palpable kidneys with tenderness over the right flank.

His investigations: Hb-12 gm/dl, TLC-11,000/cmm with 76% polymorphs and platelet count-2,25,000/cmm. B. Urea-32 mg/dl, S. Creatinine-0.78 mg/dl, Na/K/Cl-136/4.3/98 meq/l.

Urine routine: 1+proteinuria, 100-120 RBC/hpf, 15-20 WBC/hpf with no RBC casts.

USG abdomen: Bilaterally enlarged kidneys with right kidney measuring 15.5 cm and left kidney measuring 14.2 cms. Multiple cysts in both kidneys of varying size involving both cortex and medulla. There was a hyperechoic focus in a cyst in the right kidney suggestive of cyst hemorrhage.

This patient is having autosomal dominant polycystic kidney disease which presented with cyst hemorrhage with flank pain and hematuria.

Discussion

In healthy individuals, sporadic renal cysts are quite common. By USG, one cyst is present in 1.7% of healthy individuals aged 30–49 years, in 11.5% of individuals aged 50–70 years and in 22.1% of those older than 70 years. Bilateral renal cysts can be visualized in 1%, 4% and 9% of the same age groups, respectively (Flowcharts 22.1 and 22.2).

- Autosomal dominant polycystic kidney disease (ADPKD) and Autosomal recessive polycystic kidney disease (ARPKD) are always accompanied by renal cysts, both in cortex and medulla. In other disease entities such as nephronophthisis, Senior-Løken syndrome, Joubert syndrome, Bardet-Biedl syndrome, Meckel-Gruber syndrome, Von Hippel-Lindau syndrome (VHL) or Tuberous sclerosis complex (TSC), renal cysts are not an obligatory finding; moreover, in nephronophthisis and Medullary cystic kidney disease (MCKD), cysts are found predominantly at the corticomedullary junction with normal or small sized kidney.
- In VHL syndrome and TSC, kidney size is usually enlarged and presence of renal cell carcinoma and angiomyolipomas of the kidney strongly suggest towards these entities.
- If renal involvement is asymmetrical and strictly or mostly unilateral cystic localization is present, then nonprogressive localized renal cystic disease, segmental multicystic dysplasia, or cystic tumours should be considered.

Autosomal Dominant Polycystic Kidney Disease (ADPKD)

Genetics and Pathogenesis

ADPKD is most common monogenic kidney disease with incidence of 1 in 400 to 1 in 1000. It is the most common genetic cause of end stage renal disease (ESRD) with 2/3rd of the patients developing ESRD in their lifetime. It is transmitted in an autosomal dominant pattern with almost complete penetrance with only 10% being sporadic with no family history. But the phenotype in ADPKD is recessive, since it requires mutations in both the alleles. The cyst formation in the kidney and liver is presumably triggered by an additional somatic mutation of the second allele in a limited number of cells (second-hit hypothesis) leading to clinical disease.

It has a more progressive course in men than in women and women usually exhibit smaller kidney size and develop ESRD later in life than men.

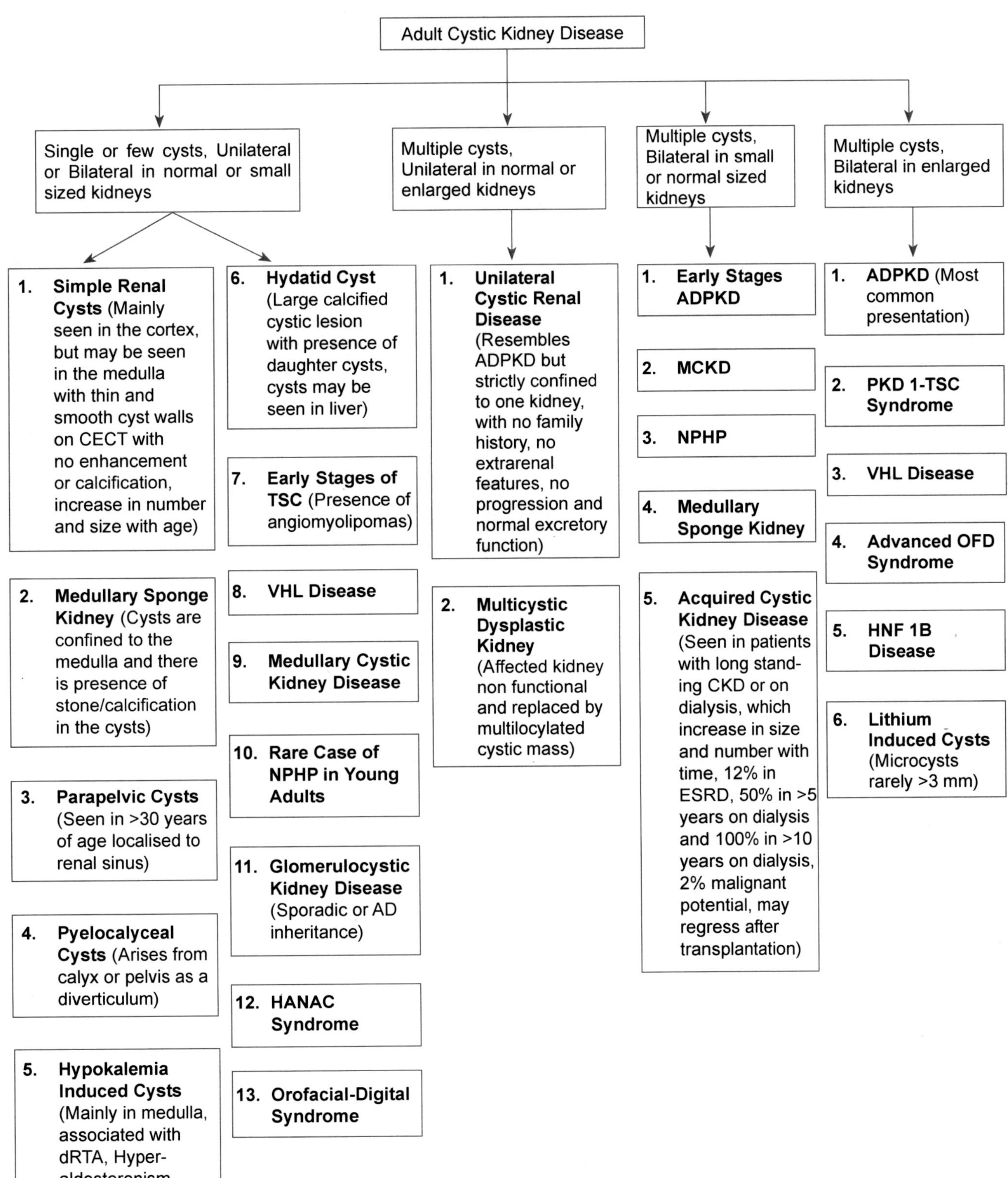

Flowchart 22.1: Adult cystic kidney disease

ADPKD: Autosomal dominant polycystic kidney disease; ARPKD: Autosomal recessive polycystic kidney disease; VHL: Von Hippel-Lindau syndrome; TSC: Tuberous sclerosis complex; NPHP: Nephronophthisis; HANAC: Hereditary angiopathy with nephropathy, aneurysms and muscle cramps syndrome; MCKD: Medullary cystic kidney disease; OFDS: Oral-facial-digital syndrome; HNF1B: Hepatocyte nuclear factor 1β.

Yet Another Approach to Cystic Kidney Disease in Adults

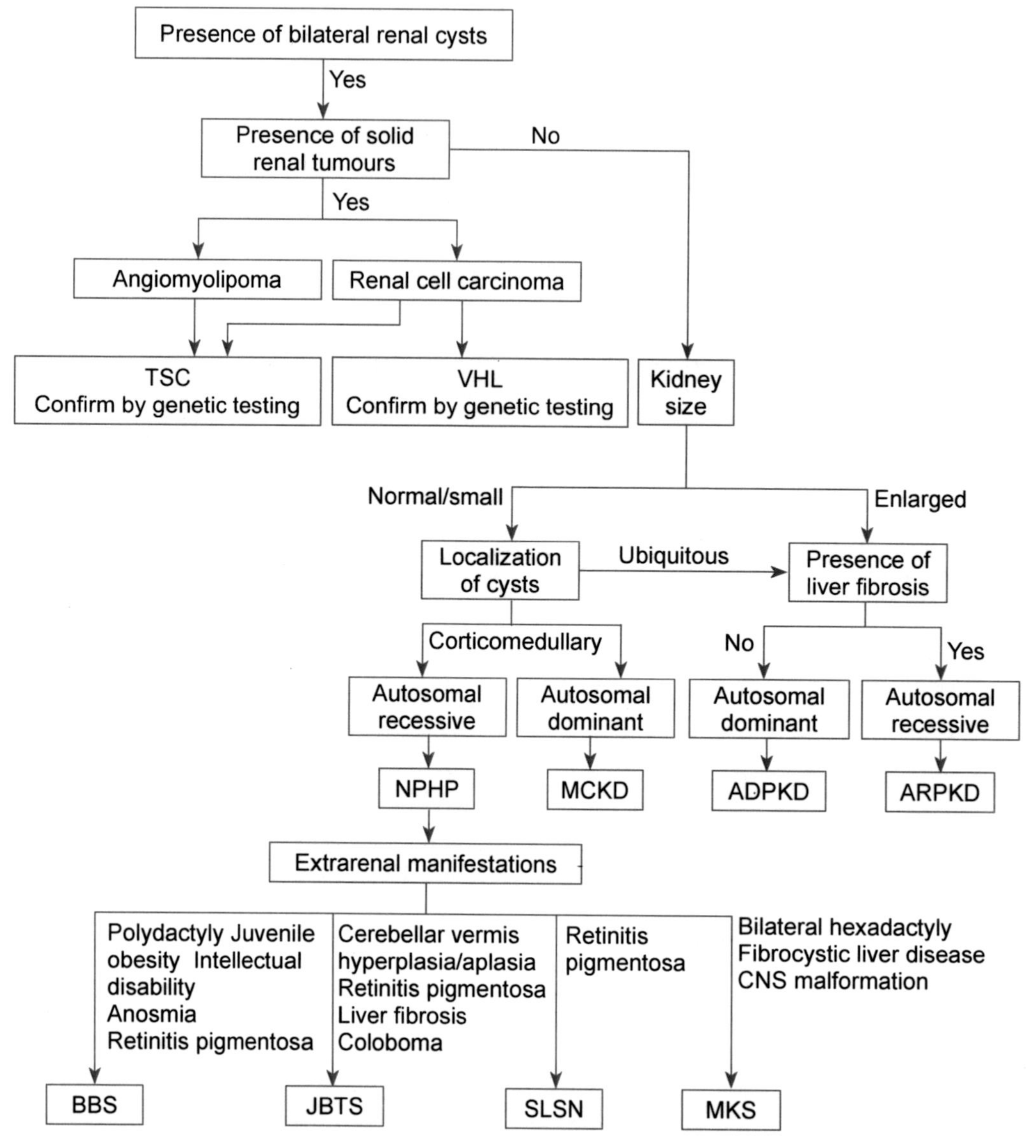

Flowchart 22.2: Cystic kidney disease in adults

NPHP: Nephronophthisis; MCKD: Medullary cystic kidney disease; ADPKD: Autosomal dominant polycystic kidney disease; ARPKD: Autosomal recessive polycystic kidney disease; BBS: Bardet-Biedl syndrome; JBTS: Joubert syndrome; SLNS: Senior-Loken syndrome; MKS: Meckel syndrome.

Almost 85% of the cases have PKD 1(Chr. 16p) gene and 15% have PKD 2 (Chr. 4q) gene. Both proteins localize to the primary cilia and are essential for their correct function. These proteins constitute a mechanosensory ion channel complex, and have an important function in tubular differentiation and maintenance. PKD 1 develop cysts at an earlier stage than those with PKD 2 and the progression to ESRD is also faster with PKD 1 (mean age 54 years) as compared to PKD 2 (mean age 74 years) and mutations in 5′ region of PKD 1 gene associated with earlier onset of ESRD as compared to 3′ mutations (53 vs 56 years).

In PKD 1, 65% are truncating mutations and 35% are non-truncating and in PKD 2, 87% truncating and 13% non truncating.

1-2% of ADPKD may manifest in utero or in infancy, may be associated with HNF1B gene, PKHD 1 gene or TSC 2 gene mutations in addition to PKD1 gene.

Cysts arise from all segments of nephron and <1% of the tubules in the kidney form the cysts.

Diagnosis

Denver Polycystic Kidney Disease Research Group (1997) found 60% of children < 5 years and 75-80% of children 5-18 years of age with PKD1 mutation had renal cysts.

Modified Ravine Criteria for Diagnosis/exclusion of ADPKD by ultrasound (US) are given in Tables 22.1 and 22.2.

Table 22.1: Modified Ravine criteria for diagnosis of ADPKD by ultrasound (Pei *et al.*, 2009)

Age (in yr)	PKD 1	PKD 2	Unknown
15-30 (≥ 3 cysts Unilateral or Bilateral)	PPV - 100% Sensitivity - 94%	PPV - 100% Sensitivity - 69%	PPV - 100% Sensitivity - 82%
30-39 (≥ 3 cysts Unilateral or Bilateral)	PPV - 100% Sensitivity - 97%	PPV - 100% Sensitivity - 95%	PPV - 100% Sensitivity - 95%
40-59 (≥ 2 cysts in each kidney Bilateral)	PPV - 100% Sensitivity - 93%	PPV - 100% Sensitivity - 89%	PPV - 100% Sensitivity - 90%
≥ 60 years (≥ 4 cysts in each kidney Bilateral)	PPV - 100% Sensitivity - 100%	PPV - 100% Sensitivity - 100%	PPV - 100% Sensitivity - 100%

Table 22.2: Ultrasound criteria for exclusion of ADPKD (Pei *et al.*, 2009)

Age (in yr)	PKD 1	PKD 2	Unknown
15-30 (≤ 1 cyst)	NPV - 99% Specificity - 98%	NPV - 83% Specificity - 97%	NPV - 91% Specificity - 97%
30-39 (≤ 1 cyst)	NPV - 100% Specificity - 96%	NPV - 97% Specificity - 94%	NPV - 98% Specificity - 95%
40-59 (≤ 1 cyst)	NPV - 100% Specificity - 94%	NPV - 100% Specificity - 94%	NPV - 100% Specificity - 94%

In those individuals where US is equivocal, presence of >10 cysts in total on MRI/CT in subjects who are at high risk for ADPKD with a positive family history, older than 15 years has a diagnostic specificity and sensitivity of 100% whereas <5 cysts may be considered as a criteria for exclusion.

In the absence of a family history of cystic kidney disease, the presence of bilaterally enlarged kidneys with multiple cysts or bilateral renal cysts as well as hepatic cysts suggest ADPKD, provided that any additional renal or extrarenal manifestations do not point towards a different disease.

Progression of Disease (Flowchart 22.3)

- The progression of the disease may be associated with the Total Kidney Volume (TKV) and the change in TKV from baseline bears a prognostic significance in terms of progression of kidney disease (CRISP study). Height adjusted TKV of 600 ml/m^2 was predicted the progression to CKD stage 3 in next 8 years.
- Factors associated with rapid increase in TKV are PKD1, high urinary sodium excretion, high urinary osmolality, low HDL-Cholesterol, lower renal blood flow and sickle cell trait.
- Renal volume >1500 ml associated with fastest decline in GFR (or a kidney size >16.5 cm in <45 years).
- Other risk factors for rapid loss of kidney functions include hypertension, age <35 years, male gender, black race, higher grades of proteinuria, onset of hematuria <30 years and multiple pregnancies.
- Once the renal function starts to decline, average decline in GFR is 4.4-5.9 ml/min/yr.
- ERA-EDTA defines rapid progression as an annual fall in eGFR >5 ml/min/1.73 m^2 in 1 yr or >2.5 ml/min/1.73 m^2 per year over 5 years or a TKV increase of >5%/year by repeated measurements (at least 3 or more each atleast 6 months apart and by MRI).

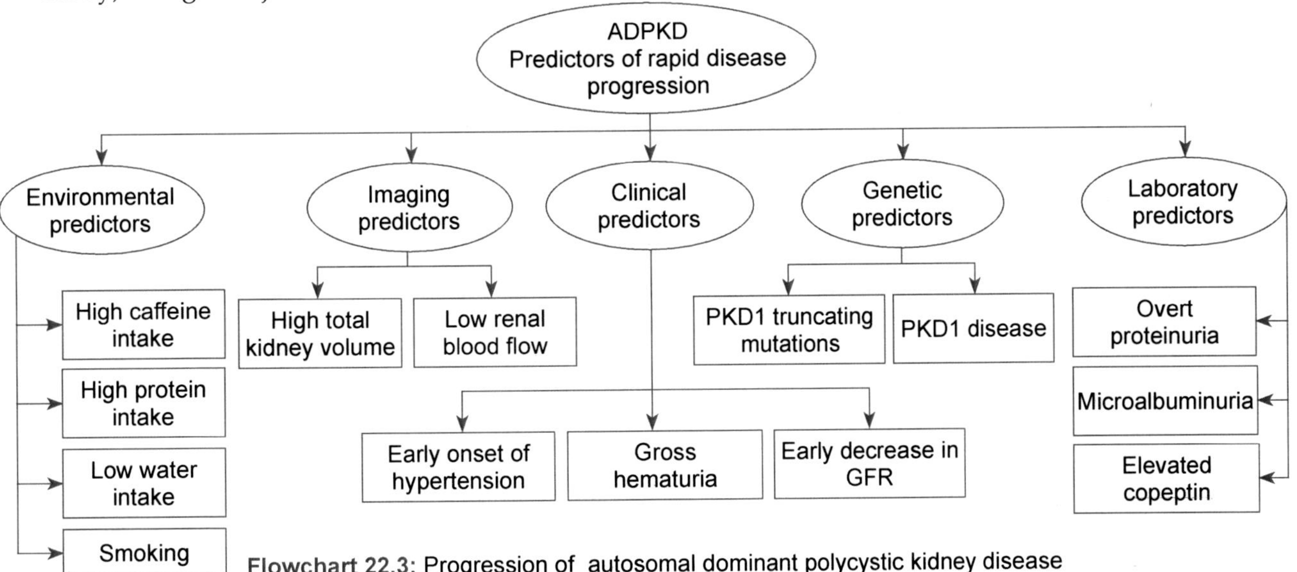

Flowchart 22.3: Progression of autosomal dominant polycystic kidney disease

- The Mayo Classification of ADPKD into typical (Class 1) and atypical (Class 2) cysts. Class 1 included bilateral diffuse cysts in both kidneys and all cysts contributing similarly to TKV with mild to severe replacement of kidney tissue by cysts. Further Class 1 was classified to 1A to 1E according to htTKV to predict progression (Fig. 22.1).
- The incidence of ESRD at 10 years increased by subclass (1A–1E), being 2.4, 11.0, 37.8, 47.1 and 66.9%, respectively. So Class 1C-1E were considered as rapid progression (Irazabel *et al.*).
- PRO-PKD score (2015) was formulated to predict the risk of progression.

> - **Being male:** 1 point
> - **Hypertension before 35 years of age:** 2 points
> - **First urological event (macroscopic hematuria, flank pain or cyst infection) before 35 years of age:** 2 points
> - **PKD2 mutation:** 0 point
> - **Non-truncating PKD1 mutation:** 2 points
> - **Truncating PKD1 mutation:** 4 points
>
> A score of ≤ 3 excludes progression to ESRD before the age of 60 years with a negative predictive value of 81.4%.
>
> A score of > 6 predicts rapid disease progression with ESRD onset before the age of 60 years with a positive predictive value of 90.9%.
>
> For those with an intermediate score (4-6 points), the prognosis is unclear.

- The initial manifestation of ADPKD is a defect in urine-concentrating capability with onset in childhood many of whom report polydipsia and polyuria at an early stage of disease.

The Important Causes of Loin Pain in ADPKD

1. **Renal cystic change per se:** May present with chronic pain, unilateral or bilateral due to distension of the renal capsule or traction on the renal pedicle or musculoskeletal pain due to large cysts.
2. **Renal cyst hemorrhage or rupture:** Present with acute pain with low grade fever and leukocytosis. CT/MRI may suggest the diagnosis, differentiation from cyst infection is difficult.
   - Hematuria may or may not be present depending on whether the ruptured cyst communicates with the pelvicalyceal system.
   - Incidence of gross hematuria in ADPKD is 42% with mean age 30 years and tendency for recurrent episodes. Risk factors for hematuria include larger TKV, renal failure, hypertension and PKD1.
   - Usually hematuria lasts for < 1 week and without hemodynamic compromise but if more severe may need embolisation or even nephrectomy.
   - Other causes of hematuria included nephrolithiasis and cyst infection.
3. **Renal cyst infection:** Present with acute pain, high grade fever and local tenderness. CT/MRI may suggest the diagnosis but the most sensitive are PET scan and culture from cyst aspirate. Galium or Indium labelled Leukocyte scans also can be helpful.

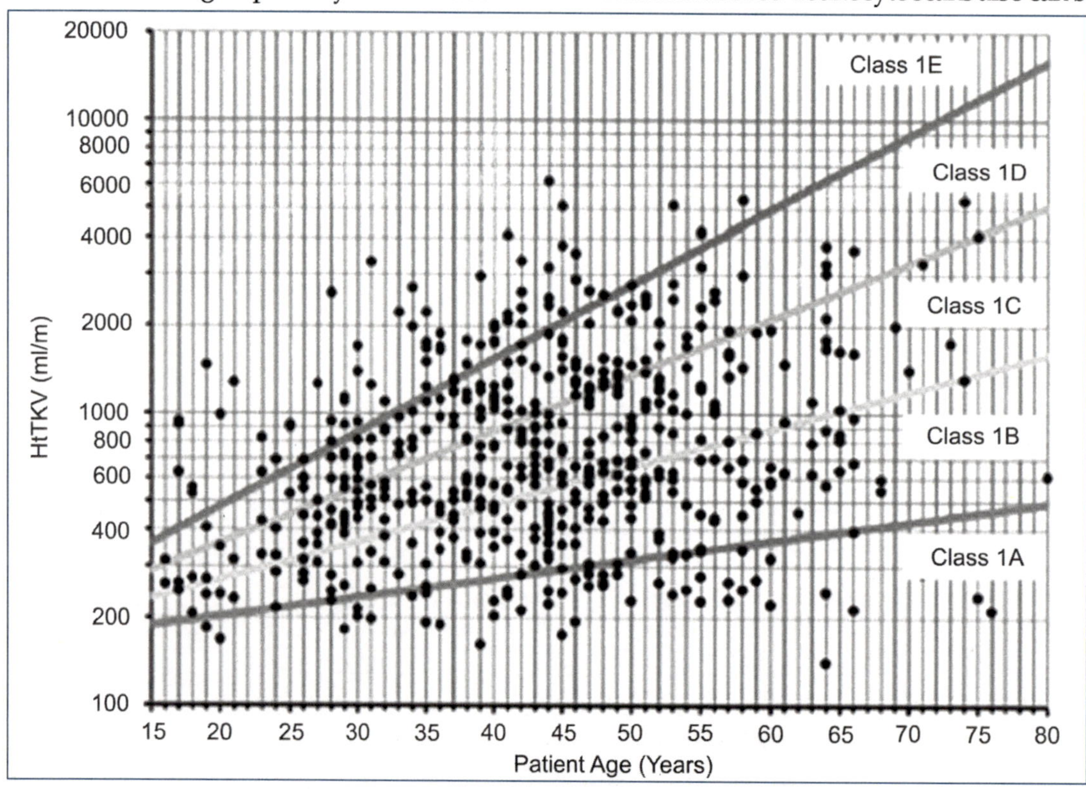

Figure 22.1: The Mayo classification of ADPKD
Class 1 was classified to 1A to 1E according to htTKV to predict progression

- Cyst infection occurs in 50% of patients in their lifetime in ADPKD and more common in women. If the infected cyst does not communicate with the pelvicalyceal system, the urine culture may be negative.
- Caused by gram negative coliforms usually and antibiotics like fluoroquinolones with good cyst penetration must be used.
- Drugs that can be detected in cysts are lipid soluble and secreted through tubules or have high pKa values. These include erythromycin, vancomycin, cefotaxime, ampicillin, and trimethoprim-sulfamethoxazole. Drugs active against anaerobes such as metronidazole and clindamycin also achieve therapeutic concentrations in cysts.

4. **Pyelonephritis:** Presents with pain which may be more diffuse and bilateral, urine and blood cultures may be positive.
5. **Nephrolithiasis:** May cause acute or recurrent loin pain or hematuria. CT scan is most sensitive. Risk factors for nephrolithiasis include large kidney size, hypocitraturia and low urinary pH. Incidence of nephrolithiasis is 30% in ADPKD and the most common stones are uric acid and calcium oxalate.
6. **Malignancy:** Although the incidence is not different from that of general population, renal cell carcinoma (RCC) can be more metastatic, bilateral, multicentric, younger age of onset and more constitutional symptoms.

Other causes of pain abdomen include:

1. **Liver Cysts:** Hepatic cysts are the most common extrarenal feature of ADPKD and are evident on MRI in 58%, 85% and 94% of patients aged 15–24, 25–34 and 35–46 years. These originate from biliary ducts and peribiliary glands.

   Liver cyst hemorrhage or infection or rupture can lead to abdominal pain and fever.

   The liver cysts are larger in females (as these cysts have estrogen receptors) and massive liver cysts are seen only in females with history of multiple pregnancies or OC pills.

   Liver function impairment is very rare. Polycystic Liver Disease is the only extra-renal manifestation for which mortality is increased in patients on dialysis.
2. **Colonic Diverticulosis:** Present with left iliac fossa pain, diarrhoea or rectal bleed, diagnosed with CT scan.
3. **Abdominal wall hernias.**

Extra Cystic Manifestations of ADPKD

1. **Hypertension:**
   - Early feature of ADPKD- 60% of patients before significant loss of renal function (median age 32-34 years). HTN is present universally in all patients on dialysis.
   - Risk factors for earlier occurrence of hypertension in ADPKD are PKD 1, larger kidney volume, family history of hypertension in parents with ADPKD and male gender.
   - Left ventricular hypertrophy (LVH)–50% of patients with hypertension.
   - Those with intensive blood pressure control have a slower increase in cyst volume and a decrease in LV mass (HALT-PKD).
   - The activation of intra-renal RAAS–important role in hypertension due to local ischemia from expanding cysts and decreased renal blood flow.
   - The leading cause of death in ADPKD is cardiovascular (CV) disease but the incidence of CV mortality in ADPKD patients on dialysis is lower than non-diabetic patients on dialysis.
2. **Valvular Heart Disease:**
   - Mitral valve prolapse (MVP) seen in 25%.
   - Mitral regurgitation (MR) may be seen which can be hemodynamically significant.
   - Aortic regurgitation (AR) may be seen in 8-20%.
3. **Aneurysmal Disease: (Flowchart 22.4)**
   - Intracranial aneurysm (ICA) seen in 8% patients (6-12% in those with a negative family history and 16-21% in those with a positive family history)–85% are in anterior circulation and mostly <6 mm.
   - PKD 1 with mutations in 5′ region have higher chance of having an ICA and rupture.
   - Other vascular abnormalities are–dolichoectasias, thoracic aorta and cervicocephalic artery dissection and coronary artery aneurysms.
   - The only risk factor for ICA is a family history of ICA.
   - **Symptoms:** Subarachnoid haemorrhage (SAH), Intracranial haemorrhage (ICH) (sudden intense worst headache), symptoms of compression of adjacent structures and focal ischemia due to embolism.
   - Average time of ICA rupture is 41 years.
   - The risk of rupture was very low (0.05%) in patients with <10 mm aneurysm without previous history of rupture vs. 0.5% in patients with previous history of SAH and the risk increased progressively with increasing size.
   - Screening in asymptomatic patients is indicated in those with a family history of aneurysm, previous history of aneurysmal rupture, before major elective surgery or in high risk professions like pilot or bus drivers.
   - If Time of flight angiography (TOF)–MRI is positive for ICA, screen annually and if negative re-screening every 5-10 years.
   - Aggressive control of BP and elimination of smoking is indicated.
   - However ischemic stroke and hypertensive non-aneurysmal hemorrhage are more common

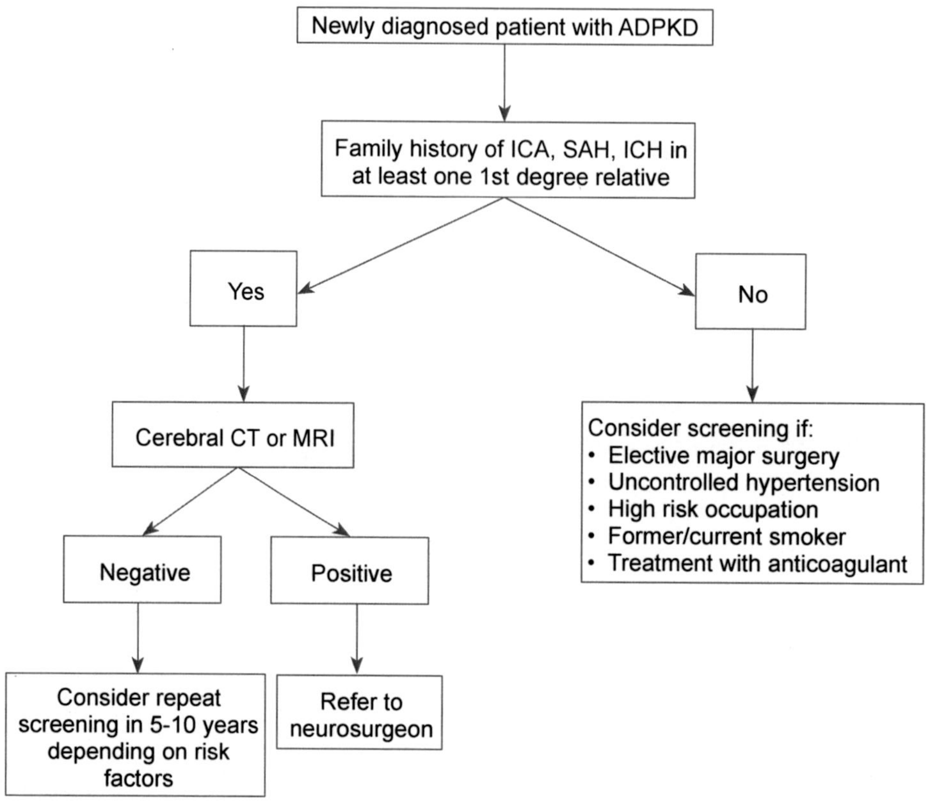

Flowchart 22.4: Aneurysmal disease in ADPKD patient

cause of neurological symptoms in ADPKD than aneurysmal bleed.

Cysts in Other Part of Body

1. Liver cyst–80%.
2. Pancreatic cysts–5%.
3. Cysts in ejaculatory ducts and seminal vesicles–50%.
4. Arachnoid cysts–8%.

Genetic Testing Indication

1. In case of diagnostic uncertainty especially when they present with early onset symptoms or severe disease with no family history.
2. In case of potential living related donors.
3. Those considering prenatal or pre-implantation diagnosis.

Linkage analysis may need large number of family members to be tested and also indirect and may be confounded by de novo disease or mosaicism. Sanger's sequencing are used. Next generations sequencing (NGS) yields better results.

Newer Concepts in Treatment of ADPKD

Care of ADPKD patients mainly involve supportive measures, due to the lack of targeted therapeutic strategies. The management is confined to symptoms and complications of ADPKD, including blood pressure and pain control, in addition to antibiotic treatment of cyst infections and treatment of renal stones.The newer targeted therapies are still evolving in clinical practice.

Blood Pressure Goals in ADPKD

The HALT PKD study, a 7-year randomized placebo-controlled interventional trial, showed benefits of rigorous blood pressure control (blood pressure target of <110/70 mm Hg) on kidney volume progression rate, left ventricular mass index, and urinary albumin excretion in patients with early ADPKD. This study changed our current treatment strategies for younger patients with early ADPKD (eGFR >60 ml/min) to target a blood pressure of <110/70 mm Hg. For patients with more advanced ADPKD (eGFR <60 ml/min) or older individuals, it is reasonable to target a blood pressure of 130/80 or below especially in the presence of proteinuria. This low blood pressure goal was well tolerated and easy to achieve.

The choice of antihypertensive is either an ACE inhibitor/ARB or calcium channel blocker. Given the mechanism of hypertension as well as the benefit of RAAS blockade in reducing proteinuria and reducing intraglomerular pressure, ACEi may be preferred. However, calcium channel blockers have been found to be equally effective in controlling hypertension.

Diet and Fluid Intake in ADPKD

Protein restriction of 0.8 g/kg for patients with CKD stage 3-5, not on dialysis is usually well-tolerated by patients. It is not known to be associated with malnutrition or other harmful effects.

A high-protein diet is believed to contribute to protein-induced hyperfiltration as in other causes of CKD. An increase in the filtered load of amino acids may enhance proximal sodium reabsorption via sodium-amino acid cotransporters in the proximal tubule. The decrease in sodium chloride delivery to the macula densa may then activate tubuloglomerular feedback, leading to an elevation in glomerular filtration rate in an attempt to restore macula densa delivery back to normal.

Another potential harmful effect of high-protein intake on ADPKD is the stimulation of vasopressin secretion associated with high-osmolar daily load in the context of fixed water ingestion.

High water intake has been proposed as a physiological approach to decrease vasopressin secretion in patients with ADPKD and patients are advised to consume 2–3 litres of fluid daily.

Higher sodium intake in subjects participating both in the CRISP and HALT cohorts was associated with more rapid progression of the disease. It is reasonable to advise all patients with ADPKD to limit sodium intake to 1500–2000 mg (65–88 mEq) per day not only for the control of blood pressure but also of cystic disease progression.

Role of V2 Receptor Blockade

One of the key strategies to slow down disease progression is the reduction of intracellular cAMP levels, which can be achieved efficiently by blocking vasopressin receptor signalling.

Tolvaptan is a potent, highly selective, orally available, V2 receptor antagonist. In 2012, tolvaptan was proven to significantly reduce both kidney growth and loss of estimated glomerular filtration rate (eGFR) in the 3-year randomized double-blinded placebo controlled TEMPO 3:4 trial, which enrolled 1445 ADPKD patients from 129 sites aged 18 and 50 years old, with a baseline TKV >750 ml and CrCL>60 ml/min.

Results at 3-year showed a reduction in the rate of kidney growth by 49% with tolvaptan during the 3-year trial; TKV increased an average of 2.8% per year in patients treated with tolvaptan versus 5.5% per year growth rate in the placebo group. Treatment effect was greatest from baseline to year 1 but continued to be significant from year 1 to year 2 and from year 2 to year 3.

The administration of tolvaptan was also associated with a reduction in the rate of renal function decline measured by the slope of the reciprocal of serum creatinine from -3.81 $(mg/ml)^{-1}$ per year on placebo to -2.61 $(mg/ml)^{-1}$ per year on tolvaptan ($p < 0.001$).

Consequently, in 2015 tolvaptan was approved by the European Medicines Agency (EMA) for the treatment of adult patients with ADPKD-CKD stages 1–3 at treatment initiation with evidence of rapid disease progression.

In the more recent REPRISE trial, 1370 patients with ADPKD who were either 18 to 55 years of age with an estimated GFR of 25 to 65 ml per minute per 1.73 m^2 of body-surface area or 56 to 65 years of age with an estimated GFR of 25 to 44 ml per minute per 1.73 m^2 were randomly assigned in a 1:1 ratio to receive tolvaptan or placebo for 12 months.

The change from baseline in the estimated GFR was -2.34 ml per minute per 1.73 m^2 in the tolvaptan group, as compared with -3.61 ml per minute per 1.73 m^2 in the placebo group ($P< 0.001$).

Safety Instructions Related to Use of Tolvaptan

- Hypersensitivity to drug.
- Liver injury.
- Volume depletion.
- Hypernatremia.
- Pregnancy/breastfeeding–not indicated.

Autosomal Recessive Polycystic Kidney Disease (ARPKD)

The incidence of ARPKD varies from 1:20,000 to 1:40,000. ARPKD is caused by mutations in the PKHD1 gene on chromosome 6p12, encoding for a multidomain integral membrane protein called fibrocystin.

The first-time finding of large polycystic kidneys in an adult patient without hepatic fibrosis makes ARPKD a highly unlikely diagnosis.The predominant characteristics in adult patients presenting with ARPKD and fairly well-preserved kidney function are hepatosplenomegaly and hepatic fibrosis.The complications of liver disease (such as due to portal hypertension) are the most frequent presentation, though chronic renal insufficiency is also present in adult patients.

As hepatocytes are not involved, hepatocellular dysfunction is rare and liver enzymes are characteristically not increased. Recurrent cholangitis is not uncommon, and adults with ARPKD are at increased risk of cholangiocarcinomas.

Affected fetuses often have oligohydramnios leading to fetal constraint and the "Potter sequence" that consists of characteristic dysmorphic facies, pulmonary hypoplasia and limb defects.

The estimated perinatal mortality rate is 30% because of respiratory insufficiency. In patients who survive the first month of life, 1-year survival rates of 92% to 95% have been reported. The kidney survival rate of neonatal survivors is 86% at 5 years and decreased to 42% at 20 years.

ARPKD kidneys in utero are hyperechoic and display "decreased" corticomedullary differentiation because of the hyperechoic medulla. In comparison, ADPKD kidneys in utero tend to be moderately enlarged with a hyperechoic cortex and relatively hypoechoic medulla causing "increased" corticomedullary differentiation.

In addition, high-resolution US can detect the fusiform dilatations of branching collecting ducts that are readily distinguished from the round cysts of ADPKD.

Also usually kidney size in ARPKD stabilizes or may decrease over time and does not show progressive enlargement as in ADPKD.

ARPKD is always associated with biliary dysgenesis, some degree of congenital hepatic fibrosis and dilatation of the intrahepatic bile ducts.

The characteristic histological features of ARPKD are fusiform dilatation of the renal collecting ducts and distal tubuli combined with defects in the ductal plate and hyperplasia of biliary ducts.

Biliary dysgenesis leads to both congenital hepatic fibrosis and Caroli disease (dilatation of the intrahepatic bile ducts).

The diagnosis of ARPKD can be established by the detection of enlarged, echogenic kidneys showing reduced corticomedullary differentiation at ultrasonography, plus at least one of the following criteria:

1. No renal cysts detected by ultrasound scanning in both parents, particularly if the parents are more than 40 years of age.
2. Radiographic, clinical or laboratory evidence of hepatic fibrosis.
3. Hepatic pathology that indicates ductal plate abnormalities.
4. Existence of a sibling with confirmed ARPKD.
5. Parental consanguinity or a family history of autosomal recessive disease.

Table 22.3: Syndromes associated with cystic kidney diseases

NPHP	Polydipsia, polyuria, urine-concentrating defects and secondary enuresis in childhood; tubulointerstitial nephropathy, corticomedullary cysts, tubular basement membrane thickening and disruption	Numerous possible extrarenal complications, largely depending upon the exact mutation. Many extrarenal complications of NPHP are described as separate syndromes	18 known subtypes (NPHP1-18), accounting for 40% of cases
MCKD	Tubulointerstitial nephritis, renal cysts, hyperuricemia, gout, small-sized kidneys	None identified to date	MUC1 mutations are associated with type 1 disease; mutations in UMOD1 account for 17.8% of type 2 disease
Senior-Løken syndrome	Similar to NPHP	Retinitis pigmentosa	Always observed in NPHP5 and NPHP6, can also occur in most other subtypes of NPHP except NPHP7
Joubert syndrome	Similar to NPHP	Cerebellar vermis hypoplasia or aplasia, liver fibrosis, retinitis pigmentosa, coloboma of the eye, altered neonatal respiration	Mutations in 21 different genes
Meckel-Gruber syndrome	Similar to NPHP	Bilateral postaxial hexadactyly, hepatobiliary ductal dysgenesis causing fibrocystic liver disease, CNS malformations, usually occipital encephalocele	Mutations in 11 different genes
Bardet-Biedl syndrome	Similar to NPHP	Polydactyly, juvenile obesity, mental retardation, retinal defects, anosmia, hypogonadism	BBS1-19 account for 80% of cases
VHL syndrome	Renal cell carcinoma, multiple renal cysts, resembling ADPKD	Hemangioblastomas in the CNS (retina, brain and spinal cord); possible pheochromocytomas, pancreatic cysts, pancreatic neuroendocrine tumors, endolymphatic sac tumors of the inner ear, cystadenomas of the epididymis and broad ligament	Autosomal dominant mutations in VHL
Tuberous sclerosis complex	Renal cell carcinoma, angiomyolipoma, sometimes multiple renal cysts	Hypomelanotic macules, epilepsy, cognitive dysfunction, behavioral disturbances, developmental disorders	Mainly sporadic TSC1 of TSC2 germ line mutations

VHL: Von Hippel-Lindau syndrome; TSC: Tuberous sclerosis complex; NPHP: Nephronophthisis; MCKD: Medullary cystic kidney disease.

Acquired Cystic Kidney Disease

Acquired cystic kidney disease (ACKD) is a condition where kidneys, often with advanced CKD, present with multiple bilateral cysts of small to medium size, which are usually <0.5 cm in diameter, but can be as large as 2–3 cm. The reported prevalence is as low as 7% in predialysis patients and as high as 80% in patients who have been on dialysis for 10 years.

Acquired cystic kidney disease can be complicated by episodes of renal pain, cyst rupture, cyst hemorrhage and malignant transformation into RCC, but most patients with ACKD are asymptomatic. The incidence of malignant transformation is 4-7% over 7 to 10 years in ESRD.

ACKD-associated RCC is the most common subtype of RCC occurring in end-stage kidneys (with a male to female ratio of 2:1) often presenting as well-circumscribed small tumors arising within cysts more likely to be multifocal. They are associated with a relatively favorable outcome but a small subset may demonstrate aggressive features. Various syndromes associated with cystic kidney diseases are shown in Table 22.3.

Suggested Reading

1. Ravine D, Gibson RN, Donlan J and Sheffield LJ. An ultrasound renal cyst prevalence survey: Specificity data for inherited renal cystic diseases. Am J Kidney Dis 1993; 22, 803-07.
2. Kurschat CE, Müller RU, Franke M, Maintz D, Schermer B and Benzing T. An approach to cystic kidney diseases: The clinician's view. Nature Reviews Nephrology 2014; 10(12), 687.
3. Harris PC and Torres VE. Polycystic kidney disease. Annu. Rev Med 2009;60, 321-37.
4. Hildebrandt F. Genetic kidney diseases. Lancet 2010;375, 1287-95.
5. Torres VE, Harris PC and Pirson Y. Autosomal dominant polycystic kidney disease. Lancet 369.
6. Grantham JJ, Torres VE, Chapman AB, *et al.* Volume progression in polycystic kidney disease. N Engl J Med 2006;354(20):2122-30.
7. O'Neill WC, Robbin ML, Bae KT, *et al.* Sonographic assessment of the severity and progression of autosomal dominant polycystic kidney disease: The Consortium of Renal Imaging Studies in Polycystic Kidney Disease (CRISP). Am J Kidney Dis 2005;46(6):1058-64.

CHAPTER

23

A Patient with Resistant Hypertension and Renal Dysfunction

Vinay Malhotra[1], Harshal Joshi[2]

[1] *Senior Professor, Department of Nephrology, SMS Medical College and Hospital, Jaipur*

[2] *Assistant Professor, Department of Nephrology, SBKS Medical Institute and Research Center, Pipariya Vadodara*

CASE

A 60-year-old man is referred for further evaluation of his blood pressure (BP). He had a past history of type 2 diabetes for 10 years and high BP for 12 years. His parents had the history of diabetes and hypertension. Recently since a month, he noticed swelling of feet that worsens as the day passes. He is also feeling fatigued these days. He had no known history of hypertension target-organ damage, and his medications included Telmisartan 40 mg BD, Metoprolol 50 mg BD, Nifedipine 20 mg TDS, Hydrochlorothiazide 25 mg OD, Atorvastatin 20 mg OD and Metformin 1000 mg BD. His examination was otherwise unremarkable apart from peripheral edema. His height is 170 cm and weight is 85 kg with BMI of 29.4 kg/m^2. Fundus examination showed mild arteriolar narrowing. His seated BP was 166/102 mm Hg and 168/100 mm Hg in the right arm and the left arm respectively, with a regular heart rate of 76 beats/min. His BP did not change on standing. His urinalysis showed +1 proteinuria on dipstick evaluation. His serum creatinine value is 2.1 mg/dl.

This case vignette shows a patient with uncontrolled hypertension despite multiple antihypertensive medications. Thorough evaluation and management of such a patient is essential to prevent target organ damage.

So how can one proceed with the evaluation of this patient?

Before evaluating a patient with resistant hypertension, it should be clear what constitutes resistant hypertension?

What is Definition of Resistant Hypertension (rHTN)?

"Drug-resistant hypertension is diagnosed when a person has a BP of more than 140/90 mm Hg in spite of taking optimal doses of three or more antihypertensive drugs, one of which is a diuretic."

This older definition of resistant hypertension has many shortcomings. According to this definition target BP is 140/90 mm Hg, but our patient is a diabetic so we could argue that the target BP should be 130/80 mm Hg instead of 140/90 mm Hg. Also, the older definition does not state about the types of antihypertensive used.

So according to AHA 2017 guidelines, the diagnosis of resistant hypertension is made "when a patient takes 3 antihypertensive medications at optimal doses with complementary mechanisms of action (a diuretic should be 1 component) but does not achieve control or when BP control is achieved but requires ≥4 medications".

Here, it must be clear that this definition is a syndromic definition (also called apparent resistant hypertension) for the initial evaluation of patient with uncontrolled hypertension and true resistant hypertension is defined only after ensuring accurate BP measurement, reinforcement of lifestyle modifications and antihypertensive medication adherence, adequate dosing and frequency, elimination of prescription and over the counter medications that may interfere with BP control, and exclusion of secondary causes.

What is Prevalence of Resistant Hypertension?

The prevalence of apparent treatment-rHTN was estimated to be 11.8% among individuals with hypertension, similar to what was reported from the ALLHAT trial, in which 12.7% of patients had apparent treatment-rHTN but it ranges from 2% to 40% according to the criteria used to define resistant hypertension. Prevalence of rHTN is higher in chronic kidney disease (CKD) population.

According to US data drug-resistant hypertension is present in about one in eight hypertensives.

Some relevant definitions are mentioned in Table 23.1.

Table 23.1: Definition of resistant hypertension	
Resistant hypertension (AHA 2017)	When a patient takes 3 antihypertensive medications at optimal doses with complementary mechanisms of action (a diuretic should be 1 component) but does not achieve control or when BP control is achieved but requires ≥4 medications
Controlled resistant hypertension	BP controlled to the patient's individualized target while receiving treatment with at least four or more antihypertensive medications, including a diuretic, maximized to optimal doses in the absence of intolerable side effects
Uncontrolled resistant hypertension	BP is not at target goal in spite of receiving four antihypertensive drugs including a diuretic.
Refractory hypertension	BP> 140/90 mm Hg despite the use of 5 or more antihypertensive agents including a diuretic and mineralocorticoid receptor antagonist in optimal dosage.

Using the American Heart Association (AHA) summary statement as a guide, we will discuss the case and approach it with the five evaluation and three management office-based steps (Figs. 23.1 and 23.2).

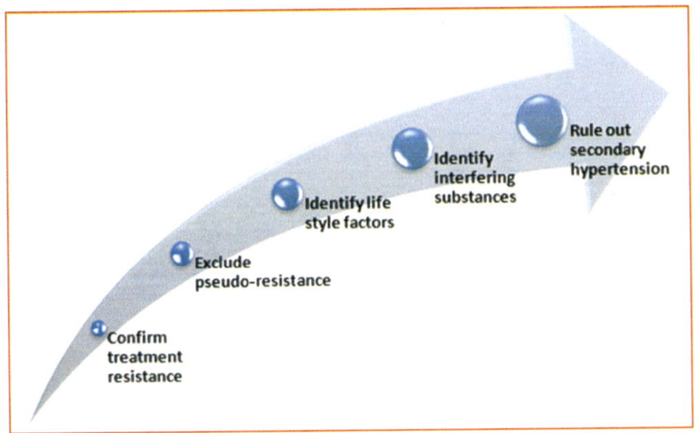

Figure 23.1: Evaluation of resistant hypertension

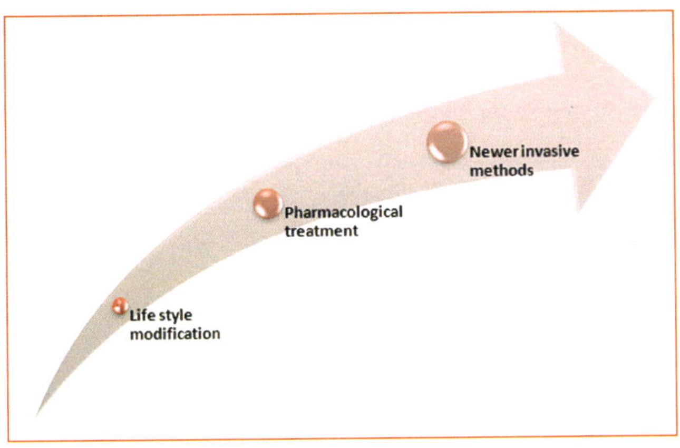

Figure 23.2: Management of resistant hypertension

Evaluation of Resistant Hypertension

Step 1: Confirm Treatment Resistance

Confirming that a patient is really drug resistant is a logical first step and could potentially avoid needless investigations and drug therapy adjustments. So as a first step, the treating physician should exclude: (i) White coat hypertension, (ii) Treatment non-adherence; and (iii) suboptimal treatment regime.

i. **Exclude white coat hypertension:** Many patients who have uncontrolled BP at the office have normal BP during home or ambulatory BP monitoring a condition known as white coat hypertension.

   Ambulatory BP monitoring (ABPM) can identify masked (Office BP-Normal, Home BP-High) and white coat hypertension and it can also assess diurnal and nocturnal patterns.

   The US Preventive Services Task Force recommends ABPM as the standard for confirmation of a hypertension diagnosis outside of the clinical setting.

   Whenever ABPM is not feasible, home BP monitoring (HBPM) records should be checked to exclude white coat hypertension.

   The advantage of ABPM over HBPM is that the former can identify patients with nondipping pattern (defined as <10% nocturnal fall in BP) which is associated with more target organ damage and poor prognosis. Nondipping occurs in 49%-82% of hypertensive patients with CKD and associated with rapid progression to ESRD (End stage renal disease).

ii. **Exclude treatment non-adherence:** Detailed history taking including the personal interview with patient and family members and review of pharmacy bills are required to ensure the compliance with medications. Medication event monitoring systems and urine screen with mass spectroscopy of antihypertensive drugs are objective methods to indicate compliance.

   One study found that only 47% of 76 patients with apparent rHTN were adherent to all prescribed medications assessed by toxicological urine analysis, that 16% did not take any prescribed medications, and that 37% took <25%.

   Non-adherence may be more common among hypertensive patients with CKD than those with normal kidney function. This is possibly related to the increased cost and complexity of medical regimens needed to treat CKD related conditions or may be a contributing cause for CKD.

iii. **Exclude suboptimal treatment regimen:** To define resistant hypertension all the medications including a diuretic should be prescribed in optimal doses. Many times uncontrolled hypertension is because of failure to prescribe medications in optimal doses.

In our patient, when queried, produced detailed reports of home BP readings that confirmed that out-of-the-office BPs were in a range slightly lower than the office values but above 150 mm Hg systolic, indicating true resistance.

On further inquiry, he and his family members denied any non-adherence to medications. He was on four antihypertensive drugs of different classes including a diuretic.

Step 2: Exclude Pseudo-Resistance

Pseudo-resistance is the false appearance of treatment resistance due to factors such as inadequate BP measurement, poor adherence, and white coat hypertension.

The accuracy of BP measurements using optimal technique needs to be established. Common pitfalls include improper patient positioning, wrong cuff size, not allowing an adequate period of rest before taking BP, poor timing of measurements, and equipment-related error.

In old aged hypertensive patient because of arteriosclerosis non-invasive, BP is falsely high (Pseudo-hypertension) as compared to intra arterial BP. This condition can be diagnosed when radial artery is still palpable with the thick wall after inflating BP cuff to supra-systolic level (Osler's sign).

Our patient reported measuring BP at home by following the instructions provided in the manual. Our patient was not pseudo-resistant.

Step 3: Identifying Lifestyle Factors Contributing Resistant Hypertension

The main lifestyle factors contributing to drug-resistant hypertension are dietary sodium exposure and excess body weight. Volume intake is also one of the contributory factors especially in a patient with CKD.

Our patient was well aware of the sodium content of the food and maintained low sodium diet. He is 170 cm tall and weighed 85 kg, yielding a body mass index of 29.4 kg/m^2. He was advised for regular exercise and diet modification for weight loss. He had lost 4 kg without major BP benefit in the last 2 months.

Step 4: Identifying Interfering Substances

At first encounter a patient with resistant hypertension should be asked about whatever they take, all prescribed and nonprescribed products and herbal preparations (Table 23.2).

Our patient has occasional alcoholic drinks and does not take prescribed or over-the-counter medications other than those listed in Table 23.2.

Step 5: Rule Out Secondary Hypertension

When to Suspect Secondary Hypertension?

Secondary hypertension is suspected in all young hypertensive, all resistant hypertensives, sudden loss of control of BP in recent times, non-dippers, hypokalemia at evaluation or on the administration of diuretics, the presence of metabolic alkalosis, target organ damage disproportionate to the level of BP.

Table 23.2: Common prescription and non-prescription drugs that can raise BP

Prescription Drugs	Non-prescription Drugs
Anabolic steroids	Anabolic steroids
Antidepressants (MAOI, SSRI, SNRI)	Caffeine
Calcineurin inhibitors	Cocaine
Glucocorticoids	Ethanol (In excess)
Erythropoietin	Glycyrrhizic acid (contained in some licorice, cough drops, and chewing tobacco)
Oral contraceptives	NSAIDs
NSAIDs	Sympathomimetic and illicit drugs (Amphetamines, cocaine, decongestant, nasal spray)
Sympathomimetics (Decongestant)	Alpha-Adrenergic herbal supplements
VEGF inhibitors	
Tyrosine kinase inhibitors	
Amphetamines (in context of ADHD)	

MAOI: Monoamino oxidase inhibitors; SSRI: Selective serotonin receptor blocker; SNRI: Selective norepinephrine receptor blocker; NSAIDs: Non-steroidal anti-inflammatory drugs; VEGF: Vascular endothelial growth factor; ADHD: Attention-deficit hyperactivity disorder.

Major causes of secondary hypertension and their diagnostic evaluation are listed in Table 23.3.

Table 23.3: Causes and diagnostic evaluation of secondary hypertension

Cause	Clinical indications	Diagnostic testing
Evaluate in all patients		
Renal parenchymal disease	Urinary tract infections; obstruction, hematuria; urinary frequency and nocturia; analgesic abuse; family history of polycystic kidney disease; elevated serum creatinine; abnormal urinalysis Abdominal mass (polycystic kidney disease); skin pallor	Basic blood chemistry, including creatinine, sodium, potassium, bicarbonate; urinalysis with microscopic examination, urine protein-to-creatinine and/or albumin-to-creatinine ratio, kidney ultrasound
Secondary causes to be considered		
Renal artery stenosis Atherosclerotic Fibromuscular dysplasia	Resistant hypertension; hypertension of abrupt onset or worsening or increasingly difficult to control; flash pulmonary edema (atherosclerotic); early-onset hypertension, especially in women (fibromuscular hyperplasia) Abdominal systolic-diastolic bruit; bruits over other arteries (carotid)	Kidney ultrasound with Duplex Doppler, magnetic resonance imaging, computed tomography angiography, conventional angiography
Obstructive sleep apnea	Resistant hypertension; snoring; fitful sleep; breathing pauses during sleep; daytime sleepiness, Obesity, Mallampati class III–IV; loss of normal nocturnal BP fall	Berlin questionnaire, overnight oximetry, polysomnography
High-aldosterone states Primary hyperaldosteronism (Adrenal adenoma, Bilateral adrenal hyperplasia) Secondary hyperaldosteronism (Renal artery stenosis, Renin-secreting tumor) Glucocorticoid remediable aldosteronism	Resistant hypertension; hypertension with hypokalemia (spontaneous or diuretic induced); hypertension and muscle cramps or weakness; hypertension and incidentally discovered adrenal mass; hypertension and obstructive sleep apnea; hypertension and family history of early-onset hypertension or stroke Arrhythmias (with hypokalemia); especially atrial fibrillation	Serum sodium and potassium concentration, serum aldosterone concentration-to-plasma renin activity ratio, BP response to mineralocorticoid receptor antagonist, genetic testing, CECT adrenal glands, adrenal vein sampling
Cushing syndrome	Rapid weight gain, especially with central distribution; proximal muscle weakness; depression; hyperglycemia Central obesity, "moon" face, dorsal and supra-clavicular fat pads, wide (1 cm) violaceous striae, hirsutism	Dexamethasone suppression test, 24-hour urine cortisol excretion, salivary cortisol
Congenital adrenal hyperplasia	Hypertension and hypokalemia; virilization (11-beta-hydroxylase deficiency [11-beta-OH]); incomplete masculinization in males and primary amenorrhea in females (17-alpha-hydroxylase deficiency [17-alpha-OH])	Clinical diagnosis, Hormonal studies
Apparent mineralocorticoid excess Liddle syndrome Gordon syndrome	Early-onset hypertension; resistant hypertension; hypokalemia or hyperkalemia	Clinical diagnosis, family history, low aldosterone and renin levels, serum electrolytes, Urinary cortisol metabolites; genetic testing

Contd.

Contd.

Pheochromocytoma	Resistant hypertension; paroxysmal hypertension or crisis superimposed on sustained hypertension; "spells", BP lability, headache, sweating, palpitations, pallor; positive family history of pheochromocytoma/paraganglioma; adrenal incidentaloma Skin stigmata of neurofibromatosis (café-au-lait spots; neurofibromas); Orthostatic hypotension	Plasma-free metanephrines, 24-hour urine metanephrines and catecholamines
Hyper- or hypothyroidism	**Hypothyroidism:** Dry skin; cold intolerance; constipation; hoarseness; weight gain, Delayed ankle reflex; periorbital puffiness; coarse skin; cold skin; slow movement; goiter **Hyperthyroidism:** Warm, moist skin; heat intolerance; nervousness; tremulousness; insomnia; weight loss; diarrhea; proximal muscle weakness, Lid lag; fine tremor of the outstretched hands; warm, moist skin	Thyroid-stimulating hormone
Aortic coarctation	Young patient with hypertension (<30 years of age) BP higher in upper extremities than in lower extremities; absent femoral pulses; continuous murmur over patient's back, chest, or abdominal bruit; left thoracotomy scar (postoperative)	BP measurements in both arms and legs, echocardiogram, thoracic CTA or MRA
Acromegaly	Acral enlargement, enlarging shoe, glove, or hat size; headache, visual disturbances; DM	Elevated age- and sex-matched IGF-1 level; MRI scan of the pituitary

Most forms of secondary hypertension fall under one of the three possibilities: Renal causes, Endocrinal causes and other causes.

Most common cause of secondary hypertension is renal which includes renal parenchymal (CKD) causes and renovascular causes (Fibromuscular dysplasia, atherosclerosis).

Therefore the initial evaluation should include measurement of electrolytes, eGFR, urinalysis, urine protein assessment and kidney imaging.

The young patient with resistant hypertension with normal renal function should be further studied using renal artery imaging by CT angiography or conventional angiography. Many studies showed that angioplasty alone in such patients may improve or totally cure hypertension.

Major endocrinal cause of secondary hypertension is hyperaldosteronism. Hyperaldosteronism is classically associated with hypokalemia and metabolic acidosis but normokalemia should not preclude the diagnosis. If hyperaldosteronism is suspected, the serum aldosterone concentration-to-plasma renin activity ratio (ARR) should be measured as an initial screening step. ARR had a sensitivity of 89% and a specificity of 71% in one study.

Few points to consider before testing serum aldosterone concentration-to-plasma renin activity ratio (ARR) are:

1. Do the testing in a daytime only after the patient has been awake and walking about for a couple of hours (stimulates renin activity).
2. Do not use the ratio unless the aldosterone exceeds a laboratory-based cutoff value for elevation, the generally accepted cutoff is 15 ng/dl.
3. The ratio can be tested even if the patient is on antihypertensive medications except for mineralocorticoid receptor antagonists, which should be stopped 4-6 weeks prior to testing.
4. When the ARR cutoff is used as >25:1, ensure that renin activity is measured in units of ng/ml/hour. Most recently laboratory measures renin concentration in mg/ml, which is a different measure of renin and not the one used in studies evaluating the role of ARR.

ARR is elevated (>25:1) in about 15-20% of resistant hypertension patients indicating pathogenesis of aldosterone excess in pathogenesis. When the ARR is elevated further contrast-enhanced CT scan of adrenals should be ordered to diagnose adrenal adenoma or adrenal tumors.

Obstructive sleep apnea (OSA) is also a common cause of secondary hypertension. Screening tools, such as the Berlin questionnaire, can be useful followed by overnight oximetry and polysomnography for confirmation. Prevalence of OSA among patients with CKD range from 22% to 33%, it is considered a contributing factor to rHTN. Treatment of OSA with continuous positive airway pressure (CPAP) therapy has variable BP reducing effect in various studies.

Other causes of secondary hypertension are considered on the clinical basis and investigated further as mentioned in Table 23.3.

Our patient is a non-smoker, with no bruits noted on examination. His records indicated that he had a serum creatinine of 2.1 mg/dl, normal serum potassium, urine protein creat ratio of 860 mg/gm and bland urine microscopy. Renal Doppler duplex ultrasound did not reveal renal artery stenosis. CT angiography of renal arteries was not done in view of decreased GFR. His plasma metanephrine assays were in the normal range. He had peripheral edema attributed to the volume overload secondary to CKD. He has no nocturnal symptoms or daytime sleepiness, although a formal sleep study was not done. Serum aldosterone and a plasma renin activity were requested. These returned the following values: (1) Renin: 0.10 ng/ml per h (normal 1.5 to 3.5 ng/ml per h), and (2) Aldosterone: 8 ng/dl (normal 3 to 15 ng/dl). The renin activity was suppressed, but the aldosterone concentration was in the middle of the normal range, the ratio was not applied. Presence of CKD should not discourage investigation for other causes if clinical suspicion exists.

Management of Resistant Hypertension

After completing the stepwise evaluation to confirm that the hypertension is actually resistant, the provider can formulate a therapeutic plan for treating resistant hypertension.

Step 1: Lifestyle Modification

Table 23.4 summarizes efficacious lifestyle modifications in hypertensive patients that are not specific to rHTN or CKD.

Step 2: Pharmacological Treatment

- **Maximize diuretic therapy to achieve volume control:** Achieving volume control is an essential part of the management of rHTN especially in patients with CKD. Use potent loop diuretics in optimal doses in patients with CKD and/or patients receiving potent vasodilators (e.g., minoxidil). Patients with CKD require higher doses of diuretics than patients with normal renal function. Regarding thiazide diuretics, Chlorthalidone is more potent than hydrochlorothiazide in patients with CKD. In patients with advanced CKD, hemodialysis may be required to achieve volume control.
- **Add a mineralocorticoid receptor antagonist:** Most of the patients with rHTN are treated with at least three anti-hypertensive agents of different classes, including a renin-angiotensin system blocker,

Table 23.4: Various lifestyle modification approaches and its effectiveness to control BP

Modification	Description	Systolic BP Reduction
Weight reduction	To attain normal weight (i.e., BMI, 25)	5–20 mm Hg/10 kg weight loss
DASH diet	Rich in fruits, vegetables, low-fat dairy, reduced saturated and total fat and reduced sodium	8–14 mm Hg
Reduced dietary sodium	To 65–100 mmol/d (1.5–2.4 g Na^+ or 3.8–6 g NaCl)	2–8 mm Hg
Increased physical activity	Regular aerobic exercise 30 min/d most days of week	4–9 mm Hg
Moderate alcohol intake	Limit to <2 drinks per day for men and <1 drink per day for women and those with lighter weight	2–4 mm Hg
Increased potassium intake	120 mmol/d (4.7 g/d; also included in DASH diet) (Not recommended in CKD)	Variable
Alternative approaches	Meditation, yoga, acupuncture and other relaxation therapies	Variable up to 2–10 mm Hg

BMI: Body mass index; DASH: Dietary approaches to stop hypertension.

One drink is equivalent to 12 oz beer, 5 oz wine, or 1.5 oz 80-proof liquor, each representing, on average, 14 g ethanol.

a calcium antagonist, a diuretic, and possibly, a β-blocker. As will be described, there are data to support the addition of a mineralocorticoid receptor antagonist as an add-on fourth or fifth agent, but it needs monitoring of potassium and creatinine especially when used along with RAAS blockers.

Addition of a Spironolactone leads to substantial reduction in BP (22/10 mm Hg) in resistant hypertension patients.

Another trial (PATHWAY-II) showed the superiority of spironolactone as an add-on therapy over placebo, doxazosin, and bisoprolol as an add-on therapy. Spironolactone (25–50 mg) was the most effective and reduced home systolic BP by 14 mm Hg, about 9 mm Hg more than placebo and 5–6 mm Hg more than doxazosin or bisoprolol.

Recently published AMBER trial showed significant reduction of BP with spironolactone. Use of Patiromer enabled more (69%) number of patients to receive higher (50 mg) dose in advanced CKD compared to placebo (51%).

- **Add other agents with different mechanisms of actions:** After optimizing diuretics and addition of spironolactone, it may be necessary to add additional antihypertensive agents like direct vasodilators, alpha-blockers, and central sympathetic agonists.

Step 3: Newer Methods

- **Renal denervation (Symplicity® System):** In earlier studies, catheter-based sympathetic renal denervation (RDN) using radiofrequency ablation reported striking reductions of office BP in patients with rHTN. The SIMPLICITY-3 Trial was the first sham treatment controlled trial using this approach, but it failed to confirm earlier findings.

  In the context of RDN, other techniques are now being developed with externally delivered focused ultrasound, which may offer safer adjunct treatment options. Apart from BP reduction, other favorable clinical effects of RDN include improvements in insulin sensitivity, microalbuminuria and apnea/hypopnea index.

- **Baroreceptor stimulation (Rheos® System):** In a study, electrical carotid sinus baroreceptor stimulation using implantable devices led to significant reductions in mean systolic BP. But, safety endpoints were not met, issues were related to surgery (nerve damage and wound healing) and uncontrolled hypertension. Unfortunately, robust controlled studies are not available. Moreover, carotid body stimulation has not been associated with the favorable metabolic effects observed for RDN.

  None of the above mentioned emerging therapies are approved by FDA.

Our patient is having treatment-resistant hypertension most probably due to chronic kidney disease (Diabetic kidney disease) with volume overload. The patient was advised to follow lifestyle changes in form of low salt diet, exercise, weight reduction and water restriction to achieve dry weight. He was started on more potent loop diuretic (Furosemide 40 mg BD) in place of hydrochlorothiazide. This change resulted in good diuresis and negative fluid balance of 4-5 kg of weight. The patient was instructed to monitor his weight daily and make necessary adjustments in water intake. His peripheral edema disappeared and he could achieve a BP of 146/86 mm Hg still higher than the target goal. To achieve a BP control, a fifth drug, Clonidine was added to the regime leading to further reduction in BP to 132/78 mm Hg (Reasonable target goal in diabetic CKD patient). Choice of central sympathetic agonist over spironolactone as a fifth drug was due to consideration of CKD in our patient. Had this patient's BP been uncontrolled despite above pharmacological treatment, what would have been the next step?

The other classes of antihypertensive drugs which can be added to the regime include mineralocorticoid receptor antagonist (Spironolactone, Eplerenone), alpha-blocker (Prazosin) and direct vasodilators (Hydralazine). It must be remembered that addition of a mineralocorticoid antagonist leads to substantial reduction in BP, but it needs monitoring of potassium and creatinine. Even though spironolactone is most effective in patients with high aldosterone renin ratio, in the patient with low renin and aldosterone level (suggesting an element of fluid and sodium surplus), like in our patient, an addition of spironolactone would result in further diuresis which can be helpful if BP remains uncontrolled on 5 drugs. However, creatinine and potassium levels must be monitored vigilantly as our patient is already having CKD. Lastly, the clinical utility of newer emerging therapies needs to be weighed against safety concerns and limited efficacy, until further robust controlled trials are available.

Suggested Reading

1. Whelton PK, Carey RM, Aronow WS, Casey DE Jr, Collins KJ, Dennison Himmelfarb C, DePalma SM, Gidding S, Jamerson KA, Jones DW, MacLaughlin EJ, Muntner P, Ovbiagele B, Smith SC Jr, Spencer CC, Stafford RS, Taler SJ, Thomas RJ, Williams KA Sr, Williamson JD, Wright JT Jr. 2017 ACC/AHA/AAPA/ABC/ACPM/AGS/APhA/ASH/ASPC/NMA/PCNA Guideline for the Prevention, Detection, Evaluation and Management of High Blood Pressure in Adults: A Report of the American College of Cardiology/American Heart Association Task Force on Clinical Practice Guidelines. J Am Coll Cardiol 2018 May 15;71(19):e127-48.

2. Chobanian AV, Bakris GL, Black HR, Cushman WC, Green LA, Izzo JL Jr, Jones DW, Materson BJ, Oparil S, Wright JT Jr, Roccella EJ: Seventh report of the joint national committee on prevention, detection, evaluation and treatment of high blood pressure. Hypertension 2003;42: 1206-52.
3. Braam B, Taler SJ, Rahman M, Fillaus JA, Greco BA, Forman JP, Reisin E, Cohen DL, Saklayen MG, Hedayati SS. Recognition and Management of Resistant Hypertension. Clin J Am Soc Nephrol 2017 Mar 7;12(3): 524-35.
4. Townsend RR. Attending rounds: A patient with drug-resistant hypertension. Clin J Am Soc Nephrol 2011;Sep;6(9):2301-06.
5. Pickering TG, Hall JE, Appel LJ, Falkner BE, Graves JW, Hill MN, Jones DH, Kurtz T, Sheps SG, Roccella EJ. Council on High Blood Pressure Research Professional and Public Education Subcommittee, American Heart Association: Recommendations for blood pressure measurement in humans: An AHA scientific statement from the Council on High Blood Pressure Research Professional and Public Education Subcommittee. J Clin Hypertens (Greenwich) 2005;7:102-09.
6. Judd E, Calhoun DA. Apparent and true resistant hypertension: Definition, prevalence and outcomes. J Hum Hypertens 2014 Aug;28(8):463-68.
7. Williams B, MacDonald TM, Morant S, *et al.* Spironolactone versus placebo, bisoprolol and doxazosin to determine the optimal treatment for drug-resistant hypertension (PATHWAY-2): A randomised, double-blind, crossover trial. Lancet 2015;386(10008):2059-68. doi:10.1016/S0140-6736(15)00257-3.
8. Agarwal R, Rossignol P, Garza D, *et al.* Patiromer to Enable Spironolactone Use in the Treatment of Patients with Resistant Hypertension and Chronic Kidney Disease: Rationale and Design of the AMBER Study. Am J Nephrol 2018;48(3):172-80. doi:10.1159/000492622.

CHAPTER

A Patient with Renal Stones and Obstructive Uropathy

Manav Suryavanshi[1], Somendra Bansal[2]

[1] *Director, Endourology and Robotic Surgery, Medanta,The Medicity, Gurugram*
[2] *Assistant Professor, SMS Medical College, Jaipur*

CASE

35 years old male with no previous comorbidities was admitted with complaints of colicky pain in the right flank for last 1 day. History of dysuria was also present. There was similar past history of renal colic. His evaluation showed normal counts however serum creatinine was 3.2 mg/dl. Urine exam revealed microscopic hematuria. USG KUB revealed right renal stone in the lower calyx and lower ureteric stone causing upstream hydronephrosis. Left kidney showed scarring at lower pole, however, there was no stone. He was treated with IV analgesics and hydration. Subsequently he underwent right ureteroscopy with DJ stenting for stone removal. Stone analysis and metabolic work up for stone formation was done. After 1 week, his renal functions started improving.

Classification of Urinary Stones According to:

1. **Etiology of stone formation:**
   (i) *Non-infection stones:* Calcium oxalate, calcium phosphate, uric acid.
   (ii) *Infection stones:* Magnesium ammonium phosphate, carbonate apatite, ammonium urate.
   (iii) *Genetic causes:* Cystine, Xanthine.
   (iv) *Drug stone:* Indinavir, triamterene, guaifenesin and ephedrine, silicate stone, topiramate, vitamin D, furosemide, acetazolamide.
2. **Stone composition:**
   (i) *Calcium oxalate monohydrate:* Whewellite.
   (ii) *Calcium oxalate dihydrate:* Wheddelite.
   (iii) *Calcium phosphate:* Apatite.
   (iv) *Calcium hydrogen phosphate:* Brushite.
   (v) *Calcium hydroxyl phosphate:* Carbonite apatite.
   (vi) *Magnesium ammonium phosphate:* Struvite.
3. **X-ray characteristics:**
   (i) *Radiopaque:* Calcium oxalate dihydrate, Calcium oxalate monohydrate, Calcium phosphate.
   (ii) *Poor radiopaque:* Magnesium ammonium phosphate, apatite, cystine.
   (iii) *Radiolucent:* Uric acid, xanthine, ammonium urate, drug stone.
4. **Shape of renal stone (Table 24.1, Fig. 24.1).**

Table 24.1: Microscopic appearance of urinary calculi

Chemical type	Appearance
Calcium oxalate monohydrate	Hourglass
Calcium oxalate dehydrate	Envelope, tetrahedral
Calcium phosphate-apatite	Amorphous
Brushite	Needle shaped
Magnesium ammonium phosphate (struvite)	Rectangular, coffin-lid
Cystine	Hexagonal
Uric acid	Amorphous shards, plates

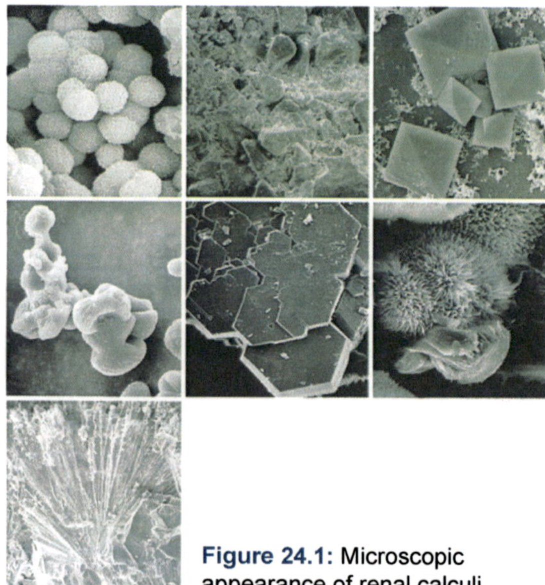

Figure 24.1: Microscopic appearance of renal calculi

Metabolic Abnormalities in Patients with Renal Stone

(A) Hypercalciuria: >200 mg/day of urinary calcium after adherence to 400 mg calcium and 100 mg sodium diet for 1 week.

Excretion of calcium > 4 mg/kg/day; or

>7 mmol/day in male and >6 mmol/day in female.

Types of Hypercalciuria and Metabolic Abnormalities are given in Tables 24.2 and 24.3.

Table 24.2: Types of hypercalciuria

Absorptive Hypercalciuria	Renal Hypercalciuria	Resorptive Hypercalciuria
1. Increase calcium absorption 2. Transient increase serum calcium 3. **Suppress serum PTH** 4. Increase renal filtration of calcium 5. Hypercalciuria 6. Serum calcium remain normal	1. Impaired renal calcium reabsorption 2. Elevated urinary calcium 3. **Secondary hyperparathyroidism** 4. Serum calcium remain normal	1. **Primary hyperparathyroidism** 2. Elevated serum and urinary calcium level and reduced serum phosphorus level *(hallmark of this disorder is persistence of increased urinary calcium during all parts of dietary calcium manipulation)*

Two Types of Absorptive Hypercalciuria

- **Type 1:** When urinary calcium remain high despite low calcium diet.
- **Type 2:** Urinary calcium normalize with restricted calcium intake.

Table 24.3: Types of metabolic abnormalities in hypercalciuria

	Absorptive Hypercalciuria	Renal Hypercalciuria	Resorptive Hypercalciuria
Serum calcium	Normal	Normal	Increased
Parathyroid function	Suppressed	Stimulated (secondary)	Stimulated (primary)
Fasting urinary calcium	Normal	Increased	Increased
Intestinal calcium absorption	Increased (primary)	Increased (secondary)	Increased (secondary)

(B) Hyperoxaluria: > 40 mg/day urinary oxalate, leads to increased urinary saturation of calcium oxalate and subsequent promotion of calcium oxalate stone.

Causes

- *Primary:* Disorder in biosynthetic pathway (oxalate overproduction).
- *Enteric:* Increased intestinal oxalate absorption (intestinal malabsorptive states associated with inflammatory bowel disease, celiac sprue or intestinal resection).
- *Dietary:* Excessive dietary intake or high substrate level (vitamin C).

(C) Hypocitraturia: < 320 mg/day urinary citrate level.

- Normal urinary citrate level can enhance inhibitory effect of Tamm-Horsfall glycoprotein.

Causes of hypocitraturia:

- Distal renal tubular acidosis (RTA).
- Chronic diarrhoeal state.
- Excessive animal protein.
- Diuretic-thiazide induce hypokalemia, intracellular acidosis.
- Enalapril.
- Chronic metabolic acidosis can lead to low urine pH, Hypercalciuria and hypocitraturia.

(D) Hyperuricosuria: > 600 mg/day urinary uric acid.

- Hyperuricosuria increases urinary level of monosodium urate which in turn promotes calcium oxalate stone formation.
- Uric acid may also reduce effectiveness of naturally occurring inhibitors of crystallization.
- At pH <5.5, undissociated form of uric acid predominates, leading to uric acid and/or calcium oxalate stone formation (uric acid not soluble at pH <5.5).
- At pH >5.5, sodium urate formation promotes calcium oxalate stone formation through heterologous nucleation (uric acid soluble at pH >5.5).

(E) Renal tubular acidosis (RTA): It is family of syndromes of normal anion gap metabolic acidosis from defect in tubular H^+ secretion and urinary acidification.

- Inability to acidify urine in response to oral acid (NH_4Cl) load confirm diagnosis of RTA.

Type 1 (Distal):

- Most common form, classic RTA.
- Failure of H^+ secretion in distal nephron.
- Hallmark is hyperchloremic metabolic acidosis with high urine pH >5.5 in face of persistently low serum HCO_3.
- Volume contraction from Na^+ loss is common which lead to secondary hyperaldosteronism and hypokalemia.
- Recurrent renal stone composed of calcium phosphate.

Type 2 (Proximal):

- Caused by failure of bicarbonate reabsorption in proximal tubule.
- HCO_3^- is replaced in circulation by Cl^- resulting in hyperchloremia.
- Acidosis is self limited.
- More common in children, it can lead to growth retardation and metabolic bone disease.

Type 4 RTA:

- Due to impairment of cation exchange in distal tubule with reduced secretion of both H^+ and K^+.
- Due to aldosterone deficiency or resistance.
- Unique feature–Hyperkalemia.
- Occasionally seen in obstructive uropathy (Table 24.4).

(F) Uric acid stone:

- 3 major pathophysiologic mechanisms that contribute to uric acid nephrolithiasis: Low urine volume, low urinary pH and hyperuricosuria.
- Most important pathogenic factor is low urinary pH because most patients with uric acid stone have normal uric acid excretion.

(G) Cystine stone: Patients are unable to reabsorb dibasic aminoacids: Cystine, ornithine, lysine and arginine (COLA).

- Cystinuria manifest when concentration exceeds 250 mg/liter.
- Stones are often yellow and waxy in appearance and relatively faint on plain radiograph.
- Historically diagnosis by sodium nitroprusside spot test which turned purple in presence of cystine.

(H) Infection calculi: Infection stones are composed primarily of magnesium ammonium phosphate hexahydrate, but may in addition contain calcium phosphate in form of carbonate apatite.

- These stones occur in association with urinary infection by urea-spiltting bacteria.
- Most common urease producing pathogens: Proteus mirabilis (most common), Klebsiella, Pseudomonas and Staphylococcus.
- Struvites stone form in presence of alkaline urine and in an environment rich in ammonia. Ammonia is produced via splitting of urea by colonization with bacteria that produce urease.
- Rarely long standing infection and obstruction produce a xanthogranulomatous pyelonephritis (XGP).

(I) Ammonium acid urate stone: Ammonium acid urate crystallization occur in laxative abuse, recurrent UTI, recurrent uric acid stone formation and inflammatory bowel disease.

Abbreviated Evaluation of Single Stone Former[1]

1. **History:**
   - Medications (Calcium, vitamin D, vitamin C, acetazolamide, steroid).
   - Dietary excess, inadequate fluid intake, fluid loss.
2. **Blood:** Sodium, potassium, chloride, carbon dioxide, blood urea nitrogen, creatinine, calcium, intact parathyroid hormone, uric acid (Table 24.5).
3. **Urine:**
   - *Urinalysis:* pH > 7.5: infection, lithiasis.
     pH < 5.5: uric acid lithiasis.
     sediment for crystalluria.
   - *Urine culture:* Urea-splitting organisms–suggestive of infection lithiasis.
   - Qualitative cystine.
4. **Radiography:**
   - *Radiopaque stones:* Calcium oxalate, calcium phosphate, magnesium ammonium phosphate (struvite), cystine.
   - *Radiolucent stones:* Uric acid, Xanthine, triamterene.
5. **Intravenous pyelography (IVP):** Radiolucent stones, anatomic abnormalities.
6. **Stone analysis:** X-ray crystallography/infrared spectroscopy.

Table 24.4: Renal tubular acidosis

	Type 1 (Distal RTA)	Type 2 (Proximal RTA)	Type 4 RTA
1. Minimum urine pH	>5.5	<5.5	<5.5
2. Serum K^+	Hypokalemia	Hypokalemia	Hyperkalemia
3. Renal stone	Present	Absent	Absent
4. Fanconi syndrome	Absent	Present	Absent

Table 24.5: Basic laboratory analysis[2]
Urine
1. Dipstick test of spot urine sample • RBCs • WBCs • Nitrite • Urine pH
2. Urine microscopy and/or culture
Blood
1. Serum blood sample • Creatinine • Uric acid • Ionised calcium • Sodium • Potassium
2. CBC
3. CRP
If intervention is likely or planned: Coagulation test (PTT and INR).

Metabolic Evaluation of Stone[3]

- Patients do not need to stone free to undergo metabolic evaluation.
- Only prerequisite is absence of gross hematuria and renal obstruction.
- 2-4 weeks waiting period after ESWL or endourological procedure is usually required before collection of 24 hours urine.
- The first step in a metabolic evaluation is to know the patient's stone analysis (stone composition by X-ray crystallography or infrared spectroscopy).
- Correction of 24 hours urine sample done by determining amount of creatinine in 24 hours urine sample (Men should have 20-25 mg/kg/day and women should have 15-20 mg/kg/day of creatinine in their 24-hour urine sample).
- Patient should stay on a self-determined diet under normal daily conditions and should ideally be stone free for at least 20 days.
- At least two consecutive 24 hours urine collection should be completed before treatment is prescribed because of additional diagnoses that multiple collection reveal.
- The first follow-up 24 hours urine measurement is suggested 8-12 weeks after starting pharmacological prevention of stone recurrence.
- Once urinary parameters have been normalized, it is sufficient to perform 24 hours urine evaluation every 12 months.
- The collecting bottles should be prepared with:

  5% thymol in isopropanol.

  Boric acid (10 g powder per urine container).

  Stored at < 8°C during collection.
- To prevent or minimize error, urine analysis should be done immediately after collection.
- In non-toilet trained children, spot urine samples is an alternative method.

Indications for Metabolic Stone Evaluation

- Recurrent stone.
- Stone composed of cystine, uric acid and struvite.
- Strong family history of stone.
- Solitary kidney.
- Anatomic abnormality.
- Renal insufficiency.
- Morbid obesity (difficult to treat).
- Multiple or bilateral stone at their first presentation.
- All children.
- Intestinal disease (chronic diarrhea).
- Pathological skeletal fracture.
- Osteoporosis.
- History of UTI with calculi.
- Personal history of gout.
- Infirm health (unable to tolerate repeat stone episodes).

No Need of Metabolic Evaluation in:

- First time.
- Adult.
- Calcium stone former without family history of stone and metabolic abnormality.

Recurrent Stone Former

1. **Blood:**
   - Serum creatinine, uric acid, sodium, potassium, chloride, calcium and phosphate.
   - Blood gas analysis: pH, pO_2, pCO_2, HCO_3, base excess.
2. **24-hour urine:**
   - *pH:* < 5.8 (suspicious of acidic arrest, uric acid stone, hypocitralluria).

     > 5.8 (suspicious of RTA).

     > 7.0 (suspicious of infection).
   - *Urine volume:* Low urine volume < 2 liter.
   - *Specific weight:* Normal >1.010.
   - Creatinine.
   - Calcium, magnesium, phosphate, ammonium.
   - Oxalate, citrate, uric acid and cystine.

Limited metabolic evaluation: 2 random 24-hour urine sample.

Table 24.6: Calcium load test

	Renal leak	Type 1 AH	Type 2 AH	Type 3 AH	Resorptive
Fasting Ca/Cr ratio	>0.11	<0.11	<0.11	<0.11	>0.11
Calcium load test (Ca/Cr ratio)	>0.22	>0.22	>0.22	>0.22	>0.22

Comprehensive Metabolic Evaluation

- 2 random 24-hour urine sample.
- 1 week restricted diet (low calcium, low oxalate, low sodium, and low purine diet) to eliminate effect of absorbed calcium on fasting calcium excretion followed by 24-hour urine sample.
- **Fast and calcium load test:** To differentiate various type of Hypercalciuria, performed on morning of second visit, routinely not required to complete metabolic evaluation because of same treatment of patients with absorptive hypercalciuria and urine leak.

Fast and Calcium Load Test

- Restricted diet for at least 7 days before test.
- To assure adequate hydration (300 ml distilled water 12 hours and 9 hours before calcium loading).
- 2 hours before calcium loading, patient empty their bladder completely and drink additional 600 ml of distilled water.
- After 2 hours fasting, from 6 AM to 8 AM, measure urinary calcium/creatine ratio.
- At 8 AM, administer 1 gm oral calcium load.
- From 8 AM to 10 AM, collect urine and measure urinary calcium/creatine ratio.
- From 10 AM to noon, collect urine and measure urinary calcium/creatine ratio.
- Fasting urinary calcium is expressed as mg/dl Glomerular filterate (GF) because it is reflective of renal function.
- To obtain this unit of measurement, urine calcium in mg/dl of creatinine is multiply by serum creatinine (mg/dl).
- Normal fasting urinary calcium is <0.11 mg/dl GF (Table 24.6).

Diagnostic Evaluation (Tables 24.7, 24.8 and 24.9)

- Ultrasound (US) should be used as the primary diagnostic imaging tool.
- NCCT can detect uric acid and xanthine stones, which are radiolucent on plain films, but not indinavir stones.

Table 24.7: Diagnostic imaging evaluation

	Sensitivity	Specificity
Ultrasound		
Ureteric stone	45%	94%
Renal stone	45%	88%
X-ray KUB	44-77%	80-87%

Table 24.8: Diagnostic evaluation

	LE	GR
Following initial US assessment, NCCT should be used to confirm stone diagnosis in patients with acute flank pain, because it is superior to IVU.	1a	A
A contrast study is recommended if stone removal is planned and the anatomy of the renal collecting system needs to be assessed.	3	A

Radiation Exposure of Imaging Modalities

Table 24.9: Diagnostic evaluation

Method	Radiation exposure (mSv)
KUB radiography	0.5-1
IVU	1.3-3.5
Regular dose NCCT	4.5-5
Low dose NCCT	0.97-1.9
Enhanced C	25-35

Medical Management (Table 24.10)

Table 24.10: Medical management of stone disease

Metabolic abnormality	Treatment
Normocalciuria	Potassium citrate (9-12 gm/day) (side effects–GI upset, hyperkalemia)
Hypercalciuria	Thiazide (25 mg/day, upto 50 mg) with potassium citrate (if decrease urine citrate)
Uric acid stone	Potassium citrate, if relapse then Allopurinol (100 mg/day)
Hyperuricosuria, hyperuricemia	Allopurinol (100 mg/day)
Cystinuria	Alpha-mercaptoacylglycine (Thiola) D-penicillamine Captopril
Infectious stone	Acetohydroxamic acid (Urease inhibitor)–15% risk of DVT Antibiotic
Urine acidification	Ammonium chloride Ascorbic acid Methenamine hippurate/ Methionine (200-500 mg TDS)

Citrate

- Complex with calcium.
- Inhibit spontaneous precipitation of calcium oxalate.
- Prevent heterogeneous nucleation of calcium oxalate.

Matrix Stone Management

Non-crystalline component, formed by mucoprotein, protein and carbohydrate. Treatment includes:

- Complete stone clearance (flexible nephroscope in all calyx).
- Kanamycin irrigation for 3 days.
- Chemoprophylaxis.
- Acidic urine (Litmus paper: Blue-Red) by ammonium chloride/ascorbic acid/methenamine hippurate.

Infectious Stone

- Complete surgical removal is mandatory to prevent recurrence. Percutaneous chemolysis (10%) hemiacridin (pH 3.5-4), suby G may be a useful adjunct.
- *Antibiotics:* Short term/long term.
- *Urine acidification:* Ammonium chloride/ascorbic acid/methenamine hippurate.
- *Urease inhibition:* Acetohydroxamic acid.

Surgical Management (Tables 24.11, 24.12 and 24.13)

Indications of Active Stone Removal of Renal Stone

- Stone growth.
- Stones in high-risk patients for stone formation.
- Obstruction caused by stones.
- Infection.
- Symptomatic stones (e.g., pain or hematuria).
- Stones > 15 mm.
- Stones < 15 mm if observation is not the option of choice.
- Patient preference.
- Comorbidity.
- Social situation of the patient (e.g., profession or travelling).
- Choice of treatment.

Indications for Active Removal of Ureteral Stones

- Stones with low likelihood of spontaneous passage.
- Persistent pain despite adequate analgesic medication.
- Persistent obstruction.
- Renal insufficiency (renal failure, bilateral obstruction, or single kidney).

Renal Stone (all but lower pole stone 10-20 mm)

Table 24.11: Surgical management renal stone

>20 mm	10-20 mm	<10 mm
1. PCNL 2. RIRS or ESWL	1. ESWL 2. Endourology (PCNL/RIRS)	1. ESWL/RIRS 2. PCNL

Lower Pole Stone (10-20 mm)

Table 24.12: Unfavorable factors for ESWL

No	Yes
ESWL/ Endourology (PCNL/RIRS)	1. Endourology (PCNL/RIRS) 2. ESWL

ESWL: Extracorporeal shock wave lithotripsy; PCNL: Percutaneous nephrolithotomy; URS: Ureterorenoscopy; RIRS: Retrograde renal surgery.

Proximal/Distal Ureteric Stone

Table 24.13: Surgical management ureteric stone

>10 mm	<10 mm
1. URS 2. ESWL	ESWL/URS

ESWL (Extracorporeal Shock Wave Lithotripsy)

Sampaio and Sabnis: Factors associated with decrease stone clearance in lower pole renal calculi in ESWL:

- Narrow lower pole infundibulum (width <4 mm).
- Acute lower pole infundibulopelvic angle (<90 degree).
- Multiple lower pole infundibular.
- Length of calyx > 3 cm.

Contraindications of ESWL

- Pregnancy, due to the potential effects of shock waves on the fetus.
- Bleeding disorders, which should be compensated for at least 24 hours before and 48 hours after treatment.
- Uncontrolled UTIs.
- Severe skeletal malformations and severe obesity, which prevent targeting of the stone.
- Arterial aneurysm in the vicinity of the stone.
- Anatomical obstruction distal to the stone.

Management of patients with residual stone: For well disintegrated stone material in lower calyx, inversion therapy with simultaneous mechanical percussion maneuver under enforced dieresis may facilitate stone clearance.

PCNL (Percutaneous Nephrolithotomy)

- Standard PCNL access tracts are 24-30 F.
- *Mini-perc:* Tract size <20 fr (12-20 fr).
- *Ultramini:* 11/13 fr.
- *Micro-perc:* 4.85 fr tract size (renal access and PCNL are performed in a single step through the all seeing optical needle). No tract dilatation.
- *Supra-perc:* 10/12 fr shah sheath with suction mechanism.

Contraindications of PCNL

- Patients receiving anticoagulant therapy must be monitored carefully pre- and post-operatively. Anticoagulant therapy must be discontinued before PCNL.
- Untreated UTI.
- Tumour in the presumptive access tract area.
- Potential malignant kidney tumour.
- Pregnancy.

During PCNL, ultrasonic, ballistic and Ho:YAG devices are recommended for intracorporeal lithotripsy.

Indications of Open Surgery

- *Anatomical abnormalities:* Infundibular stenosis, diverticuli, PUJ obstruction, stricture.
- Concomitant open surgery or complex stone burden.
- Cost consideration and need for single stage clearance–patient choice.
- Comorbid illness, skeletal deformities.
- Morbid obesity.
- Non-functioning lower pole or non-functioning kidney.
- Ectopic kidney where laparoscopic procedure may fail.
- Failure of ESWL/PCNL.

Operative Procedures

- *Simple pyelolithotomy:* For 1-2 cm pelvic calculus.
- *Extended pyelolithotomy:* For stone in renal pelvis and multiple extensions into calyces.
- *Pyelonephrolithotomy:* Large stone in a lower calyceal system.
- *Radial nephrolithotomy:* For calyceal calculi not amenable to pyelolithotomy.
- Anatrophic nephrolithotomy.

Bilateral Simultaneous Renal Stones

It is recommended that either the side that is more symptomatic or side that is more difficult, be treated first.

Second side should be perused only.

- No significant bleeding is encountered on first side.
- First side did not take an undue amount of time.
- Patient is clinically stable.
- Anesthesia team is agreeable.

Suggested Reading

1. Campbell-Walsh Urology, 11th edition.
2. European guideline 2017.
3. Urol Clin N Am 2007;34:315-22.
4. The Urology Masterclass-2017 (6th annual CMC Vellore postgraduate course, May 26th-27th, 2017).

CHAPTER

25 A Chronic Kidney Disease Stage 5 Child with Metabolic Bone Disease

Aliza Mittal[1], Sidharth Kumar Sethi[2]

[1] *Associate Professor, Department of Pediatrics, All India Institute of Medical Sciences (AIIMS) Jodhpur*

[2] *Senior Consultant, Pediatric Nephrology and Pediatric Kidney Transplantation, Kidney and Urology Institute, Medanta, The Medicity, Gurugram*

Metabolic bone disease is a common complication of chronic kidney disease (CKD) and is part of a broad spectrum of disorders of mineral metabolism that occur in this clinical setting and result in both skeletal and extraskeletal consequences.

CASE 1

11-year-old boy presented to orthopedics OPD with bowing of legs progressively increasing since last 1 year. He was evaluated for rickets and found to be deficient in Vitamin D which was prescribed in therapeutic doses. However, 6 months later the child still had persistently increasing deformities. An osteotomy was advised.

He was referred to Pediatric OPD for opinion. On evaluation the child was found to have obvious bowing of both lower limbs. He was pale and had hypertension (BP >95th Centile for age and height).

There was no preceding history of bladder problems, polyuria, salt craving. However, the child had been taking over the counter pain medications for headache which had been there since last 1 year.

On investigations, the child was found to have metabolic acidosis (pH-7.21, HCO_3-12.3, Base excess - 8.2). There was anemia (Hemoglobin-6.8 g/dl, MCV- 82.5, Peripheral smear; Normocytic normochromic picture), Blood Urea was 156 mg/dl and Creatinine was 4.3 mg/dl. Serum Sodium-145 mEq /dl and Potassium- 5.1 mEq/dl. The chest was clear and no features of fluid overload.

CASE 2

A 16-year-old presented to Nephrology OPD for opinion.

He is a known case of Chronic Kidney Disease (CKD) on conservative management as the family has no long-term plans for transplant. At age 3 years this child found to have urinary tract infection with obstructive uropathy, for which he underwent ureterostomy on both sides.

At 4 years he underwent right nephrectomy due to recurrent non-resolving pyelonephritis and later left uretrostomy was closed. This child was lost to follow-up for next 8 years when he was readmitted elsewhere with another episode of UTI. This time he was found to have a deranged Urea and Creatinine as a result of CKD V (Blood Urea 126 mg/dl, Creatinine 3.2 mg/dl) and short stature. The parents were counselled regarding need for Renal Replacement Therapy for which the parents did not consent.

The child also started developing progressive deformities of both lower and upper limbs thereafter and presented at 14 years of age to our hospital with a pathological fracture (Fig. 25.1). The above cases

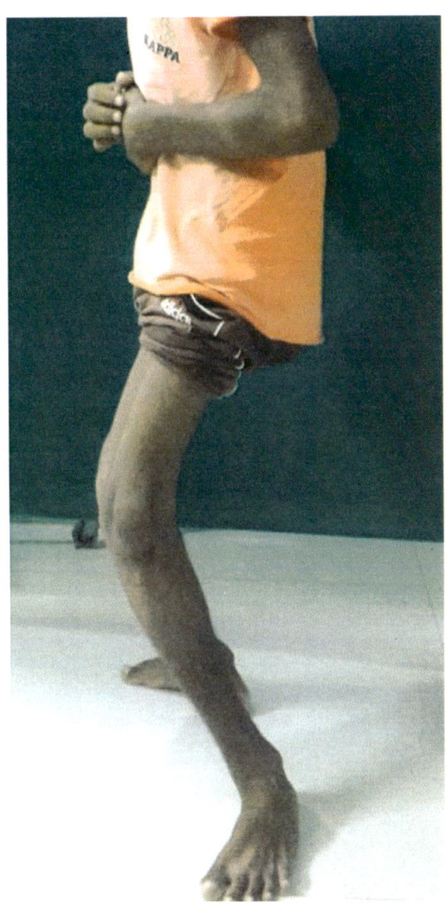

Figure 25.1: Severe bony deformities due to osteomalacia secondary to severe acidosis and hypocalcemia in a child with CKD 5, not on dialysis

represent the gravity of CKD–MBD as a morbidity in practice of pediatric nephrology and multiple complex issues in their management.

CKD-Mineral Bone Disease

CKD-Mineral bone disease sets in as early as CKD stage 3 and we should start monitoring for the same right from stage 2 CKD. There may be features associated with increased morbidity and mortality such as bone pains, fractures, vascular calcifications and adverse cardiovascular events.

The primary aim while treating a child with mineral bone disorder is to maintain a normal serum calcium and phosphrous level, while simultaneously preventing hyperparathyroidism and maintaining normal bone metabolism. This however gets complicated by the fact that a positive calcium balance is required in childhood for adequate growth.

To realise the above objectives, various principles of management may be used, like vitamin D therapy, phosphate control, calcium supplementation and parathyroid suppression. Each strategy has its own pros and cons and needs a careful balancing act to attain optimal management.

Let us look at each of them one by one while approaching a child with CKD.

Evaluation of a Child with Mineral Bone Disorder

We know, that monitoring for development of mineral bone disorder should start right from CKD stage 2, and the target for calcium, phosphorous, PTH and Ca × P product would vary with age of the child.

Table 25.1 shows the frequency of monitoring for various parameters for development of CKD-MBD.

However the same may not apply to infants who require more frequent assesments.

The KDIGO guideline (Updated in 2017) recommends measurement of Vitamin D levels at the baseline and then testing further as needed based on individual requirement and whether the patient is on replacement or conservative management.[1] Deficiency and insufficiency are to be corrected using same treatment strategies as recommended for general population.

Bone Radiographs

These are indicated in children who present with clinical features suggestive of rickets, avascular necrosis, slipped capital femoral epiphysis or while evaluating for skeletal maturation.

Dual-Energy X-Ray Absorptiometry (DEXA) only gives an estimate of bone mineral content and bone mineral density (BMD) and does not provide any information on bone structure like thinning of cortical shell, bone microarchitechture, increased cortical porosity and neither estimates a risk of fracture. Newer techniques like micro MRI and high resolution peripheral quantitative CT are more promising, but not yet established in clinical setting.[2]

Bone biopsy is rarely required. The indications for same include: Fractures with minimal or no trauma, suspected aluminium bone disease and persistent hypercalcemia with PTH between 400-600 pg/ml.

Screening for *valvular or vascular calcifications* may be done by performing an Echocardiography or a lateral abdominal radiograph respectively.[3]

Newer diagnostic tools for assessment of CKD MBD status are being evolved, owing to the limitations of iPTH as a marker, as there are considerable inter-assay differences (upto 150%) specially in patients on dialysis. The newer generations of PTH assays are being developed which facilitate measurement of biologically active form of Parathyroid hormone rather than intact PTH only. This may be accomplished by measuring oxidised and non-oxidised form of PTH. The T50 test is yet another tool that measures integrated functional status of this systemic calcium phosphate buffering system by measuring the transformation time from primary calciprotein particles.[4]

Biomarkers of bone turnover such as osteocalcin, procollagen type 1, C-Terminal peptides, type 1 collagen cross-linked telopeptide or osteoprotegrin have been evaluated, but none of them is robust enough to ameliorate the diagnostic dilemma in children with CKD.

FGF-23: The levels of this protein increase as the GFR starts declining below 90 ml/kg/min and its increase precedes that of PTH. It helps to maintain serum levels of phosphorous in normal range. It, however, suppresses the synthesis of 1,25-OH Vitamin D3 and stimulates its turnover and metabolism. Measurement of FGF-23 may

Table 25.1: Frequency of monitoring for various parameters for development of CKD-MBD

Stage of CKD	Biochemistry	Vitamin D/PTH
CKD Stage 2 and 3	6-12 monthly	At baseline and then annually or as per need and supplementation
CKD Stage 4 and 5	6-3 monthly	3 to 6 monthly
CKD Stage 5D	1-3 monthly	3 monthly

be an early biomarker of phosphorous metabolism in patients with CKD. High levels of FGF-23 in children with CKD have been correlated with high levels of osteoprotegrin, receptor activator of nuclear factor κβ ligand (RANKL), PTH and phosphorous and might indicate a need for improved control of mineral and bone homeostasis.[2]

Let us now Examine Certain Aspects of Managing these Patients

Dietary Counselling should begin as early as stage 2 CKD. Daily intake of phosphorous may be reduced to 80% of recommended dietary allowance, i.e., 800-1000 md /day, of which 60-70% is likely to get absorbed. This dietary restriction does not entail restriction of protein alone, but also products such as dairy, soft drinks, sausages, chocolates, Bengal gram etc.

The daily protein intake multiplied by 15 gives an approximate of phosphate intake of the child. A food containing 10 gram protein otherwise contains approximately 100 mg of phosphate. Boiling and prolonged soaking helps to leach out phosphate content of foods such as lentils and vegetable proteins. Food such as cottage cheese, pulses, egg and chicken have a lower phosphate content. Extreme reduction of dietary phosphate is to be avoided as it would result in restriction of growth, hence the use of phosphate lowering agents is of utmost importance.[1]

How to Manage Hyperphosphatemia?

The normal serum phosphate value is 3.5-5.5 mg%. However, this represents only a small fraction of total body phosphate which is stored in the body in form of organic, inorganic, intra and extracellular stores, phospholipids and bones.[2] The control of hyperphosphatemia also directly impacts secondary hyperparathyroidism (Fig. 25.2).

KDIGO 2017 Update recommends that in patients with CKD G3a to 5D decisions on phosphate lowering should be based on progressively and persistently elevated levels of serum phosphate. This is to emphasise that preventive phosphate lowering strategy is not supported by the current data.

The various phosphate lowering strategies are as follows:

1. Calcium based phosphate binders (e.g., Calcium acetate with 25% elemental calcium and calcium carbonate with 40% elemental calcium).
2. Non-calcium based phosphate binders, Metallic (e.g., Lanthanum, Aluminium, or Non-Metallic, e.g., Sevelamer).

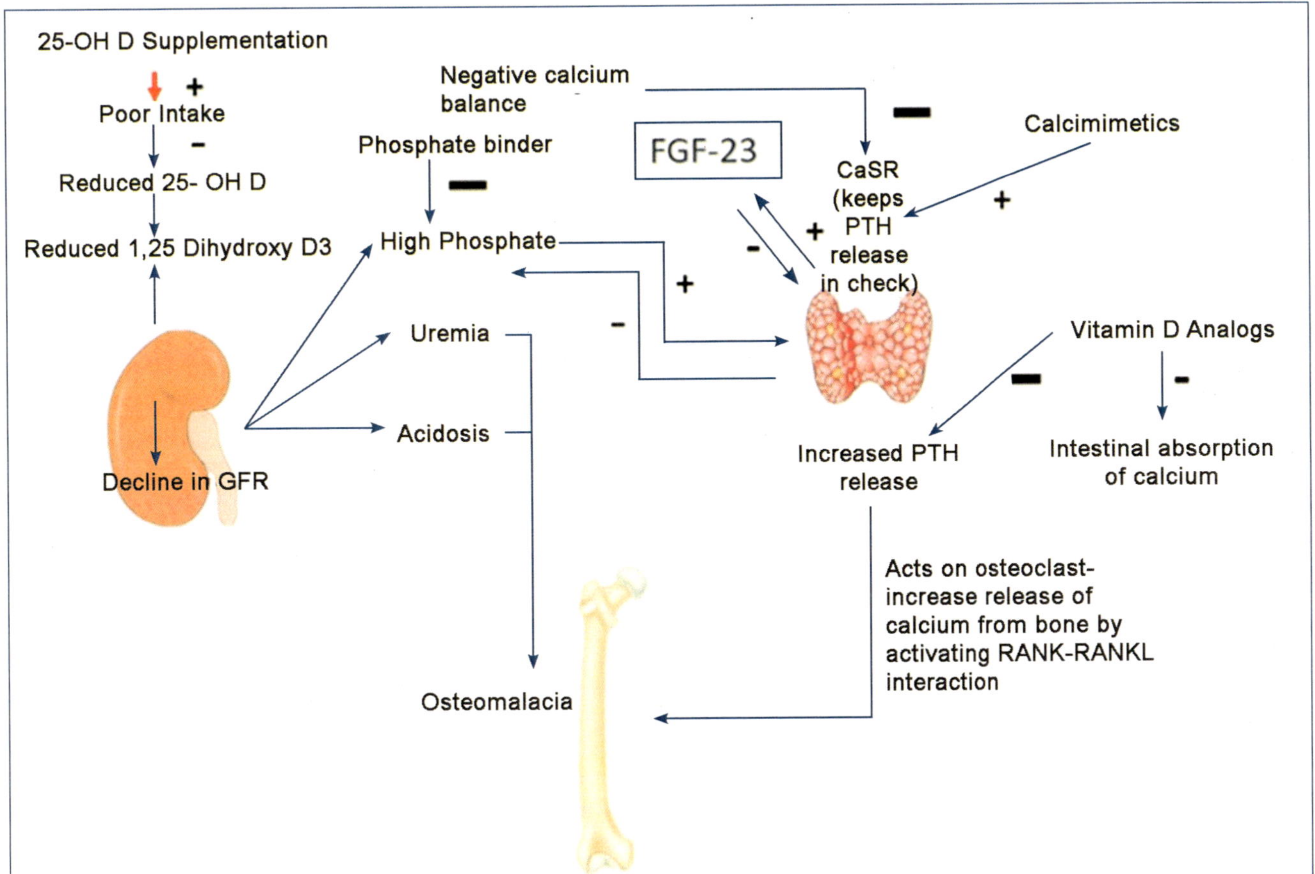

Figure 25.2: Control of bone mineral metabolism and action of various therapeutic agents

3. Dietary restriction.
4. Dialysis.

The KDOQI guidelines recommended a maximal dose of 1500 mg/day of elemental calcium with total elemental calcium intake from diet and binders not to exceed 2000 mg/day. KDIGO recommends that in children it is reasonable to base the choice of phosphate lowering treatment based on serum calcium levels.

They may be administered at a dose of 30-50 mg/kg of elemental calcium. In general *calcium acetate* is considered to have better phosphate binding capacity and lower risk of hypercalcemia than *calcium carbonate*. The recent data from various RCTs has shown that there is benefit of restricting the use of calcium based phosphate binders across all severities of CKD in view of the risk of hypercalcemia. Overall the data is limited to suggest the use of one type of binder over the other, but if there is evidence of arterial calcification or adynamic bone disease or recurrent hypercalcemia, it is prudent to avoid using calcium based binders.

There is a risk of toxicity associated with metal based binders.[3]

Metal based phosphate binders are approved for use in adults. However, one should be careful to avoid using *aluminum based binders* for more than 6 weeks owing to toxicity which may cause neurological dysfunction and adynamic bone disease. *Lanthanum* again is not licenced for use in children and there are concerns of its deposition in skeleton and liver. *Magnesium carbonate* may cause diarrhea and is hence not preferred.

The newer potential binders are *ferric citrate* based binders, however the experience with these is limited. Non metallic phosphate binders such as *Sevelamer* is currently not recommended for use in infants and young children, and cannot be added to tube feeds due to propensity to form a thick insoluble gel. For these children one may mix sevelamer to the milk, allow the solution to stand till a thick sediment containing sevelamer bound to phosphate is formed. The supernatant that is free of phosphate may be fed to the baby.

Sevelamer is available in both hydrochloride and carbonate forms. The former carries a risk of metabolic acidosis and hence the carbonate preparation is preferred. Practically one needs to add approximately 3 pills, i.e., 1200 mg of sevelamer to bind 100 mg of phosphorous.[3]

The advantage of using sevelamer is that it reduces the calcium load and incidence of episodes hypercalcemia and improves plasma lipid profile in children with stages 3-5 CKD.

Sucroferric oxohydroxide has also been approved for use in adults. However, all citrate preparations carry the risk of aluminum toxicity by enhancing absorption and keeping aluminum soluble. It has the advantage of providing benefit in anemia, decreased iron and ESA requirement. The advantage of using calcium free binders is that it allows increased doses of active Vitamin D to be administered without increasing the chances of hypercalcemia.

Dialysis

While dialysing children with hyperphosphatemia, it is recommended to use a dialysate calcium of 1.25 to 1.5 mmol/l.[1] Though dialysis is not very effective in removing phosphates, one may use extended diffusive hemodialysis and nocturnal dialysis for effective phosphate clearance. A routine hemodialysis session removes only about 2.3 to 2 gm of phosphorous which rises to 80% pre-dialysis levels within 12 hours after hemodialysis. Intermittent hemodialysis removes 1000 mg of phosphorous and since a same amount of phosphorous is also absorbed each day, the net balance is 4000 mg/day.[3]

Vitamin D and Its Analogues

Vitamin D supplementation are required once blood level of 25-OH Vitamin D is <30 ng/ml. Upto 80% children are deficient in Vitamin D across all ages. Therefore, in the absence of serum levels one may empirically treat with vitamin D supplements if PTH and alkaline phosphatase is elevated. Vitamin D therapy in CKD has also been shown to be effective in attenuation of inflammation, reduced dosing of erythropoiesis stimulating agents and possibly improvement of cardiac dysfunction. The goal of Vitamin D therapy is to keep parathyroid suppressed, maintain normal bone metabolism and normocalcemia. It is important to monitor for any evidence of hypercalcemia for a child on Vitamin D therapy or oversuppression of Vitamin D. The common available preparations contain 60,000 IU in a sachet or 5 ml syrup. The calcium preparations contain up to 200 IU of 25-OH Vitamin D in 5 ml syrup and 400 IU in a tablet. 200,000 to 400,000 IU are given over 2-3 months, or 60,000 twice weekly for 3 weeks, weekly for 4 weeks or fortnightly for 8 weeks followed subsequently by RDA for Vitamin D in a calcium or multivitamin preparation.

However, one should keep in mind that patients with CKD 5 are not able to convert 25-OH Vitamin D and hence they require 1,25 dihydroxy Vitamin D3 for management of hyperparathyroidism persisting despite lowering serum phosphorous below 5.5 mg/dl while serum calcium is normal.[5]

High doses of calcitriol (1,25 dihydroxy Vitamin D) have been used, sometimes even in supraphysiological doses in order to keep PTH suppressed, even at the cost of having an increased calcium phosphorous product and extraosseous calcification. In children with CKD 2-4 such therapy should be administered only if metabolic abnormalities persist despite correcting 25-OH Vitamin D levels. A child weighing <10 kg may receive 0.25 μg calcitriol twice a week and the dose may be titrated upwards based on weight of the child. In a child weighing 10-20 kg-0.25 μg on alternate days may be adequate and for weights above that 0.25 μg daily.

In a child on dialysis the dose may be adjusted with PTH levels such as 300-500 pg/ml-7.5 ng/kg (maximum 0.25 µg/d), 500-1000 pg/ml-15 ng/kg (maximum 0.5 µg/d) and >1000 pg/ml-25 ng/kg (maximum 1 µg/d). One should temporarily stop administration of alpha-calcitriol if blood PTH level is low or there is hypercalcemia (serum calcium >10.2 mg/dl) or raised phosphorous (>5.5 mg/dl).

Vitamin D analogues and calcitriol traditionally are used for their PTH-lowering effects and are effective in patients receiving dialysis. They inhibit PTH secretion without affecting intestinal calcium absorption.

They may be required in patients with CKD who develop hypercalcemia. Agents available include Doxercalciferol (1 α hydroxyl Vitamin D_2) and Paracalcitol (1,25-dihydroxyvitamin D_2) and are indicated in patients with persistently elevated PTH despite normal serum calcium. They are not approved for use in children as yet. It should be borne in mind that one should not use Vitamin D analogs to treat Vitamin D deficiency.

The KDIGO recommendation states that calcitriol and Vitamin D analogues may be used in children to maintain serum calcium in age appropriate normal range, however in adults it was suggested that calcitriol and Vitamin D analogues should not be routinely used as data from recent RCTs have failed to demonstrate any improvements in clinically relevant outcomes but increased the risk of hypercalcemia. However, KDIGO Guidelines do not recommend one Vitamin D analogue over another.

Parathyroidectomy

The acceptable level of serum PTH may vary by the degree of CKD. If GFR is >50 ml, the PTH upto upper limit of normal range may be acceptable, while if GFR is between 20-50 ml/kg/hr PTH-1-1.5 times the normal may be acceptable. If GFR is <20 ml, the values in the range of 1.5-2 times the normal may be present and in patients on dialysis it may be upto as high as 2-3 times the normal.

Indications of parathyroidectomy–If PTH >1000 pg/ml, with recurrent persistent hypercalcemia with or without persistent hyperphosphatemia refractory to other measures. Some other uncommon indications are calciphylaxis and metastatic calcifications, refractory pruritis, debilitating hyperparathyroid bone disease. One needs to perform an Ultrasound Scan of the neck to look for any adenoma in parathyroids and a nuclear scintigraphy to evaluate parathyroid glands. Subsequently a subtotal or a total parathyroidectomy with auto-transplantation is performed.[4] The advantage of parathyroidectomy is the lack of adverse effects that occur secondary to prolonged use of Vitamin D or its analogues. A recent data from the USRDS showed lower mortality risk in patients who underwent parathyroidectomy. KDIGO does not recommend any specific PTH level as an absolute indication of performing parathyroidectomy.[3,6]

Use of Calcimimetics

These agents are allosteric activators of extracellular calcium sensing receptors that sensitize the parathyroid gland to extracellular calcium, thereby mimicking calcium in suppressing the release of parathyroid hormone, independent in their actions from Vitamin D. The administration of *Cinacalcet* thereby causes dose dependent decrease in serum PTH levels. It also has the potential to reverse parathyroid gland hyperplasia and slow the progression of cardiovascular calcification. The side effects include nausea, vomiting and hypocalcemia, and currently the drug is not approved for use in children in view of the absence of information on drug safety. The KDIGO guidelines state that, depending on the serum calcium and phosphorous levels, one may use calcitriol, Vitamin D analogues or calcimimetics.[3,6]

Conclusion

Despite an armamentarium of therapeutic options, the clinical management of mineral and bone metabolism in children with CKD remain difficult. Adequate monitoring of the levels of 25-OH Vitamin D and providing supplementation when needed, avoiding episodes of hypercalcemia and hyperphosphatemia by using calcium free binders and altering dialysate calcium would yield positive results. One may use analogs of vitamin D which will have a positive impact on cardiovascular outcomes and with approval of use of cinacalcet in children, the available tools for management would expand.

References

1. Ketteler M, Block GA, Evenepoel P, Fukagawa M, Herzog CA, McCann L, Moe SM, Shroff R, Tonelli MA, Toussaint ND, Vervloet MG, Leonard MB. Executive summary of the 2017 KDIGO Chronic Kidney Disease-Mineral and Bone Disorder (CKD-MBD) Guideline Update: What's changed and why it matters. Kidney Int 2017 Jul;92(1):26-36. doi: 10.1016/j.kint.2017.04.006. Review. Erratum in: Kidney Int 2017 Dec;92(6):1558. PubMed PMID:28646995.
2. Schmitt CP and Mehls O. Nat. Rev. Nephrol 2011; 7,624-34.
3. Srivastava RN, Bagga A (2016). Pediatric Nephrology. Ed 6. New Delhi: Jaypee.
4. Hocher B, Pfasch A. Hope for CKD-MBD Patients: New Diagnostic Approaches for Better Treatment of CKD-MBD. Kidney Dis 2017;3:8-14.
5. Hruska KA, Sugatani T, Agapova O, Fang Y. The chronic kidney disease. Mineral bone disorder (CKD-MBD): Advances in pathophysiology. Bone 2017;Jul;100:80-86. doi: 10.1016/j.bone.2017.01.023. Epub 2017 Jan 22. Review. PubMed PMID: 28119179; PubMed Central PMCID: PMC5502716.
6. Moorthi RN, Moe SM. CKD-mineral and bone disorder: Core curriculum 2011. Am J Kidney Dis. 2011 Dec;58(6):1022-36. doi: 10.1053/j.ajkd.2011.08.009. Epub 2011 Oct 21. PubMed PMID: 22018457; PubMed Central PMCID: PMC3983665.

CHAPTER

26

An Adult Patient with Neurogenic Bladder

Nikhil Khattar[1], Deepanshu Gupta[2], Laxmikant Sharma[3]

[1] *Consultant, Urology, Medanta, The Medicity, Gurugram*

[2] *Consultant, Urology, Dr. RML Hospital and ABVIMS, New Delhi*

[3] *Fellow, Urology, Medanta, The Medicity, Gurugram*

CASE

Mr. X is a 25-year-old male graduate student. Two years ago, he suffered a complete spinal cord injury (SCI) at T4 as a result of a motor vehicle accident. Although paraplegic and confined to a wheelchair, he has recovered sufficiently to return to graduation. He has good health overall, with strong upper body function and lives independently. He is having urinary incontinence and has had two recent episodes of febrile urinary tract infection (UTI) managed with IV antibiotics by physician. Today when he presented to nephrology OPD, he was found to have a raised creatinine of 4 mg/dl.

With this initial picture a urology consult was sought and an ultrasound was ordered which showed thickened, irregular bladder wall with bilateral hydroureteronephrosis with loss of parenchymal thickness on either side.

As a nephrologist, the concerns involved in management of this and similar cases are dealt within the following sections with frequent reference to this index patient of ours.

The Immediate Management of Incontinence in Neurogenic Bladder (NGB)

The neurogenic conditions such as a cerebrovascular accident, parkinsonism or a brain tumor can also present with neurogenic urinary incontinence, but usually the type of incontinence in such cases is an overactive detrusor causing urge incontinence and usually the upper tracts are safe and such patients will rarely be attending a nephrology outpatient department.

On the other hand, *patients with spinal cord injury, transverse myelitis or a meningomyelocele when presenting with lower tract symptoms or incontinence, are at the risk of upper tract damage* because of high bladder pressures and can present with febrile UTIs, obstructive uropathy and even urosepsis.

All patients with neurogenic conditions presenting with Urinary incontinence (UI) should be screened for the risk to upper tracts. A proper history/going through the available papers from neurology consult and an *ultrasound of the KUB* region are generally enough to recognise these *'at risk'* patients. *Presence of a thickened, irregular bladder wall with or without floating internal echoes, a high postvoid residual urine or bilateral hydroureteronephrosis are the pointers to identify patients who would require further evaluation.*

Our index patient has already presented with a yet unrecognised damage to the upper tracts and has deranged renal function. Such a condition requires an immediate decompression of the bladder by an indwelling catheter. This will help to drain any infected urine and also to put bladder to be at low pressures to allow the renal units to pour urine in the bladder which was till now blocked due to a high pressure gradient between the ureter and bladder at the vesicoureteric junction and was leading to bilateral hydronephrosis and renal parenchymal damage (Note that the *upper tract dilatation is not because of reflux in these cases but by accumulation of urine in the upper tracts because of this pressure gradient caused by high storage pressures in the bladder,* although secondary reflux may also be coexisting). *Persistent storage pressures above 20 cm of H_2O are dangerous for the kidneys.*

Since the patient already has deranged renal parameters, he is also likely to develop a *post obstructive diuresis* soon after drainage of the bladder is established. An hourly urine output measurement is enough to identify this condition which may cause severe loss of body water and sodium leading to dangerous hyponatremia if not properly managed. A production of more than 4 ml/kg/hour of urine may indicate this condition and should prompt management of the same.

A continuous bladder drainage for 2-3 weeks brings the creatinine to the nadir level for the patient. Once that level is achieved, it is time to assess the bladder storage and voiding functions by a urodynamic study to plan for further management in such a case.

Urodynamic Study (UDS) for Categorisation of Neuro-urologic Dysfunction, Prognostication and Choosing Appropriate Therapy

As urodynamics is a subjective test and findings depend on the focus of the person performing the study, before any urodynamic study we need to know the question for which we are looking for an answer through that study (Formulation of a Urodynamic question).

Principally, the bladder has two functions/phases in the micturition cycle:

1. **The storage phase:** The bladder spends most of its time in storing the urine being poured each minute from the kidneys. For a safe storage the bladder should be *silent* (not having any detrusor contractions) *and compliant* to maintain low pressures that are not a threat to the kidney, should have an *adequate capacity* and at the same time should have *normal sensation* to send timely signals for awareness of bladder filling. *The outlet (which includes the functional sphincteric mechanisms at bladder neck and external sphincter and the physical channel of the urethra) should be competent* not to allow urinary leak during this phase.
2. **The voiding phase:** This phase is 'switched on' when a person finds a suitable place to void. The outlet (sphincteric mechanisms) relaxes and bladder generates a coordinated contraction, the pressure of which is proportional to the resistance the outlet provides (thereby being higher in males, because of the presence of a prostate and longer urethra, than in females), that empties the bladder to completion without any residual urine.

In the context of a neurogenic bladder presenting with already deranged renal parameters, the most important urodynamic question will be: *"Is the bladder providing safe storage of urine without further threat to the native kidneys or a transplanted kidney?"* and *"Are the voiding pressures safe for the native/transplanted kidney?"*

A urodynamic study would typically consist of:

- **A Uroflowmetry with Postvoid Residual Volume:** The volume of urine voided per unit of time. It is primarily used to screen for bladder outlet obstruction. A high residual suggests either a poorly contractile bladder or bladder outlet obstruction.
- **Filling and Voiding Cystometrogram (with or without electromyogram):** Evaluates bladder capacity, compliance and the presence of detrusor overactivity, while a voiding test records voiding detrusor pressure along with the rate of urinary flow.
- **Electromyography:** Can help determine the presence of coordinated or uncoordinated voiding, and allows for an accurate diagnosis of detrusor sphincter dyssynergia that is common in suprasacral SCIs.
- **Videourodynamic study with fluoroscopy:** Combines the radiographic findings of voiding cystourethrogram with urodynamics.

Normal micturition involves autonomic and somatic pathways from the lumbosacral spine to the urethral outlet, bladder neck and detrusor muscle and a change in any of these can produce symptoms of NGB.

Neurologic disorders often damage and disrupt the central or peripheral pathways involved in the central control of the lower urinary tract. Damage to areas of the nervous system may result in detrusor overactivity, with or without detrusor-sphincter dyssynergia, detrusor underactivity, detrusor areflexia and impaired contractility. The causes of neurologic conditions leading to NGB include supraspinal, spinal, peripheral or mixed.

Supraspinal disorders involve central nervous system lesions that occur above the pontine micturition center. They include conditions such as Parkinson's disease, Shy-Drager Syndrome, cerebral palsy, frontal lobe lesions, stroke, cerebral trauma and multiple sclerosis (MS). *Bladder dysfunction at this level usually presents as neurogenic detrusor overactivity combined with synergistic activity between the bladder and sphincter (i.e., when the bladder contracts, the sphincter appropriately relaxes). These conditions generally do not pose a threat to the kidneys.*

Suprasacral spinal neurologic conditions include SCI, spinal stenosis, spinal cord infarction, multiple sclerosis (MS), transverse myelitis, cervical spondylosis and intervertebral disk disease. Patients with complete cord transections above the level of the sacrum *generally present with detrusor overactivity (DO) and striated sphincter dyssynergia* (i.e., when the bladder contracts, the external sphincter inappropriately contracts at the same time). Detrusor external sphincter dyssynergia (DESD) is associated with *a high risk for other urologic complications such as hydronephrosis, vesicourethral reflux, urosepsis* and *urolithiasis*.

In addition, patients with lesions at *T6 and higher are also at risk for symptoms of autonomic dysreflexia.*

Lesions in the sacral spinal cord, including those in patients with spina bifida, diabetes mellitus, herpes zoster and herniated lumbar disk disease, often lead to an *acontractile detrusor. In addition, poor bladder compliance can be seen, which places the patients at risk for upper urinary tract damage if bladder storage pressures are too high.* These patients are at risk for poor sphincteric activity as well.

Among patients with *peripheral nerve lesions* caused by diabetes mellitus, herpes zoster and herniated lumbar disk disease, bladder dysfunction generally manifests as detrusor areflexia.

As a general rule, persistently high storage phase pressures between 30-40 cm H_2O pose a risk to the upper *tracts* and all measures should be taken to keep them in a safe range. Bladder relaxants (anticholinergics, beta agonists), Botulinum toxin injections, Clean intermittent catheterisation and bladder size augumentation using ileal patch are all strategies to keep the storage pressures safe.

Our index patient was evaluated by a urologist and urodynamics revealed poorly compliant bladder and DESD with a detrusor pressure (Pdet) of 50 cm H_2O at 165 ml, of storage volumes. Further filling of bladder reproduced the symptom of overflow incontinence and the leakage started at a volume of 185 cc and Pdet of 60 cm H_2O (leak point pressures). This meant that the trigger of urinary leakage as a reminder for passing urine would also be subjecting him to prolonged periods of unwarranted high storage pressures thereby causing renal deterioration. This also meant that he has to be either on a permanent indwelling catheter or be on *Clean Intermittent Self Catheterisation (CISC)* to remain dry and maintain some quality of life.

Clean Intermittent Self Catheterisation (CISC): A Friend and not an Enemy!

Although intermittent catheterization instead of a continuous indwelling catheter as a modality to treat emptying failure was around since 1940s, it was Lapides work in 1972 which emphasized that catheterization could be done at home using proper hygiene rather than aseptic precautions, that lead to the concept of CISC. *The basic premise was that before the bacterial doubling time is reached, the next catheterization empties the bladder again reducing the bacterial load and so on managed with anticholinergic medication and clean intermittent catheterisation (CIC), which his schedule, hand function, and mobility permit.*

Diagnosis and Assessment of NGB

Appropriate management relies on an accurate diagnosis.

Presenting symptoms (chief complaints) can be roughly divided into failure to empty or failure to store. Typical symptoms of disrupted *bladder emptying* include feelings of fullness and difficulty emptying the bladder, such as a slow stream while straining to void. Other patients report hesitancy, an interrupted or diminished stream, a sensation of incomplete emptying, lower abdominal discomfort, nocturia and recurrent UTIs. *Failure to store* usually presents as frequency, urgency and UI. Depending on the level and severity of the neurologic lesion, patients may not have any bladder sensation; symptoms therefore may not be a reliable indicator of significant NGB dysfunction in certain patients.

In history current medication use should be evaluated, as certain drugs can impact bladder function. In addition, issues related to bowel and sexual function are commonly seen in patients with NGB and may have to be addressed. Loss of genitourinary and gastrointestinal function are important sequelae of SCI. Constipation can affect voiding function, leading to incontinence or retention. When taking a history, it is important to realize that some patients may have coexisting problems such as stress UI or benign prostatic hyperplasia, in addition to lower urinary tract dysfunction from NGB.

Physical examination should include a focused neurourologic evaluation. In addition to standard evaluation of the abdomen, back, rectum, pelvis, and genitalia, clinicians need to evaluate the sacral dermatomes, including perianal sensation and anal sphincter tone. The neurologic evaluation should be primarily focused at the sacral 2-4 level and assess the bulbocavernosus reflex, voluntary external sphincter control, and reflexes in the sacral dermatome levels. Deep tendon reflexes in the lower extremities, clonus and plantar responses should be included.

Investigations

Urinalysis with or without a urine culture, should be done to rule out UTI, glucosuria indicative of diabetes, and blood or protein in the urine that might indicate renal disease. If the results suggest an associated condition, the patient may need further diagnostic testing.

Urodynamic assessment can help determine the underlying neurologic issues, categorize the vesicourethral dysfunction, and provide a basis for appropriate therapy. Patients *at high upper tract risk should undergo a UDS despite whether or not they are having symptoms. Such patients are mainly with spinal level pathologies like spinal cord injury, transverse myelitis.* In these patients, UDS is not only diagnostic but also prognostic.

In patients with *minimal upper tract risk (which includes mainly supraspinal pathologies like CVA, Parkinson's disease, brain tumor etc.),* UDS may be used selectively if there are symptoms or signs that suggest failure of empiric treatment and change in bladder condition.

After entire evaluation one should try to conclude whether the problem belongs predominantly to store or to void. All attention must be paid to make the storage safe even if it is at the cost of voiding ability (treatments like Augmentation, Botulinum toxin, high doses of anticholinergics etc. are all directed to make the storage safe) on the premise that emptying can be taken care of with teaching self-catheterisation.

Goals of Treatment (In Order of Priority)

1. Prevention or worsening of upper tract damage.
2. Prevention of recurrent/severe UTI.

3. Maintaining the patient dry.
4. Ability to self void.

In patients with elevated bladder storage pressures or vesicoureteral reflux at higher risk for renal complications, the primary goal is to protect kidney function and prevent further complications. Conversely, in patients not at high risk for kidney damage, quality-of-life issues such as UI and self voiding may be of greatest concern.

Treatment

Failure to Empty

- Behavioral modification, i.e., pelvic floor exercises.
- Intermittent catheterization.
- Botulinum toxin A injection into the sphincter.
- Suprapubic catheter.
- Indwelling catheter.
- Sphincterotomy.
- Urethral stent.
- Urinary diversion.

Failure to Store

- Lifestyle modifications, i.e., diet and fluid intake, timed voiding.
- Antimuscarinics.
- Botulinum toxin A injections into the detrusor.
- Indwelling catheter.
- Reconstruction.

Clinicians need to consider the patient's degree of disability, mobility, hand function, cognitive status, general condition, likelihood of progression of the neurologic disease goals and concerns, and available resources.

Behavioral/Non-pharmacologic Interventions

Behavioral/nonpharmacologic interventions include lifestyle interventions, the use of external appliances such as pads and/or portable urinals and the use of CIC or condom or indwelling catheters for patients with incomplete bladder emptying. These conservative approaches are often used in combination with medications.

Lifestyle intervention includes timed voiding, fluid alterations, pelvic floor muscle exercises, biofeedback, toileting assistance and bladder education/retraining.

Intermittent Catheterization

Intermittent catheterization is the preferred method for patients with NGB who cannot adequately void volitionally. CIC decreases the risk of infection and lowers the risk for long-term complications such as hydronephrosis, bladder and renal calculi and autonomic dysreflexia. However, for patients with poor hand function or who lack a caregiver, CIC is not an option. It also may be less than optimal in patients with bladder capacity <200 ml, abnormal urethral anatomy such as bladder neck obstruction and strictures, poor cognition or who cannot adhere to a catheterization schedule. Using a hydrophilic coated catheter (12-16 fr) reduces and delays the onset of symptomatic UTIs and can also decrease the risk of complications related to UTIs.

Teaching Catheterisation

Intermittent catheterisation is best taught with the patient admitted to the hospital as this gives an opportunity to closely observe the patient during the learning process. Clear diagrams help the patient in understanding the anatomy. The support of a fellow user of intermittent catheterisation is invaluable. A booklet or a list of "do's and don'ts can be a very useful aid.

The lesson starts with emphasis on thorough cleaning of the hands and perineal area/penis with soap and water. The catheter is then washed with water. After washing the hands and catheter, the patient must be instructed not to touch any contaminated area. The female subject sits on the examination table with feet on the table, lower limbs flexed and knees held apart. In the sitting position the patient is able to visualise the perineum in a mirror at the foot of the table. The labia are separated and the subject is instructed to insert the catheter through the urethral meatus into the bladder holding the catheter 2 cm from the tip. With practice the patient learns to locate the meatus without the mirror by just feeling for the meatus. Male patients may learn the technique in the sitting or standing position and are advised to use a water-soluble lubricant for easy catheterisation. Once urine starts to flow out the patient is instructed to pass the catheter in for 2 cm more. Once urine has stopped flowing the catheter should be rotated and suprapubic pressure given. Then the catheter is withdrawn slowly. If urine starts to drain during withdrawal, the patient is instructed to wait with the catheter at that level till the urine stops flowing. These simple measures ensure that the bladder is completely emptied. The patient is warned never to forego catheterisation even when soap and water are not available but to catheterise at the prescribed time with the best available measures.

How often to Catheterise?

Catheterisation must be frequent enough to prevent the bladder becoming overdistended and to keep the patient dry. Patients should normally catheterise at least four times a day, more frequently in children, in patients with a high fluid intake, and in patients with a small capacity bladder. The volume obtained on catheterisation gives an estimate of bladder capacity and suggests how much can be drunk between catheterisation if the patient is to remain dry. This volume should ideally be kept around 300 ml. Patients soon learn to balance fluid intake with frequency of catheterisation in order to remain dry. To ensure timely catheterisation the technique is kept simple. No bedtime drink is to be taken, unless the patient catheterises during the night. A daily intake of 2 litres is sufficient.

Catheters and Catheter Care

Plastic (Polyvinyl chloride) catheters are commonly used. In India, plastic catheters such as "K90", "Safe-flo" are available. Foley catheters have been successfully used by patients, but some feel more comfortable with the stiffer plastic catheter. In the West hydrophilic (Polyvinyl pyrrolidone) coated "low fric" catheters are available, but they are expensive. The use of stainles steel catheters by females and also red rubber tubes has been reported. Adults use 10-14 F catheters while children use 6-10 F catheters. For small babies, a 4-6 F infant feeding tube is ideal.

The care of catheters is varied: Some authors have advocated a new catheter for each use. Some have advocated keeping the catheter in antiseptic solutions (Sodium hypochlorite, Povidone iodine, etc.) Some have advocated boiling or microwave sterilisation of the catheter. *But even with the most casual catheter use, symptomatic UTI are not more than what is commonly reported. Infections are more of a problem in patients who catheterise infrequently, in patients with faulty techniques, and in those with established renal damage. Keeping the catheter clean and dry is all that is required,* and has been compared to the care of the toothbrush. After use, the outer surface of the catheter may be washed with soap and water and the inside with clean water. Water inside the catheter is then thoroughly wrung out and the catheter carried in a dry state in a clean container. *The catheter may be re-used,* and there is no fixed period of time for usage. A common sense approach is applied and the catheter is changed when it gets dirty or damaged.

Complications of CISC

Urinary tract infection (UTI). *(Actually, CISC reduces UTIs because it reduces the amount of residual urine in the bladder and reducing reflux.)* Urinary bladder calculi, bleeding from urethra because of trauma to asensate urethra leading to occasional stricture urethra with or without false passages. Urethritis or Epididymo-orchitis are not very uncommon complications of CISC. *These complications can be reduced when CISC is being learned well and performed under supervision for sometime.*

Indwelling Catheterization

Indwelling catheters, *often considered a last resort,* may still be the best option for certain patients. These can cause UTIs and may lead to reduced compliance and a thickened bladder. Over time, patients may develop vesicoureteral reflux that leads to bladder stones, a higher risk for kidney stones and renal damage. *A suprapubic catheter is less traumatic to the urethra and more hygienic.*

Pharmacologic Treatment Options

Anticholinergic/antimuscarinic agents, the standard therapy for patients with neurogenic detrusor overactivity, are often used in conjunction with CIC to allow for optimal storage and emptying.

More Invasive Procedures

An intraurethral stent may be an option for the long-term management of detrusor-sphincter dyssynergia inpatients with SCIs. Potentially reversible, it can circumvent urethral obstruction while avoiding surgery.

Bladder augmentation uses an intestinal segment (usually ileum) to enlarge the bladder and increase bladder capacity. The aim is to restore continence and preserve upper urinary tracts by lowering intravesical storage pressures and minimizing the risk of reflux and hydronephrosis.

Ileovesicostomy uses a section of ileum to create a channel leading from the urinary bladder upward to the abdominal wall. It provides for a low-pressure storage.

Renal Transplantation in Neurogenic Bladder Patients

Neurogenic bladder is not a contraindication for renal transplant. An appropriate selection makes graft outcome not different from other general transplant patients.

It is difficult to assess the filling and voiding dynamics of a defunctionalized bladder (daily urinary output is less than 300 ml) or a bladder that has not been used for several years. Before the patient develops oligoanuria, if the voiding was normal than after transplantation bladder will regain its normal capacity within few weeks. However it is mandatory to maintain intravesical pressure less than 20 cm H_2O during filling phase to prevent upper urinary tract damage and this should be ensured before transplant and at frequent intervals initially after a transplant.

Pretransplant evaluation should ensure that the bladder can store urine at safe pressures so as not to harm the transplanted kidney. Bladders known to be fibrotic or which remain smaller even after transplant may require an augmentation. Less than favourable outcome of the transplanted kidney may put these augumented bladders to risk of metabolic acidosis due to urinary absorption from the intestinal mucosa which is now part of bladder. A permanent catheter or ilial conduit non retentive diversion may be considered in such patients. Patients with very high voiding pressures are also at risk of complications and may require outlet reduction surgeries like TURP or bladder neck resection before or after a transplant. Patients with poor complaint bladder needs bladder rehabilitation before transplant. Anticholinergic drugs can be used to decrease unstable contractions and to reduce filling pressures.

MCU is recommended to diagnose the presence of VUR. Vesicoureteric reflux per se without voiding dysfunction post transplant does not correlate with subsequent graft function, hypertension, rejection or the number of UTI episodes. Neurogenic bladders with severe reflux may need augmentation prior to transplant. Both native dilated ureters can be used for augmentation cystoplasty in such cases to avoid any ileal segment which promotes urinary absorption and metabolic complications. Due to postoperative UTI the outcomes are compromised in patients with high grade reflux.

Suggested Reading

1. Cambell-Walsh Urology, 11th edition.
2. Urologic Clinic of North America. The Impact of Neurologic Disease on the Urinary Tract, August 2017; Volume 44, Issue 3, 333-516.
3. Kidney Transplantation–Principles and Practice, 7th Edition. Editor Peter Morris.
4. Mishra SK *et al.* (review article). Kidney Transplantation in Abnormal bladder. Indian J Urol 2007 Jul-Sep;23(3): 299-304.

CHAPTER

27

A Child with Vesicoureteric Reflux and Reflux Nephropathy

Rana Saha[1], Rajiv Sinha[2]

[1] *Consultant, Paediatrician and Paediatric Nephrologist, Institute of Child Health, Kolkata*

[2] *Professor and Head, Division of Paediatric Nephrology, Institute of Child Health, Kolkata*

CASE 1

AG 1.6 years old girl was admitted with fever, chill, rigor and persistent vomiting. She had a past history of culture positive urinary tract infection (UTI) at 9 months of age which responded to oral antibiotic. Initial investigation showed normal creatinine, high white cell count and elevated C-reactive protein (CRP). Urine routine revealed plenty of pus cells. She was started on intravenous ceftriaxone. AG remained febrile and urine culture came back as multi drug resistant Escherechia Coli only sensitive to carbapenem, nitrofurantoin, amikacin/gentamycin and colistin. Antibiotic was switched to meropenem and amikacin. Ultrasound revealed mild bilateral hydronephrosis [Right pelvis anteroposterior diameter (APD) 1.2 mm and left pelvis APD 1.1 mm]. Fever subsided and AG was discharged after completing 7 days of Meropenem and 5 days of Amikacin. In view of abnormal ultrasound as per Indian Society of Paediatric Nephrology guideline (ISPN) a micturating cystourethrography (MCUG) was ordered. MCUG revealed right grade 4 reflux (Fig. 27.1). AG was started on prophylactic cephalexin. Technetium 99m dimercaptosuccinic acid scan (DMSA) done after 4 months was reported normal. Despite being on prophylactic antibiotic she had two further febrile UTI within next 6 months. DMSA was done three months after her third UTI and it revealed scar on right kidney. Her prophylactic antibiotic was switched to cotrimoxazole and she has also been referred to the pediatric surgeons.

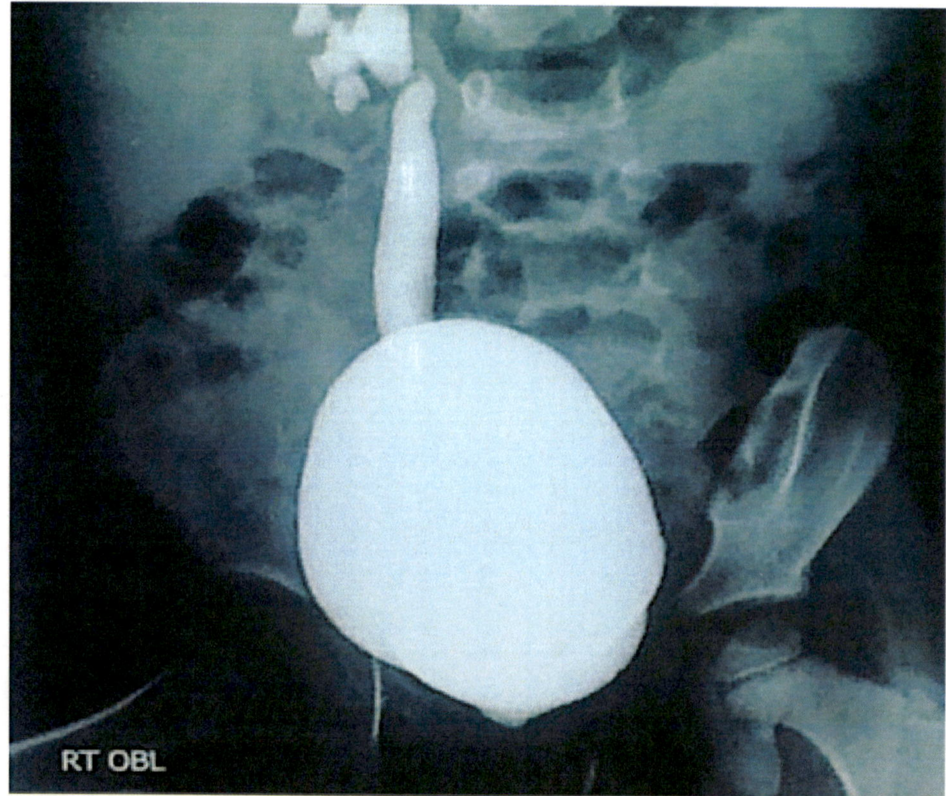

Figure 27.1: Micturating cystourethrogram of Case 1

CASE 2

DS 3.6 years old boy was admitted with UTI. Investigation revealed elevated creatinine of 1.67 mg/dl (eGFR = 56) and ultrasound scan revealed bilateral gross hydronephrouretrosis (Left kidney smaller than right) with normal bladder. DS was started on cefoperazone – sulbactum combination and the klebsiella grown in the urine culture was found to be sensitive to it. Despite hydration and treating the UTI successfully with appropriate antibiotics creatinine only dropped to 1.5 mg/dl. DS was discharged on prophylactic cotrimoxazole. Subsequent MCUG showed bilateral gross grade 5 reflux (Fig. 27.2) and DMSA showed poorly functioning both kidneys without any definite scars. DS did not have any further UTI but at one year follow up creatinine remained elevated at 1.6 mg/dl (Chronic Kidney Disease, Stage 3). He is being managed as per CKD protocol.

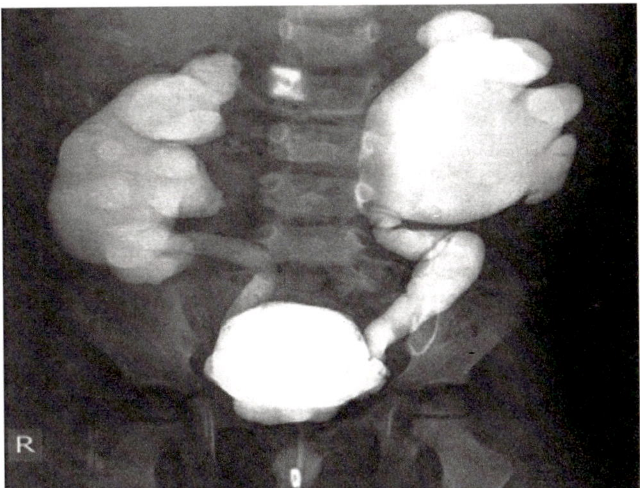

Figure 27.2: Micturating cystourethrogram of Case 2

CASE 3

PS 18 days old boy was admitted with dribbling of urine and high grade fever. Investigation was consistent for urosepsis (urine plenty of pus cells and CRP grossly elevated) with elevated creatinine (2.4 mg/dl). Rest of the biochemistry showed sodium 130 mmol/l, potassium 5.4 mmoml/l and bicarbonate 16 mmol/l. Ultrasound showed bilateral gross hydronephroureterosis with thick trabeculated bladder wall. The child was put on intravenous antibiotic (ceftriaxone) along with fluids and urinary catheter drainage. Urosepsis responded to the antibiotic and creatinine dropped to 1.2 mg/dl. MCUG done once child was stable and urine free of infection revealed posterior urethral valve, small trabeculated bladder and right grade 4 VUR (Fig. 27.3). Cystoscopy and fulgration was done and the child was discharged with creatinine of 0.8 mg/dl. He subsequently had another UTI at 6 months of age. At follow-up of 1 year

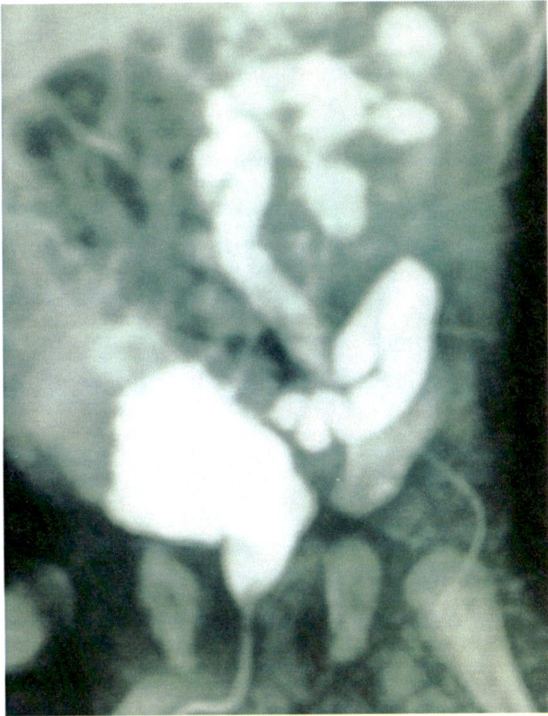

Figure 27.3: Micturating cystourethrogram of Case 3

his creatinine was 1.1 mg/dl (eGFR 48) and ultrasound still showed bilateral hydronephroureterosis with trabeculated thick bladder wall. He was on bicarbonate supplement as well as cotrimoxazole. Urodynamic (Fig. 27.4) study revealed high pressure bladder for which oxybutanin was started.

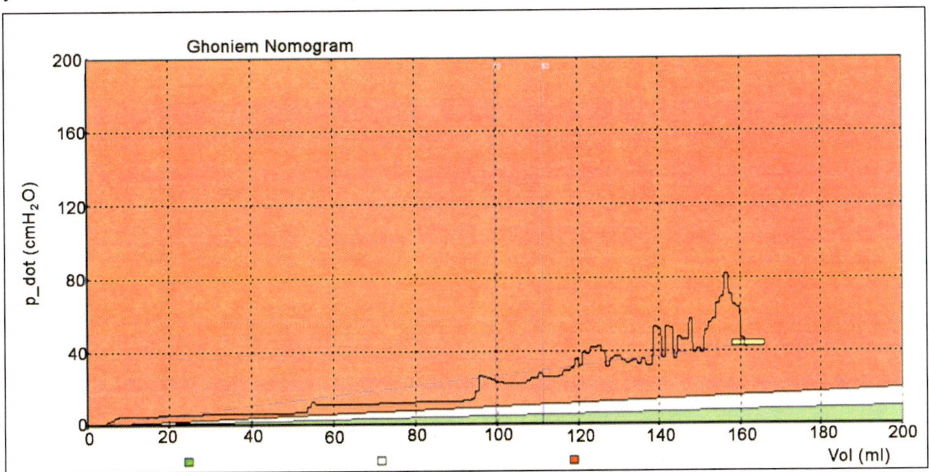

Figure 27.4: Urodynamic of case 3

What is Vesicoureteric Reflux (VUR)?

VUR is defined as the back flow of urine from the urinary bladder into one or both ureters, the renal pelvises, or both. Its severity is graded using the International Reflux Study in Children Classification from grade I to V, based on the appearance of the urinary tract on MCUG (Fig. 27.5), each ureter is graded separately and classification is usually based on the worse side.

Lower grades of reflux (grade I-III) are more likely to resolve. The presence of moderate to severe VUR, particularly if bilateral, is an important risk factor for pyelonephritis and renal scarring, with subsequent risk of hypertension, albuminuria and progressive kidney disease. The risk of scarring is highest in the early years of life. The presence of intrauterine VUR has been associated with renal hypoplasia or dysplasia.

What is Reflux Nephropathy (RN)?

The term RN is generally used for scenario wherein there is kidney damage associated with VUR. Based on current knowledge RN can be classified as following:

- **Acquired RN** *(Prototype Case 1)*–Renal scarring due to intra renal reflux of infected urine (pyelonephritis) in the presence or absence of a VUR emphasizing the role of other factors like bacterial virulence and host defence in its development. This is more commonly seen in females and is frequently mild.
- **Congenital RN** *(Prototype Case 2)*–Renal damage can occur with VUR even in the absence of a UTI particularly in infants in whom prenatal hydronephrosis and VUR results in development of focal renal dysplasia. This occurs mostly in males and is severe. The renal damage may be identified after work up for an UTI but the damage is nowadays often thought to be acquired antenatally.
- **Secondary RN** *(Prototype Case 3)*–Nephropathy associated with secondary VUR is often related to bladder outflow obstruction, as with posterior urethral valves, neurogenic bladder or a functional voiding disorder.

In majority of cases there is an association between reflux nephopathy and primary VUR but there is a need to distinguish between acquired and congenital RN and separately consider RN in association with obstruction. In addition there is often an overlap with congenital renal dysplasia being present not only in cases like Case 2 but also in obstructive uropathies such as Case 3.

Epidemiology

Incidence of primary VUR in children is 12-50%, this is much greater than the incidence in general population (0.1 to 1%). Black girls with UTI have much lower incidence of VUR when compared to white girls. In the majority (80%), VUR resolves with time and hence most frequently manifests in childhood.

Exact incidence of RN in children is unknown but there is evidence that increasing age at the diagnosis of VUR correlates with increasing incidence of renal scarring (10% in preterm, 26% in < 8 years and 47% in > 8 years).

Risk Factors for RN in Children

a. VUR–Children with VUR of gr III and above, particularly with other urological malformations, are more likely to develop renal damage compared to children with lower grade VUR.
b. UTI – VUR related renal scarring is more common with UTI.
c. Constipation.
d. Bowel bladder dysfunction–Rate of febrile UTI is much more common in this group.
e. Delay in treatment of febrile UTI–Mixed evidence.
f. Young age–Mixed evidence.

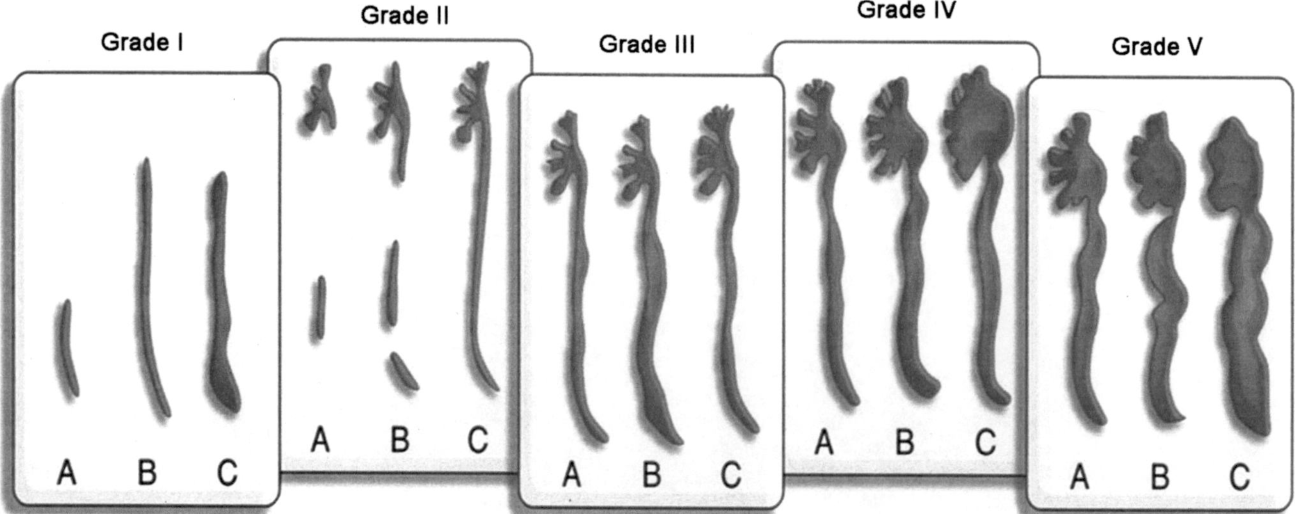

Figure 27.5: International reflux study grading system

A. Pathogenesis of VUR

Primary VUR has been postulated to be secondary to abnormal positioning of the ureteral orifice. This can be a result of either abnormal ueteric budding or dysfunctional interaction between ureteric bud and metanephric mesenchyme or a combination of both. Apart from this VUR can also arise from physical stresses resulting from obstruction on bladder outflow or dysfunction of the bladder.

B. Pathogenesis of Acquired RN

1. **Intra Renal Reflux:** Scars seen in acquired RN usually follow an episode or repeated episodes of UTI. It occurs primarily in areas with intra-renal reflux of infected urine into the collecting ducts and into the renal periphery.

   Histopathology studies have shown that the scarred segment usually have compound papillae with open gaping orifice allowing intra renal reflux in contrast to simple papillae in unscarred segments with slit shaped orifice, which do not allow intra renal reflux. It has to be remembered that non-refluxing papillae can be converted to refluxing one due to physical distortion from hydronephrosis, high pressure voiding or adjacent renal scarring.
2. **Role of Infection:** Renal scarring occurs more often when both VUR and infection are present. It is presumed that VUR compromises the host defence mechanisms, which then allow the direct invasion of bacteria in to collecting duct. Infection activates a cascade of mediators, which leads to renal epithelial cells damage.

C. Pathogenesis of Congenital RN

Two theories have been proposed to explain the pathogenesis of renal damage in the presence of VUR but in the absence of infection.

1. **Abnormal Bladder Dynamics and Water–Hammer Effect:** It has been observed in animal studies that with increased bladder pressure due to obstruction, the non-refluxing simple papillae start to show gaping ductal opening and free intra renal reflux.
2. **Abnormal Ureteric Bud-Metanephric Mesenchyme Interaction:** In congenital RN affected kidney appears small and smooth with histopathologic features of dysplasia and or hypoplasia resulting from anomalous metanephric development.

   VUR in humans is genetically heterogeneous. The majority of reported pedigrees have shown dominant inheritance patterns, but cases of recessive and X-linked inheritance are also reported. There is evidence of a 20-50 times increased risk of VUR in children with family history of VUR.

   However, in relation to scar formation in RN as opposed to VUR itself, it seems angiotensin-converting enzyme gene polymorphism may play some important role.

Natural History of VUR

VUR has a high chance of spontaneous resolution. Non-dilating reflux disappears more quickly than dilating ones. Studies have shown median time to resolution for grade I-II reflux as 38 months, whereas for grade IV-V it was around 156 months.

Complications

The complications of RN are well-known but poorly defined because of their insidious onset and slow progression. These include:

- Hypertension.
- Proteinuria.
- Urine concentration defects.
- Hyperkalemia.
- Acidosis.
- Focal segmental glomerulosclerosis.
- Chronic kidney disease with progressive renal failure, including end-stage renal failure (ESRF) in some patients. Variable registry reports have attributed RN to be responsible for 12% to 21% of all children with chronic renal failure.
- Pregnancy related complications.

Of these, hypertension and proteinuria are the most common ones that have a significant bearing on long-term renal outcome and both are amenable to medical intervention.

Investigations

Common methods available to investigate VUR in children are as below:

- MCUG remains the gold standard investigation for detection of VUR and also provides anatomical details regarding the bladder and the urethra. There is no need for delay of MCUG following an UTI and can be done at earliest convenient time once urine is sterile. Disadvantages of MCUG are distress in child during catheterisation, risk for infection and radiation burden.
- Ultrasound provides information on kidney size, number and location, presence of hydronephrosis, urinary bladder anomalies and post-void residual urine.
- Renal cortical Scintigraphy–DMSA is a sensitive technique for detecting renal parenchymal infection and cortical scarring. DMSA should be done 2-3 months after a UTI to show permanent scarring reliably. Role of acute DMSA for diagnosing pyelonephritis is not yet routinely accepted.

Other investigations include:

- **Indirect voiding cystography through MAG 3:** It has the advantage of low radiation and not needing bladder catheterisation. It is generally used for the reassessment of children with known reflux, or as a screen in older children presenting with a UTI, who have normal USG. It cannot be done in younger children as the child must be co-operative and must have bladder control.
- **Direct radionuclide cystography (DRC):** Though carries less radiation exposure, still has the disadvantage of needing bladder catheterisation. Moreover it does not give anatomical details and is unable to grade reflux as per the international classification.
- **Still in research domain:** Voiding urosonography, analysis of ureteric Doppler waveforms, MR urography etc.

National Institute of Clinical Excellence (NICE) and American Academy of Pediatrics (AAP) no longer recommends extensive radiological investigations to detect VUR in most children with uncomplicated febrile UTI. There is limited evidence that extensive imaging and subsequent management alters the long-term outcome of children with reflux nephropathy diagnosed following a UTI. In contrast Indian Society of Paediatric Nephrology (ISPN) recommends a more aggressive approach (Table 27.1). This has been justified because of variable availability of health infrastructure in India increasing the chance of missed or delayed diagnosis of UTI as well as any underlying urinary tract malformations.

Management of VUR and RN

Evidences are inconclusive regarding the optimum management of VUR and RN, and clinical trials have usually failed to come up with a clear conclusion. Once proteinuria, hypertension, or renal dysfunction has developed, it is unlikely that surgical correction of VUR can reverse the renal damage.

The aims of the management are to:

- Prevent recurrent febrile UTI/ pyelonephritis.
- Reduce the risk of further renal scarring.
- Reduce the morbidity associated with medical treatment and follow-up.
- Identify and manage children with bowel bladder dysfunction.

Treatment Options for Primary VUR (Table 27.2)

1. **Surveillance and Prompt Treatment of Inter-Current Episodes of UTI:** This approach may be suitable only in toilet trained, verbal children, and compliant families who understand the need for regular follow-up and recognition of further UTI.
2. **Medical Management:** Antibiotic prophylaxis to prevent recurrent (or sometime first) UTI and consequent renal scarring while waiting for VUR to resolve with time. Though various studies have reported no benefit of antibiotic prophylaxis in reducing UTI and renal scarring the recently published Randomized Intervention for VUR (RIVUR) trial did show a significant reduction in risks of recurrent febrile UTI primarily among girls with VUR. However even in RIVUR trial there was no difference in scar formation between the antibiotic and the placebo group. As per the ISPN guideline antibiotic prophylaxis is usually given to

Table 27.1: Evaluation following initial urinary tract infection (ISPN guideline)

Age < 1 year	Age 1-5 years	Age > 5 years
Ultrasound	Ultrasound	Ultrasound
MCU	DMSA scan	If ultrasound abnormal: MCUG and DMSA scan
DMSA renal scan	MCUG if ultrasound or DMSA scan is abnormal	

All patients with recurrent UTI need detailed evaluation with ultrasonography, DMSA scan and MCUG

Table 27.2: Management based on severity of reflux

Grade I-II VUR	Grade III-V VUR
Observation if compliant family (ISPN guidelines advocates antibiotic till 1 year of age)	Prophylaxis with antibiotic
Prophylaxis with antibiotic specially in:	*Surgery if:*
• Child with BBD	• Breakthrough infection
• Child not toilet trained	• Grade IV/V VUR persisting beyond 2-3 years of age
Surgery if breakthrough infection	Serious adverse effect from prophylaxis

children who are not toilet trained or those with high grade reflux and to children with BBD. Antibiotic commonly used are:

- Trimethprim–sulphamethoxazole (TMP-SMZ) or TMP alone–dose is based on TMP 2 mg/kg.
- Nitrofurantoin–1-2 m/kg.
- Amoxycillin (10 mg/kg) and Cephalexin (10-15 mg/kg) in infant less than 3 months old in whom first two groups are contraindicated or for those children where TMP-SMZ or Nitrofurantoin cannot be given.

This is typically single dose and given at bed time.

Optimum duration of prophylaxis is not known particularly when VUR does not resolve but it is usually discontinued when VUR resolves spontaneously or is surgically corrected.

3. **Surgical Treatment:** This involves correcting the anatomy at the refluxing ureterovesical junction. Although various guidelines contradicts each other surgical intervention is usually reserved for the following children:
   - Children with Grade IV/V VUR persisting beyond 2-3 years of age.
   - Children with grade III to IV VUR:
     - Who cannot tolerate prophylactic antibiotic?
     - Who are not compliant with medical treatment?
     - Who is having breakthrough febrile UTI even on antibiotics?

   The Surgical Options are:

   - **Open or laparoscopic ureteral reimplantation:** Basic principle is lengthening of intramural part of the ureter. Open procedure has two approaches intra vesical and extra vesical. Surgical success in curing VUR with re-implantation is high, greater than 98% in grades of reflux I to IV, dropping to 80% with grade V. Open procedure is a major surgical endeavour requiring a stay of several days in hospital. Skills pertaining to laparoscopic or robotic ureteric reimplatation are currently evolving.
   - **Endoscopic sub-ureteric transurethral injection of bulking agents:** Injection of tissue augmenting substance is done under anesthesia and requires short stay in hospital. The most commonly used agent is combined dextranomer and hyaluronic acid (Dx/HA or DEFLUX). Resolution rate varies with degree of reflux (79% in Grade I and II and 51% for grade V reflux). There are concerns regarding long-term effects, including migration of foreign material. Also the longevity of treatment and need for repeat treatment are not fully known.
   - Circumcision is a treatment option in the management of male infants with VUR as this has shown to reduce the risk of acute pyelonephritis and subsequent scarring.

4. **Management of Bowel Bladder Dysfunction (BBD):** Appropriate management of BBD is important as it helps in preventing recurrent UTI, improves chances of resolution of the VUR, and even increases success rate of surgical correction. The treatment options include use of laxative and fibre for constipation, timed frequent and complete voiding, pelvic floor exercise, biofeedback and or use of anti-cholinergic medication or alfa-blockers for bladder, and continuous intermittent catheterization in extreme cases.

   Treatment options for secondary VUR: This includes treating any underlying cause such as those for obstructive uropathy.

Treatment Options for RN

Renal Impairment

Management of renal failure due to RN should be done along the lines of other causes of renal failure. Aggressive treatment of hypertension, use of angiotensin-converting enzyme (ACE) inhibitors and prevention of breakthrough infection can slow down further renal damage.

Hypertension

Timely diagnosis and adequate control of hypertension is essential as it curtail the progression to end stage renal disease.

- **ACE inhibitor and/ or angiotensin receptor blocker (ARB):** These agents are beneficial in presence of scarring and proteinuria to preserve renal function.
- **Nephtrectomy:** When hypertension is severe and uncontrollable despite multiple anti-hypertensive medication removal of affected small scarred kidney may be considered but one needs to keep in mind that it may not cure the problem, as disease is often bilateral.

Long-Term Follow-up

Long-term follow-up clinically and radiologically should be planned for all children with persisting VUR as well as those with renal scarring/dysplasia.

Follow-up assessment should include:

- Assessment of linear growth.
- Measurement of blood pressure.
- Renal parameters including urinalysis to detect proteinuria or infection.

Families should be counselled regarding the association of VUR and increased risk of chronic kidney disease (e.g., hypertension, renal impairment or proteinuria).

Key Points

- Most of VUR resolves with time although higher grades take longer time to resolve.
- Prophylactic antibiotic does help in maintaining urine sterility although its utility in preserving renal function is still debatable.
- There are controversies about best investigations and management strategies in the prevention of recurrent UTI and renal scarring.
- Timely diagnosis and treatment of UTI, hypertension and proteinuria remains mainstay in preserving renal function.
- Multiple interactions between genetic factors, environmental factors and anatomical factors results in the unpredictability of outcome measures even despite aggressive management. This to a large extent explains the fact that despite increased awareness of VUR and UTI the overall incidence of end stage renal disease secondary to reflux nephropathy has remained constant.

Suggested Reading

1. Mattoo TK. Vesicoureteral Reflux and Reflux Nephropathy. Adv Chronic Kidney Dis 2011 September;18(5):348-54. doi:10.1053.
2. Dillon MJ and Chulananda D, Goonasekera S. Reflux Nephropathy, J Am Soc Nephrol 1998;9:2377-83.
3. Tullus K, Vesicoureteric reflux in children. Lancet 2015 Jan 24;385(9965):371-79.
4. Williams G, Fletcher JT, Alexander SI and Craig JC. Vesicoureteral reflux. J Am Soc Nephrol 2008;19:847-62.
5. Fernando F. Fonseca, Fabio Y, Tanno, Hiep T. Nguyen. Current options in the management of Primary Vesicoureteral reflux in children, PediatrClin N Am 2012; 59:819-34.

CHAPTER

28 A Patient with Hepatorenal Syndrome

Suman Lata[1], Manoj Kumar Sharma[2], Tarun Kaushik[3]

[1] *Director, Nephrology, Dharamshila Narayana Superspecialty Hospital, New Delhi*

[2] *Professor, Hepatology, ILBS, New Delhi*

[3] *Consultant, Nephrology, Dharamshila Narayana Superspecialty Hospital, New Delhi*

CASE

34 years old male known alcoholic cirrhosis with ascites presented with complains of abdominal distension and pain abdomen for past 3 days. Examination revealed icterus, ascites and pedal oedema. Investigation results are as follow:

Hb=10.6 gm%; TLC=14500/cumm; Platelet=2.0 l/cumm; Reticulocyte count=2.1%; Peripheral smear= Normocytic RBC. Bilirubin= 4.2 mg/dl; AST=370 IU/l; ALT=107 IU/l; Total Protein=7.0 g/dl; albumin=1.9 g/dl; Alkaline phosphatase=145 IU/l; PT= 3 sec prolonged, Serum creatinine=2.3 mg/dl.

USG abdomen: Shrunken and Coarse echotexture of liver, Moderate ascites.

Ascitic fluid analysis: TLC 1000 cells/cumm, Poly 90%.

Introduction

Acute kidney injury (AKI) is a frequent complication in patients with cirrhosis which is associated with significant mortality and morbidity in these patients. Acute Kidney Injury Network (AKIN) and Kidney Disease: Improving Global Outomes (KDIGO) criteria define AKI as an increase in serum creatinine (sCr) of more than 0.3 mg/dl ($\geq$ 26.5 μmol/l) within 48 hours, percentage increase in sCr of more than 50% from the baseline, which is known, or presumed, to have occurred within the previous 48 hours to 7 days or urine output <0.5 ml/kg/hour for greater than 6 hours. This definition for AKI has resulted prompt diagnosis of AKI resulting in early interventions. An incremental change in serum creatinine to diagnose AKI is more relevant in chronic liver failure (CLF) patients who have low baseline serum creatinine due to reduced muscle mass. Hence serum creatinine within normal laboratory range could still represent AKI in a CLF patient. Case example given above shows a typical presentation of a CLF patient presenting with AKI.

AKI is a known complication in patients with cirrhosis and acute on chronic liver failure (ACLF). ACLF is a distinct syndrome where an acute insult on the chronic liver disease leads to liver failure which is associated with an extremely high mortality in the absence of liver transplant. AKI is known to have higher frequency, more rapid progression, a different spectrum and higher mortality in patients with ACLF as compared to decompensated cirrhosis. This chapter details the unique features of AKI in patients with cirrhosis and ACLF, diagnosis, prognosis and management of AKI, the outcomes of different forms of AKI including the potential role of novel biomarkers. AKI is universally present in patients with ACLF according to the definition by the EASL-CLIF consortium while on the contrary the APASL definition of ACLF does not incorporate kidney dysfunction or failure in its definition.

Pathophysiology of AKI

The pathophysiology of AKI (Fig. 28.1) is the same as that of ascites and hyponatremia in cirrhotic patients. In fact, AKI rarely occurs in the absence of ascites or edema in these patients. The main abnormality is systemic and splanchnic vasodilatation secondary to portal (or sinusoidal) hypertension which leads to decreased effective arterial blood volume. This in-turn causes activation of neurohormonal systems, i.e., the renin angiotensin aldosterone system (RAAS), the sympathetic nervous system and non-osmotic release of antidiuretic hormone (ADH). This results in salt and water retention by the kidneys causing ascites, edema and dilutional hyponatremia. The cause of this vasodilatation is excessive production of nitric oxide (NO) which is the main mediator of vasodilatation. Nitric oxide via increased cGMP production also causes negative inotropic effects on the heart causing cardiac dysfunction what is termed as cirrhotic cardiomyopathy. This leads to a state of relative hypovolemia which in the

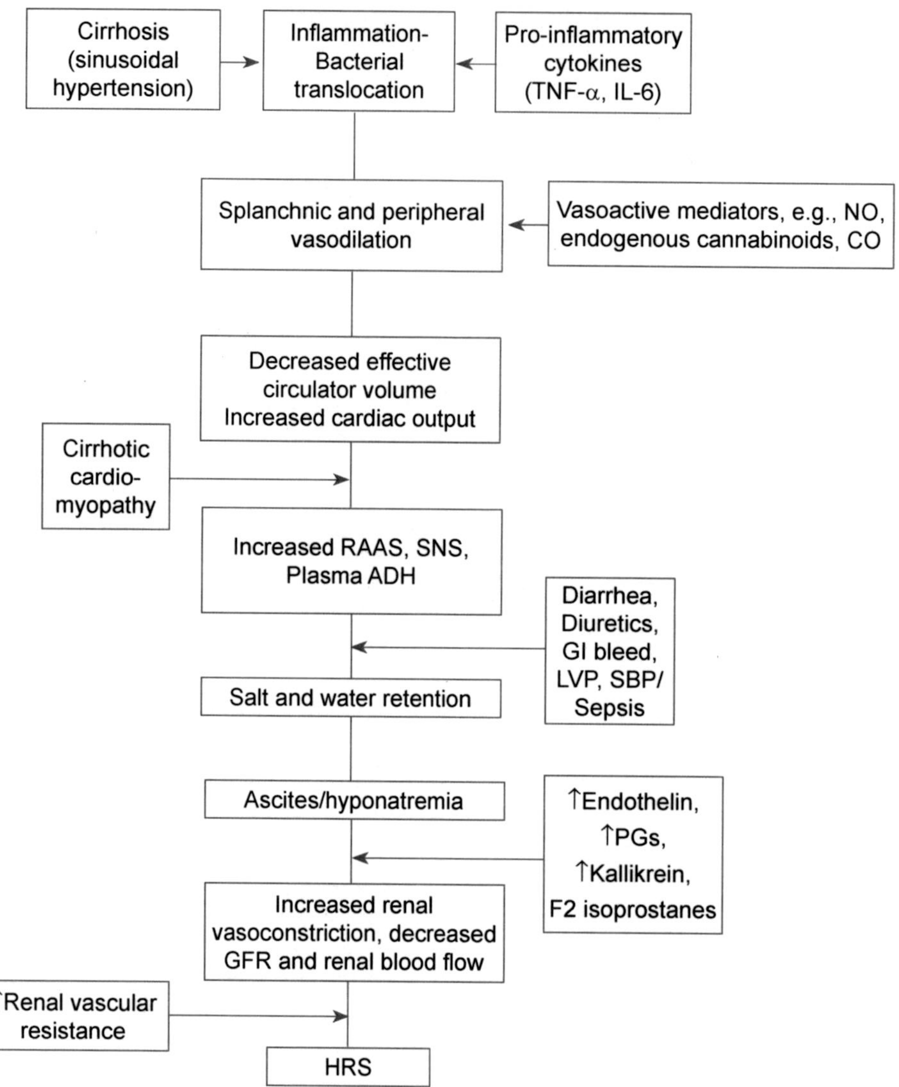

Figure 28.1: Pathophysiological basis of hepatorenal syndrome (HRS) in cirrhosis

RAAS: Renin angiotensin aldosterone system; SNS: Sympathetic nervous system; ADH: Antidiuretic hormone; NO: Nitric oxide; SBP: Spontanous bacterial peritonitis; LVP: Large volume paracentasis.

initial stages of cirrhosis is compensated by an increased cardiac output and heart rate as well as compensatory renal vasoconstriction. However, with the progression of cirrhosis there is a perturbed balance between the vasoconstrictive forces mediated by endothelin, prostaglandins, kallikreins in the kidney and the systemic and splanchnic vasodilatation which leads to a decreased renal blood flow and glomerular filtration and increased renal vascular resistance contributed also by an impaired cardiac output because of cirrhotic cardiomyopathy. AKI can also occur because of any acute event like sepsis, diarrhoea, gastrointestinal bleed, spontaneous bacterial peritonitis, large volume paracentesis or nephrotoxic drugs which disturb the state of balance between the renal and the systemic hemodynamics leading to a rapid decline in renal function. Furthermore, it has been shown that patients with bacterial infection have an increased severity of cardiac and renal dysfunction secondary to an exaggerated systemic inflammatory response with increased levels of pro-inflammatory cytokines like TNFα and IL-6. In cases with spontaneous bacterial peritonitis, studies in both laboratory animals and patients have shown that bacterial translocation (mostly gram negative bacteria) from the intestinal lumen to the mesenteric lymph nodes elicits an inflammatory response with increased production of pro-inflammatory cytokines (TNFα and IL-6) and vasodilatation factors (e.g., nitric oxide) causing vasodilatation of splanchnic vessels impairing the circulatory function and cause renal failure which is mostly severe in these cases.

Spectrum of AKI in Cirrhosis

AKI in patients with cirrhosis can be either functional or structural. Functional group comprises of volume responsive (Pre renal) and the unresponsive state (Hepatorenal syndrome).

Structural group comprises acute tubular necrosis (ATN) and other renal parenchymal disorders.

Functional AKI

Volume Responsive (Pre Renal Azotemia)

It is the most common type of AKI in cirrhotic patients, accounting for up to 68% of patients with a multifactorial etiology. A number of factors can cause renal hypoperfusion mainly secondary to intravascular volume depletion which responds promptly by improving the renal perfusion. In patients with cirrhosis and upper gastrointestinal bleeding, the prevalence of renal failure is approximately 11%. However, in patients with ongoing volume losses pre-renal AKI can progress to a structural type lesion in the kidney such as ATN. The later may not respond well to intravascular fluid replacement compared to pre renal AKI.

Diuretics induced volume depletion can also lead to an AKI and has been reported in up to 30% of patients. This is usually reversible after withdrawal of diuretics and or with expansion of intravascular volume unless complicated by another contributory factor.

Infections are among the most important contributing factors in development of AKI in patients with liver cirrhosis. The incidence of renal failure in liver cirrhosis and spontaneous bacterial peritonitis is about 30%.

Volume Unresponsive (Hepatorenal Syndrome)

HRS is a unique type of syndrome exclusively seen in advanced liver failure and characterized by acute and rapidly progressive renal failure. The median survival of patients with type 1 HRS is 2–3 weeks if not treated. HRS is usually precipitated by infections such as spontaneous bacterial peritonitis (SBP) and UTI. There are some noninfectious events which can precipitate HRS although, less frequently such as viral or alcoholic hepatitis, gastrointestinal bleeding; and major surgical procedures. However, in some patients no obvious precipitating event is found.

Structural AKI

It mainly includes acute tubular necrosis and renal parenchymal diseases. Patients who do not respond to vasoconstrictors and albumin develop ATN although in such group of patients, further histology is needed to prove the diagnosis. ATN secondary to HRS carries a bad outcome and renders patients dialysis dependent.

Apart from ATN, patients with liver cirrhosis for instance secondary to chronic Hepatitis B and C infections may also have renal involvement, which primarily manifests as proteinuria (>500 mg/day) and microscopic hematuria. The most common form of glomerular diseases being membranous nephropathy and membranoproliferative glomerulonephritis. There is an association between alcoholic cirrhosis and IgA nephropathy leading to microscopic hematuria. Also, both liver and kidney may be involved in multisystem autoimmune disorders. This group of patients require renal biopsy to establish the diagnosis correctly. Structural diseases involving both liver and kidneys also include adult polycystic kidney disease and amyloidosis, both of which can progress to end stage renal and liver diseases.

Spectrum of AKI in ACLF

The spectrum of AKI in ACLF is different from that of decompensated cirrhosis. As for patients with decompensated cirrhosis, AKI in patients with ACLF can be precipitated by hypovolemia secondary to diuretic use, large volume paracentesis or variceal bleed, systemic inflammation, bacterial infection or use of nephrotoxic medications. The most common cause of AKI in two-thirds of patients with decompensated cirrhosis is functional while structural AKI is noted in rest one-third of patients. However, patients with ACLF more often have structural AKI secondary to circulatory dysfunction, bacterial infections and systemic inflammation which is responsible for renal hypoperfusion, alteration in renal microcirculation and increased incidence of tubular dysfunction. Furthermore, a significantly higher prevalence of "bile pigment nephropathy" in postmortem kidney biopsies has been reported in patients with ACLF as compared to decompensated cirrhosis. This entity also called as "cholemic nephrosis" is proposed to be secondary to direct toxic damage to the renal tubules by the elevated levels of bilirubin and bile acids.

Moreover, the clinical diagnosis of ATN as well as its differentiation from HRS is notoriously the most difficult in patients with ACLF as these patients have impaired coagulation profile with ascites. Hence, trans-jugular kidney biopsies are not feasible in these patients. Preliminary data from prospective studies in decompensated cirrhotics have highlighted the potential role of biomarkers in differentiating functional from structural AKI. However, there are no studies specifically addressing diagnostic AKI biomarkers in patients with ACLF. The differentiation of HRS and ATN in patients with ACLF is also important while contemplating liver transplant as functional AKI or HRS is likely to resolve following liver transplantation alone. On the other hand established severe ATN and its sequela may necessitate the need of simultaneous liver-kidney transplant.

Diagnosis of AKI

Traditionally, renal failure in patients with cirrhosis was defined by the "conventional criteria", i.e., an increase in serum creatinine (sCr) of more than 50% from baseline to a final value of 1.5 mg/dl. The diagnosis of HRS also relied on stringent criteria based on absolute value of sCr of 1.5 mg/dl. Based on this, Type 1 HRS was defined as a rapidly progressive decline in renal function, characterized by doubling of the initial creatinine to a level of more than 2.5 mg/dl in 2 weeks and type 2 HRS was characterized by an insidious clinical course, associated with a moderate increase in sCr to more than 1.5 mg/dl with a median survival of 4-6 months.

In the most recent revised consensus of the International Club of Ascites (ICA) a modified version of the KDIGO criteria was used to define AKI in patients with cirrhosis. According to the revised consensus criteria, AKI was defined either by an increase in sCr of more than 0.3 mg/dl (≥26.5 μmol/l) within 48 hours or by a percentage increase in sCr of more than 50% from the baseline, which is known, or presumed, to have occurred within the previous 7 days.[1]

The modifications considered in the revised criteria when compared to the KDIGO criteria included first, consideration of sCr within the last 3 months before admission as baseline value for the diagnosis of AKI, in case of non-availability of baseline value of sCr within the previous 7 days. Second, calculation of baseline sCr by the reverse application of the Modification of Diet in Renal Disease (MDRD) formula, using an arbitrarily defined normal value of GFR of 75 ml/min/1.73 m^2. Third, the abandonment of urine output criteria from the diagnosis of AKI in patients with cirrhosis. This is because urine output correlates poorly with the severity of renal dysfunction in patients with cirrhosis as these patients are mostly on diuretics. Further, patients with cirrhosis despite being oliguric still may have a relatively normal glomerular function. The problem is further compounded by the inaccuracies in urinary collection in these patients. Further, in the revised consensus, the previous type 2 HRS was proposed to be considered as a type of chronic kidney disease (CKD) called as HRS-CKD. The other major change that was considered in the revised consensus criteria was removal of any cut-off value for sCr both from the definition of AKI and HRS. Type 1 HRS according to the revised criteria is now defined as "HRS-AKI" (Tables 28.1 and 28.2). This is because even though sCr remains the most practical biomarker for the assessment and management of renal failure in patients with cirrhosis it is associated with several limitations. First, it lags behind the onset of disease process and is affected by numerous extrarenal factors such as body weight, race, age, sex, total body volume, drugs, muscle metabolism, and protein intake and is falsely recorded low in sarcopenic patients with advanced cirrhosis. Levels of sCr are also affected by increased tubular secretion of creatinine and presence of hyperbilirubinemia in these patients. Second, sCr does not provide any relevant information regarding the etiology of kidney injury, i.e., the presence of underlying structural kidney damage and therefore the response to various treatment modalities.

Glomerular Filtration Rate (GFR)

Various methods have been used to estimate the GFR which include either creatinine-based equations or real time estimation by DTPA scan, iothalamate and inulin clearance. Though cockroft Gault and the simplified "modification of diet in renal disease" formula of GFR are simple to estimate however they are not true reflective

Table 28.1: International Club of Ascites (ICA-AKI) new definitions for the diagnosis and management of AKI in patients with cirrhosis

Subject	Definition		
Baseline sCr	A value of sCR obtained in the previous 3 months, when available, can be used as baseline sCr. In patients with more than one value within the previous 3 months, the value closest to the admission time to the hospital should be used In patients without a previous sCr value, the sCR on admission should be used as baseline		
Definition of AKI	• Increase in sCr ≥ 0.3 mg/dl (≥26.5 μmol/l) within 48 hours; or • A percentage increase sCr ≥50% from baseline which is known, or presumed, to have occurred within the prior 7 days		
Staging of AKI	• **Stage 1:** Increase in sCr ≥0.3 mg/dl (26.5 μmol/l) or an increase in sCr ≥1.5-fold to 2-fold from baseline • **Stage 2:** Increase in sCr >2-fold to 3-fold from baseline • **Stage 3:** Increase of sCr >3-fold from baseline or sCR ≥4.0 mg/dl (353.6 μmol/l) with an acute increase ≥0.3 mg/dl (26.5 μmol/l) or initiation of renal replacement therapy		
Progression of AKI	**Progression** Progression of AKI to a higher stage and/or need for RRT	**Regression** Regression of AKI to a lower stage	
Response to treatment	**No response** No regression of AKI	**Partial response** Regression of AKI stage with a reduction of sCR to ≥0.3 mg/dl (26.5 μmol/l) above the baseline value	**Full response** Return of sCr to a value within 0.3 mg/dl (26.5 μmol/l) of the baseline value

AKI: Acute kidney injury; RRT: Renal replacement therapy; sCR: Serum creatinine.

Table 28.2: Diagnostic criteria of hepatorenal syndrome (HRS) type of acute kidney injury (AKI) in patients with cirrhosis

HRS-AKI
ICA-AKI criteria for HRS-AKI in patients with cirrhosis and ascites
No improvement in serum creatinine after 2 consecutive days of withdrawal of diuretics and plasma volume expansion with albumin (1 g per kg of body weight, maximum 100 g/day)
Absence of shock
Exclusion of recurrent or recent use of nephrotoxic agents (e.g., NSAIDs, aminoglycosides, contrast media)
Exclusion of parenchymal kidney disease:
• Absence of proteinuria (>500 mg/day)
• Absence of microhematuria (>50 RBCs per high-power field)
• Normal renal ultrasonography
**Patients who fulfil these criteria may still have structural damage such as tubular damage. Urine biomarkers will become an important element in making a more accurate differential diagnosis between HRS and acute tubular necrosis.*

of GFR as creatinine is used in both as a variable. Newer serum markers such as cystatin C are promising; and studies in advanced cirrhotics awaiting liver transplantation have shown that equations incorporating both creatinine and cystatin C performed better than the creatinine-based equations and were equivalent to the gold-standard methods of GFR estimation.

Urinary Indices

These indices are traditionally used to differentiate structural from functional renal failure in acute kidney injury. The commonly used variables are spot urinary sodium, fractional excretion of sodium and ratio of blood urea nitrogen to creatinine. Prerenal azotemia and HRS are classically described as sodium avid states with low (20 mEq/l) urinary sodium (UNa), low (1%) fractional excretion of sodium (FENa), and elevated (> 500 mOsm/kg) urine osmolality. Conversely, patients with ATN have high UNa (40 mEq/l), high FENa (2%), and urine osmolality under 350 mOsm/kg. However clinical presentation doesn't match with classical paradigms because of various confounding factors. Most of these patients are on diuretics therefore urine Na and FENa does not carry any significance. Muddy brown granular casts are typically seen in ATN and the presence of active sediment differentiates between structural and functional renal failure. Recent studies have highlighted the significance of urinary albumin and protein to creatinine ratio in the context of AKI to differentiate HRS from ATN and have shown to be more reliable than urinary spot sodium which is influenced by use of diuretics in patients with cirrhosis.

Kidney Biopsies

As already mentioned, kidney biopsies even though gold-standard for the diagnosis of AKI are usually difficult in patients with cirrhosis because of presence of ascites and coagulopathy. The diagnosis of ATN, bile-cast nephropathy and other renal parenchymal diseases can be reliably obtained by transjugular kidney biopsies in these patients.

Role of Biomarkers

Biomarkers of Glomerular Injury

Serum Cystatin C

Cystatin C (CysC) is a non glycosylated protein with low molecular weight (13 kDa), belongs to the cystatin superfamily of cysteine endopeptidase inhibitors which catabolize enzymes and proteins. Because of its constant rate of production, concentration of cystatin C is determined by glomerular filtration and therefore it is considered as an early marker of glomerular dysfunction. In patients with ACLF, because of the marked hyperbilirubinemia, serum creatinine can also be spuriously low for the extent of renal impairment. In a large cohort study in patients with cirrhosis, serum cystatin C was shown to be marker of renal reserve to predict development of new AKI episode after recovery from AKI. The incorporation of cystatin C into the MELD score, i.e., MELD-Cystatin was shown to be superior for prediction of mortality as compared to the MELD and CTP scores. In case of damage to proximal tubules there is decreased reabsorption and increased urinary secretion of CysC. Studies in patients with advanced liver cirrhosis have shown CysC to be more accurate in estimating GFR as compared to the creatinine based equations. Further, in patients with hepatitis-B virus (HBV) related ACLF, CysC was shown to accurately predict AKI even in patients with normal serum creatinine. Belcher *et al.* also showed a better predictive ability of cystatin C as compared to serum creatinine. Changes in CysC were more closely associated with eventual requirement of RRT as well as mortality.

Proximal Tubular Damage

Kidney Injury Molecule (KIM-1)

Kidney injury molecule-1 is a type 1 transmembrane glycoprotein which is comprised an immunoglobulin and mucin domain. Under normal conditions, KIM-1 protein is only minimally expressed in kidney tissue or urine but is shed from the proximal tubules with tubular dysfunction wherein it can be detected in the urine by immunoassay. It is known to be upregulated in response to renal ischemia or nephrotoxic insult and is also believed to participate in the regeneration process after epithelial injury.

Liver Fatty Acid Binding Protein (L-FABP)

Fatty-acid protein bindings (FABPs) facilitate transfer of fatty acids between intra and extracellular membranes. They also have a role in the amelioration of cellular oxidative stress by inhibition of the toxic effects of oxidative intermediates on cellular membranes. In the normal healthy state, urinary L-FABP is undetectable; however, under states of renal ischemia there is decreased proximal tubular reabsorption of L-FABP which is detected as increased excretion in urine.

Interleukine-18

Interleukine-18 (IL-18) is a proinflammatory cytokine which is synthesized in renal proximal tubular epithelial cells as well as monocytes and macrophages. The concentrations of IL-18 have also been demonstrated to be increased in post ischemic AKI following renal hypoxia. It can therefore be considered as an early biomarker of AKI in critically ill patients. It has also been shown to correlate with poor clinical outcomes (death or requirement of renal replacement therapy) in patients with sepsis.

Distal Tubular Damage

Neutrophil Gelatinase-Associated Lipocalin

Neutrophil gelatinase-associated lipocalin (NGAL) NGAL belongs to the lipocalin superfamily (lipocalin 2, siderocalin). Both plasma and urine NGALs are increased after an episode of AKI. Elevated urine NGAL originates from both proximal and distal nephron after a nephrotoxic insult. Injury to proximal renal tubules precludes NGAL reabsorption and/or increase de novo NGAL synthesis secondary to upregulation of NGAL mRNA in the distal nephron segments (especially in the thick ascending limb of Henle's loop and the collecting ducts).

Studies Assessing Markers of Tubular Injury in Patients with Cirrhosis

In a prospective multicentric study by Belcher *et al.* in patients with cirrhosis and AKI a panel of biomarkers for differential diagnosis of clinically adjudicated AKI were studied. Median values for neutrophil gelatinase associated lipocalin (NGAL), interleukin-18 (IL18), kidney injury molecule 1 (KIM 1), liver type fatty acid binding protein (L-FABP) and albumin were noted to be different amongst various etiologies of AKI and were significantly higher in patients adjudicated with ATN. The fractional excretion of sodium (FENa) was lowest in patients with HRS, but did not differentiate pre-renal AKI from ATN. The likelihood of ATN diagnosis was accurate with the panel of these biomarkers and increased step-wise with number of biomarkers above optimal cut-offs and hence helped in delineation of structural AKI, i.e., ATN from other forms of AKI. In an earlier study by Fagundes *et al.*, it was reported that urinary N-GAL levels were significantly higher in patients with cirrhosis and ATN; however, these levels could not differentiate ATN from HRS associated with bacterial infections.[2]

The major challenge in patients with ACLF is to differentiate HRS associated with bacterial infections from ATN as it evolves through a continuous spectrum. In fact, HRS patients who are non-responders to vasoconstrictors are known to have tubular dysfunction requiring prolonged RRT. In another prospective study in patients with cirrhosis and bacterial infections, measurement of urinary NGAL at infection diagnosis was reported to be useful in predicting clinical outcomes, persistent AKI and type of AKI. Interestingly, N-GAL also accurately predicted development of a second infection and 3-month mortality. Barreto *et al.*, demonstrated that a significantly higher uNGAL titre was noted in patients who developed persistent AKI and amongst these patients was able to discriminate type-1 HRS from other causes of AKI with accuracy. In another study done in 55 patients with an acute decompensation of cirrhosis a panel of 12 biomarkers was studied to differentiate ATN from other causes of AKI. In this study also, NGAL was identified as the best biomarker, others being IL-18, albumin, trefoil-factor-3 (TFF-3) and glutathione-S-transferase-π (GST-π).[3]

Management of AKI

According to the new consensus by the ICA for AKI, a new algorithm for the management of AKI based on the revised criteria has been proposed. Based on this algorithm it is recommended that patients with initial AKI stage 1 should be managed by removal of all precipitants (careful review of medications, diuretics, nephrotoxic drugs, vasodilators or non-steroidal anti-inflammatory drugs). Second step is to consider plasma volume expansion in patients with hypovolemia (the choice of fluid could either be a crystalloid or albumin or even blood as indicated) along with identification and early treatment of bacterial infections. Patients who respond with a decrease in sCr value of 0.3 mg/dl of the baseline value should be subsequently followed up for any new episodes of AKI. Patients who have progression, should be managed as ICA-AKI stage 2 and 3. In this group of patients, along with the institution of all measures as recommended for patients with stage 1 AKI a work up for the differential diagnosis should be done on an immediate basis to identify whether it is HRS-AKI, intrinsic AKI or post-renal cause. It was further decided by the panel of experts that for patients with stage 1 AKI who do not improve but have no progression further management can be decided based on the absolute value of sCr and if the sCr is more than 1.5 mg/dl it was recommended to consider the same protocol as for management for stage 2 and 3 AKI. Patients with HRS-AKI are recommended to be managed with early use of vasoconstrictors based on the revised criteria for HRS-AKI (either with terlipressin or norepinephrine or midodrine plus octreotide). Management of non-responders to vasoconstrictors which constitute a large group of patients therefore still remains an ongoing challenge. There is paucity of data on dialysis in patients with cirrhosis therefore there are no specific recommendations regarding the dose, the intensity, duration and time of initiation of dialysis in these patients (Fig. 28.2).

Albumin

Albumin has an important role both in the diagnosis as well as treatment of HRS. Normal liver synthesizes 11-15 g of albumin, however this capacity is reduced by 60-80% in patients with cirrhosis. Albumin previously known for its colloid osmotic functions has recently been identified with important properties like carrying different substances, anti-inflammatory and anti-oxidant property as well as maintenance of capillary permeability. Prospective studies have shown that albumin when combined with vasoconstrictors is superior to albumin use alone in patients with hepatorenal syndrome. Its beneficial effect in improvement of renal functions is attributed to its property of both an increase in plasma blood volume and a vasoconstrictive effect on peripheral blood circulation. For the treatment of hepatorenal syndrome a bolus of 1g/kg/day on presentation (maximum dose, 100 g daily) and subsequently continued dose of 20-60 g daily as needed to maintain central venous pressure between 10 and 15 cm H_2O is administered.[4]

Vasoconstrictors

Terlipressin, noradrenaline and octreotide-midodrine are the key vasoconstrictors which have been used for the management of HRS. Till date, there are various trials which have assessed the efficacy of terlipressin in reversal of HRS, majority of which have used terlipressin in combination with albumin while others have compared its efficacy against other vasoconstrictors.

Terlipressin

It is the preferred vasopressin analogue because of its ease of administration and low incidence of side-effects. It causes vasoconstriction of systemic and splanchnic circulation by binding to V1 receptors on the vascular smooth muscle, reduces the portal inflow causing reduction in porto-systemic shunting and also causes decreased intrahepatic resistance by causing dilatation of intrahepatic vessels. Hence the treatment with terlipressin is associated with improved cardiac

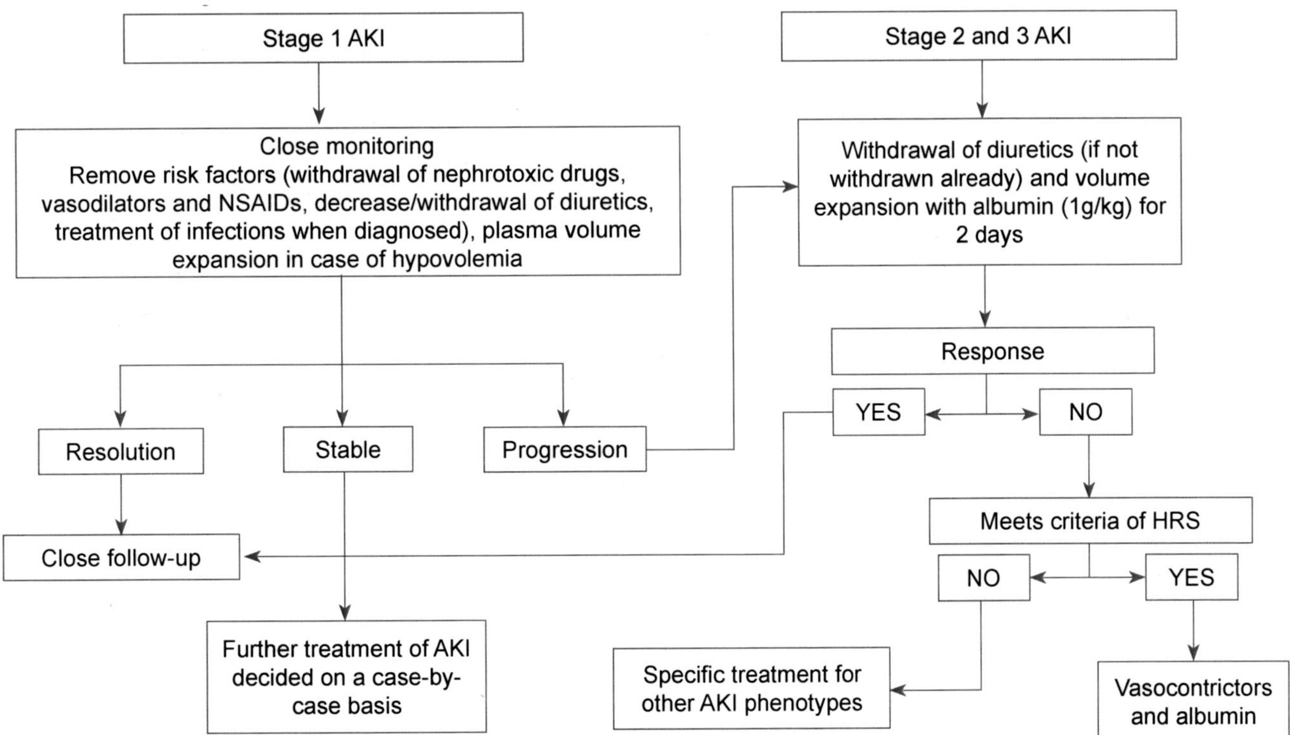

Figure 28.2: Proposed algorithm for the management of acute kidney injury (AKI) according to International Club of Ascites—AKI (ICA-AKI) classification that combines Kidney Disease Improving Global Outcomes (KDIGO) criteria and conventional criteria in patients with cirrhosis and ascites (Paolo Angeli *et al.* Gut 2015;64:531-537)

and urinary output, lower serum creatinine and rennin levels, improved renal blood flow and improvement in mean arterial pressures. Terlipressin is given at a dose of 2 mg/24 hours and gradually increased to a maximum infusion dose of 12 mg/24 hours. Dosage of terlipressin is doubled every 48 hourly in case of no response to the maximum dosage of 12 mg/hour. Recent studies have shown a superior efficacy of continuous infusion of terlipressin as compared to bolus dosing in HRS which is not only associated with better resolution but also associated with fewer incidence of side-effects and better tolerability.[5]

α-1 Adrenergic Agonists

These include norepinephrine (NE) and midodrine. These act by binding to the α-1-adrenergic receptors on the vascular smooth muscle cells, which in turn leads to an increase in the intracellular calcium, thereby causing smooth muscle cell contraction and vasoconstriction. NE is not inferior to terlipressin in the management of HRS.[6]

NE is given at 0.1-0.7 µg/kg/min as an IV infusion and increased by 0.05 µg/kg/min every 4 hours to titrate to a MAP increase of at least 10 mm Hg. At doses of 1.5 mg/h, NE has been associated with ventricular arrhythmias (7%) and myocardial hypokinesia (5%), which reverse with dose reduction. Given the lower cost and wider availability of NE, it can be considered a safe and effective alternative to terlipressin for HRS.

Midodrine: It is a selective α-adrenergic agonist which when taken together with octreotide improves GFR, increases urinary volume and creatinine levels in patients with type 1 HRS. It also reduces mortality in these patients. The combination of midodrine, octreotide and albumin has been shown to improve renal functions as well as survival in both patients with type 1 and type 2 HRS. However, in a randomized controlled trial, a significantly higher rate of recovery of renal function was noted with terlipressin (19/27, 70.4%) compared to the octreotide and midodrine (6/21, 28.6%). The trial had to be stopped early after the interim analysis reported a superiority of the intervention (terlipressin) compared to the standard therapy (midodrine+ octreotide). Importantly, terlipressin was administered as a continuous infusion which may have accounted for superior response rates of HRS reversal as noted in this trial.[4]

Renal Replacement Therapy

The indications of renal replacement therapy are the same as those for other conditions, i.e., metabolic acidosis, volume overload, uremic complications and electrolyte abnormalities. It should be considered in patients who are candidates for orthotopic liver transplantation (OLT) or those with ATN, hypovolemia related renal failure or where renal functions are likely to be reversible. The leading indication identified in these patients has been volume overload. Continuous RRT is better tolerated than intermittent hemodialysis because of improved cardiovascular stability and less effect on intracranial pressure. However, superiority of continuous RRT has not been established in a controlled trial. There are no studies comparing renal replacement therapy with the vasoconstrictors and ideal method is also still not known. Complications like hypotension, bleeding secondary to coagulopathy and catheter-related sepsis are commonly encountered with renal replacement therapy when used in patients with advanced liver disease. Hence, a multidisciplinary approach involving a hepatologist, a nephrologist and an intensive care specialist is needed to decide the exact timing and modality of renal replacement therapy in patients of HRS. Considering an extremely poor response to vasoconstrictors in only 35% of patients with HRS in patients with ACLF and higher prevalence of structural AKI in patients with ACLF, the utility of RRT remains to be explored. There is paucity of data on dialysis in patients with ACLF and decompensated cirrhosis therefore there are no specific recommendations regarding the dose, the intensity and the duration of dialysis in these patients. The definitive indications for initiation of dialytic support include failure of standard medical management with complications of fluid overload, metabolic acidosis, hyperkalemia refractory to medical therapy and uremia. It has been shown by various studies in the past that patients with cirrhosis with deteriorating kidney function who require renal replacement therapy while awaiting liver transplantation have a high mortality in the absence of transplantation and only few patients survive on renal replacement therapy alone for long. There is emerging data to suggest that initiation of RRT early may attenuate both kidney-specific and non-kidney-specific organ dysfunction as well as counteract systemic inflammation in critically ill patients. However, unfortunately complications like hypotension, coagulopathy-related bleeding and catheter-related sepsis are frequently encountered with RRT in patients with cirrhosis and therefore in the absence of absolute indications it's a daunting task for the clinicians to decide initiation of early RRT in such a group of critically unwell patients. Randomized controlled trials are therefore needed to decide the timing of initiation of RRT (that is, "early" versus "late") in patients of ACLF who have structural kidney damage or have non-response to vasoconstrictors awaiting liver transplantation.[7]

Extracorporeal Liver Support Systems

These can be non-cell based or cell-based systems. Non-cell based systems do not incorporate tissue and provide only detoxification functions using membranes and adsorbents which allow removal of both water-soluble and protein bound substances as against conventional hemodialysis which removes only water-soluble toxins. These newer developing therapies have demonstrated benefits in biochemical parameters, hemodynamics, hepatic encephalopathy and also renal functions but are expensive and still considered experimental. They can be considered as a bridge to liver transplantation or as a bridge to recovery in patients with acute on chronic liver failure who are not candidates for liver transplantation. The Molecular Adsorbents Recirculatory System (MARS), single-pass albumin dialysis (SPAD) and the Fractionated Plasma Separation and Adsorption (FPSA or Prometheus) have been introduced into clinical practice however only limited data are available regarding their efficacy. The utility of artificial liver support in the management of patients with ACLF and HRS also remains questionable because of the lack of adequately powered trials. In the HELIOS trial survival of patients with type 1 HRS when treated with FPSA was better as compared to SMT (28-day survival 62% vs 39%; 90-day survival probability, 42% vs 6%, respectively; log-rank test, P=.04).[8]

Similarly in the RELIEF trial with MARS it was seen that the proportion of patients with a serum creatinine below 1.5 mg/dl at day 4 in patients with HRS at baseline tended to be higher in patients who were treated with MARS (p=0.07).[9] Artificial liver support with its ability to transiently improve renal function could be used as a bridging therapy to liver transplantation in these patients.

Transjugular Intrahepatic Portosystemic Shunt

The role of TIPS in management of HRS is still investigational as it is not feasible in many patients with advanced liver disease because of hepatic encephalopathy or high bilirubin and MELD scores.

Liver Transplantation

OLT remains as the most definitive treatment till date for HRS and has also demonstrated a survival benefit. Hence, it should be considered as early as possible in all patients in the absence of any contraindications. It has also been shown that renal insufficiency, including HRS, has a negative impact on OLT outcomes, with a higher mortality and higher posttransplantation end-stage renal disease. Patients who are transplanted with HRS have more complications and a higher in-hospital mortality rate than those undergoing transplantation without HRS.[10]

Combined Liver-Kidney Transplantation (CLKT)

The presence of HRS alone is not an indication for combined liver-kidney transplant however it should be considered in patients who have irreversible renal failure, requirement of dialysis of more than 6-8 weeks, uncontrolled or progressive primary kidney disease. There is also emerging data to suggest that HRS which was once thought to be functional is no more functional but associated with structural kidney damage. The previous HRS-2 has now been retermed as HRS-CKD considering an underlying structural component. Therefore identification of patients for a liver transplant alone versus a combined liver-kidney transplant should be considered after a careful assessment of renal functions. The current recommendations for considering simultaneous liver-kidney transplant includes end-stage renal disease associated with cirrhosis and symptomatic portal hypertension or a hepatic venous pressure gradient of 10 mm Hg or higher, acute renal failure or the hepatorenal syndrome with a serum creatinine level of 2.0 mg per deci-liter (177 μmol per liter) or higher and treatment with dialysis for longer than 8 weeks, and liver failure and chronic kidney disease with a GFR below 30 ml per minute or more than 30% glomerulosclerosis or fibrosis in a renal-biopsy specimen.

Prevention of AKI

As AKI is associated with a grim prognosis in patients with ACLF and cirrhosis, every effort should be made to prevent this complication. Adequate measures to prevent volume depletion or vasodilatation should be taken in patients with advance liver disease who are at risk of HRS. Albumin should be considered with large-volume paracentesis to prevent post-paracentesis circulatory dysfunction.

Judicious use of diuretics and nephrotoxic drugs and administration of albumin especially in patients with SBP has been shown to prevent HRS. However, the benefit of albumin infusion in the context of non-SBP AKI has still not been established.

In patients with ACLF, akin to patients with cirrhosis, judicious use of diuretics and repletion of intravascular volume by albumin during large volume paracentesis to prevent paracentesis induced circulatory dysfunction (PICD), avoidance of nephrotoxic drugs and importantly appropriate dose modifications of antibiotics according to creatinine clearance as well as early diagnosis and management of bacterial infections with prompt initiation of antibiotics should be instituted. Prevention of second infections, administration of albumin for prevention of HRS in patients with SBP and also use of prophylactic antibiotics have shown reduction in the incidence of kidney failure. Use of norfloxacin for primary prophylaxis of SBP also holds promise in prevention of AKI.

Future studies are needed to explore the management of non-responders. Possible options considering the proposed mechanisms of non-response include dialysis (no data regarding the timing (early versus late), dose, modality and duration), artificial liver support (ALS), or using cardiac intropes. Finally, all patients with HRS should undergo a liver transplantation (LT) alone or alternatively combined liver-kidney transplantation (SLK) in patients who have already developed structural kidney damage. Further, because prevention of AKI is an unmet need it is important to explore further the role of biomarkers (i.e., Cystatin C, Neutrophil gelatinase-associated lipocalin (NGAL), Liver Fatty Acid Binding Protein (L-FABP), Interleukin-18 (IL-18), Kidney-Injury Molecule (KIM-1)) in these patients with risk factors before development of AKI.

References

1. Angeli P *et al.* Diagnosis and management of acute kidney injury in patients with cirrhosis: Revised consensus recommendations of the International Club of Ascites. J Hepatol 2015;62(4):968-74.
2. Fagundes C *et al.* Urinary neutrophil gelatinase-associated lipocalin as biomarker in the differential diagnosis of impairment of kidney function in cirrhosis. J Hepatol 2012;57(2):267-73.
3. Barreto R *et al.* Urinary neutrophil gelatinase-associated lipocalin predicts kidney outcome and death in patients with cirrhosis and bacterial infections. J Hepatol 2014; 61(1):35-42.
4. Cavallin M *et al.* Terlipressin plus albumin versus midodrine and octreotide plus albumin in the treatment of hepatorenal syndrome: A randomized trial. Hepatology 2015;62(2):567-74.
5. Cavallin M *et al.* Terlipressin given by continuous intravenous infusion versus intravenous boluses in the treatment of hepatorenal syndrome: A randomized controlled study. Hepatology 2016;63(3):983-92.
6. Mattos AZ, AA Mattos and RA Ribeiro. Terlipressin versus noradrenaline in the treatment of hepatorenal syndrome: Systematic review with meta-analysis and full economic evaluation. Eur J Gastroenterol Hepatol 2016;28(3):345-51.
7. Ikegami T *et al.* The impact of renal replacement therapy before or after living donor liver transplantation. Clin Transplant 2012;26(1):143-48.
8. Kribben A *et al.* Effects of fractionated plasma separation and adsorption on survival in patients with acute-on-chronic liver failure. Gastroenterology 2012;142(4): 782-89, e3.
9. Banares R *et al.* Extracorporeal albumin dialysis with the molecular adsorbent recirculating system in acute-on-chronic liver failure: The RELIEF trial. Hepatology 2013; 57(3):1153-62.
10. Northup PG *et al.* Pretransplant predictors of recovery of renal function after liver transplantation. Liver Transpl 2010;16(4):440-46.

CHAPTER

29 A Patient with Pulmonary Renal Syndrome

Sree Bhushan Raju

Professor and Head, Department of Nephrology, Nizams Institute of Medical Sciences, Hyderabad, Telangana

CASE

56-year-old female with no significant comorbidities presented with on and off history of low grade fever, dry cough and occasional serosanguinous nasal discharge of 3 months duration. She also had history of insignificant weight loss and loss of appetite. She was evaluated elsewhere and found to have–Hb-11 gm/dl, TLC-12500/cmm, Platelets-2.5 lakh/cmm, creatinine 1.4 mg/dl, blood urea-35 mg/dl, urine albumin-2+, urine RBC-5-6/HPF, serum bilirubin-0.6 mg/dl, AST 25 IU/ml, ALT-20 IU/ml, serum albumin-2.9 gm/dl, total protein 6.3 gm/dl. Radiograph of the chest was normal. Patient was empirically started on antitubercular therapy. She complained of difficulty in breathing and hematuria after five days. At the time of admission into this institute, her vitals were stable and there was no icterus or lymphadenopathy. She had mild pedal edema, excessive nasal crusting and deformed nose. Investigations revealed - Hb-9.5 gm/dl, TLC-12000/cmm, S. creatinine-3.2 mg/dl, urine albumin 3+, RBC-15-20/HPF, S. alb-2.7 gms/dl, Total bilirubin - 0.7 mg/dl, ALT 20 IU/ml, AST 22 IU/ml, C3, C4-normal, HIV, HbsAg, HCV were negative. ANA, dsDNA-Neg, C-ANCA +, ELISA for PR3 +, chest radiograph showed bilateral middle and lower lobe infiltrates, HRCT chest showed multiple nodules, cavitatory lesions and diffuse infiltrates in middle and lower lobes. BAL analysis negative for tuberculosis. A Percutaneous renal biopsy was performed which showed Pauci immune crescentic glomerulonephritis, with 50% crescents. Immediately patient was started on pulse methyl prednisolone, cyclophosphamide and therapeutic plasma exchange (TPE) with 60 ml/kg. Total 7 sessions of TPE were done. Infiltrates in CXR improved. Patient was discharged with S. creatinine 1.3 mg/dl and advised to come for follow-up for cyclophosphamide doses.

Pulmonary Renal Syndrome

Pulmonary renal syndrome (PRS) describes the occurrence of renal failure in association with respiratory failure, characterised by autoimmune-mediated rapidly progressive glomerulonephritis (RPGN) and diffuse alveolar hemorrhage (DAH), occurring simultaneously or one after the other. PRS is an emergency situation associated with significant morbidity and mortality, and which requires prompt diagnosis and treatment for better outcomes. Prompt diagnosis of PRS requires a high index of suspicion, as clinical features are non-specific, and immunological testing aids the diagnosis in many cases.

The diagnostic evaluation of DAH and RPGN is outlined in the context of the important differential diagnoses.The most common causes of PRS include antineutrophil cytoplasm antibody (ANCA)-associated vasculitis (AAV) and anti-glomerular basement membrane (Anti GBM) disease.

As such, more emphasis has been placed on AAV, in addition to an overview of the less common causes of PRS. We provide a practical review of the diagnostic evaluation, current treatment strategies and clinical outcomes of PRS.

Lungs and kidneys are intricately related, physiologically as homeostatic organs controlling the cellular electrolyte and acid-base status that guarantee the best microenvironment for cellular function.

Pulmonary abnormalities may arise as a direct consequence of renal disease like pleural effusion, pulmonary edema or through generalized systemic processes that specifically involve both organ systems concomitantly, so-called pulmonary renal syndrome, is classically exemplified by the vasculitidis, intoxications and infections (Table 29.1). The term 'Pulmonary-Renal Syndrome' (PRS), as first described by Goodpasture[1] in 1919, is used to describe the occurrence of renal failure in association with respiratory failure, characterised by rapidly progressive glomerulonephritis (RPGN) and diffuse alveolar hemorrhage (DAH) secondary to an underlying autoimmune process, occurring simultaneously or one after the other within days to weeks' time gap.

Table 29.1: Causes of pulmonary renal syndrome

1. Antineutrophil cytoplasm antibody (ANCA)-associated vasculitis (AAV)
   - Granulomatous Polyangiitis, previously Wegener's granulomatosis
   - Microscopic Polyangiitis
   - Eosinophilic Granulomatous Polyangiitis, previously Churg-Strauss syndrome
2. Anti-glomerular basement membrane (Anti GBM) disease
3. Collagen vascular disease related
   - Systemic Lupus Erythematosus
   - Primary Antiphosholipid antibody syndrome (APLA)
   - Polymyositis
   - Systemic sclerosis
4. Other vasculitis
   - IgA Vasculitis (Henoch-Schönlein purpura and IgA nephropathy)
   - Mixed cryoglobulinaemia
   - Behcet's disease
5. Drug-induced vasculitis
   - Hydralazine, propylthiouracil, D-penicillamine, phenytoin, mitomycin
   - Allopurinol, sulfasalazine
6. Toxins
   - Acute silicoproteinosis, trimetallic anhydride (epoxy resin) toxicity, Paraquet poisoning
7. Infections
   - Leptospirosis, malaria, hanta virus syndrome, scrub typhus, Infective endocarditis
8. Pneumonia with renal failure
   - Metastatic hematogenous bacterial infections: Staphylococcus aureus, others
   - Sepsis with disseminated intravascular coagulation
9. Thrombotic microangiopathy
   - Thrombotic thrombocytopenic purpura, Hemolytic uremic syndrome
10. Pulmonary malignancy associated glomerulopathy
11. Congestive cardiac failure with acute renal failure

Pathology of Pulmonary–Renal Syndrome

Small vessel vasculitis, necrotic pulmonary capillaritis, as well as focal proliferative glomerulonephritis are the characteristic pathological features of PRS. Among the histopathologies of DAH (pulmonary capillaritis, pulmonary hemorrhage, diffuse alveolar damage, and various histologies), pulmonary capillaritis the most common. Pulmonary capillaritis differs from pulmonary vasculitis in the size of the vessel it affects, i.e., pulmonary vasculitis refers to inflammation of lung vessels of any size, whereas pulmonary capillaritis is restricted to the microcirculation of the lung (arterioles, venules and alveolar capillaries). Both may be encountered in systemic vasculitides and in connective tissue disorders. Pulmonary capillaritis has an exclusive histopathologic appearance consisting of an interstitial mainly neutrophilic infiltration, fibrinoid necrosis of the alveolar capillary walls, and leukocytoclasis. The infiltrating neutrophils undergo cytoclasis; nuclear debris accumulates within the interstitium, causing interstitial and alveolar edema with hyaline membrane formation. After recurrent attacks or episodes of DAH, interstitial fibrosis may develop. These injuries disrupt perfusion and increase pulmonary capillary permeability, causing flooding of blood into the alveoli, resulting in hypoxemia and hypocapnia with impairment of oxygen transfer.

Extensive glomerular crescent formation (crescentic glomerulonephritis) is the fundamental pathologic finding of RPGN that is observed by light microscopy and electron microscopy. The pathological aspect of crescentic glomerulonephritis is a focal rupture of glomerular capillaries, basement membranes, and blood extravasations, followed by an invasion of macrophages and fibrinogen with the development of extracapillary cellular proliferation (crescents formation). Fibrinoid necrosis is commonly encountered, in addition to microvascular thrombi.

AAV leads to focal necrotising glomerulonephritis (FNGN) with crescents and a marked tubulointerstitial nephritis in small number of cases only. Necrotising arteritis is seen in 10-30% of cases. Infiltration with neutrophils, macrophages, lymphocytes is common. Interstitial granulomas present in granulomatous polyangiitis (GPA), eosinophilic granulomatous polyangiitis (EGPA), but not in microscopic polyangiitis (MPA).

Crescents and fibrinoid necrosis, the hallmark histologic lesions occur at same frequency irrespective of the presence or absence of systemic vasculitis. The extent of crescent formation is not different between PR3-ANCA and MPO-ANCA (Fig. 29.1).

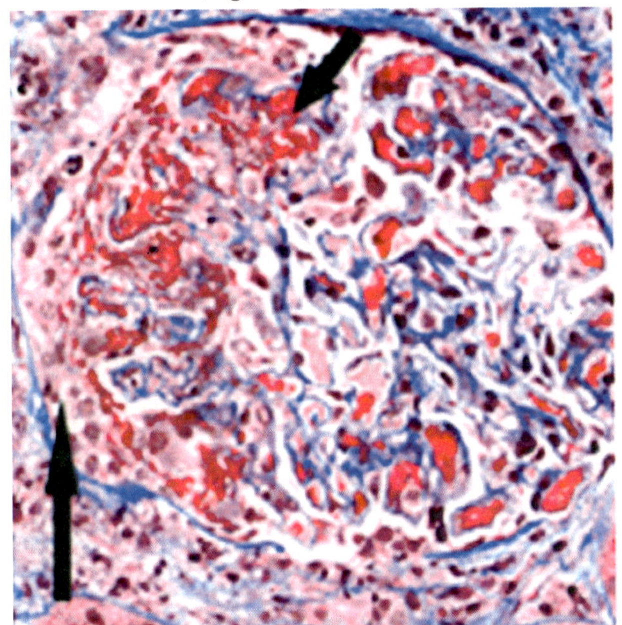

Figure 29.1: The glomerulus has a small cellular crescent (long arrow), and a break in Bowman's capsule in the upper left corner. (Masson trichrome stain)

Based on studies from CYCAZAREM study, MEPEX-trial, a classification system for ANCA-associated glomerulonephritis was launched in 2010.[2] The classification scheme has four general categories, named focal, crescentic, sclerotic and mixed (Fig. 29.2).

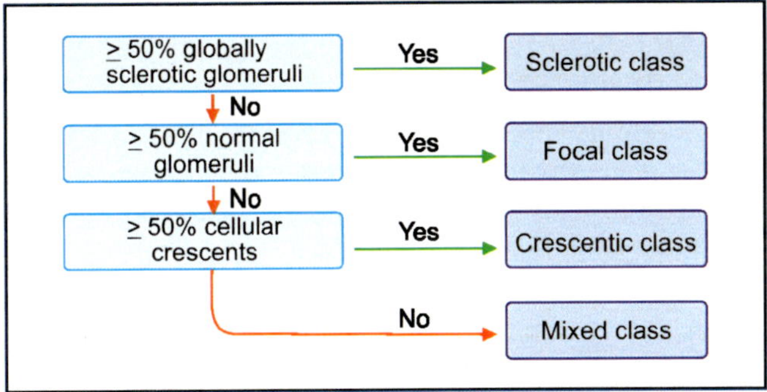

Figure 29.2: BERDEN-EUVAS renal biopsy classification. Biopsies should be scored for glomerular lesions in the following order: Globally sclerotic glomeruli, normal glomeruli and cellular crescentic glomeruli. Any biopsies that do not fit into one of the categories on the basis of a predominant glomerular phenotype will automatically be included in the mixed category

Focal class has the least progression to ESRD, sclerotic class has the worst progression, and crescentic class and mixed class have intermediate progression. A caveat is that in patients with eGFR<15 ml/min per 1.73 m^2, the Berden class does not predict renal outcome.[3] In this setting, number of normal glomeruli and higher overall chronicity score are risk factors for ESRD (Table 29.2).

On IF examination, the type and deposition pattern of Immunoglobulins differ (either linear, capillary, granular, or mesangial). In Goodpasture syndrome, linear IgG deposits along the glomerular and/or the alveolar basement membrane. The granular pattern deposit of complement and Ig is observed in lupus and post infectious glomerulonephritis, and also in necrotizing vasculitis (Pauci-immune glomerulonephritis).

The definition of "Pauci-immune" is somewhat arbitory. Most pathologists use a staining intensity of 2+ or less as the cut-off point. The term Pauci-immune rather than non-immune staining is used because many patients have low level of staining for Ig as well as complements. Roncho *et al.*[4] were among the first investigators to report this observation.

Diagnostic Workup of Pulmonary Renal Syndrome

1. The diagnosis of PRS in the ICU is challenging. There is no single specific test and the symptoms and signs are usually vague.

Table 29.2: Differentiation of various crescentic glomerulonephritis

	Anti-GBM	AAV	Immune Complex GN
Glomerular lesions in various phases	-	+	+
Granulomatous periglomerular inflammation	+	+	-
Un-involved segments	Normal	Normal	Thick capillary walls, endocapillary hypercellularity +

AAV: ANCA-associated vasculitis; Anti-GBM: Anti-glomerular basement membrane disease.

There is an overlap with other common ICU presentations such as sepsis and cardiorespiratory morbidity.

2. The clinical presentation of PRS is variable, and could be related to acute respiratory and/or renal failure, a common symptom of systemic vasculitis, as well as the underlying pathology.
3. Acute exacerbation of the underlying pathology or infectious complications secondary to severe immunosuppressive therapy of the underlying cause are the most common triggering factors of PRS.

   The three basic steps for the diagnosis of PRS as with any systemic vasculitis involve the following:
   - Careful clinical history and evaluation of present and past illnesses.
   - Confirmation of the diagnosis by laboratory investigations and examinations of biopsy samples.
   - Exclusion of an alternative diagnosis for vasculitis.

Clinical Manifestations

1. Breathlessness is a common clinical presentation of PRS.
2. Presentation of patients with DAH can range from fever and cough, often acute or sub acute (<1 week), with or without hemoptysis, to severe respiratory distress. Many patients show rapid deterioration and are admitted to the ICU with an acute respiratory and/or renal failure.
3. Clinically apparent hemoptysis (absent in 1/3 of patients) may be present; 2/3 have at least mild haemoptysis (<200 ml/24 hours).
4. In patients with hemoptysis, bleeding from the upper respiratory tract and gastrointestinal bleeding sources must be excluded. Alternative diagnoses such as pulmonary embolism, pneumonia, congestive heart failure, severe mitral stenosis, and drug exposure, that is, propylthiouracil and cocaine as possible causes should also be excluded.
5. Patient usually have nephritic presentation with rapid impairment of renal function, presence of proteinuria and active urinary sediments. These features have diagnostic as well as prognostic value.
6. Flu-like illness is an early common symptom of ANCA-related vasculitis and involves fever, generalized body ache, myalgias, malaise, bonyache, and loss of appetite and weight. These are reported in more than 90% of cases and usually occur within days to months of development of vasculitis or nephritis. Migratory polyarthropathy, painful cutaneous nodules or ulcerations, and abdominal pain are the most common complaints following the vasculitis attack.
7. Otitis media, sinusitis, nasal mucosal ulceration, and subglottic stenosis are the most common presenting clinical manifestations of vasculitis of the upper respiratory tract.
8. An accurate ophthalmology examination for the suspicion of retinal vasculitis or episcleritis, and a dermatological examination for leukocytoclastic vasculitis and the nasopharynx for saddle nose deformities or nasal septal erosion should be considered (Table 29.3).

Laboratory Studies

All available specimens, that is, sputum, blood/urine cultures, and serological investigations have to be obtained to exclude bacterial or viral infectivity.

1. **ABG** for the assessment of oxygenation and acid base status.
2. **CBC with DLC:** Evidence of hemolysis with damaged erythrocytes on the blood film may possibly reveal causal factors, that is, thrombotic thrombocytopenic purpura, Thrombocytopenia reported secondary to cytotoxic drugs, anti-phospholipid syndrome, or SLE. Eosinophilia of 13% or more is indicative of Churg-Strauss syndrome.

Table 29.3: Comparison of approximate frequency of manifestations of microscopic polyangiitis to several other forms of small-vessel vasculitis[5]

	MPA (%)	GPA (%)	EGPA (%)	IgA vasculitis HSP (%)	Cryoglobulinemic vasculitis (%)
Renal	90	80	45	50	55
Pulmonary	50	90	70	5	5
Cutaneous	40	40	60	90	90
ENT	35	90	50	5	5
Musculoskeletal	60	60	50	75	70
Neurologic	30	50	70	10	40
Gastrointestinal	50	50	50	60	30

GPA: Granulomatous polyangiitis; EGPA: Eosinophilic granulomatous polyangiitis; MPA: Microscopic polyangiitis.

3. Increased ESR and C-reactive protein may occur in active vasculitis, but may be nonspecific.
4. Serum creatinine can be normal at presentation, but may be abnormally elevated with disease progression. Abnormally elevated tissue enzyme (i.e., lactate dehydrogenase, creatine phosphokinase) levels may suggest significant inflammation causing myalgia.
5. Abnormal PT, INR, aPTTare reported in SLE, DIC.
6. Serological markers for the underlying cause:
   (a) Determination of serum antibodies, that is, anti-GBM and/or ANCA is the most important step.
   (b) SLE should be considered with high titres of ANA, ds DNA.
   (c) *ANCA serology:* Pauci-immune crescentic glomerulonephritis is almost synonymous with ANCA crescentic glomerulonephritis, because 85% to 90% of pauci-immune crescentic glomerulonephritis occurs in ANCA-positive patients and 80% to 90% of the crescentic glomerulonephritis that occurs in ANCA-positive patients is pauci-immune. Approximately 90% to 95% of patients with active untreated GPA or MPA, and approximately 45% of patients with EGPA, are ANCA positive. Thus, ANCA serology is least sensitive for EGPA; however, three quarters or more of EGPA patients with evidence for glomerulonephritis have ANCA.

   ANCA are specific for proteins in the cytoplasmic granules of neutrophils and the lysosomes of monocytes. Davies *et al.*[6] first reported ANCA in the serum of patients with systemic small-vessel vasculitis and pauci-immune necrotizing glomerulonephritis.

   ANCA are identified in the serum of approximately one third of patients with anti-GBM disease. Compared with patients with anti-GBM alone, patients with both autoantibodies are older, often have features of systemic small-vessel vasculitis, and have a better prognosis for renal survival with treatment. The concurrent anti-GBM and ANCA specificity of serum is the result of two different antibody populations rather than one cross-reacting population, and the antigen specificities of anti-GBM antibodies are the same in patients with anti-GBM antibodies alone compared to those with ANCA and anti-GBM antibodies.

   ANCA are detected by indirect immunofluorescence microscopy using alcohol-fixed neutrophils as substrate. The perinuclear distribution of antigen is an artefact of substrate preparation that results from redistribution of the antigen from the cytoplasm to the nucleus during substrate preparation.

   Extremely high titres of proteins myeloperoxidase (MPO)-ANCA, proteinase 3 (PR3)-ANCA and ANCA specific for elastase. Dual positivity for MPO-ANCA and PR3-ANCA should raise the possibility of drug- induced disease. Drugs, such as hydralazine, propylthiouracil, penicillamine and illicit cocaine adulterated with levamisole can induce ANCA vasculitis.[7] Penicillamine can induce membranous glomerulopathy, some patients with penicillamine-induced ANCA and crescentic glomerulonephritis also have concurrent membranous glomerulopathy. ANCA titers are more predictive of renal disease activity than nonrenal disease activity.[8] Patients with ANCA GN who become ANCA negative during follow-up have low risk for relapse, and a rise in ANCA titre increases the likelihood of relapse 11 times.[8]

   ANCA specificity independently predicts relapse among patients with ANCA vasculitis more effectively than classification systems that use only the clinicopathologic phenotype, with PR3-ANCA–positive patients approximately twice as likely to relapse compared with MPO-ANCA–positive patients.[9] ANCA serotypes correlate with different predilections for organ involvement.[9] Patients with pulmonary capillaritis and no nodules or cavities have a similar frequency of MPO-ANCA and PR3-ANCA, whereas patients with lung nodules or cavities more often have PR3-ANCA. Approximately 5% of patients with ANCA vasculitis also have anti-GBM antibodies, and approximately 35% of patients with anti-GBM disease have ANCA (usually MPO-ANCA).[10] These patients have kidney disease that more closely resembles anti-GBM disease, i.e., it is more severe pathologically and clinically, and the risk of progression to ESRD is greater than for ANCA GN in the absence of anti-GBM (Table 29.4).

   Positive ANCA serology at the time of transplantation does not increase the risk of recurrent disease in the transplant. A negative ANCA result by no means rules out these diseases and patients who are ANCA negative have the same prognosis and should receive the same treatment as ANCA-positive patients.

   ANCA positive is observed in 90% of patients with WG and the majority of them have C-ANCA with PR3 specificity, particularly when the lung is affected. Also, ANCA-positive was

Table 29.4: Comparing the serotypes

PR3	MPO
More common in northern Europe, northern North America and Australia	More common in southern Europe, southern United Statess and Asia
HLA-DP genetic association	HLA-DQ association
More upper respiratory tract disease	More renal disease
More granulomatous inflammation	Less granulomatous inflammation
At the time of biopsy, PR3-ANCA GN has more necrosis	At the time of biopsy, MPO-ANCA GN has more sclerosis
PR3-ANCA–positive patients approximately twice as likely to relapse compared with MPO-ANCA–positive patients	
More likely to have refractory disease	

MPO: Myeloperoxidase and PR3: Proteinase 3.

reported in 80% of patients with MPA, and most of them reveal P-ANCA with MPO specificity. On the other hand, ANCA type and specificity is not specific for these disorders, as few cases of WG are P-ANCA positive, as well as C-ANCA-positive were observed in few patients with MPA. According to the International Consensus Statement on Testing and Reporting of ANCA, combining indirect IF assays and ELISAs for PR3 and MPO is more accurate than the use of either assay alone. It is important to note, however, that not all patients with ANCA-associated vasculitis will test positive for ANCA, and therefore, ANCA are not considered a diagnostic criterion. However, ANCA have also been observed in numerous other autoimmune nonvasculitic disorders, that is, inflammatory bowel disease, rheumatoid arthritis, and autoimmune hepatitis and infectious and neoplastic diseases.

(d) Cryoglobulin titer should be negative in patients with ANCA-related diseases as symptoms of cryoglobulinemia are similar to those in ANCA-related disease.

(e) **Hepatitis markers:** Hepatitis C is linked to mixed cryoglobulinemia, whereas hepatitis B is linked to polyarteritis nodosa.

(f) Tests for antiphospholipid antibodies.

7. **Urine analysis:** Proteinuria is almost constantly present, but is seldom more than 2-3 g/24 hours. Also, microscopic hematuria is always detected. Microscopic hematuria with proteinuria are most commonly detected early in WG and MPA.
8. **Urine and serum protein electrophoresis:** This may be considered a key investigation in patients with RPGN with the aim of confirming or excluding the light-chain disease or overt multiple myeloma as a reason for the presenting symptoms.

Imaging Studies

Chest X-Ray and HRCT Chest

1. There may be radiologic signs even without clinically significant symptom. Near normal chest radiography is recorded in 25% of cases, and in such cases, pulmonary embolic disease should be excluded.
2. The most common radiologic findings include (Fig. 29.3):

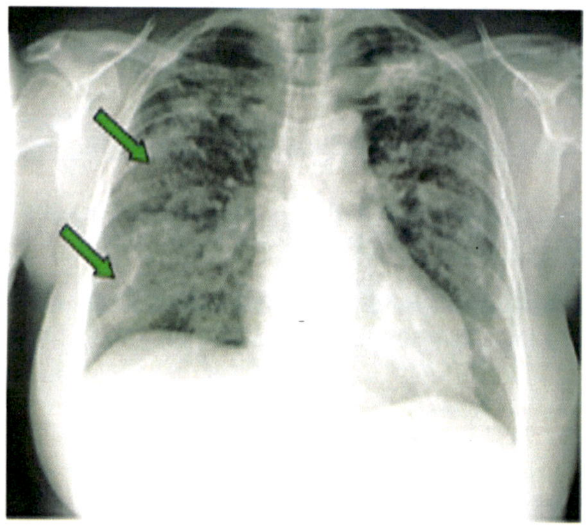

Figure 29.3: A chest radiograph revealed diffuse interstitial opacities with relative sparing of the periphery consistent with pulmonary hemorrhage. This sparing of the peripheries is typical for alveolar hemorrhage and is due to gravity-dependent density gradients

   a. Bilateral diffuse alveolar infiltrates, mainly perihilar infiltrates, toward the lower zones.
   b. Areas of consolidations with air bronchogram with preserved normal areas.
   c. Diffuse consolidation mimic an adult respiratory distress syndrome picture.
   d. Rarely DAH radiographic pictures appear as ground glass opacities. The presence of interstitial opacities might be a result of an underlying cause or may indicate the presence of primary pulmonary hemosiderosis, caused by chronic or repeated episodes of DAH.
3. Vasculitis as a cause of DAH is highly suggested by multiple cavities, diffuse ground glass infiltrations and nodules. Wegener's granulomatosis (WG) is

commonly associated with cavitations; diagnostic workup should be performed for exclusion of alternative diagnoses, that is, cavitating pneumonia, mycobacterial, or malignant disease.

4. Lymphadenopathy is usually not present in DAH, but usually add suspicious of infectivity or malignancy.
5. The finding of Kerley A, B, or C shadows with diffuse alveolar infiltrate indicates an alternative diagnosis, that is, veno-occlusive disease of the lung, cardiogenic pulmonary edema, or mitral valve stenosis.
6. Pleural effusion is not feature of AAV, may have mild effusion secondary to associated renal failure.
7. Renal ultrasound is definitely performed to exclude obstructive uropathy in any patient with acute renal failure and also to establish the presence of two functioning kidneys before a percutaneous renal biopsy.
8. Nuclear imaging, like gallium tagged red blood cell studies, are rarely performed in the evaluation of DAH and have additionally not been shown to be useful.

Pulmonary Function Tests in Stable Patients

1. Diffusion lung capacity for carbon monoxide (DLCO) – this is significant if there is an increase of >30%.

   Recent alveolar hemorrhage increases DLCO, whereas DAH that occurs more than 2 days before the test is unlikely to cause a significant increase in DLCO.

   Continuous increase in DLCO may be a sign of progressive alveolar hemorrhage.

   DLCO measurement maneuvers require breath-holding on an air, carbon monoxide and helium mixture for around 10 seconds. The major disadvantage of this maneuver is that it is difficult and not practical in patients with marked dyspnea or hemoptysis.
2. Restrictive changes, that is decrease in total lung capacity and forced vital capacity (FVC), with a preserved FEV1/FVC, may characterize DAH.

   Frequent attacks of DAH can cause interstitial fibrosis.
3. Obstructive changes, that is, ↓FEV1 and ↓ratio of FEV1/FVC are less commonly observed in patients with DAH, but if present, may indicate airflow obstruction. Many authors attributed this possibly to flooding of alveolar spaces by blood, which causes neutrophilic infiltration that sequentially releases proteolytic enzymes and reactive oxygen species, which in turn may result in parenchymal destruction and small airway disease, for example, emphysema and bronchiolitis.
   - A mixed pattern of obstructive and restrictive lung disease associated with DAH is suggestive of a differential diagnosis causing airflow obstruction and parenchymal destruction, that is, commonly, sarcoidosis, MPA, or WG, occasionally idiopathic pulmonary hemosiderosis, or, less frequently, lymphangioleiomyomatosis, or histiocytosis X.

Bronchoscopic Examination

Visual inspection of airway sources of bleeding, exclusion of infection, and obtain lavage samples for various laboratory investigations that is, bacterial, viral, mycobacterial, and fungal cultures, in addition to pneumocystis stains. Evidence supporting DAH is continual or increase blood quantity on three sequential lavage aliquots from a single affected area. Prussian blue staining for bronchioloalveolar lavage shows hemosiderin-laden macrophages (siderophages). The diagnostic yield is enhanced if the bronchoscopy is carried out within the first 2 days of manifestations instead of later.

Tissue Biopsy

The gold standard for the diagnosis of PRS is renal and/or pulmonary biopsy when the lung is involved.

Transbronchial biopsy specimens are small and unlikely to help establish a diagnosis. Thoracoscopic lung biopsy or open lung biopsy, although invasive and involving considerable risk, is more definitive. In general, lung biopsy should only be used as a last option if the diagnosis cannot be confirmed in a different way.

Renal biopsy is favoured and should be performed as soon as possible keeping in mind the end goal of assessment of a renal biopsy, the pathologist should correlate complete clinical and laboratory research facility data with light microscope and IF, and the electron microscopic examinations should be carried out as soon as appropriate.

In those patients whom can't tolerate or at high-risk operative interference for lung or renal biopsy, biopsies from other organs (i.e., skin, sinuses or nerves) can be replaced. Proper treatment should be initiated rapidly even in the absence of histopathological proof to reduce morbidity and mortality in patients with a high clinical suspicion of ANCA-associated or anti-GBM-associated vasculitis and with a positive ANCA or anti-GBM antibody result, respectively.

Radiological clearance, and improvements in arterial blood gases, renal function, neurologic signs, and other signs (such as purpura) can be expected within a few days of initiation of therapy.

If this diagnostic workup is not conclusive or if is the patient's condition worsens, refractory PRS with a differential diagnosis should be considered, for example:

1. Drug reactions, sepsis syndrome, or septicemia or exacerbation of the underlying cause.
2. Antiphospholipid syndrome with vasculitis.
3. Mixed connective tissue diseases, that is, systemic-sclerosis, polymyositis.
4. Thrombocytopenic purpura.
5. Infectious complications of the lung and kidney (e.g., sepsis, mycoplasma, legionella, cytomegalovirus, hantavirus, leptospirosis).

Treatment

1. The primary goal of therapy for patients with PRS is to induce remission as fast as possible to minimize irreversible organ damage as well as to prevent further antibody formations. In addition, treatment plans should be focused on causal factors with the prevention of treatment related toxicity.
2. Once the induction–remission phase has occurred, the secondary goal of therapy is to maintain remission with as few side effects as possible.
3. Supportive therapies and care should be provided throughout the duration of illness. Therapy is subdivided into the induction–remission phase and the maintenance phase. Attempts have been made to subgroup patients at diagnosis according to disease extent and severity in order to design treatments of ascending strength (Flowchart 29.1).

Cyclophosphamide was first used in GPA by Novack and Pearson in 1967 and subsequently by Fauci and colleagues at the US National Institutes of Health (NIH) (Novack and Pearson, 1971). Cyclophosphamide is equally effective as a daily oral or pulsed intravenous (IV) administration for the induction of remission (deGroot *et al.*, 2009). However, the IV protocols expose the patient to a lower cumulative cyclophosphamide dose and permit bladder protection. Leucopenia is more common with daily oral cyclophosphamide and is an important risk factor for severe infection (Little *et al.*, 2010). The leucocyte nadir after IV cyclophosphamide occurs at 10–14 days and subsequent cyclophosphamide dosing is reduced if leucopenia occurs. Cyclophosphamide is continued for 3–6 months, by which time remission will have been achieved in 80–90%. IV methyl prednisolone is widely used for severe presentations at total doses of 1000–3000 mg. Daily oral prednisolone commences at 1.0 mg/kg/day, maximum 80 mg/day, for 1–4 weeks, then reduces in steps to 10–15 mg/day by 12 weeks (Jayne *et al.*, 2003; WGET Research Group 2005).

Plasma exchange improves the chances of renal recovery in those presenting in renal failure, creatinine above 500 µmol/l but does not influence the high mortality risk of this subgroup (Jayne *et al.*, 2007). A meta-analysis failed to confirm a significant benefit of plasma exchange on the composite outcome of death and ESRD. MEPEX study showed effectiveness with TPE with 60 ml/kg plasma volume. Volume replacement with albumin is recommended but plasma or coagulation factor-rich plasma fractions are used in the setting of increased bleeding risk, such as after a renal biopsy or in the presence of alveolar hemorrhage.

Cyclophosphamide dosing for IV pulsed and daily oral regimens as defined in the EUVAS CYCLOPS protocol (From de Groot *et al.* 2009) (Table 29.5).

Rituximab

The RITUXVAS trial, RAVE trial studied the rituximab as induction agent (Table 29.6).

Rituximab can be recommended for remission induction when cyclophosphamide is contraindicated,

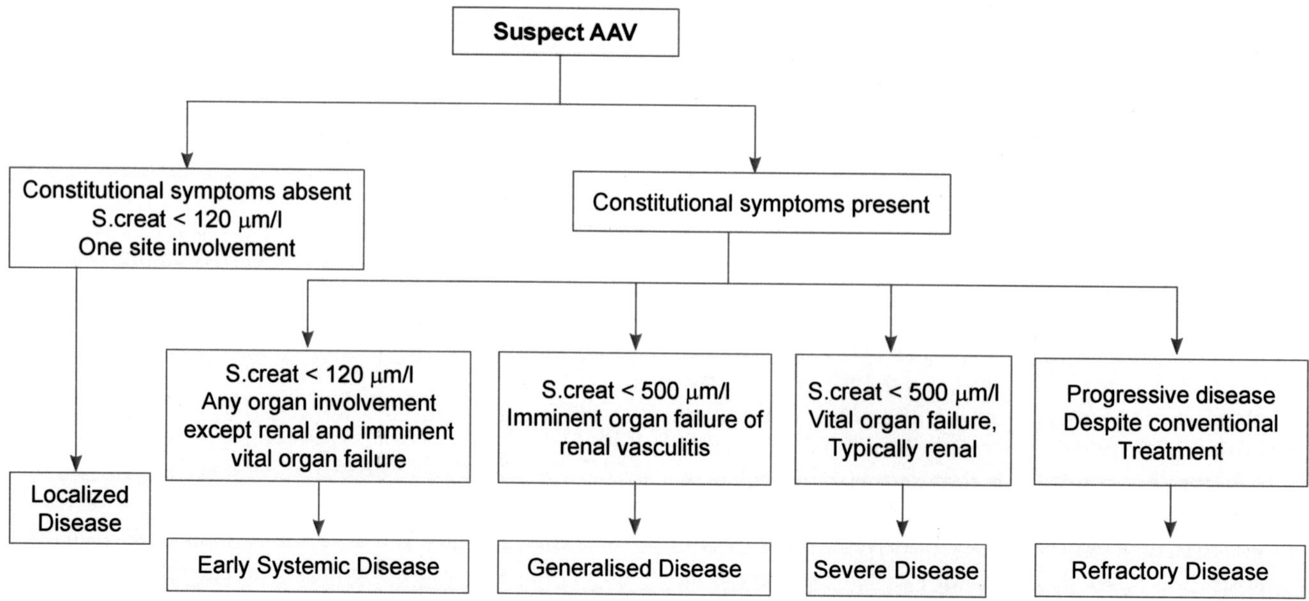

Flowchart 29.1: Staging of ANCA associated vasculitis (AAV)

Table 29.5: Pulsed cyclophosphamide dosing (mg/kg/pulse) with reductions for impaired renal function and age

Age (years)	eGFR > 30 ml/min	eGFR ≤ 30 ml/min
< 60	15	12.5
60-70	12.5	10
>70	10	7.5
Timing of cyclophosphamide pulses		
Weeks: 0, 2 and 4, then every 3 weeks (weeks 7, 10, 13, 16, 19, 21 and 24)		
Daily oral cyclophosphamide dosing		

Age (years)	Dose (mg/kg/day)
< 60	2.0
60–70	1.5
> 75	1.0

Table 29.6: Trials using rituximab

RITUXVAS trial	RAVE trial
2 pulses of cyclophosphamide along with rituximab 375 mg/m^2 /week × 4 weeks	No concurrent cyclophosphamide Same dose of rituximab
Relapse 26%	40% at 2 years
	In relapses, high rate of response than to cyclophosphamide

for example, cytopenia, intolerance, malignancy, or fertility protection (Guerry *et al.*, 2012). A simpler regimen of rituximab 1 g repeated after 14 days appears to be similar in efficacy to the four-dose regimen (Jones *et al.*, 2009).

The time to achieve remission of renal vasculitis, and the renal outcomes were the same for rituximab or cyclophosphamide in the RAVE trial. The latter excluded patients with creatinine > 360 μmol/l. Because rituximab is removed by plasma exchange when both therapies are employed, at least 48 hours should elapse between rituximab infusion and the next plasma exchange and atleast 50% of the rituximab total dose should be administered after the plasma exchange course has been completed.

Assessing Response

Control of renal vasculitis is judged by improvement or stability of renal function, absence of extrarenal vasculitis and normalization of C-reactive protein (CRP). Microscopic haematuria persists for many months after the onset of therapy and proteinuria typically increases during the recovery period, occasionally to levels sufficient to cause the nephrotic syndrome especially in those uncommon patients with evidence of immune complex deposition. The level of proteinuria during the recovery phase indicates the degree of glomerular injury and is associated with worse renal outcomes (Bakoush *et al.*, 2006) (Table 29.7).

Remission Maintenance Therapy

Disease relapse occurs in 75% of GPA and 30% of MPA and EGPA cases by 5 years (Booth *et al.*, 2003; Walsh *et al.*, 2012). Predictors of relapse include anti-proteinase 3 (PR3) antibodies, lung and upper respiratory involvement, age, nasal carriage of Staphylococcus aureus (Stegeman *et al.*, 1994), and absence of severe renal involvement (Koldingsnes and Nossent, 2002; Pierrot-Deseilligny Despujol *et al.*, 2010).

Factors Increasing Relapse Risk in ANCA-Associated Vasculitis (Table 29.8)

Changes in ANCA do not correlate closely with disease activity and rises should not trigger increases in therapy on their own. A persistent ANCA after induction therapy, a rise in ANCA during remission therapy and ANCA positivity at the time of treatment withdrawal indicate a higher relapse risk (McKinney *et al.*, 2006; Tomasson *et al.*, 2012).

The goals of maintenance therapy are to prevent disease relapse while minimizing drug toxicity. Cyclophosphamide is withdrawn after 3–6 months and substituted by azathioprine 2 mg/kg/day, or methotrexate, up to 25 mg/week. They were equally effective for remission maintenance with similar safety risks in the WEGENT trial (Pagnoux *et al.*, 2008). Methotrexate is excreted by the kidneys and should be avoided in the presence of renal impairment, glomerular filtration rate (GFR) < 50 ml/min.

Table 29.7: Consensus disease state definitions (From Hellmich *et al.* 2007)

Activity state	Definition
Remission	Absence of disease activity attributable to active vasculitis qualified by the need for ongoing stable relapse prevention therapy. 'Active disease' is not restricted to vasculitis only, but includes other inflammatory features, such as granulomatous inflammation in GPA or tissue eosinophilia in CSS
Response	50% reduction of disease activity score and absence of new manifestations
Relapse	Reoccurrence or new onset of disease attributable to active vasculitis
Major relapse	Reoccurrence or new onset of potentially organ-or life-threatening disease
Minor relapse	Reoccurrence or new onset of disease which is neither potentially organ-threatening nor life-threatening
Refractory	1. Unchanged or increased disease activity in acute AAV after at least 4 weeks treatment with standard induction therapy, or 2. Lack of response, defined as ≤ 50% reduction in the disease activity score, after at least 6 weeks of treatment, or 3. Chronic, persistent disease defined as the presence of at least one major or three minor items on the disease activity score list, after ≥ 12 weeks of treatment
Low-activity disease state	Persistence of minor symptoms (e.g., arthralgia, myalgia) that respond to a modest glucocorticoid increase and do not necessarily warrant an escalation of other therapies

Table 29.8: Factors increasing relapse risk in ANCA associated vasculitis

Clinical presentation	Serology	Treatment related
Diagnosis of GPA (Wegener's)	PR3-ANCA positive at Diagnosis	Steroid withdrawal
Ear, nose and throat involvement	Persistent ANCA positivity after induction therapy	Immunosuppressive withdrawal
Serum creatinine < 200 µmol/l	Rise in ANCA during remission	Lower cyclophosphamide exposure

Mycophenolate mofetil was less effective than azathioprine for relapse prevention after cyclophosphamide induction therapy (Metzler *et al.*, 2007; Hiemstra *et al.*, 2010).

Prednisolone is either continued in conjunction with an immunosuppressive at doses of 5–10 mg/day or is withdrawn at the end of the induction phase. There is an increased relapse risk following steroid withdrawal which has to be balanced against the toxicity of long-term administration (Walsh *et al.*, 2010). Long-term steroids are often required in patients with EGPA due to persistent asthma.

There is no clear guidance as to how long remission maintenance treatment should be continued. The IMPROVE trial withdrew therapy 42 months after diagnosis, but withdrawal after 24 months has also been suggested (Table 29.9).

Table 29.9: Overview of key trials ANCA associated vasculitis

Study	Induction or maintenance	Agents used	Key comments
RAVE	Induction	Rituximab vs. cyclophosphamide	Rituximab was not inferior to cyclophosphamide in induction of remission and may be more effective than cyclophosphamide in relapsing disease. Excludes patients with severe kidney disease
CYCLOPS	Induction	Pulse cyclophosphamide vs. daily oral cyclophosphamide	Less cumulative dose and lower rates of leukopenia in the pulse group compared with daily oral cyclophosphamide with no difference in time to remission. Under-powered study therefore of limited utility
NORAM	Induction	Cyclophosphamide vs. methotrexate	Methotrexate was non-inferior to cyclophosphamide in remission rates in early AAV. It was less effective in extensive disease. Early withdrawal of treatment in both arms was associated with high relapse rate. Limited applicability to those with significant kidney disease

Contd.

Contd.

RITUXIVAS	Induction	Rituximab vs. cyclophosphamide	Rituximab-based regimen was not superior to cyclophosphamide in achieving remission and had similar rate of adverse events. Small trial. Highlights the fact that the role of rituximab in severe disease is not known
Plasma exchange in focal necrotizing glomerulonephritis without anti-GBM antibodies	Induction	Plasma exchange vs. no plasma exchange	Higher rate of recovery of renal function in dialysis-dependent patients when treated with plasma exchange and immunosuppression compared to treatment with immunosuppression alone. Small, single-center, unblended study with no clear power calculations for cohorts who were dialysis dependent
MEPEX	Induction	Plasma exchange vs. high-dose methyl prednisolone	Plasma exchange improved renal survival in patients with AAV and serum creatinine >500 μmol/l when compared to high-dose methyl prednisolone. However, there was no difference in ESRD or dialysis rates at 3 years
RAVE maintenance study	Maintenance	Rituximab vs. cyclophosphamide + azathioprine	Rituximab was non-inferior to conventional therapy with cyclophosphamide and azathioprine in maintaining remission. This was a steroid withdrawal study, so efficacy of rituximab in those maintained on long-term, low-dose steroids not clear
CYCAZAREM	Maintenance	Azathioprine vs. cyclophosphamide	Azathioprine was as effective as cyclophosphamide in maintaining remission
WEGENT	Maintenance	Azathioprine vs. methotrexate	Methotrexate was not safer than azathioprine as a maintenance therapy
IMPROVE	Maintenance	Mycophenolate vs. azathioprine	Higher relapse rates with mycophenolate compared to azathioprine

References

1. Goodpasture E. The significance of certain pulmonary lesions in relation to the etiology of influenza. Am J Med Sci 1919;158:863-70.
2. Berden AE, Ferrario F, Hagen EC *et al.* Histopathologic classification of ANCA-associated glomerulonephritis. J Am Soc Nephrology 2010;21:1628-36.
3. Lee T, Gasim A, Derebail VK, Chung Y, McGregor JG, Lionaki S, Poulton CJ, Hogan SL, Jennette JC, Falk RJ, Nachman PH. Predictors of treatment outcomes in ANCA-associated vasculitis with severe kidney failure. Clin J Am Soc Nephrol 2014;9:905-13.
4. Ronco P, Verroust P, Mignon F, *et al.* Immunopathological studies of polyarteritis nodosa and Wegener's granulomatosis: A report of 43 patients with 51 renal biopsies. Q J Med 1983;52:212.
5. Jennette JC, Falk RJ. Small-vessel vasculitis. N Engl J Med 1997;337:1512.
6. Davies DJ, Moran JE, Niall JF, *et al.* Segmental necrotising glomerulonephritis with antineutrophil antibody: Possible arbovirus aetiology? Br Med J (Clin Res Ed) 1982;285:606.
7. Pendergraft 3rd WF, Niles JL. Trojan horses: Drug culprits associated with anti-neutrophil cytoplasmic autoantibody (ANCA) vasculitis. CurrOpinRheumatol 2014;26:42-49.
8. Kemna MJ, Damoiseaux J, Austen J, Winkens B, Peters J, van Paassen P, Cohen Tervaert JW. ANCA as a predictor of relapse: Useful in patients with renal involvement but not in patients with non renal disease. J Am Soc Nephrol 2015;26:537-42.
9. Lionaki S, Blyth ER, Hogan SL, Hu Y, Senior BA, Jennette CE, Nachman PH, Jennette JC, Falk RJ. Classification of anti-neutrophil cytoplasmic auto antibody vasculitides: The role of anti-neutrophil cytoplasmic auto antibody specificity for myeloperoxidase or proteinase 3 in disease recognition and prognosis. Arthritis Rheum 2012;64: 3452-62.
10. DE Zoysa J, Taylor D, Thein H, Yehia M. Incidence and features of dual anti-GBM-positive and ANCA-positive patients. Nephrology (Carlton) 2011;16:725-29.

CHAPTER

30 A Patient with Cardiorenal Syndrome

K Praveen Kumar [1], S Raghavendra[2]

[1] Professor and Head, Department of Nephrology, Narayana Medical College, Nellore
[2] Assistant Professor, Department of Nephrology, Narayana Medical College, Nellore

CASE 1

A 60 years old diabetic male presented with acute myocardial infarction (MI). On evaluation, he was found to have hypotension with elevated renal parameters with serum creatinine of 3 mg/dl. He was treated with inotropic support along with loading doses of aspirin and clopidogrel and acute peritoneal dialysis support. In the next 3 days blood pressures normalised and renal function improved. It comes under category cardiorenal syndrome (CRS) type 1 where in acute heart failure cause acute renal failure and it improves with treatment of cardiac failure.

CASE 2

A 32 years old female known case of dilated cardiomyopathy with severe left ventricular dysfunction since 6 years and slowly increasing serum creatinine for the past 2 years admitted with generalised oedema and severe shortness of breath. Laboratory reports revealed serum creatinine 3.5 mg/dl and LV ejection fraction 20%. She was managed conservatively with fluid and salt restriction, intravenous diuretics with which patient became symptomatically better and discharged in a stable condition. It comes under CRS type 2 where in chronic cardiac dysfunction cause chronic kidney disease.

CASE 3

A 42 years old man previously fit and well presented with two weeks history of malaise and a 2 days history of hemoptysis. Laboratory reports revealed serum creatinine of 9 mg/dl. Bedside echocardiography revealed moderate global systolic dysfunction indicating probable uremic cardiomyopathy. Renal biopsy confirmed the diagnosis of glomerulonephritis and after repeated sessions of hemodialysis echocardiography revealed normal systolic function. It comes under CRS type 3, where in acute renal failure causes acute heart failure, which improves once renal function improve.

CASE 4

A 32 years old female with type 1 diabetes developed end stage renal failure. 2D ECHO revealed severe impaired systolic function. She was initiated on hemodialysis, 3 months later echocardiography showed mild systolic dysfunction rather than severe. It comes under CRS type 4 where in chronic kidney problem cause left ventricular dysfunction.

CASE 5

A 30-year-old man with no past medical history, was admitted with fever for the past 3 days, on examination patient was extremely ill with temperature of 40°C, BP 80/50 mm Hg and pulse rate of 130/minute. Laboratory tests revealed leucocytosis (36,000/cmm) and elevated serum creatinine of 2.5 mg/dl. 2D ECHO revealed severely impaired systolic function. With inotropic support and IV antibiotics in less than 72 hours he was feeling significantly better and renal function had returned to normal. Repeat echocardiography revealed normal systolic function. It belongs to CRS type 5 where in systemic condition cause both cardiac and renal dysfunction and treatment of infection results in improvement of both cardiac and renal function.

All of these patients had coexisting cardiac and renal dysfunction, but clearly with grossly different underlying pathophysiology and therefore different prognosis.

What is Cardiorenal Syndrome?

The heart is responsible for supplying the organs and tissues of the body with blood and the kidneys play an integral role in fluid balance and salt homeostasis. It should therefore come as little surprise that renal dysfunction frequently accompanies cardiac failure and that cardiac dysfunction frequently accompanies renal failure. This interdependent relationship has come to be known as the "cardiorenal syndrome". [1] The definition of cardiorenal syndrome was first proposed by the ADQI to describe disorders of the heart and kidney where by acute or chronic dysfunction in one organ may induce acute or chronic dysfunction of the other (Ronco *et al.* 2010).[2] The incidence of heart failure has been steadily increasing due to the ageing of the general population and the availability of better treatment. The incidence of acute kidney injury (AKI)/worsening renal function varies between 25-33% and 9-19% in acute decompensated heart failure (ADHF) and acute coronary syndrome (ACS) respectively. Inconsistent definitions for AKI caused broad range in incidence, limit standardization of data and make epidemiologic studies difficult (Table 30.1).

What are the Predisposing Factors for Cardiorenal Syndrome?

Obesity

Obesity without diabetes can cause hyperfiltration that ultimately leads to CKD and CRS, particularly type II and type IV and also has been associated with a 3- to 7-fold increased risk of CRS type I in a variety of clinical settings.[3,4] The adipocytes secrete cytokines such as interleukin (IL)-6 and tumour necrosis factor alpha, which are implicated in the progression of both cardiac and renal disease.

Anemia and Nutritional Deficiencies

Anemia, cachexia and nutritional deficiencies result in elevated tumour necrosis factor alpha and other pro-inflammatory cytokines associated with either heart failure (HF) or chronic kidney disease (CKD) and may contribute to further damage and fibrosis of the other organ.[5]

Hypertension

Elevated blood pressure reflects increased sympathetic activation and it causes direct cardiac and renal injury and is also associated with increased incidence of worsening renal failure in patients with decompensated congestive heart failure (CHF).[6]

Diabetes Mellitus

Diabetes mellitus (DM) through many mechanisms contributes to glomerular dysfunction and damage and ultimately loss of functioning filtration units and further contributes to CKD. Endothelial, mesangial, and podocyte injury in the presence of hypertension and DM results in excess quantities of albumin in Bowman's space, thus the proximal tubular cells have an increased reabsorption workload. This phenomenon has been suggested to result in apoptosis of renal tubular cells, further nephron loss, and progression of kidney disease. Indeed, albuminuria and gross proteinuria has been consistently associated with the risk of AKI in a variety of settings.[7]

What is Pathophysiology of Cardiorenal Syndrome?

The pathophysiology of CRS is complex and includes neurohormonal activation, abnormal endothelial activation and release of pro-inflammatory cytokines. These pathophysiological adaptive mechanisms operate simultaneously and sequentially, later become maladaptive leading ultimately to cardiac and renal dysfunction (Fig. 30.1).

Neurohormonal Dysfunction

In type I and type II CRS, reduction in cardiac output causes venous congestion and systemic hypoperfusion which simulates intravascular volume depletion. This activates the renin–angiotensin–aldosterone system (RAAS) and nonosmotic release of arginine–vasopressin and sympathetic nervous system leading to renal injury.[9]

Studies have shown that plasma catecholamine levels were elevated in patients with renal dysfunction indicating sympathetic hyperactivity in type III and type IV CRS. It contributes to hypertension, cardiac injury and further deterioration in renal function.

Angiotensin II, aldosterone and sympathetic nervous system (SNS) also has direct trophic effects on cardiomyocytes and renal tubular cells that promote cellular hypertrophy, apoptosis, and fibrosis (Burns and Thomas 2011).

Table 30.1: Schematic of the classification system proposed by Ronco *et al.*[8] for subdivision of CRS into 5 subtypes based upon etiology of dysfunction

CRS Type	Name	Description	Example
1.	Acute cardiorenal	Acute cardiac dysfunction leading to acute kidney injury	Acute coronary syndrome causing acute heart failure and then renal dysfunction
2.	Chronic cardiorenal	Chronic heart failure leading to renal dysfunction	Congestive cardiac failure
3.	Acute reno cardiac	Acute kidney injury leading to acute cardiac dysfunction	Uremic cardiomyopathy secondary to acute renal failure
4.	Chronic reno cardiac	Chronic renal failure leading to cardiac dysfunction	Left ventricular hypertrophy and diastolic heart failure secondary to renal failure
5.	Secondary	Systemic condition causing cardiac and renal function	Septic shock, vasculitis

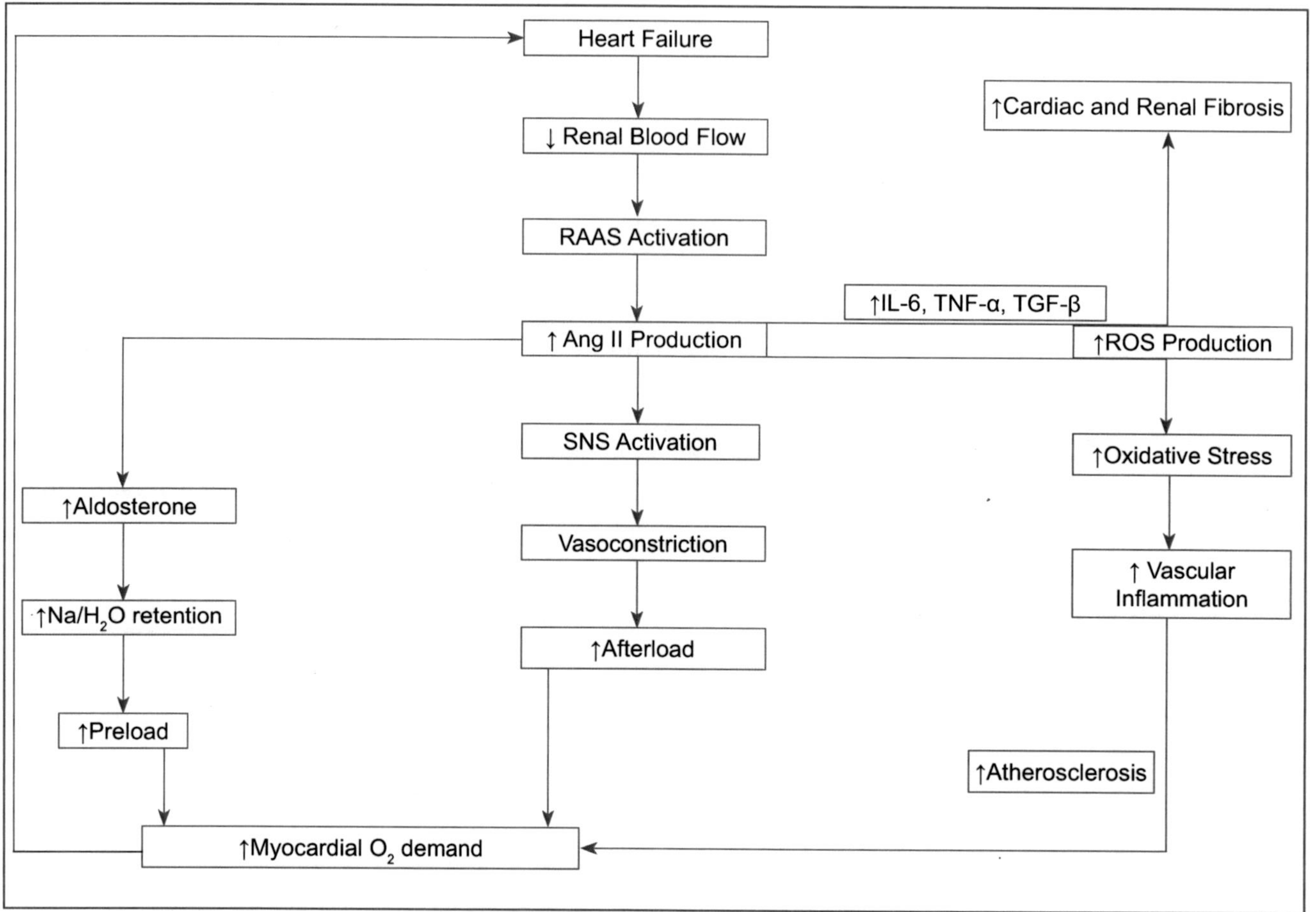

Figure 30.1: Illustration of the pathophysiological pathways activated by angiotensin II. Both preload and afterload are ultimately increased, leading to worsening cardiac and renal function

IL-6: Interleukin; TNF–α: Tumour necrosis factor alpha; TGF–β: Transforming growth factor beta; ROS: Reactive oxygen species.

Abnormal Endothelial Activation

Volume overload resulting from either cardiac or renal dysfunction causes circumferential stretch of endothelial cells. The activated endothelial cells changes their synthetic profile from a quiescent state toward an activated state, which is pro-oxidant, pro-inflammatory, and vasoconstricting. This impairs myocardial function, renal function and accelerates HF progression.[10]

Endotoxemia, Infection and Inflammation

Cardiac and renal dysfunction causes intestinal hypoperfusion and congestion leading to intestinal translocation of lipopolysaccharides in to systemic circulation (Ronco *et al.* 2012). It activates circulating immune cells with release of cytokines, such as tumour necrosis factor alpha, IL-1 and IL-6, that can exacerbate myocyte and renal dysfunction.[11] Inflammation seems to be more than just accompanying feature during HF and it may have a role in organ damage in particular AKI (Friedwaid and Rabb 2004, Cantaluppi *et al.* 2012). However, randomized placebo controlled trials of anti-tumour necrosis factor alpha therapies in patients with CHF (i.e., Randomized Etanercept North American Strategy to Study Antagonism of Cytokines [RENAISSANCE], Etanercept Cytokine Antagonism in Ventricular Dysfunction [RECOVER], and Anti-Tumor Necrosis Factor Therapy Against Congestive Heart Failure [ATTACH] have been disappointing and showed no clinical benefit.

Role of Venous Congestion

There is a common belief in the medical community that hypoperfusion is the cause for worsening renal function. While it is not the only mechanism by which HF leads to renal dysfunction. Mullens *et al.* showed that in low output decompensated HF venous congestion was the strongest determinant for the development of cardiorenal syndrome. If interstitial hydrostatic pressure exceeds tubular hydrostatic pressure, tubules will collapse and decrease net ultrafiltration pressure, causing renal dysfunction.[12]

Drugs

Drugs that are commonly used for the treatment of acute heart failure can also contribute to renal injury. Diuretics are the cornerstone in the management of AHF. These cause resolution of congestion and provide rapid relief from symptoms, but overdiuresis can cause arterial underfilling and worse kidney function. Drugs acting on RAAS have proven efficacy in stabilized HF, however during AHF may cause CRS type 1. Patients with heart failure can be exposed to various nephrotoxic medications like NSAIDs, antibiotics, contrast material.

How to Manage a Case of Cardiorenal Syndrome?

Prevention

As there is no definite therapy available to directly treat any one type of CRS, prevention should be a key strategy. In patients with heart failure with reduced ejection fraction ACE inhibitors have been showed to reduce the incidence of CHF decompensation and HF related hospitalization and overall is associated with improved mortality.[13]

Drugs that can cause renal injury such as NSAIDs and contrast agents should be avoided in patients with or who are at risk for CHF (Table 30.2).

Table 30.2: Practical recommendations for the management of acute decompensated heart failure patients with cardiorenal syndrome (Katerina Koniari *et al.*)

- Restrict fluid and sodium intake
- Increase furosemide dose
- Use continuous intravenous furosemide
- Add thiazides or metolazone
- Add renoprotective dopamine at 2–3 mcg/kg/min
- Add inotrope or vasodilator (according to systolic blood pressure)
- Start ultrafiltration
- Insert intra-aortic balloon pump
- Insert another device

Treatment of Congestion

Guidelines are currently available for management of heart failure (McMurray *et al.* 2012) and AKI (KDIGO); however specific recommendations are not there for cardiorenal syndrome. Diuretics, inotrope, vasopressors and vasodilators can all be used according to the clinical presentation.

Congestion is treated with diuretics and salt restriction. Diuretic dosing is based on renal function and pharmacokinetic properties of diuretics and patients volume status. Biomarker guided therapy and the use of bioelectric impedance vector analysis to assess hydration status could be helpful to monitor diuretic therapy and avoid unwanted iatrogenic complications (Aspromote *et al.* 2011). Monitoring natriuretic peptides can be helpful for assessing volume status and target diuretic therapy. The DOSE-AHF study demonstrated no significant differences in prognosis or serum creatinine levels between high doses of furosemide (2.5 times their outpatient dose) and lower doses (equal to outpatient dose) in patients hospitalized for ADHF. There was also no benefit of continuous infusion over bolus dosing.[14]

Once-daily dosing of loop diuretics, such as furosemide, can lead to rebound increase in sodium absorption. Hence, twice-daily dose of loop diuretics should be used. Intravenous loop diuretics should be used in hospitalized patients with ADHF to overcome decreased absorption caused by splanchnic congestion.

When diuretic resistance is encountered, addition of thiazides or mineralocorticoid receptor antagonists (MRAs) can promote diuresis by decreasing the enhanced sodium reabsorption in the distal tubule.

Ultrafiltration

In UNLOAD trial ultrafiltration (UF) produced a greater weight and fluid loss and resulted in lower HF rehospitalisation rates compared to IV diuretics (Costanzo *et al.* 2007). The Cardiorenal Rescue Study in Acute Decompensate Heart Failure (CARRESS-HF), a multicenter randomized trial, compared veno-venous ultrafiltration therapy vs. diuretic escalation in patients with either systolic or diastolic HF and worsening renal function (creatinine increase >0.3 mg/dl and evidence of volume overload). When compared with diuretic therapy, ultrafiltration in patients with type I CRS did not show a significant difference in weight loss, mortality, or the rate of hospitalization for HF during the 60-day follow-up period. There was a trend towards increased mortality in the ultrafiltration arm. However, patients requiring inotropes or vasodilator therapy and those with admission creatinine levels >3.1 mg/dl were excluded in this trial. Cardiopulmonary hemodynamics measurements were not made. Hence, it is not known if ultrafiltration has any role in patients who are diuretic resistant. In patients with significant ascites, paracentesis might be useful to reduce intra-abdominal pressure and improve renal hemodynamics and function.[15]

RAAS Blockade

Excess salt and water retention from activation of RAAS, affects cardiac preload and afterload which further worsens cardiac and renal function. Breaking this cycle prevents further cardiorenal injury.

MRAs inhibit neurohumoral surge and prevent worsening of both cardiac and renal function in CRS. However patients should be monitored carefully for hyperkalemia when given alone or with ACE inhibitors particularly in the setting of pre-existing renal dysfunction. These drugs can also help overcome loop diuretic resistance when used for hypervolemia.

LV Assist Devices

An LV assist device (LVAD) is an implantable mechanical circulatory support device that has revolutionized the treatment of end-stage HF. Pre-LVAD implant renal dysfunction predicts higher mortality after LVAD implantation.[16]

Hence, it is important that patients receive timely referral for LVAD therapy before HF worsens and leads to CKD. Renal function usually improves after LVAD implantation if decreased GFR is due to renal hypoperfusion before implantation. Most of the recovery tends to occur in the first month after LVAD placement and no further improvement in renal function occurs from about 1 month after pump placement.

What the Future Holds?

Implantable devices to measure intravascular volume in real time are being developed. The COMPASS-HF.[17] Trial showed that increases in intracardiac pressures often arose independently of weight changes, such that monitoring of weight alone was inadequate to identify congestion in time to avert the events associated with HF. This provides an opportunity to provide early intervention by targeting these pressures, which might reduce the risk of CHF decompensation and reduce the incidence of CRS.

Aldosterone plays a major role in cardiac, vascular, and renal remodelling by promoting oxidative stress, inflammation, fibrosis and hypertrophy. Clinical trials are underway using finerenone, a novel nonsteroidal MRA, in CRS.

Recently serelaxin was tested in RELAX AHF[18] trial and has shown promising results in CRS. Serelaxin is a recombinant form of human relaxin-2. Relaxin, a peptide hormone secreted during pregnancy, is associated with increase in cardiac output and decrease in systemic vascular resistance.

Recent research has focused on enhancing the effects of natriuretic peptides (NPs). Neprilysin is an enzyme that degrades these NPs. The *PARADIGM-HF* trial showed that the novel drug, LCZ696 (sacubitril/valsartan) that inhibits both the Angiotensin II and Neprilysin, was found to be more effective in reducing the risk of death from cardiovascular causes or hospitalization for HF than was ACE inhibition with enalapril. Sacubitril/valsartan is being increasingly used in this setting.

Pilot trials are underway to study the effect of renal denervation on the heart and kidney in CHF.[19]

Conclusion

CRS is a well established entity relating to the complex interaction that exists between the heart and the kidney.

The prevention and treatment still remains a challenge to the treating physicians. As there is no definite treatment that reverses the established CRS, key focus is on the prevention strategies like modifications of risk factors such as obesity, hypertension, DM, and tobacco use are important. Treatment modalities like hemodynamic support in low output states, judicious use of diuretics for congestion, and suppression of neurohumoral activation remain the cornerstone. Novel devices and therapeutics such as intracardiac pressure monitoring, Neprilysin inhibition, third-generation MRAs, and sympathetic denervation are being investigated.

References

1. JT Heywood. "The cardiorenal syndrome: Lessons from The ADHERE database and treatment options", Heart Failure Reviews, Vol. 9, 2005;3:195-201.
2. Ronco C, McCullough PA and Anker SD, *et al.* Cardiorenal syndromes: An executive Summary from the consensus conference of the Acute Dialysis Quality Initiative (ADQI). Contrib Nephrol 2010;165:54-67.
3. Glance LG, Wissler R, Mukamel DB, *et al.* Preoperative outcomes among patients with the modified metabolic syndrome who are undergoing noncardiac surgery. Anaesthesiology 2010;113(4):859-72.
4. Hunley TE, Ma LJ, Kon V. Scope and mechanisms of obesity-related renal disease. Curr Opin Nephrol Hypertens 2010;19(3):227-34.
5. Cicoira M, Bolger AP, Doehner W, *et al.* High tumour necrosis factor-a levels are associated with exercise intolerance and neurohormonal activation in chronic heart failure patients. Cytokine 2001;15(2):80-86.
6. Forman DE, Butler J, Wang Y, *et al.* Incidence, predictors at admission, and impact of worsening renal function among patients hospitalized with heart failure. J Am Coll Cardiol 2004;43(1):61-67.
7. Warnock DG, Muntner P, McCullough PA, *et al.* Kidney function, albuminuria and all-cause mortality in the REGARDS (Reasons for Geographic and Racial Differences in Stroke) study. Am J Kidney Dis 2010;56(5):861-71.
8. Ronco M, Haapio A A, House N, Anavekar and R Bellomo. "Cardiorenal syndrome", Journal of the American College of Cardiology 2008;Vol 52,19:1527-39.
9. Schrier RW. Role of diminished renal function in cardiovascular mortality: Marker or pathogenetic factor? J Am Coll Cardiol 2006;47(1):1-8.
10. Braunwald E. Biomarkers in heart failure. N Engl J Med 2008;358(20):2148-59.
11. Kraut EJ, Chen S, Hubbard NE, *et al.* Tumor necrosis factor depresses myocardial contractility in endotoxemic swine. J Trauma 1999;46(5):900-06.
12. Burnett JC JR, Knox FG. Renal interstitial pressure and sodium excretion during renal vein constriction. Am J Physiol 1980;238(4):F279-82.
13. Effect of enalapril on survival in patients with reduced left ventricular ejection fracti\ons and congestive heart failure. The SOLVD Investigators. N Engl J Med 1991;325(5): 293-302.
14. Felker GM, Lee KL, Bull DA, *et al.* Diuretic strategies in patients with acute decompensated heart failure. N Engl J Med 2011;364(9):797-805.
15. Bart BA, Goldsmith SR, Lee KL, *et al.* Ultrafiltration in decompensated heart failure with cardiorenal syndrome. N Engl J Med 2012;367(24):2296-304.
16. Kirklin JK, Naftel DC, Kormos RL, *et al.* Quantifying the effect of cardiorenal syndrome on mortality after left ventricular assist device implant. J Heart Lung Transplant 2013;32(12):1205-13.
17. Bourge RC, Abraham WT, Adamson PB, *et al.* Randomized controlled trial of an implantable continuous hemodynamic monitor in patients with advanced heart failure: The COMPASS-HF study. J Am Coll Cardiol 2008;51(11): 1073-79.
18. Metra M, Cotter G, Davison BA, *et al.* Effect of serelaxin on cardiac, renal and hepatic biomarkers in the Relaxin in Acute Heart Failure (RELAX-AHF) development program: Correlation with outcomes. J Am Coll Cardiol 2013;61(2): 196-206.
19. McMurray JJ, Packer M, Desai AS, *et al.* Angiotensin-neprilysin inhibition versus enalapril in heart failure. N Engl J Med 2014;371(11):993-1004.

CHAPTER 31

Immunological Work-Up for Renal Transplant Recipient

Aseem Kumar Tiwari[1], Abhishek Saini[2]

[1] *Director, Department of Transfusion Medicine, Medanta, The Medicity, Gurugram*

[2] *Scientist, Molecular and Transplant Immunology, Medanta, The Medicity, Gurugram*

Introduction

Besides improved surgical techniques, advanced immunosuppression, improved dialysis care, transplant immunology plays a pivotal role in ensuring successful renal transplantation in most patients with end-stage renal disease (ESRD). In India, an Act for the regulation of removal, storage and transplantation of human organs for therapeutic purposes was enacted in 1994 and was known as The Transplantation of Human Organs Act, 1994. In 2011, Government of India amended the Act and this was then called The Transplantation of Human Organs (Amendment) Act, 2011, which also included a provision of swapping of organs among recipient-donor pairs and increased the donor pool by including grandparents and grandchildren to the list of potential donors. This Act was again revised in 2014 and termed as "The Transplantation of Human Organs and Tissues Rules (THOT), 2014" which has now included several provisions to remove the impediments to organ donation while curbing misuse/misinterpretation of the rules. The major revision in 2014 was creation of the national registry of donors and recipients of Human Organ and Tissue, accessible on-line through dedicated websites having national, regional/state level specificities. Thereafter, The National Organ and Tissue Transplant Organization (NOTTO), under the Ministry of Health and Family Welfare, came into existence and NOTTO has also issued guidelines for allocation criteria for a deceased donor kidney transplant.[1]

The renal transplantation markedly improves quality of life. Advances in immune-suppression and plasma apheresis have led to an incremental improvement in the outcome, not just limited to ABO compatible cases but ABO-incompatible as well. Enhanced efforts are now being directed toward improving long-term outcomes in renal transplantation and it is in this context, that transplant immunology plays a crucial role. The two major categories of tests essential for pre-transplant immunology testing are:

1. Test(s) to confirm the kinship as per THOT.
2. Test(s) to evaluate compatibility of the recipient-donor pair.

To confirm the kinship, HLA (Human Leucocyte Antigen) typing is done routinely, and if required, further advanced tests like Mitochondrial DNA (Deoxyribose Nucleic Acid) analysis, Y-STR (Short Tandem Repeats) DNA analysis, or Autosomal DNA analysis are performed. For evaluation of compatibility testing, the algorithm that is usually followed by most tertiary health centers in India is to perform CDCXM (Complement Dependent Lymphocyto-toxicity Crossmatch), FCXM (Flowcytometric crossmatch), and PRA (Panel Reacting Antibodies). If these tests are negative, then nephrologist would proceed for transplant. While CDCXM positivity is an absolute contraindication to transplant. If either CXM or PRA is positive, Single Antigen Bead (SAB) assay is performed to identify the DSA (Donor Specific Antibodies). The decision to transplant depends on DSA along with other clinical parameters. All the tests for proving kinship and ascertaining compatibility of donor organ with recipient are discussed in the subsequent sections.

Tests to Confirm the Kinship

HLA Typing Tests

HLA Typing can be performed either by PCR or by DNA Sequencing. There are two PCR based methods: Sequence-Specific Priming (SSP) Typing and Sequence-Specific Oligonucleotide (SSO) Typing. These methods are discussed briefly here:

Sequence-Specific Priming (SSP) Typing

Genomic DNA (gDNA) is isolated from the whole blood collected in EDTA vacutainers. Now the HLA regions of interest let say A, B, DR loci are amplified using small oligonucleotide sequences specific primers (oligos).

These 'oligos' bind to an exact location of a DNA as per complementarity, and act as the starting point for the amplification of the intermediate region and generate multiple complimentary copies. These primers can either be used for single locus or multiple loci in a single PCR reaction, depending on the requirement, in generally typing of HLA–A, B and DR loci are done in renal transplant cases. The polymorphic-specific primers are used for amplification, to ensure that they only extend and amplify if the targeted polymorphism is present. Furthermore, amplified products of specific lengths are produced depending on the polymorphism and the primer design. Afterward, these are visualized using gel electrophoresis. PCR/SSP may become a time and labor-intense technique. This technique is also prone to false-positive bands and false-negative results, especially for not-so-fresh (degraded) samples.[2]

Sequence-Specific Oligonucleotide (SSO) Typing

In this procedure, after the genomic DNA extraction, the locus-specific (A, B, or DR) amplification of the polymorphic sites of HLA alleles is carried out. The ratio of forward and reverse primers is adjusted in such a way that in the amplified product single strands of DNA are obtained. These DNA strands are then hybridized with a set of sequence-specific oligonucleotide probes (SSOP). These oligonucleotides probes are coated onto beads of the same size but different colors to distinguish them with the help of flow cytometer, usually in PE channel. The beads which get hybridized with the amplified product are detected through the fluorochrome. The probe that completely matches with the target sequence amplified will hybridize and give a positive signal. The next step is to identify the alleles by matching it with the database. All these steps are carried out by the new era instruments.

Sequence-Based Typing (SBT)

Other than conventional methods, High-resolution HLA typing can also be done by the sequencing of the genomic DNA. Here the HLA locus-specific DNA sequences are amplified using the primers that specifically amplify the different HLA genes. After amplification, the locus-specific amplicons are pooled for library generation followed by clonal amplification. Once each DNA fragment is amplified using adapter specific primers, the sequencing is carried out, and then the data is analyzed by using the software which has the potential to separate sequences of each locus from the other loci to form an unambiguous typing result. Sequence-based typing is more automated, user-friendly thus, reducing the technical and interpretational errors.[3]

HLA Compatibility Testing between Donor and Recipient

These tests can be broadly divided into Antibody screening and cross match. The immunological factors affecting the graft survival are Anti-HLA antibodies are generally defined as panel reactive antibody (PRA). Identification of such antibodies can be carried out either by cell-based methods or HLA bead-based method known as solid-phase immunoassays.

In cell-based methods recipient's serum is incubated with donor's cells followed by cell-bound antibody detection. The simplest one is complement-dependent-lymphocytotoxicity crossmatch (CDCXM), used with or without the addition of an antihuman globulin (AHG), detects complement-activating antibodies. The more sensitive test is flow cytometric crossmatch (FCXM), where fluorochrome-conjugated AHG is used to detect all cell-bound antibodies.

Antibody screening and characterization are currently done mainly by Luminex-based assays. The targets are suspension arrays of differentially fluorescently labeled microbead populations coated with soluble HLA antigens. After incubation with the patient's serum and addition of AHG conjugated with a reporter fluorochrome, HLA bound antibody is detected by analyzing the beads with a flow cytometry based Luminex analyzer. The mean fluorescence intensity (MFI) of the reporter signal is used to make a semi-quantitative estimation of the antibody level.

Antibody Tests

Panel Reactive Antibody (PRA) Screening

The affinity-purified HLA class I and class II antigens of known HLA type, either pooled or specific, are bound directly to wells of microtiter plates. Antibody reactivity is detected by the addition of secondary antibody, an enzyme-conjugated antihuman immunoglobulin that induces a color change upon addition of the enzyme-substrate, detected by measuring optical density. This is a quick, objective, semi-quantitative assay that detects both complement and non-complement-fixing HLA antibodies with a reported higher sensitivity than CDC tests.

PRA detection using methods based on enzyme-linked immunosorbent assay (ELISA) and fluorescence-based flow cytometry or Luminex technologies offer higher sensitivity and specificity. PRA screening consists of two main incubation steps. First of all, patient and control sera are incubated with PRA screening beads containing HLA Class I and Class II (except DQ) coated onto them. In the second step, fluorescence-conjugated anti-human secondary antibodies are added. The fluorescence peak is detected by the detectors, which determines the result based on MF.

Single Antigen Bead (SAB) Assay (Luminex Single Antigen Assay; LSA)

This test is mostly used to carry out a virtual crossmatch, where the HLA alleles of donor are virtually cross-matched with the antibodies present in the patient's serum. To start with this test, multiple beads, each coated with a single HLA antigen for either HLA class I or class II are incubated with the recipient's serum. In the second step fluorescence-conjugated anti-human secondary antibodies are added to the reaction mix. After incubation, the reaction well is read by Luminex plate reader, and a fluorescence peak is analyzed for the presence or absence of the antibodies with their mean fluorescence index (MFI).[4]

Compatibility Testing Assays

Complement Dependent Lymphocytotoxicity Crossmatch (CDCXM)

The long-established CDC assay is over 30 years old and is still widely used. In this technique, donor lymphocytes (cadaveric/living) are incubated recipient's serum. The humoral immunological response is mediated through the activation of the complement system by the classical pathway. Rabbit complement is added externally to the reaction, and the addition of anti-human immunoglobulin (AHG) helps increase the sensitivity of CDC as multiple AHGs bind to a single donor-specific antibody, amplifying its complement activation response at smaller titers.

Although CDC is criticized for its low sensitivity, the pattern of CDC panel reactivity as a measure of anti-HLA sensitization (*in vivo*) is a useful indicator of an increased risk of rejection and potential hyperacute rejection. CDC is subjective, and it requires manual reading of the test and expert analysis, and can't detect non-complement-fixing antibodies.

Flow Cytometry Cross-Match (FCXM)

FC-XM test is a highly sensitive antibody-binding assay. Following incubation of donor lymphocyte targets with recipient serum, a fluorescent-labeled detecting antibody is used to tag any bound alloantibody. Following the passage of the target cells through a flow cytometer, a semiquantitative assessment can be made of the degree of binding of alloantibody to donor lymphocytes, leading to an assessment of XM positivity.[5,6]

Testing Algorithms

As discussed earlier, in India usually, CDCXM, FCXM, and PRA are performed initially; if these tests are negative, then nephrologist would proceed for transplant. In case CDCXM is positive, the donor is deferred; in case FCXM or PRA is positive, then SAB assay for class I and Class II (as per the requirement) is performed to identify the DSA present. A virtual crossmatch is carried out by looking for the HLA typing of the prospective donor and antibody profile of the recipient.[7]

References

1. Government of India. Transplantation of Human Organs Act, 1994. Central Act 42; 1994. Available from: https://mohfw.gov.in/acts-rules-and-standards-health-sector/acts/transplantation-human-organs-acts-and-rules [Last accessed on 09/11/2019].
2. Erlich H. HLA DNA typing: Past, present and future. Tissue Antigens 2012;80(1):1-11.
3. Spinola H, Bruges-Armas J, Brehm A. Discrepancies in HLA typing by PCR-SSOP and SBT techniques: A case study. Human Biology 2007;79(5):537-43.
4. Bettinotti MP, Zachary AA, Leffell MS. Clinically relevant interpretation of solid phase assays for HLA antibody. Current opinion in organ transplantation 2016 Aug;21(4):453.
5. Kerman RH, Susskind B, Buelow R, Regan J, Pouletty P, Williams J, *et al.* Correlation of ELISA-detected IgG and IgA anti-HLA antibodies in pretransplant sera with renal allograft rejection. Transplantation 1996;62:201-05.
6. Lobashevsky AL. Methodological aspects of anti-human leukocyte antigen antibody analysis in solid organ transplantation. World J Transplant 2014:24:4(3):153-67. doi:10.5500/wjt. v4. i3.153.
7. Susal C, Pelzl S, Simon T, Opelz G. Advances in pre- and post-transplant immunologic testing in kidney transplantation. Transplant Proc 2004;36:29-34.

CHAPTER 32

A Post Renal Transplant Patient with Acute Graft Dysfunction

Shyam Bihari Bansal[1], Ashwini Gadde[2]

[1] *Director, Department of Nephrology, Medanta, The Medicity, Gurugram*

[2] *Associate Consultant, Department of Nephrology, Medanta, The Medicity, Gurugram*

Introduction

Acute allograft dysfunction is a common and complex problem and appropriate management is critical for short term and long-term graft survival. Acute graft dysfunction has been defined differently in various studies but most transplant physicians consider a 15% decrease in eGFR or 0.3 mg/dl increase in serum creatinine level as significant and worthy of further investigation. We would be discussing various causes of graft dysfunction by a case based approach.

CASE

24-year-old male, steroid resistant focal segmental glomerulosclerosis (FSGS) diagnosed 5 years ago, now progressed to end stage renal disease (ESRD), on maintenance hemodialysis since last 4 months. He underwent a live related renal transplant with mother as a donor, no induction. His urine output was good for next 2 days and serum creatinine came down to 1.9 mg/dl on post operative day (POD) 2, however on POD2, he developed decrease in urine output and on POD3, his creatinine increased to 2.5 mg/dl. He also developed swelling and gained 2 kg wt. His renal doppler was normal and tacrolimus (TAC) level was 11 ng/ml on day 1 and 9 ng/ml on day 3. What is our next step in terms on diagnosis and management?

Most Nephrologist would have experienced above mentioned scenario. Differential diagnosis in this case are many, however in the post-transplant scenario in addition to the common causes of acute kidney injury (AKI), there are few causes which are specific to transplant. This review will predominantly discuss this transplant specific causes and approach to such cases.

Differential Diagnosis of Acute Graft Dysfunction According to Timeline

Timeline of acute graft dysfunction is important as list of differential diagnosis differs in early (< 3 months post transplant) or late (> 3 months post transplant) graft dysfunction.

Causes of Acute Graft Dysfunction

Early (< 3 months).

Prerenal

- Volume depletion.
- Hypotension.
- *Drugs:* Nonsteroidal anti-inflammatory drugs (NSAIDs), calcineurine inhibitors (CNIs).
- Vascular thrombosis or compression.

Intrinsic Renal Diseases

- Acute tubular necrosis (ATN) due to prolonged ischemia (deceased donor transplant, donation after cardiac death), perioperative and post-operative hypotension.
- Hyperacute/accelerated acute rejection-although rare now-a-days but might be seen in sensitized patients like previous transplant, multiple blood transfusions, pregnancies and ABO incompatible (ABOi) transplant etc.
- Acute rejection (AR) (cellular, humoral or both).
- Thrombotic microangiopathy due to – acute rejection, calcineurin inhibitor (CNI), everolimus or some infections like CMV etc.
- Graft pyelonephritis.
- Calcineurine inhibitors toxicity.
- Cytomegalovirus (CMV)/BK virus (BKV) infections.
- Recurrent glomerular disease (FSGS, aHUS).

Post Renal Obstruction

- Foley catheter obstruction.
- Perinephric fluid collection (urine leak, hematoma, lymphocele).
- Ureteral obstruction (kinking, stricture, blood clots).
- Neurogenic bladder.
- Enlarged prostate (BPH, prostate cancer).

A proper history and knowledge about background of patient is very important part of evaluation of acute graft dysfunction, so as to get the baseline information and to make differential diagnosis accordingly:

- **Pre-transplant immunological workup** including sensitization history (history of multiple blood transfusion, multiple pregnancies, previous transplant) – for possible preformed antibodies and predict chances of antibody mediated rejection.
- **Basic disease** and degree of pre-transplant proteinuria–to predict disease recurrence.
- **Native urine output:** In patients with pre-emptive kidney transplant or patients with chronic interstitial nephritis might have substantial urine output despite graft kidney not functioning as compared to patients with little or no urine output from native kidneys.
- **Deceased donor transplant:** As they are more likely to have delayed graft function (DGF).
- **Warm and cold ischemia time:** As longer warm or cold ischemia time would lead to ATN.
- **Induction agent:** If patient has got induction with Anti thymocyte globulin (ATG), the chances of developing cellular rejection is less as compared to patient with IL2RA induction which is again better as compared to no induction.
- **Maintenance immunosuppression:** There are higher chances of acute rejection if tacrolimus levels are low in patients without induction and conversely there are more chances of CNI toxicity if levels are too high initially, however it may not always correlate as patients with high tacrolimus levels may also develop acute rejection.

Approach to Patient with Acute Graft Dysfunction in Immediate Post-Transplant Period

The earliest step in evaluation of any patient with oliguria within few hours to days of transplant is to check the patency of Foley's catheter and flush it and if this is clear then patient should get a trial of bolus administration of fluid to correct any dehydration. If the patient's volume status is good then he can be given a trial of intravenous furosemide. Meanwhile in early transplant period one should always get a renal doppler to rule out graft venous or arterial thrombosis and if there is any suspicion, it should be confirmed by an experienced radiologist well versed with doing renal doppler. In the event of high suspicion of vascular event, the patient should be re-explored and one might salvage a graft sometimes. After excluding vascular cause, one should look for other causes of graft dysfunction, e.g., acute rejection, ATN, CNI toxicity, thrombotic microangiopathy and recurrence of basic disease. Urinary leak is very uncommon now-a-days with routine use of double J stents in most transplant centres. One needs to remember that chances of delayed graft function (DGF) is high in patients with deceased donors (30-40%) and more in DCD (donor after cardiac death) donors (50-60%), however in living donation, the DGF is less than 5%.

Unless contraindicated, a kidney biopsy must be done in all patients with graft dysfunction in early post-transplant period. There are some clinical clues, which might suggest a particular diagnosis more likely than other, however, it is not always correct and one might miss a chance of treating an acute rejection under the mask of ATN.

Renal Dysfunction–Immediate Post-Transplant

Graft dysfunction or oliguria

↓

Check volume status–hydrate if necessary, trial of diuretics after that. If still oliguric

↓

Urgent renal doppler–if suspicion of arterial or venous thrombosis then urgent rexploration needed If normal

↓

Check Tacrolimus levels. If High, reduce it and wait only if graft dysfunction is mild or no oliguria

↓

If persistent graft dysfunction of oliguria

↓

Kidney biopsy

Renal dysfunction – after discharge

↓

Patient does not have any acute infection, dehydration etc.

↓

TAC/cyclosporine level, if high–reduce dose and repeat creatinine after 48 hours

↓

USG graft, if any hydronephrosis or compression then manage accordingly

↓

If normal

↓

Persistent graft dysfunction

↓

Kidney biopsy

Acute Rejection

Acute rejection (AR) can occur in early as well as in late post-transplant period. AR can be mediated by T cells (Acute cellular rejection) or by preformed or de novo antibodies (Acute antibody mediated rejection). AR can be further classified according to the severity and time of rejection:

1. **Hyperacute rejection:** Severe rejection usually on table leading to mottling of kidney due to preformed antibodies either anti-HLA or ABO. It is rare now-a-days with universal use of cross match before transplant, however, it might still be seen especially in highly sensitized recipients and ABOi transplant. It is advisable to go for more sensitive cross match, i.e., flow cytometry cross match and/or luminex cross match in sensitized/ABOi patients before going for transplant.
2. **Accelerated acute rejection:** Which is also severe acute rejection not on OT table, however within 24 hours of transplantation is mostly due to acute antibody mediated rejection (AMR) and occurs in sensitized recipients.
3. **Acute cellular rejection:** Most commonly seen within first few months of transplant. Now-a-days the incidence of acute cellular rejection (ACR) during the first year post-transplant has decreased to 10% or less. This decline can be attributed to use of T cell depleting induction agents and better and potent maintenance triple immunosuppression protocol having tacrolimus as CNI. Now-a-days more than 90% transplant patients are discharged on TAC based maintenance immunosuppression.

ACR after 1 week post-transplant usually presents as asymptomatic rise in serum creatinine. Graft biopsy is required for diagnosis and classification as per BANFF (from Revised 2017):

Borderline TCMR: Foci of tubulitis (t > 0) with minor interstitial inflammation 10-25% (i0 or i1), or with mild (t1) tubulitis.

Grade IA: Interstitial inflammation involving >25% of nonsclerotic cortical parenchyma (i2 or i3) with moderate tubulitis (t2) involving 1 or more tubules, not including tubules that are severely atrophic.

Grade IB: Interstitial inflammation involving >25% of nonsclerotic cortical parenchyma (i2 or i3) with severe tubulitis (t3) involving 1 or more tubules, not including tubules that are severely atrophic.

Grade IIA: Mild to moderate intimal arteritis (v1), with or without interstitial inflammation and/or tubulitis.

Grade IIB: Severe intimal arteritis (v2), with or without interstitial inflammation and/or tubulitis.

Grade III: Transmural arteritis and/or arterial fibrinoid necrosis of medial smooth muscle with accompanying mononuclear cell intimal arteritis (v3), with or without interstitial inflammation and/or tubulitis.

ACR is treated with pulse Methylprednisolone 7 to 15 mg/kg, intravenously for 3 to 5 days. Steroid-resistant ACR is defined as lack of improvement in renal function within a week of intravenous pulse steroids. These steroid resistant ACRs and severe ACR with vascular involvement, such as Banff class 2A or above, often needs anti thymocyte globulin (ATG) therapy, the typical dose of thymoglobulin is 1.5 mg/kg per day for 3-5 days. The FDA approved total dose of thymoglobulin for treatment of steroid resistant acute rejection is 10 mg/kg. But considering the side effect profile, lower doses are preferable especially in Indian population.

Acute rejection after day 2 may be AMR or ACR, the distinction becomes difficult, however, AMR has more vigorous course.

Most of the acute rejections occur in early post-transplant period. Late acute rejections, i.e., rejections 3 months post-transplant are predominantly caused by non-adherence to immunosuppressive therapy, or suboptimal immunosuppression especially lower doses of CNIs. Nonadherence is more commonly seen in adolescence age group. Use of electronic devices reminders is found to be effective (TAKE-IT trial).

Acute Antibody Mediated Rejection

Early AMR generally occurs in the setting of preformed antibodies like ABO incompatible or HLA incompatible transplant or patient has previous transplant, multiple pregnancies and multiple blood transfusions. Though advances in desensitization protocols (with use of Rituximab, Plasmapheresis, IVIG) have made HLA incompatible transplants possible, rejection rates still remains high ranging from 20-40%, because of presence of memory B cells. Late AMR are caused by de novo antibodies formed chiefly because of inadequate immunosuppression. Clinical presentation of AMR is similar to ACR, so biopsy is required for differentiation as management and outcome differs. Revised BANFF (2017) criteria is used to define ABMR which require 3 criteria.

Active ABMR; all 3 criteria must be met for diagnosis:

1. **Histologic evidence of acute tissue injury, including 1 or more of the following:** Microvascular inflammation (g > 0 and/or PTC > 0), in the absence of recurrent or de novo glomerulonephritis, although in the presence of acute TCMR, borderline infiltrate, or infection, PTC ≥ 1 alone is not sufficient and g must be ≥ 1.

   Intimal or transmural arteritis (v > 0)1.

   Acute thrombotic microangiopathy, in the absence of any other cause.

Acute tubular injury, in the absence of any other apparent cause.

2. **Evidence of current/recent antibody interaction with vascular endothelium, including 1 or more of the following:** Linear C4d staining in peritubular capillaries (C4d2 or C4d3 by IF on frozen sections, or C4d > 0 by IHC on paraffin sections).

   At least moderate microvascular inflammation ([g + PTC] ≥ 2) in the absence of recurrent or de novo glomerulonephritis, although in the presence of acute TCMR, borderline infiltrate, or infection, PTC ≥ 2 alone is not sufficient and g must be ≥ 1.

   Increased expression of gene transcripts/classifiers in the biopsy tissue strongly associated with ABMR, if thoroughly validated.

3. **Serologic evidence of donor-specific antibodies (DSA to HLA or other antigens):** C4d staining or expression of validated transcripts/classifiers as noted above in criterion 2 may substitute for donor specific antibody (DSA); however, thorough DSA testing, including testing for non-HLA antibodies if HLA antibody testing is negative, is strongly advised whenever criteria 1 and 2 are met.

Treatment of AMR usually involves combination of pulse steroids, plasmapheresis, and intravenous immunoglobulin. Rituximab has been found to be useful in some cases of acute AMR. There are case reports of successful treatment of acute AMR with bortezomib, eculizumab, and splenectomy, however they are more often used as rescue therapy. Rejection is an important cause of death censored graft loss but early diagnosis and management is crucial as complete recovery can avoid these long-term deleterious effects on graft.

Early recognition even before the clinical manifestation (Subclinical rejections) by either protocol biopsies or by transplant genomics or proteomics is the recent area of interest as subclinical rejections are found to have poorer long-term graft outcome. Several urine proteomics and biomarkers have been reported, such as CXCL 9, CXCL 10, mRNA levels of grazyme B, perforin, TIM-3, FOXP3 and others. A three-gene signature of CD3ε mRNA, IP-10 mRNA and 18 SrRNA levels in urinary cells has been reported to be diagnostic and prognostic of acute cellular rejection in kidney transplant grafts.

Vascular Thrombosis

Rare but serious complication presents in early post-transplant period seen in as few as 1% to 3% of transplants. Several transplant specific factors may be involved in the pathogenesis of graft thrombosis in addition to usual thrombophilias contributing to vessel thrombosis.

- Paediatric recipients (dehydration, donor-recipient vessel size mismatch).
- Technical errors–like kinks, vascular clamp injury or perfusion cannulation injury.
- Vascular abnormalities in the donor kidney (thrombosis is reported in up to 36% of allografts with multiple renal arteries, atheroma).
- Vascular rejection.
- Cadaveric paediatric 'en bloc' transplantation.
- Kidney transplants from elderly donors because donor hypotension together with ischaemia-reperfusion injury may cause the activation of a procoagulant surface from cytokines and the recipient immune response in atherosclerotic vessels.
- The risk is increased in patients pretreated with OKT3, high-dose intravenous methylprednisolone, which may activate the tissue factor/factor VII pathway.
- Patients with hypercoagulable states such as–antiphospholipid antibody syndrome.

It is usually heralded by oliguria followed by anuria within hours and by tenderness and severe pain over the graft region. Thrombocytopenia may occur after a few hours because of platelet accumulation in the thrombus.

Color doppler is a simple and reliable technique and is generally used to detect renal artery or vein thrombosis. Additional imaging modalities have also been used to detect or confirm renal vascular thrombosis, including angiography, scintigraphy, computed tomography and magnetic resonance but these modalities add little to the information required and might delay the management.

If there is strong suspicion of graft thrombosis than patient should be reexplored as soon as possible and the graft can be saved sometimes by doing this. It is important to remember that the therapeutic window from diagnosis to management for successful graft rescue is small, around 2 hours. Considering the high chances of graft loss despite intervention, prevention is better. But protocol for prevention is unclear. Ponticelli *et al.* have suggested following protocol:

Weak clinical risk factors
(history of recurrent miscarriages, history of vascular access thrombosis, SLE, history of previous graft loss by thrombosis, history of superficial vein thrombosis)

↓

Thrombobophilia workup

↓

If negative–standard protocol–Heparin for 3-5 days followed by Aspirin.

If positive–intensive protocol–Heparin for 4 weeks followed by aspirin (decision for long-term anticoagulation should be taken on individual basis.

Patients with history of deep vein thrombosis (DVT), pulmonary thromboembolism or known thrombophilia–intensive protocol to be followed.

Renal allograft vein thrombosis may be induced by renal vein kinking or by renal vein compression caused by lymphocele or other fluid collection, and often results from extension of deep vein thrombosis to the renal allograft vein. Treatment with streptokinase or urokinase may be useful particularly in case of acute or partial vein thrombosis. Percutaneous mechanical thrombectomy and localized catheter-directed thrombolysis may also allow the return of kidney function in some patients. Prognosis is poorer in cases of chronic graft vein thrombosis.

Acute Calcineurine Inhibitor (CNI) Toxicity

Since late 1970s, CNI have revolutionised transplant medicine. Currently, around 94% of renal transplant recipients are discharged on CNI based immunosuppression. CNI toxicity is supposed to be one of the important contributor of acute as well as chronic graft dysfunction and interstitial fibrosis and tubular atrophy (IFTA).

Due to their vasoconstriction effect of afferent arterioles (Acute arteriolopathy), CNIs reduce GFR and impair autoregulation of kidney which make graft kidney more prone for hemodynamic insult caused by volume depletion, hypotension, NSAIDs etc. causing acute tubular injury.

Other histological features include isometric vacuolisation in proximal tubules caused by enlargement of endoplasmic reticulum and increased lysosomes (toxic tubulopathy), TMA though these are not very specific.

Differential Diagnosis of Tubular Vacuolisation: Ischemic injury, hyper osmotic fluids (mannitol, radiocontrast), intravenous immunoglobulins. Acute CNI toxicity is well proven in animal as well as human.

Differential Diagnosis of Post-Transplant TMA: Recurrent disease (primary HUS/TTP), ischemia-reperfusion injury, Antibody mediated rejection, other drugs (mTOR inhibitors) anticardiolipin antibodies, malignancies, viral infections.

The toxicity is dose dependent and responds to dose reduction or withdrawal. Usually reducing the dose of CNI by 25% would lead to improvement, however, if the levels are very high than temporary withholding the drug and restarting at lower doses should be done. In chronic CNI toxicity, change to mTOR inhibitors (Convert trial, transform trial) Or belatacept (BENEFIT trial) are the possible options available but may be associated with higher rejection rates.

Acute Tubular Necrosis

Graft kidney is very prone to acute tubular injury because of ischemia reperfusion injury, effect of CNIs and any insult like hypotension, dehydration, infection might lead to ATN. Severe ATN can present as slow or delayed graft function (DGF), which is defined as requirement of dialysis within first week of transplant and is very common in deceased donor transplant where cold ischemia time is prolonged. Observed DGF rate in cadaveric transplant is around 25%, as per 2016 OPTN/SRTR data and long-term graft survival in these patients is poor as compared to living donor kidney transplant.

It is important to note that the clinical setting required for ATN like hypotension, severe volume depletion may not be very obvious in transplant patients and even slight volume depletion due to diarrhoea, vomiting or mild hypotension can cause ATN in these kidneys. Therefore it is important to give fluid challenge to these patients except when they are in obvious fluid overload. ATN in early post-transplant period can be due to acute antibody mediated rejection. So biopsy should be reviewed thoroughly for other histological evidence of AMR like glomerulitis, PTC capillaritis, TMA and IF with C4d staining is essential so not to miss AMR associated ATN. Donor specific antibodies (DSAs) should be done in the setting of unexplained ATN/nonrecovering ATN. In patients with prolonged ATN in early post-transplant period, weekly kidney biopsy should be done to rule out any rejection.

Perinephric Collections

Common etiologies of perinephric fluid collection in early post kidney transplant period include; urinomas, hematomas, lymphoceles, seromas. They can cause renal dysfunction either by causing pressure effect on graft or pelviureter or graft vessels.

Whenever there is evidence of large perinephric collection on ultrasound or causing compression, aspiration and analysis of the content should be done for correct diagnosis.

Urinomas

Urinary leaks are seen within the first few weeks following kidney transplant. The incidence now-a-days is approximately 1%. Leaks often arise from the site of ureteroneocystostomy. Urinary leaks are unlikely in presence of DJ stents which is the routine practice in most of the transplant centres, but can become apparent after stent removal. Common causes for urinary leaks are ischemia to the distal ureter (usually from ligating an artery to the lower pole of the kidney that simultaneously supplies the distal ureter), surgical trauma, or tension from a short ureter and rejection of donor ureter.

Diagnosis can be made by estimation of drain fluid creatinine which will be much higher than the serum creatinine. Confirmation of site of urinary leak can be made by radionuclide imaging, voiding cystogram, antegrade nephrostogram, or cystoscopy. The first step in management of urinary leak is placement of a Foley`s catheter and a ureteral stent if possible. Small urinary leaks may heal without further intervention, but large or persistent leaks may require operative intervention. Operative treatments of a urinary leak include reimplantation of the transplant ureter into the bladder or ureteroureterostomy, using the native ureter.

Lymphocele

Lymphoceles develop from surgically disrupted lymphatic vessels and are usually small and asymptomatic. Most develop within 2 to 6 weeks after a transplant. Reported incidence vary, can be as high as 20%. Aspiration shows high triglyceride content. Small lymphoceles resolve spontaneously. Lymphocele requires intervention only if it is large and symptomatic sometimes causing graft compression. Percutaneous image-guided aspiration is not preferred as it is associated with high recurrence rate. The standard surgical approach is creation of a peritoneal window either by laparoscopic or open technique. Injecting a sclerosing agent after inserting a drainage catheter is an option but is associated with risk of infection and recurrence and is not uncommon.

Recurrence of Primary Diseases

The possibility of recurrence of the original disease after transplantation was described in a seminal paper 50 years ago.

It is now clear that all forms of glomerulonephritis (GN) may recur after kidney transplantation and reduce the long-term graft survival. Recurrent GN is the third most common cause of allograft loss after death with a functioning graft and chronic allograft nephropathy.

Clinical manifestations of GN recurrence has wide range from mere histological recurrence to full blown RPGN like picture causing graft loss. Clinically important and frequent recurrences occur with FSGS, IgA nephropathy, MPGN (DDD >C3 glomerulonephritis), membranous glomerulopathy. Secondary GN can also rarely recur. Recurrence should always be suspected in patient with acute or chronic graft dysfunction with proteinuria with or without hematuria. The timeline of recurrence for each glomerular disease varies. The clinical manifestation of recurrent IgA nephropathy varies from asymptomatic microscopic hematuria to proteinuria and graft dysfunction to rapidly progressive GN. Recurrent MPGN and FSGS usually presents as significant proteinuria and renal impairment.

Several factors including male gender, younger recipient age, rapid progression of basic disease, living related donors, and better HLA matching have been shown to be associated with disease recurrence in the transplanted population, but the risk factors identified have also been inconsistent except younger recipient age. ATG induction, continued steroid maintenance have been associated with reduced recurrence in some studies.

There is no definitive management of recurrent diseases and management depends upon clinical severity. Patients with early recurrence of FSGS should be managed with plasmapheresis and rituximab. Patients presenting with mild proteinuria or hematuria in IgAN or membranous or MPGN, better blood pressure control, optimization of ACEi/ARBs should be done. Patients presenting as RPGN, needs aggressive management like pulse steroids and cyclophosphamide etc. The role of phasmapheresis and rituximab is not well proven. Details of each glomerulonephritis is beyond the scope of this article.

Other than these glomerular diseases, other important renal disease having significant recurrence are diseases of alternative pathway in the form of atypical HUS (varying from 20-90% recurrence as per the type), C3 glomerulapathy, and primary hyperoxaluria (almost 100% recurrence). In these diseases, primary genetic defect causes defect in complement synthesis in liver or enzyme defect in liver in oxaluria. Combined liver kidney transplant is the treatment of choice in these patients (except MCP deficiency as it's the membrane bound complement regulatory protein, levels of which are normal in transplanted kidney).

BKV Nephropathy

BK virus is a common post-transplant opportunistic viral infection, affecting ~5-10% of renal transplant recipients in the first post-transplant year and lacking an effective prophylaxis strategy. BKV is near ubiquitous in adults with a seroprevalence of >80%.

After primary infection, the virus establishes latency in the uroepithelium and renal tubular epithelial cells, and reactivation occurs in the setting of immunosuppression causing viruria. Approximately one-third of patients with viruria will develop BK viremia (BKV) and, without intervention, 1-10% could progress to BKV nephropathy presenting as interstitial inflammation, tubular cytopathic changes, atrophy, and interstitial fibrosis which can be semiquantitatively assessed by various histological grading systems given by BANFF working group. Sometimes BKV can present as ureteric stricture causing upstream hydroureteronephrosis.

Most important risk factor for BKV is overall net state of immunosuppression. Other inconsistent risk factors are male gender, older recipient age, rejection episodes, degree of human leukocyte antigen (HLA) mis-matching, prolonged cold ischemia, BK serostatus and ureteral stent placement.

As management strategies for BKVN are limited, screening for early diagnosis of viremia before overt nephropathy is crucial. BK virus is detectable in both blood and urine. After BK re-activation, the virus is first detectable in the urine, with viremia developing several weeks later. BKV viremia has a higher positive predictive value for BKVN (50–60%) than BK viruria, hence it is a preferred screening modality. Viral load is measured by PCR. BK viral load >4 log copies/ml is strongly associated with finding BKVN on biopsy, so at this viral load kidney biopsy is ideally indicated even if clinically asymptomatic. Other screening modalities are decoy cells in urine, Haufen by EM in urine, urine mRNA profile etc.

Reduction of immunosuppression is the mainstay of BKVN treatment. Discontinuation of the anti-metabolite such as mycophenolate/azathioprin is the most common approach and reduction in CNI levels to lower therapeutic levels should be done. CNI withdrawal/minimization/substitution with mTOR has also been tried. Other treatment alternatives with inconsistent benefit include use of leflunomide, cidofovir, ciprofloxacin, or intravenous immunoglobulin.

Going back to the case discussed earlier, patient had early graft dysfunction.

There was no scope for hydration as he was infact hypervolumic considering swelling and weight gain.

His TAC levels were optimal. Graft doppler ruled out any obstructive/vascular pathology.

So possible causes of his graft dysfunction were acute rejection (considering no induction and young recipient) or early recurrence of FSGS. (At POD 3, proteinuria from native kidneys is persistent, hence it's difficult to estimate graft proteinuria unless patient was anuric pretransplant or his proteinuria has significantly increased than before). He underwent a graft kidney biopsy which showed ACR IB. He responded to 3 doses of pulse steroid and discharged on POD 8 with creatinine of 1.5 mg/dl.

Summary

Acute graft dysfunction after kidney transplant is common. Early identification of cause is very important for the timely and right treatment of acute graft dysfunction. It is important to know the history and type of kidney transplant as ATN is very common in deceased donor transplant especially with prolonged cold ischemia time, similarly sensitized patients are more prone to rejection. ABOi transplant is also associated with higher incidence of hyperacute and early AMR. Graft Doppler is crucial in early oliguria as prompt re-exploration might lead to graft salvage sometimes. Early kidney biopsy is essential for most patients for correct diagnosis and treatment.

Suggested Reading

1. OPTN/SRTR 2012 annual data report. Rockville (MD): 2014.
2. Kwaku Marfo, Amy Lu, Min Ling and Enver Akalin. Desensitization Protocols and Their Outcome Clin J Am Soc Nephrol 2011;6:922-36.
3. RA Montgomery A, Loupy, DL Segev. Antibody-mediated rejection: New approaches in prevention and management Am J Transplant 2018;18 (Suppl 3):3-17.
4. El-Zoghby ZM, Stegall MD, Lager DJ, *et al.* Identifying specific causes of kidney allograft loss. Am J Transplant 2009;9:527-35.
5. Srivastava A, Kumar J, Sharma S, Abhishek, Ansari M S, Kapoor R. Vascular complication in live related renal transplant: An experience of 1945 cases. Indian J Urol 2013;29:42-47.
6. Ponticelli C De novo. Thrombotic microangiopathy. An underrated complication of renal transplantation Clin Nephrol 2007 Jun;67(6):335-40.
7. Di Carlo HN, Darras FS. Urologic considerations and complications in kidney transplant recipients. Adv Chronic Kidney Dis 2015;22:306-11.
8. Penelope J Allen, Steve J Chadban, Jonathan C Craig, Wai H Lim, Richard DM Allen. Recurrent glomerulonephritis after kidney transplantation: Risk factors and allograft outcomes Kidney International 2017;92,461-69.
9. Deirdre Sawinski and Simin Goral BK. Virus infection: An update on diagnosis and treatment Nephrol Dial Transplant 2015;30:209-17.

CHAPTER 33

A Renal Transplant Recipient with Anuria in Immediate Post Renal Transplant Period

Punit Gupta[1], Pankaj Bansal[2], Sulakshna Dahiya[3]

[1] *Director and Head, Department of Nephrology and Organ Transplantation, Sharda University Hospital Greater Noida*

[2] *Professor of Medicine, Sharda University Hospital, Greater Noida*

[3] *Senior Resident, Sharda University Hospital, Greater Noida*

CASE

A 31-year-old female patient, with history of end stage kidney disease due to chronic glomerulonephritis, underwent a one haplomatch, living related kidney transplant from her mother. Donor kidney was retrieved by laparoscopic surgery, which was uneventful. It had single artery and vein which were anastomosed end to side to external iliac artery and vein, respectively. She received no induction except for one gram of intravenous methylprednisolone just before the release of the vascular clamps. A standard ureterovesicular anastomosis was performed with a stent in situ. Graft functioned immediately with an intraoperative urine output of 800 millilitres (ml), followed by 700 ml/hour. Mild hematuria was noted in the urinary bag. In the following half hour there was absolute anuria. A bedside Doppler ultrasound showed an empty bladder with very good perfusion to the transplanted kidney. A decision for open exploration was taken. Exploration revealed a pink and turgid transplanted kidney with a good bruit in the main renal artery and good flow in the renal vein. In contrast, the ureter appeared dusky in its entire length. Upon release of ureteric anastomosis a clot was found in the entire length of the transplant ureter. Brisk urine output was noted following removal of the clot. Patient's serum creatinine decreased to 0.8 milligrams/decilitre (mg/dl) on postoperative day 3 with excellent urine output. Patient is currently on prednisolone, tacrolimus, and mycophenolate mofetil with excellent allograft function three years after transplant. A timely intervention saved the graft and avoided further unnecessary investigations including a renal biopsy.

What is Early Graft Dysfunction?

Kidney transplantation is the preferred mode of renal replacement therapy for end stage renal disease, with dramatic improvements in patient and graft survival over the last 50 years. In the modern era of immunosuppression, one year patient survival is close to 98%, and one-year allograft survival rates have improved to 90% for deceased donor kidney transplants and 95% for living donor kidney transplants with some inter-center variability. However, fluctuations in serum creatinine, which is the primary method for monitoring graft function, are frequent, particularly in the first year of transplantation.

Definition: Early Graft Dysfunction

A rise in serum creatinine of 15% or more above baseline defines allograft dysfunction. Urine output, especially in the first few days of transplantation, may also be monitored and a decline to levels of oliguria or anuria may also define early graft dysfunction.

What are the Causes of Sudden Anuria in Early Post Transplant Period?

These raises the possibility of hyperacute rejection, kinking of the renal artery, vascular thrombosis, urinary leak, or ureteric obstruction. Rarely tight closure of the abdomen may lead to sudden drop in urine output. Undetected calculi in the donor kidney obstructing the transplant ureter, after transplant, are known in deceased donor transplantation.

What is Hyperacute Rejection?

Hyperacute rejection is characterized by ischemia and necrosis of the graft that occurs from the time of transplant to 48 hours after transplant. It is believed to be caused by cytotoxic antibodies present in the recipient that respond to tissue antigens on the donor organ.

What are the Pathological Changes in Hyperacute Rejection?

Histologically, the fully developed cases are characterized by widespread glomerular capillary thrombosis and necrosis. Frequent areas of interstitial hemorrhage are noted. In early periods, the changes may be subtle and limited to endothelial reactivity with associated sparse polymorphonuclear infiltrates. A diffuse margination of neutrophils is seen throughout the peritubular and glomerular capillaries. The presence of five or more neutrophils present in any glomerulus is distinctly abnormal.

Immunofluorescence examination is a very helpful corroborative technique in establishing the diagnosis: immunoglobulin and complement deposits can be seen in the glomeruli, peritubular capillaries, and interlobular arteries. IgG present in serum permeating the interstitial compartment can give an annoying background in the tissue being examined. IgM and C3 staining is often present non-specifically in vessels affected by arteriosclerosis or hypertensive vasculopathy. Indeed IgG, IgM and C3 deposits within arterioles have been found in baseline kidney biopsies from healthy living related donors. In acute vascular rejection, linear deposits outlining individual cells are typical. Finally a negative immunofluorescence does not exclude vascular rejection.

What is the Clinical Presentation?

The manifestations of hyperacute rejection include general malaise and high fever.

Antibody mediated rejection of the kidney generally occurs hours to days after transplantation (hyperacute rejection), but may be delayed by several weeks if sensitization to donor antigens has occurred in the remote past (delayed accelerated acute rejection).

In the worst case scenario it begins immediately after perfusion of the allograft is established.

The transplanted kidney becomes grossly mottled and cyanotic. The capsule bulges out due to marked edema and rupture of the graft may occur. The transplanted kidney never functions, and the patient returns to dialysis.

Delayed cases of antibody mediated rejection present as an acute rise in the serum creatinine with or without graft tenderness.

How to Manage Hyperacute Rejection?

Plasmapheresis may be used to attempt to remove circulating antibodies from the blood. Antibody mediated rejection is frequently associated with graft loss. However early and less severely affected cases can be salvaged by increasing the dosage of cyclosporine/tacrolimus and administration of anti-lymphocyte antibodies. In highly presensitized cases with high levels of circulating antibodies plasmapheresis can be tried. In most transplant centers donor specific cross-matches are performed using peripheral blood lymphocytes. Such tests do not detect anti-endothelial antibodies, and this accounts for at least some cases of the antibody mediated rejection reported in lymphocyte crossmatch negative patients. However, usually hyperacute rejection is unresponsive to treatment and removal of the rejected organ is required.

When does Renal Artery/Vein Thrombosis Occur?

Thrombosis of renal vessels usually occurs in the first 48-72 hours and is one of the most devastating complications leading to graft loss.

What is the Incidence of Renal Vessel Thrombosis?

The reported incidence varies from 0.6-3.4% of transplants.

What are the Causes of Renal Vessel Thrombosis?

Thrombosis usually occurs as a result pre-existing hypercoagulable state, surgical technique, thrombocytosis or hyperacute rejection.

How does the Patient of Renal Artery Thrombosis Present Clinically?

- Renal artery thrombosis usually presents with oliguria or sudden anuria, rapidly increasing creatinine, graft swelling and pain over the allograft.
- Hyperkalemia, elevated serum LDH and thrombocytopenia may also seen.
- As rapidly increasing serum creatinine may be the only sign of thrombosis in patients with oliguria or anuria due to poor graft function due to reperfusion injury.

What are the Investigation Recommended for Renal Artery Thrombosis?

Renal imaging is important in these patients. Diagnosis is often made by use of duplex ultrasonography or isotope renal scan.

What are the Outcome of this Post Transplant Complication?

Transplant kidney does not have any collateral supply, so unless repaired emergently, thrombosis can result in graft loss requiring allograft nephrectomy. In some case reports, kidney allografts have been salvaged by emergent thrombectomy and use of fibrinolytic agents.

What is the Occurrence of Urinary Leak in Immediate Post Renal Transplantation?

Urine leak occurs in 1–10% of kidney transplants.

How the Patient Presents Clinically?

Clinical presentation depend on the location and degree of leak, DJ stenting and graft function.

1. Early extraperitoneal high-volume leak with good graft function may present with high output through

drains or wound, especially if DJ stent was selectively not used. Low urine output through the transurethral catheter and elevated serum creatinine owing to reabsorption may be perceived as DGF. Imaging may show perinephric collection with or without pelvicalyceal dilatation. High drain fluid creatinine and potassium compared with corresponding serum values confirm the leak. Often this presentation is owing to technical failure, anastomotic (most common), or bladder dehiscence, which may be confirmed on antegrade pyelogram or cystogram and requires surgical repair.

2. Early extraperitoneal small leak presents with persistent low output through the drains or wound, urinoma, graft site swelling, pain, and low urine output. Imaging may reveal a urinoma with or without pelvicalyceal dilatation and can be used for guidance for fluid aspiration and sampling. High fluid creatinine and potassium compared with serum confirm the leak and may be localized with CT pyelogram or scintigraphy. Such a presentation is often owing to downstream urinary obstruction (blocked transurethral catheter or DJ stent) and stabilizes with catheter change. Undrained urinomas may get infected, forming perinephric abscesses, requiring percutaneous or surgical drainage.
3. Late (1–2 weeks) leak after a transplant is often owing to ureteric necrosis presents insidiously with reduced urine output and requires surgical resection of the necrotic ureter and re-implantation.
4. **Intra-abdominal leaks:** Intra-abdominal leaks may present with acute abdomen, shock, prolonged ileus or insidiously and always requires surgical re-exploration.

How to Approach for Investigation of Suspected Urine Leak?

1. Drain/aspirate creatinine and potassium levels in comparison with serum.
2. Ultrasonography (most commonly used) for nature and size of perinephric collection and pelvicalyceal dilatation and Doppler for perfusion defects, and vascularity.
3. **Computed Tomography (CT)/MRI:** A non-contrast study for nature and size of perinephric collection and pelvicalyceal dilatation; contrast pyelogram may localize the leak; and an angiogram for graft vascularity, although uncommonly done with high creatinine. Very rarely, a migrated DJ stent may be seen with longer (> 20 cm) DJ stents or with their delayed (> 6 weeks) removal either incidentally or on investigation for presenting symptoms such as pain.
4. **Scintigraphy:** Focal tracer imaging using MAG3 or Tc99 may localize the leak, although not useful with DGF or ureteral stasis.

   Cystography: Retrograde contrast may demonstrate bladder or anastomotic dehiscence.
5. Antegrade pyelogram through a nephrostomy to accurately localize the leak, possible even with DGF, but is difficult without pelvicalyceal dilatation.

What is the Management Strategy for Urinary Leak?

Conservative management consists of maximal decompression by diversion from the leak, prevention of obstruction, and urinoma drainage to prevent infection and depends on the presence of the transurethral catheter and transanastomotic DJ stent.

The transurethral catheter is changed if blocked and removed after 2 weeks in high-risk cases.

If DJ stent is not present, it is placed either retrograde cystoscopically, which is technically challenging, or antegrade through a nephrostomy, which is more accessible and safer, although owing to lack of backpressure, fixation of nephrostomy tube may be difficult, warranting the expertise of an experienced radiologist or endo-urologist.

A blocked DJ stent can be changed cystoscopically over a guidewire. Conservative management is effective in approximately 60% of cases, especially for small, distal, late leaks.

Large-volume or proximal leaks not responding to conservative management require surgery with resection of the necrosed ureter and tension-free re-implantation of well-vascularized ureter over a DJ stent, closure of a perforated bladder, or others.

Reconstructing a short ureter may be challenging requiring anastomosis with the native ureter a bladder (Boari) flap, or ileal neo-ureter.

How Many Patients Develop Ureteral Obstruction?

Approximately 1%–4.5% of renal transplant recipients will develop ureteral obstruction at some time after surgery. Distal obstruction is most common.

What are the Causes of Ureteral Obstruction?

Ureteral devascularization leading to intrinsic stricture formation is the principle cause in nearly 90% of cases. Technical errors during the ureteroneocystostomy, extrinsic compression (e.g., hematoma, lymphocele, abscess), kinking of a redundant ureter, collecting system hematoma, a stone transplanted with the kidney, and anastomotic edema can be causes of obstruction during the early postoperative (< 3 months) period.

What are Predictors of Ureteral Obstruction Following Transplantation?

Allografts with more than two renal arteries and from donors older than 65 years of age are at increased risk.

Prolonged ischemia time and ureteroneocystostomy without ureteral stent placement have also been correlated with stricture formation.

What is the Clinical Presentation of Ureteral Obstruction?

Recipients typically present with an asymptomatic decline in renal function and a decrease in urine output. Less commonly, patients will complain of a dull ache or feeling of fullness over the allograft due to irritation of adjacent peritoneum.

Which Investigations are Recommended for the Diagnosis of Ureteral Obstruction?

Renal ultrasonography (US) is an excellent study to screen for hydroureteronephrosis.

If present, computed tomography (CT) should be considered, especially in the early postoperative period, because of its ability to identify both intrinsic (e.g., ureteral calculus) and extrinsic (e.g., lymphocele, hematoma) sources of obstruction.

Collecting system dilation without a clear etiology should prompt a nuclear medicine scan with furosemide washout to confirm the presence of obstruction (Tip: be certain the bladder is empty during the study). Hydroureteronephrosis without blockage is concerning for VUR and a voiding cystourethrogram (VCUG) should be done.

What are the Treatment Modalities?

Decompression of the collecting system to minimize allograft injury is the initial priority in recipients with ureteral obstruction. Both ureteral stent and nephrostomy tube placement are options.

Following decompression, the cause of obstruction must be fully characterized unless it is obvious. Obstruction from blood clots within the collecting system and edema of the ureteroneocystostomy will resolve with conservative management.

Nephrostomy tube drainage is continued until the patient's hematuria has resolved. The nephrostomy tube is then capped and removed 48 to 72 hours later if the urine output remains appropriate and there is no decline in renal function. A similar strategy may be employed for obstruction due to anastomotic edema.

Fluid collections that cause extrinsic ureteral obstruction should be drained percutaneously. The aspirate is sent for cell count, gram stain, culture, and creatinine determination.

Small lymphoceles may resolve following percutaneous drainage but conservative management fails in over 50% of recipients. Improved success rates following sclerosis of the lymphocele cavity with doxycycline, ethanol, povidone-iodine, bleomycin, talc and fibrin glue have been reported, but periureteral fibrosis is a potential risk. Persistent or recurrent lymphoceles are treated with either laparoscopic or open unroofing into the peritoneal cavity. Success rates with both techniques exceed 88%. However, laparoscopic drainage is usually not feasible for lymphoceles lateral to the renal allograft.

What is the Percentage of Acute Tubular Necrosis (ATN) in Post Renal Transplant?

Post transplant acute tubular necrosis (ATN) is responsible for approximately 90% of acute renal failure episodes occurring within the first few weeks following renal transplantation.

This phenomenon is observed in 34% of cadaver transplant recipients and 9% of those with live donor kidneys.

What is the Cause of Acute Tubular Necrosis?

Although the exact cause of post transplant ATN remains unknown, the following factors are thought to be associated with a higher incidence of ATN: (1) Donor hypotension, (2) Prolonged "warm ischemia time", (3) Increased vascular resistance with poor perfusate flow, (4) Presence of "ligandin" or excess lactate in the renal perfusate, (5) Reduced allograft blood flow, (6) Cold lymphocytotoxins in the patient's serum, and (7) Administration of nephrotoxic drugs particularly to the hypovolemic graft recipients.

Therapeutic maneuvers such as hydration of the donors and recipients, harvesting the kidneys from heart beating cadavers, donor pretreatment with massive doses of corticosteroids and alpha-adrenergic blocking agents and warming of the graft immediately after vascular anastomosis, seem to reduce the incidence of ATN.

What are the Differential Diagnosis?

Since the management differs significantly, post transplant ATN has to be distinguished from other causes of acute renal failure such as the renal artery thrombosis, hyperacute rejection and obstruction of the urinary tract.

What are the Tests Required?

The tests which are of use in the differential diagnosis include, 131-I Hippuran renogram, transplant ultrasound, renal angiogram, retrograde pyelogram and renal transplant biopsy.

Patients with established ATN should undergo every other day dialysis, under low dose or regional heparinization, until the creatinine clearance improves to 20 ml/min. Even though there are short-term disadvantages, the post transplant ATN does not appear to exert any detrimental effects in the long run. However, this issue remains controversial in the published reports.

Suggested Reading

1. A Srivastava, J Kumar, S Sharma, MS Ansari and R Kapoor, "Vascular complication in live related renal transplant: An experience of 1945 cases", Indian Journal of Urology 2013;Vol 29,No. 1,42-47.
2. JM Peter and JK Stuart, Kidney Transplantation Principles and Practice, Saunders Elsevier, Philadelphia, Pa, USA, 7th edition, 2014.
3. Porter KA. Renal transplantation. In: Pathology of the Kidney Ed. RH Heptinstall. Little Brown and Co. Boston 1992;1799-1934.
4. Hamouda M, Sharma A, Halawa A. Urine leak after kidney transplant: A review of the literature. Exp Clin Transplant 2018;16:90-95.
5. Streeter EH, Little DM, Cranston DW, Morris PJ. The urological complications of renal transplantation: A series of 1535 patients. BJU Int 2002;90:627-34.
6. Lempinen J, Stenman J, Kyllonen L, Salmela K. Surgical complications following 1670 consecutive adult renal transplantations: A single center study. Scand J Surg 2015; 104:254-59.
7. Singer J, Gritsch HA, Rosenthal JT. The transplant operation and its surgical complications. In: Danovitch GM, ed. Handbook of kidney transplantation, 5th ed. Philadelphia, PA: Lippincott Williams and Wilkins 2005. 193-212.
8. Neri F, Tsivian M, Coccolini F, Bertelli R, Cavallari G, Nardo B *et al.* Urological complications after kidney transplantation: Experience of more than 1,000 transplantations. Transplant Proc 2009;41:1224-26.

CHAPTER

34 A Renal Transplant Patient with Thrombotic Microangiopathy

Pranaw Kumar Jha

Senior Consultant, Division of Nephrology and Renal Transplant Medicine, Medanta Institute of Kidney and Urology, Gurugram

CASE

Ms SM, 23 years old female, with no previous comorbidities, was admitted with accelerated hypertension. On evaluation, she was found to have deranged renal function (serum creatinine of 4 mg/dl). Further evaluation showed bilaterally small kidneys. Over the next five months she progressed to end stage renal disease. After discussion about various renal replacement therapy options she opted for renal transplant with her mother as the prospective donor. After routine evaluation of the recipient and donor, complement dependent cytotoxicity and flow cytometry crossmatch was done which was negative. Renal transplant was done. Immunosuppression consisted of antithymocyte globulin as induction and tacrolimus, mycophenolate, prednisolone as maintenance immunosuppression. She had brisk diuresis in immediately post transplant. Serum creatinine reduced to a nadir of 0.9 mg/dl by post-operative day (POD) 5. She was discharged on POD7 with serum creatinine of 1.1 mg/dl. During outpatient department follow-up, on POD20 her serum creatinine increased to 1.4 mg/dl and further to 1.6 mg/dl on POD22. Tacrolimus level was 14 ng/ml. Tacrolimus dose was reduced. But her serum creatinine increased to 1.7 mg/dl on POD25 with a repeat Tacrolimus level of 10 ng/ml. Hemoglobin, which was 10 g/dl on POD2, reduced to 7.5 and she developed thrombocytopenia (platelet count dropped from 1.75 to 1.2 lakh/cu mm). Renal transplant ultrasound and doppler was normal. Peripheral smear showed schistocytes with increased reticulocytes and LDH was 780 IU/l. Graft renal biopsy showed capillary thrombi in glomeruli but no evidence of rejection. C4d was negative in peritubular capillaries. There was subendothelial swelling and features of acute tubular injury. Single antigen bead testing was done which did not show any anti-human leucocyte antigen antibody. Tacrolimus was withheld and the dose of prednisolone was increased. She received total five sessions of alternate day plasma exchanges. Serum creatinine reduced to 1.3 mg/dl. Hb also improved to 8.5 g/dl and platelets increased to 1.68 lakh/cu mm. LDH reduced to 150 IU/l. Meanwhile, genetic mutation analysis for complement pathway proteins was negative. Cyclosporine was added with close monitoring of Hb, platelets and serum creatinine over next few days. Serum creatinine remained stable and there were no further episodes of hemolysis.

What is Thrombotic Microangiopathy?

Thrombotic microangiopathy (TMA) is a pathological description. Clinically it presents as microangiopathic hemolytic anemia, thrombocytopenia and organ injury. It can involve kidneys leading to acute kidney injury that can progress to end stage renal disease if timely supportive and specific management is not initiated. Significant advances have been made in the understanding of TMA pathogenesis, which has enabled development of specific targeted therapy.

How to Classify Thrombotic Microangiopathy?

Traditionally TMA has been classified as thrombotic thrombocytopenic purpura (TTP) or hemolytic uremic syndrome (HUS) based on the clinical picture. The classification has evolved over years. Although there is an overlap, Figure 34.1 gives the current classification of TMA.[1] HUS is the one, which involves the kidneys commonly. TTP is commoner in adults, has a female preponderance, more neurologic manifestations, more severe thrombocytopenia and lesser incidence of acute kidney injury (AKI).

Classification of Thrombotic Microangiopathy

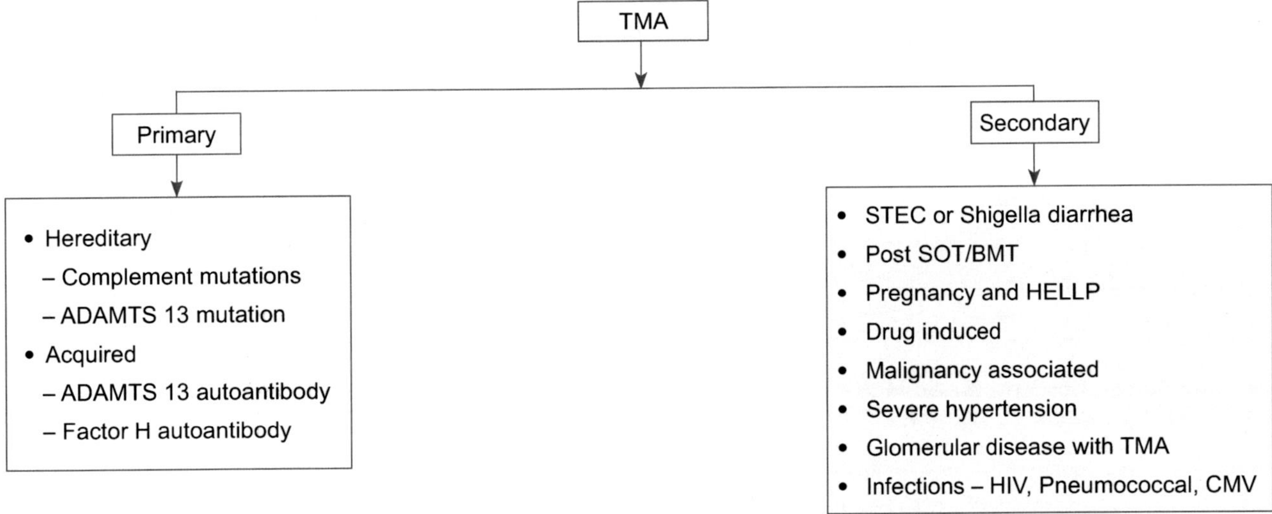

Figure 34.1: Classification of Thrombotic microangiopathy

TMA: Thrombotic microangiopathy; ADAMTS13: A disintegrin and metalloproteinase with a thrombospondin type 1 motif, member 13; STEC: Shiga toxin-producing Escherichia coli; SOT: Solid organ transplant; BMT: Bone marrow transplant; HELLP: Hemolysis, elevated liver enzymes, low platelet; HIV: Human immunodeficiency virus; CMV: Cytomegalovirus

What is Pathophysiology of Thrombotic Microangiopathy?

Complement activation as a line of defense against microbes occurs by classical, lectin and alternative pathways. While the binding of complements to immune complexes or microorganism activates the classical pathway, the lectin pathway is activated by binding of mannose binding lectin (MBL) to pathogen cell surface carbohydrates. The alternative pathway activation is antibody independent.

Alternative pathway is in a continuous state of activation at low level and works as a positive feedback (the amplification loop). The presence of complement regulatory proteins in plasma and on host cell regulates it and it is the lack of this regulation that leads to alternative pathway activation and amplification on microbial agents leading to its destruction (Fig. 34.2). Defect in these regulators or the components of alternative pathway can lead to complement dysregulation. This dysregulation occurs mainly on the surface of endothelial cells.[2]

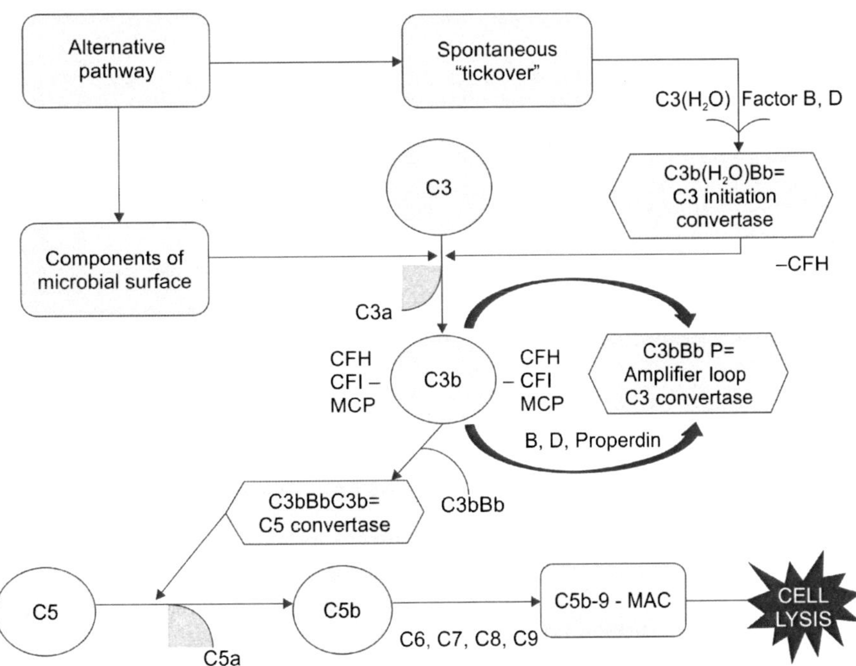

Figure 34.2: Alternative complement pathways

CFH: Complement factor H; CFI: Complement factor I; MCP: Membrane cofactor protein; MAC: Membrane attack complex.

Loss of function mutation of regulator (such as FH, FI, CD46) encoding genes or activating mutation of factor B, C3 are associated with hereditary atypical HUS. But mutations are not always causative but rather predisposing with incomplete penetrance. In acquired atypical HUS anti-FH autoantibody may be seen.

TTP occurs due to a disintegrin and metalloproteinase with a thrombospondin type 1 motif, member 13 (ADAMTS13) deficiency due to ADAMTS13 gene mutation or the presence of autoantibody. This leads to formation of unusually large vWF multimers and platelet aggregation.

What are Causes of Thrombotic Microangiopathy in Post-Renal Transplant Patients?

TMA in renal transplant may be caused due to similar factors as in a non-transplant recipient as well as factors limited to renal transplant recipients such as drugs calcineurin inhibitors (CNI), mammalian target of rapamycin (mTOR) inhibitors, antibody mediated rejection etc. Renal transplant associated TMA can be divided into recurrent or de novo disease. The rate of recurrence in patients having TMA as the primary cause of ESRD undergoing renal transplant, is 25-50%.[3,4] Recurrent disease is usually seen in patients with TMA due to a complement defect. Patients with non-complement mediated disease rarely recur post transplant. De novo disease may be due to factors commonly seen in general population or may be transplant specific (Fig. 34.3).

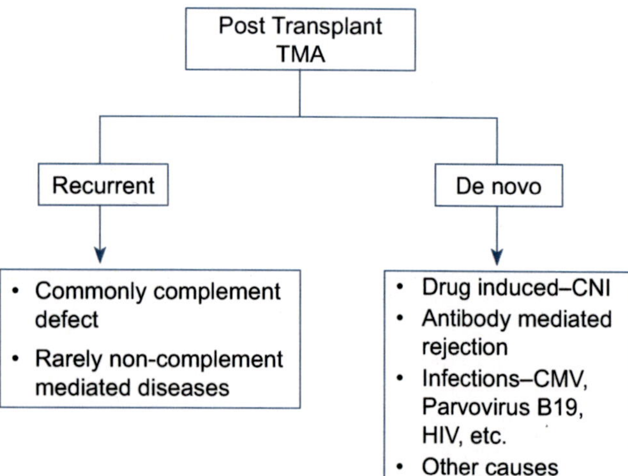

Figure 34.3: TMA in renal transplant recipients
TMA: Thrombotic microangiopathy; CNI: Calcineurin inhibitors; CMV: Cytomegalovirus; HIV: Human immunodeficiency virus.

What are Clinical Features and Laboratory Findings of Microangiopathy?

TMA usually presents within one year post transplant. Many a times it can present as early as within few days to weeks. Although presentation can be anytime in the post transplant period.

Thrombotic microangiopathy presents clinically as microangiopathic hemolytic anemia with thrombocytopenia and graft dysfunction. Blood tests reveal evidence of hemolysis such as increased reticulocyte count, schistocytes on peripheral smear and raised lactate dehydrogenase with reduction in hemoglobin. Platelet count is low. Serum creatinine and blood urea nitrogen is increased and urine analysis may show hematuria and minimal proteinuria. In 30% of the cases TMA is localized to the graft and the classical findings of thrombocytopenia and hemolysis are absent. The diagnosis in such cases is by a graft biopsy.

What are Renal Biopsy Findings in Thrombotic Microangiopathy?

Renal biopsy in a case of TMA reveals thrombosis in glomeruli and arterioles, endothelial cell swelling and detachment from basement membrane, intracapillary erythrocytes and fragments. Glomeruli ischemia progressing to typical onion-skin changes of arteriolar wall may be seen. In chronic lesions double contouring of basement membrane can be seen. Depending upon the etiology other features may be seen such as proximal tubular vacuolization indicating calcineurin toxicity, although this is not specific. In cases of TMA accompanying acute humoral rejection, peritubular capillaritis and C4d staining of peritubular capillaries may be seen (Figs. 34.4a and b).

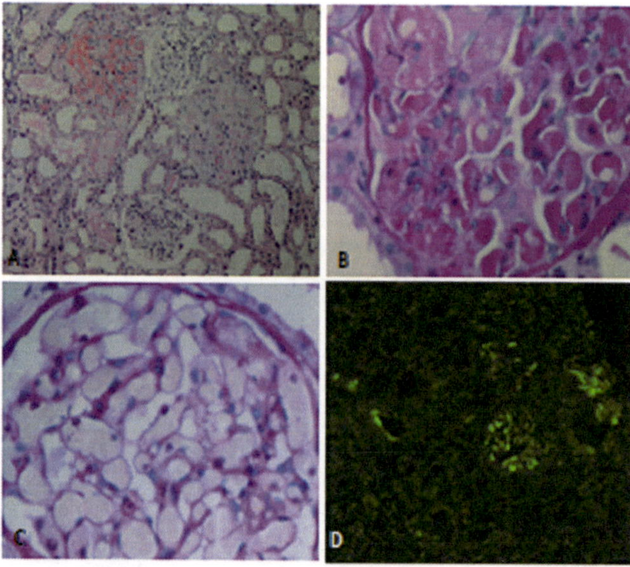

Figure 34.4a: Photomicrograph panel show CNI induced thrombotic microangiopathy. (A) Low power magnification show presence of thrombi within glomerular capillary loops. (B) High power magnification highlights these fibrin thrombi. (C) Image showing mesangiolysis with glomerular capillary loop dilatation and congestion. (D) C4d is negative in peritubular capillaries. Glomerular mesangial C4d staining act as a positive control

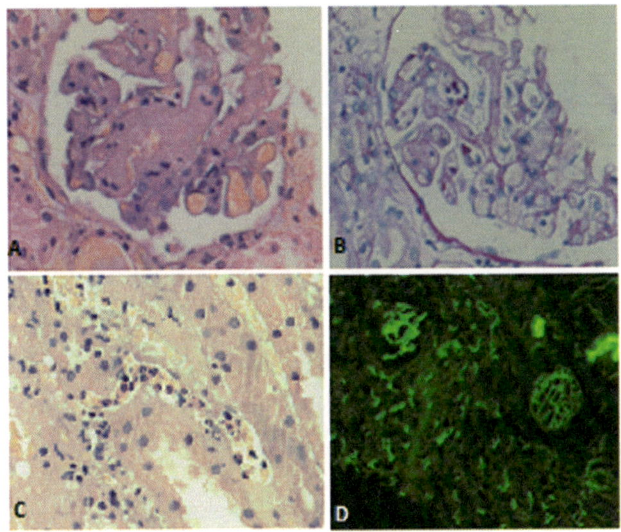

Figure 34.4b: Photomicrograph panel show antibody-mediated rejection with thrombotic microangiopathy. (A) High power magnification show fibrin thrombi within glomerular capillary loops. (B) Along with evidence of neutrophilic glomerulitis. (C) Majority of the peritubular capillaries show severe peritubular capillaritis. (D) C4d is diffusely positive in peritubular capillaries

What is the Risk of Recurrence of Thrombotic Microangiopathy Post-Transplant?

The incidence of post transplant recurrent TMA has been reported to range from 4 to 60% in the literature. This huge variability can be explained by the fact that difference in recurrence rates depend upon the cause of TMA leading to ESRD. In those with TMA associated with diarrheal prodrome the chances of recurrence are very low while in those with atypical HUS the chances of recurrence are as high as 60% with almost 90% graft failure rate.[5]

The recurrence risk and graft outcome also depends upon the type of complement abnormalities. High risk mutations include complement factor H (CFH), complement factor I (CFI), C3, complement factor B (CFB). These mutations lead to abnormalities in complement proteins produced by liver. Despite the kidney transplant these abnormalities persist, thereby causing recurrence rate as high as 92% depending upon the type of mutation.[6] Low risk mutations include membrane cofactor protein (MCP) and thrombomodulin (THBD) mutations. Recurrence rate for cases with MCP gene mutation has been reported to be about 15-20%.[7] The low rate of recurrence may be due to the fact that MCP is highly expressed in the kidneys and the graft kidney has normal MCP. Outcomes have been reported to be better with anti-CFH autoantibodies as well. Recurrence rate is difficult to quantify in those with rare cases of combined mutations. Table 34.1 shows the post transplant recurrence frequency for various genetic mutations.[8]

Table 34.1: HUS recurrence risk post transplant according to genetic mutation

Genetic mutation	Recurrence risk post transplant
CFH	70-80%
CFI	70-80%
CFB	100%
C3	40%
MCP	15-20%
THBD	Low
Anti-CFH antibodies	40-70%
Combined mutations	Variable

CFH: Complement factor H; CFI: Complement factor I; CFB: Complement factor B; MCP: Membrane cofactor protein; THBD: Thrombomodulin.

Various other risk factors for recurrence include living related donor, use of CNI (especially cyclosporine) and adult recipients.

Time to recurrence has been variably reported to range from initial few days upto 2 years post transplant. Almost 60% of them recur in the first month. There may be few triggers, which increase the recurrence risk such as infections, rejections etc. This occurs due to endothelial injury, inflammation and complement activation.

What is Risk of De Novo Thrombotic Microangiopathy in Post-Transplant?

As per the published literature incidence of de novo TMA is 4-14%.[9] Apart from all the causes of TMA in general population there are etiologies unique to transplant recipients. The three most important causes being drugs, infections and humoral rejection.

Drug induced TMA have been reported with mainly CNIs although even mTOR inhibitors have been associated with TMA. TMA incidence has been found to be higher in those treated with cyclosporine vs. tacrolimus (4-15% vs. 1%).[2,6,10] CNIs cause endothelial damage and vasoconstriction. They also have prothrombotic and antifibrinolytic actions. The combined result is TMA. mTORi traditionally were not considered as a risk factor but de novo TMA have been reported with mTORi as well.[11] Switching from one medication to the other has been shown to help in TMA resolution and improvement of the graft function.

Infections such as HIV, CMV, parvovirus B_{19} have been reported to cause TMA. Other important cause being antibody mediated rejection (AMR) where the TMA also accompanies other features of AMR such as glomerulitis, peritubular (PTC) capillaritis and C4d staining in PTCs in renal biopsy.

How to Manage Post Transplant Thrombotic Microangiopathy?

Pretransplant Evaluation and Donor Choice

All the patients with TMA as the recognized cause of ESRD should undergo TMA genetic mutation screening. It may not be required in case of Shiga toxin-producing Escherichia coli (STEC) associated diarrheal HUS but one needs to be careful as many patients with atypical HUS may also have diarrheal prodrome. Patients should be counseled about high chances of disease recurrence and living related donors should be avoided. This is important as these donors might carry similar genetic mutation and are at high risk of getting TMA due to the nephrectomy surgery. Such transplants also have high risk of recurrence.

Prophylactic Strategies

Strategies to prevent the recurrence of HUS in patients with pretransplant disease include:

- Eculizumab–Eculizumab has revolutionized the treatment of TMA and has been used as a prophylactic therapy in patients undergoing renal transplant to prevent recurrence.[12] Availability of the drug and cost is an important concern though as the drug has to be continued lifelong. Following protocols have been used.
  - For deceased donor–900 mg IV on postoperative day 3 followed by weekly three doses and then 1200 mg every two weeks thereafter.
  - For living unrelated–900 mg intravenous 24 hours pretransplant and then followed by on days 7, 14, 21 post transplant. After this it is given every 2 weeks post transplant lifelong.
  - Other protocols – In few protocols eculizumab is repeated within 24 hours of first dose. Then 900 mg of Eculizumab is given for 3 weeks. A next dose of 1200 mg is given after one week. After this 1200 mg dose is continued once in 2 weeks.
- Simultaneous kidney and liver transplantation combined with plasma-exchange preoperatively and plasma infusion intraoperatively along with post-transplant anticoagulation has been used.[13]
- Kidney alone transplant along with intensive plasma-exchange starting just before surgery and then daily for at least one week followed by tapering to once a week schedule which is maintained life-long has been used. But there may be recurrence despite the prophylaxis.[14-16]

Treatment of Thrombotic Microangiopathy

One of the first steps in treating post transplant TMA patients is to remove the most common offending drugs, which is commonly CNI or mTOR inhibitor.[17] Antimetabolites and prednisolone is continued. Switching from one CNI to the other has been shown to work. This is usually not enough and further treatment is needed.

Eculizumab is the drug of choice in patients with recurrent HUS. It is administered IV in dose of 900 mg weekly for four weeks and then 1200 mg once in two weeks thereafter.[18-20] The optimal duration of treatment is unknown and usually it is continued indefinitely. The major drawback with eculizumab is its prohibitive cost and unavailability in many countries.

While administering eculizumab, the disease response is monitored by hemoglobin, LDH and platelet count. Hemolytic complement CH50 is also monitored prior to Eculizumab for first 4 doses, targeting CH50 < 10%.

In resource constraint settings where eculizumab is unavailable or where TMA is persistent despite eculizumab administration, plasmapheresis or plasma infusion is given (1.5 volume of fresh frozen plasma) every 48 hours. This may be tapered to weekly therapy.[21,22]

In patients with de novo HUS, the CNI/mTOR inhibitor is stopped. In case of progressive disease, plasmapheresis is done.[9] In patients refractory to plasmapheresis, eculizumab is given in schedule as mentioned above. As these patients have not undergone a genetic analysis pre-transplant, a genetic testing for complement mediated HUS should be done. Those with pathogenic mutation require lifelong treatment while in those without any mutations and having a clear precipitating event, it may be stopped cautiously while monitoring for recurrence of disease.

Management of post transplant TMA is shown in Figure 34.5.

Overall outcome is poor, more so with the recurrent rather than the de novo disease although availability of eculizumab has significantly improved the outcome.

Concluding, recurrent TMA is an important cause of graft loss in renal transplant recipient. Timely diagnosis and intervention is important for preserving the graft function. The outcome depends upon the cause of TMA and those with genetic mutations have worse outcome. Eculizumab has revolutionized the treatment of TMA but cost and availability of this drug remains an important issue.

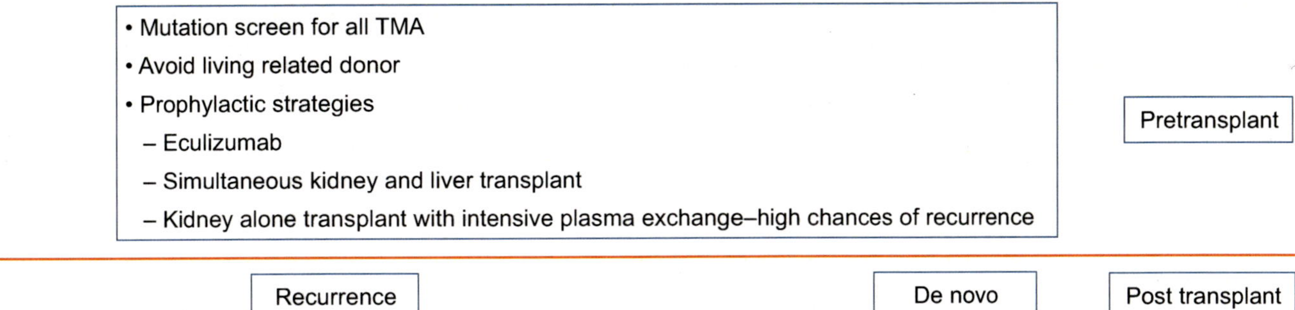

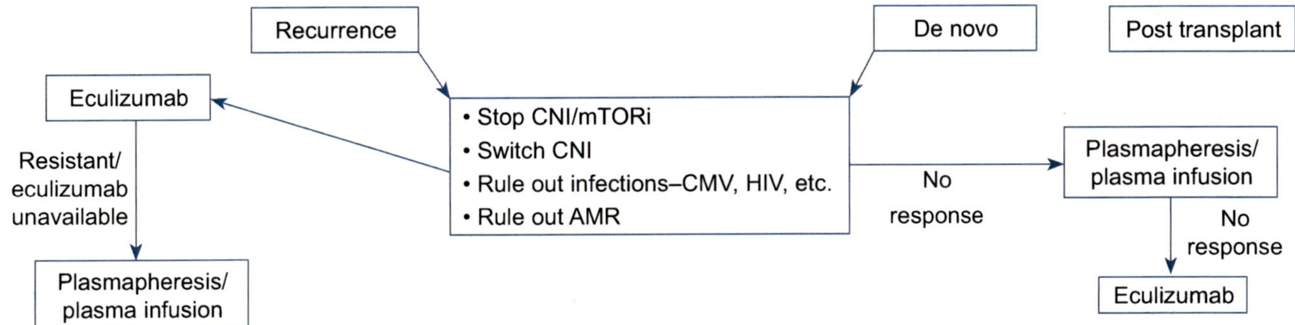

Figure 34.5: Management of post transplant thrombotic microangiopathy

Key Points

- Thrombotic microangiopathy is characterized by features of hemolysis, thrombocytopenia and renal dysfunction.
- TMA patients undergoing renal transplant have high chances of recurrence, specially those with complement genetic mutations.
- Post transplant TMA can be recurrent or de novo and can present with classical features of TMA or only graft dysfunction.
- All patients with TMA as the cause of ESRD should undergo genetic mutation screening.
- Living unrelated or deceased donor rather than living related donor should be preferred for transplantation.
- Prophylactic Eculizumab is advocated for patients with genetic mutation or dysfunction of CFH or CFI.
- Patients with post transplant recurrent TMA require cessation of CNI, ruling out infections and administration of eculizumab and/or plasmapheresis.
- Patients with post transplant de novo TMA require cessation of CNI, ruling out infections and performing plasmapheresis in cases not responding to drug cessation. Eculizumab is given in cases resistant to plasmapheresis.

Acknowledgements

The author would like to thank Dr Rajan Duggal (Associate Director, HOD Histopathology and Cytopathology, BLK Super Speciality Hospital, New Delhi) for providing the photographs of TMA in renal transplant.

References

1. Brocklebank V, Wood KM, Kavanagh D. Thrombotic Microangiopathy and the Kidney. Clin J Am Soc Nephrol 2018;13(2):300-17.
2. Noris M, Remuzzi G. Atypical hemolytic-uremic syndrome. N Engl J Med 2009;361(17):1676-87.
3. Agarwal A, Mauer SM, Matas AJ, Nath KA. Recurrent hemolytic uremic syndrome in an adult renal allograft recipient: Current concepts and management. J Am Soc Nephrol 1995;6(4):1160-69.
4. Artz MA, Steenbergen EJ, Hoitsma AJ, Monnens LA, Wetzels JF. Renal transplantation in patients with hemolytic uremic syndrome: High rate of recurrence and increased incidence of acute rejections. Transplantation 2003;76(5):821-26.
5. Bresin E, Daina E, Noris M, *et al.* Outcome of renal transplantation in patients with non-Shiga toxin-associated hemolytic uremic syndrome: Prognostic significance of genetic background. Clin J Am Soc Nephrol 2006;1(1):88-99.
6. Noris M, Remuzzi G. Thrombotic microangiopathy after kidney transplantation. Am J Transplant 2010;10(7):1517-23.
7. Zuber J, Le Quintrec M, Sberro-Soussan R, *et al.* New insights into postrenal transplant hemolytic uremic syndrome. Nat Rev Nephrol 2011;7(1):23-35.
8. Alasfar S, Alachkar N. Atypical hemolytic uremic syndrome post-kidney transplantation: Two case reports and review of the literature. Front Med (Lausanne) 2014;1:52.
9. Karthikeyan V, Parasuraman R, Shah V, Vera E, Venkat KK. Outcome of plasma exchange therapy in thrombotic microangiopathy after renal transplantation. Am J Transplant 2003;3(10):1289-94.
10. Zarifian A, Meleg-Smith S, O'Donovan R, Tesi RJ, Batuman V. Cyclosporine-associated thrombotic microangiopathy in renal allografts. Kidney Int 1999;55(6):2457-66.
11. Reynolds JC, Agodoa LY, Yuan CM, Abbott KC. Thrombotic microangiopathy after renal transplantation in the United States. Am J Kidney Dis 2003;42(5):1058-68.
12. Zimmerhackl LB, Hofer J, Cortina G, *et al.* Prophylactic eculizumab after renal transplantation in atypical hemolytic-uremic syndrome. N Engl J Med 2010;362(18):1746-48.
13. Saland J. Liver-kidney transplantation to cure atypical HUS: Still an option post-eculizumab? Pediatr Nephrol 2014;29(3):329-32.

14. Hirt-Minkowski P, Schaub S, Mayr M, *et al.* Haemolytic uraemic syndrome caused by factor H mutation: Is single kidney transplantation under intensive plasmatherapy an option? Nephrol Dial Transplant 2009;24(11):3548-51.
15. Davin JC, Strain L, Goodship TH. Plasma therapy in atypical haemolytic uremic syndrome: Lessons from a family with a factor H mutation. Pediatr Nephrol 2008;23(9):1517-21.
16. Kwon T, Dragon-Durey MA, Macher MA, *et al.* Successful pre-transplant management of a patient with anti-factor H autoantibodies-associated haemolytic uraemic syndrome. Nephrol Dial Transplant 2008;23(6):2088-90.
17. Bren A, Pajek J, Grego K, *et al.* Follow-up of kidney graft recipients with cyclosporine-associated hemolytic-uremic syndrome and thrombotic microangiopathy. Transplant Proc 2005;37(4):1889-91.
18. Zuber J, Le Quintrec M, Krid S, *et al.* Eculizumab for atypical hemolytic uremic syndrome recurrence in renal transplantation. Am J Transplant 2012;12(12):3337-54.
19. Greenbaum LA, Fila M, Ardissino G, *et al.* Eculizumab is a safe and effective treatment in pediatric patients with atypical hemolytic uremic syndrome. Kidney Int 2016;89(3):701-11.
20. Fakhouri F, Hourmant M, Campistol JM, *et al.* Terminal Complement Inhibitor Eculizumab in Adult Patients With Atypical Hemolytic Uremic Syndrome: A Single-Arm, Open-Label Trial. Am J Kidney Dis 2016;68(1):84-93.
21. Le Quintrec M, Zuber J, Moulin B, *et al.* Complement genes strongly predict recurrence and graft outcome in adult renal transplant recipients with atypical hemolytic and uremic syndrome. Am J Transplant 2013;13(3):663-75.
22. Noris M, Remuzzi G. Managing and preventing atypical hemolytic uremic syndrome recurrence after kidney transplantation. Curr Opin Nephrol Hypertens 2013;22(6):704-12.

CHAPTER

35 A Renal Transplant Patient with Post Transplant Proteinuria

Umapati Hegde

Vice Chairman, Department of Nephrology, Muljibhai Patel Urological Hospital Nadiad, Gujarat

With the understanding of immunology and introduction of new immunosuppressant medications has led to an improvement in short- and medium-term graft survival. Proteinuria is a common problem post renal transplant, which may account for 7.5% to 45% depending on the definition.[1] Proteinuria from the native kidney after transplant reduces over 3-5 weeks. New onset and persistent proteinuria is associated with poor long-term outcome. The causes of proteinuria may be the same as general population and specific to renal transplant.

How to Measure/Quantify Proteinuria?

Quantification of proteinuria is a standard practice and upper limit of normal proteinuria in general population is 150 mg/day and of albuminuria is 30 mg/day. 24 hours collection of urine is the gold standard for measurement of proteinuria. As 24 hours collection is cumbersome and prone to collection errors, spot protein measurements corrected for creatinine excretion such as urine protein creatinine ratio (UPCR) or urine albumin protein creatinine ratio (UACR) are more commonly used. Although UPCR correlates to 24 hours proteinuria, UPCR may underestimate or overestimate protein excretion and hence it is recommended to collect 24 hours proteinuria before major decision such as graft biopsy.

What is the Prevalence of Proteinuria?

Proteinuria is common in renal transplant population as in the non-transplant chronic kidney disease population. Prevalence of proteinuria varies depending on the threshold used. If the cut of proteinuria is 150 mg/day (general population) then the prevalence is 45%. If the proteinuria of > 1 gm/day is considered to be significant, then the prevalence of proteinuria is 7.5-40%[1] with average of 19%. Nephrotic range proteinuria after renal transplant is about 13%. Urinary protein excretion greater than 300-500 mg/24 hours for at least 3-6 months should be considered significant and proteinuria value to be above 1000 mg/24 hours needs urgent evaluation.

Types of Proteinuria

Proteinuria may be caused by a defective tubular reabsorption of small proteins or by abnormalities of the glomerular barrier shown in Table 35.1.

Table 35.1: Glomerular vs Tubular proteinuria

	Tubular proteinuria	Glomerular proteinuria
Definition	Urinary exceretion >150 mg/24 hours of low molecular weight (<60 kDa) proteins	Urinary loss of proteins with molecular weight exceeding 60 kDa
Etiopathogenesis	Excessive production of small proteins exceeding the reabsorption capacity of proximal tubular cells (multiple myeloma, tumorlysis, leukemia etc.)	Primary or secondary glomerular diseases that alter the morphology and function of the actin cytoskeleton of podocytes and foot processes eventually leading to a reduced permselectivity and increased passage of proteins into the tubular lumen. The size of filtered proteins may indicate the degree of permselectivity loss (albumin 68 kDa, immunoglobin G 150 kDa)
Causes	**Congenital proximal tubular defects:** Fanconi syndrome, renal tubular acidosis **Acquired proximal tubular defects:** Ischemia-reperfusion-injury Acute kidney injury, Acute rejection, Aminoglycoside toxicity, Antiviral drugs, CNI toxicty, mTOR inhibitors	Recurrent glomerular diseases De novo glomerular or systemic diseases Transplant glomerulopathy Chronic rejection Calcineurin inhibitors, mTOR inhibitors Obesity Arterial hypertenion Hepatitis C or B

Tubular proteinuria may result from a huge excretion of low molecular weight proteins that pass through the glomerular barrier and exceed the reabsorption capacity of proximal tubular cells.

Glomerular proteinuria is usually consequent to podocyte injury, frequently caused by immunological, toxic, or microbial injuries may directly alter the actin cytoskeleton leading to foot processes effacement, slit diaphragm disruption, loss of selective permeability and passage of proteins in the tubular lumen. The severity and reversibility of proteinuria largely depends on the nature of the injury and the treatment.

Source of Proteinuria: Native or Graft Kidney

The proteinuria post renal transplant may be due to the native kidney or from the graft kidney. If the transplant recipient had good urine output pretransplant, quantification of proteinuria helps to differentiate the proteinuria from the native or from the graft. D'Cunha PT *et al.*[2] showed that proteinuria normalized in all patients to a value of 0.2 UPCR from average UPCR 2.9 (0.5-9.2 PCR) by 10 weeks after transplantation (average time to normalization 4.5 weeks). This shows that native kidney proteinuria usually resolves within the first month after transplantation and persistent of proteinuria or increasing amounts of proteinuria should be assumed to be from the renal transplant.

Risk Factors and Causes for Proteinuria

There are several risk factors for proteinuria post transplant. Amer *et al.*[3] noticed that systolic and diastolic blood pressure, serum creatinine, female donor, male recipient, and acute rejection episodes were found to be risk factors for post transplant proteinuria. Patients with acute rejection were found to have greater levels of proteinuria. Sancho-Calabuig *et al.*[4] found older donor age, greater HLA mismatch, tacrolimus use, anti-hypertensive use, and delayed graft function were considered as also risk factors for new onset proteinuria (Tables 35.2 and 35.3).

Table 35.2: Etiology of proteinuria post renal transplant

1. Residual proteinuria from native kidneys
2. Glomerular disease in the graft
   a. Recurrent glomerular diseases
   b. De Novo glomerular diseases
   c. Effects of anti-HLA class II antibodies
   d. Post transplant glomerular disease
3. Interstitial fibrosis and tubular atrophy of the graft (post transplant chronic nephropathy)
4. Effect of m-TOR inhibitor drugs: Everolimus/Sirolimus

Table 35.3: Risk factors for recurrence for primary glomerular disease

Glomerular disease	High risk of recurrence
FSGS	Second transplant after loss from recurrence Childhood Rapid progression to uraemia < 3 years Mesangial proliferation in the original disease Living donation White race Elderly donor
IgA nephropathy	Younger patients Specific HLA genotypes Zero mismatch kidneys High serum IgA levels Choice of induction therapy and Duration of follow-up after transplant
Membranous GN	Male sex Rapid course of initial disease High PLA2R antibody and LRD kidneys
MPGN	HLA-B8DR3 LRD and Previous graft loss due to MPGN Hepatitis C virus (HCV) infection Genetic abnormality in alternate complement pathway

FSGS: Focal segmental glomerulosclerosis; MPGN: Membrano proliferative GN.

CASE 1

24 years old male started developing oedema feet for 3 months at the age of 21 years, underwent renal biopsy which showed minimal change disease (MCD). He was given steroids initially partially responded but had become steroid-non-responsive over 1-1.5 years. His repeat biopsy revealed focal segmental glomerulosclerosis (FSGS). He had proteinuria more than 10 gm/day and was treated with oral steroid and cyclophosphamide initially, then cyclosporin along with steroid. There was no response to immunosuppressant medication, his renal function slowly started deteriorating. Repeat biopsy after 1 year of cyclosporin therapy showed IFTA +2 with > 50% glomerulosclerosis. He was continued on ARB and immunosuppression was reduced. He was planned for live related renal transplant with mother donor. His pretransplant proteinuria was 3.3 gm per day with hypoalbuminuria. He underwent renal transplant with Basiliximab induction. Post transplant he developed proteinuria on 2nd post operative day onwards and it was serially increasing. On 4th post operative day he underwent biopsy which showed, no evidence of rejection, but mild podocyte proliferation. He was given 500 mg methyl prednisolone for 3 days to reduce

proteinuria. He was started on ARB and blood pressure controlled to 130/70 mm Hg. He was given Inj Rituximab 500 mg IV weekly for 4 doses and underwent 10 sessions of plasmapheresis. His creatinine increased by 0.35 mg with ARB didn't return back to baseline after stopping and hence repeat graft biopsy done showed no rejection but 2 glomeruli showed focal segmental sclerosis. His tacrolimus level was maintained at 9-10 ng/ml and his blood pressure was well controlled. In view of persistent proteinuria he was given oral galactose 0.25 gm/kg twice day for 28 days. His proteinuria stabilised to 5 gm and creatinine is maintained at 2.0 mg/dl after 4 years.

Patient had baseline proteinuria 3.0 gm per day which increased serially and hence graft biopsy was done which showed no focal lesion, mild podocyte proliferation. As his original renal disease was FSGS with > 10 gm proteinuria and rapid progression, it was thought to be recurrence of FSGS. Early biopsy may not show the lesion. In the graft biopsy FSGS may be primary or secondary. Primary FSGS will have nephrotic range proteinuria and electron microscopy showing diffuse foot process effacement on the contrary, secondary FSGS will have non-nephrotic proteinuria, no oedema, normal albumin and cholesterol and electron microscopy showing segmental foot process effacement. Repeat biopsy in spite of Rituximab and plasmapheresis showed FSGS in 2 glomeruli. Galactose combines with permeability factor and reduces proteinuria even when they are resistant to plasmapheresis. His proteinuria stabilised and graft is still functioning even after 4 years (Fig. 35.1).

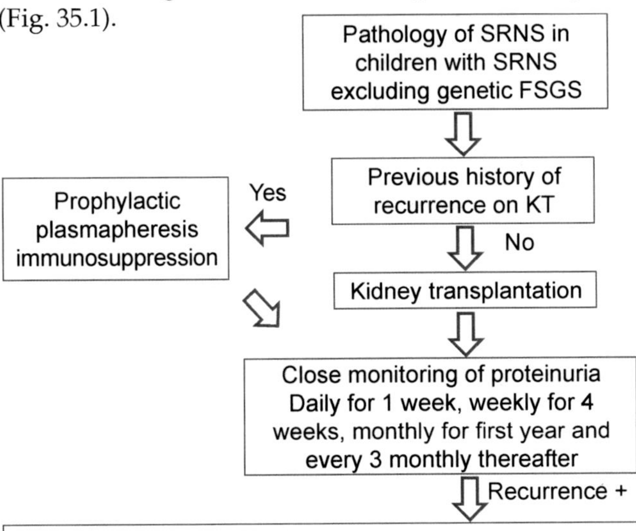

Figure 35.1: Planning renal transplant in FSGS

Different glomerular diseases have different recurrent rates MPGN II being highest of 80-100%. As FSGS is a common glomerular disease, we notice more number of recurrence of FSGS cases. Table 35.4 shows the recurrence of glomerular disease and graft loss due to recurrence of disease.

Table 35.4: Risk factors for recurrent glomerular disease

Histological type	Risk of recurrence (% patients)	Graft loss due to recurrence (% patients)
FSGS	30	50
Membranous Nephropathy	40	11
IgA Nephropathy	15-50	5
MPGN I	30-50	17
MPGN II	80	30

FSGS: Focal segmental glomerulosclerosis; MPGN: Membrano proliferative GN

Membranous nephropathy, MPGN usually present with de novo glomerular disease. Secondary FSGS usually can present with de novo. Renal damage by immunological, viral mechanical, oxidative and ischemia may lead to inflammation and immune reactivation. The antibodies produced lead to acute or chronic damage and cause proteinuria (Fig. 35.2 and Table 35.5).

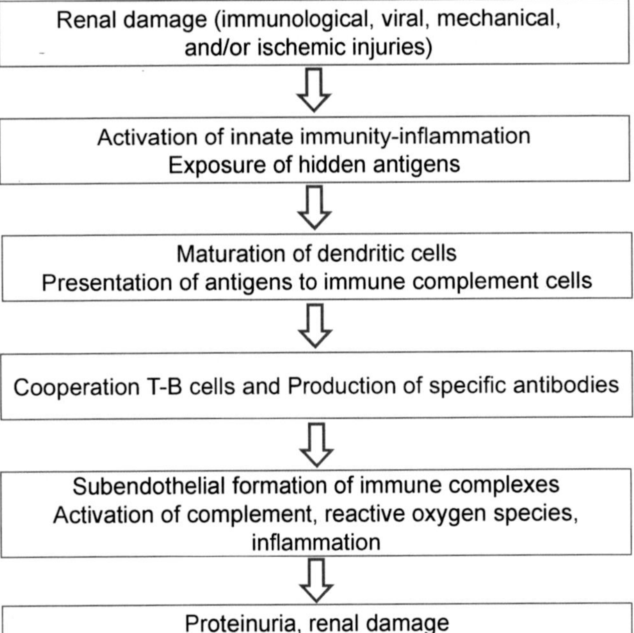

Figure 35.2: Kidney injury causing tissue damage

CASE 2

55 years old male CKD 5 due to diabetic nephropathy with retinopathy, hypertension, underwent renal transplant with wife donor (6/6 mismatch) with ATG induction. His nadir creatinine was 0.8 mg/dl on 4th post operative day. His proteinuria was 340

Table 35.5: Characteristics of de novo glomerular diseases after renal transplantation

Disease	Presentation	Time of onset	Different with native GN	Treatment	Prognosis
MN	Proteinuria, sometimes in nephrotic range	Late after transplant	Associated with transplant complications; IgG1 deposits instead of IgG4	No specific treatment	Slowly progressive
MPGN	Proteinuria, hematuria, NS, nephritic sediment	Months or years after transplant	Often associated with HCV or with other diseases	Steroid + cytotoxic drugs if Crescentic GN	Slowly progressive; poor prognosis
FSGS	Proteinuria, rarely in nephrotic range	Months or years after transplant	NS is rare; signs of rejection or CNI toxicity at biopsy	Removal of associated events	Usually poor, particularly in collapsing FSGS
MCD	NS	Early after transplant	Mild mesangial sclerosis, hypercellularity	Steroids	Good

MCD: Minimal change disease; NS: Nephrotic syndrome; MN: Membranous nephropathy; MPGN: Membrano proliferative GN; HCV: Hepatitis C virus. Ponticelli *et al.*, Clin J Am Soc Nephrology 2014;9:1479-87.

mg/day at 3 months post transplant. In view of high level of tacrolimus level, he was shifted to cyclosporin. His had asymptomatic increase in creatinine to 1.9 mg/dl at 7 months post transplant with UPCR 0.2; and his renal biopsy revealed no evidence of rejection or cause of rise in creatinine. His cyclosporin dose was reduced and he was hydrated started following which his creatinine improved to 1.1 mg/dl. At 2 years post transplant he had rise in creatinine from 1.3 mg to 2.38 mg/dl with proteinuria of 1295 mg/day. His graft biopsy showed Acute Cellular rejection with interstitial fibrosis+, Capillaritis C4d was negative. He was treated with ATG and his creatinine improved to 1.36 mg/dl. His proteinuria stabilised to 500 mg after the treatment of rejection.

Proteinuria may be the presentation of antibody mediated rejection. Clinically and histopathologically, many of the features of presentation were similar to that seen in post-transplant FSGS, but may have donor specific anti-HLA antibody. Proteinuria is an early marker of damage produced to the glomerular capillaries by anti-HLA class II antibodies, before histological signs of peri-glomerular capillaritis are visible. Treatment of rejection with high dose steroid reduces the excretion of proteins including albumin but not tubular proteins. In a retrospective study of patients having proteinuria and rejection showed poor long-term survival of the graft. A study by Arnol M *et al.* showed that increase in proteinuria after acute rejection is associated with decreased graft function and survival and could be used as a surrogate marker for poor outcomes, specifically after antibody mediated rejection.

CASE 3

42-year-old lady with ADPKD presented with flank pain, hematuria, vomiting with S. creatinine of 7 mg/dl. She was initiated on dialysis and underwent bilateral nephrectomy in view of large kidney and bleeding in the cyst. She underwent renal transplant with sister donor using Basiliximab induction. Her immediate graft function was good. She had a symptomatic rise in creatinine, biopsy showed ATN, C4d was negative and hence tacrolimus level was reduced. She was discharged with 0.9 mg/dl creatinine. After 7 months post transplant she had increase in creatinine and graft biopsy revealed tacrolimus toxicity. Dose of tacrolimus was reduced and graft function improve. She had diabetes post transplant and needed OHA. She has fever in 8th month due to CMV infection with AKI (Creatinine 3.04 mg/dl). She was treated with Intravenous Ganciclovir. Her fever reduced and graft function improved to 1.24 mg/dl. In view of 2 episodes of graft dysfunction due to tacrolimus toxicity and CMV infection with proteinuria <300 mg/dl she was put on sirolimus 1 mg per day. After 4 years of transplant she has proteinuria of 9 gm per day. She underwent renal biopsy which showed FSGS, no diabetic change. Her sirolimus was stopped and restarted on tacrolimus. Her proteinuria reduced to 3.1 gm from 9 gm per day.

The use of sirolimus or everolimus has been associated with post transplant proteinuria in numerous studies. It was suggested that the proteinuria with sirolimus associated proteinuria was the result of uncovering the hemodynamic effects of CNI. Proteinuria may be caused at least partially by glomerular hyperfiltration. m-TOR inhibitors may directly affects protein filtration in the glomerulus and specifically in the podocyte. Letavernier *et al.*[5] showed that sirolimus affects the VEGF, which is essential for podocyte and endothelial cell survival. Sirolimus can exert anti-proliferative and apoptotic effects on epithelial tubular cells and may interfere with the protein endocytosis in the tubular epithelial cell causing tubular proteinuria. There is no clear evidence that sirolimus is harmful to the graft in patients that maintain a low and stable proteinuria level (<500 mg/day). If it increases progressively, m-TOR inhibitor withdrawal should be considered. In a retrospective study by Verhave J *et al.*[6], 219 patients who were switched to sirolimus a median of 3 years after transplantation. At the time of conversion, 6.8% already had significant proteinuria (>1 g/l). New or worsening proteinuria occurred in 23%. Proteinuria was difficult to manage and required discontinuation of sirolimus in 33%.

What You Expect in Post Tx-Proteinuria; Correlation of Proteinuria with Biopsy?

Earlier articles by Seron *et al.* found a poor correlation between the amount of proteinuria and underlying disease. Biopsy lesions on renal biopsy tend to appear before clinical manifestations such as decline in renal function or proteinuria.

More recently Amer H[3] *et al.* assessed the prognostic significance of different forms of urinary protein (both high and low molecular weight proteins) with biopsy findings at 1 year after transplantation. 39% of grafts had normal histology, 36% had interstitial fibrosis and tubular atrophy (IFTA) without inflammation, 6% had inflammation (acute cellular or antibody-mediated rejection [AMR]), 5% had vascular changes, and 15% had glomerular pathology (transplant glomerulopathy, IgA nephropathy, membranous nephropathy, focal segmental glomerulosclerosis). Urine albumin level was significantly higher in those with glomerular disease compared to those with normal pathology (median ACR 24.9 mg/g vs 12.0 mg/g).

Consequences of Post Transplant Proteinuria (Fig. 35.3)

In a kidney transplantation setting, proteinuria has been associated with poor graft and patient survival. Roodnat *et al.* found that proteinuria doubled the risk of graft failure in comparison with non-proteinuric transplant patients. The relative risk of graft failure increased with increasing amounts of proteinuria, being 2.33 for proteinuria 0.5–1 g/day and 3.46 for proteinuria >1 gm/day. Even low-grade proteinuria, whatever the cause, has been reported to be a potent predictor of graft loss. Even proteinuria of 151-500 mg per day showed 4 times increased risk of graft loss. 500 mg proteinuria reduce the survival by 50% in a Korean study.[7] Low levels of proteinuria can indicate:

1. The first stage of a glomerular disease recurrence.
2. The effect of anti-HLA class II inhibitors; or
3. Interstitial disease due to drug or infective aetiology.

Residual proteinuria and m-TOR inhibitor-induced proteinuria don't affect the long-term prognosis of the graft.

Not only proteinuria but also microalbuminuria and mild increase of C-reactive protein in transplanted patients may indicate an underlying subtle systemic endothelial inflammatory damage, that could contribute to reduced graft and patient survival. A study by Lam NN *et al.*,[9] showed that reduced eGFR (increasing stage of CKD) and heavier albuminuria in kidney transplant recipients are associated with an increased risk of mortality and graft loss. However, proteinuria is not only associated with graft failure but also with an increased risk of mortality. A meta-analysis of cohort studies in non-transplant population showed a strong and continuous association between proteinuria and subsequent risk of coronary heart disease, and suggested that proteinuria should be incorporated into the assessment of an individual's cardiovascular risk.

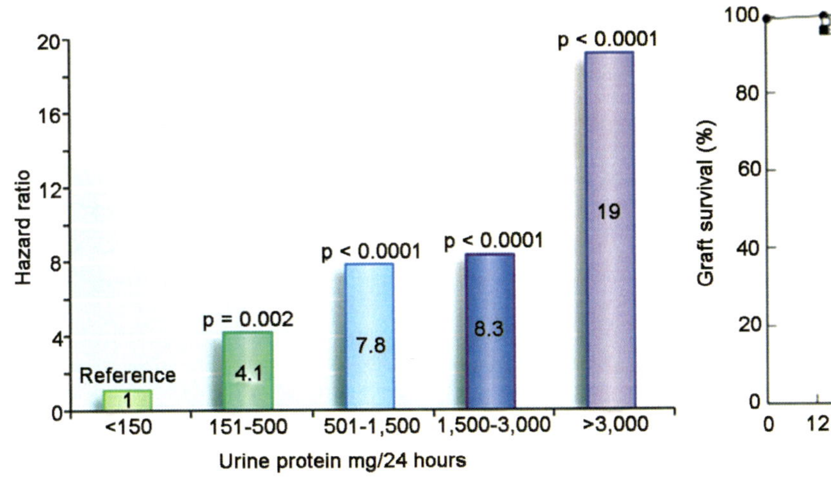

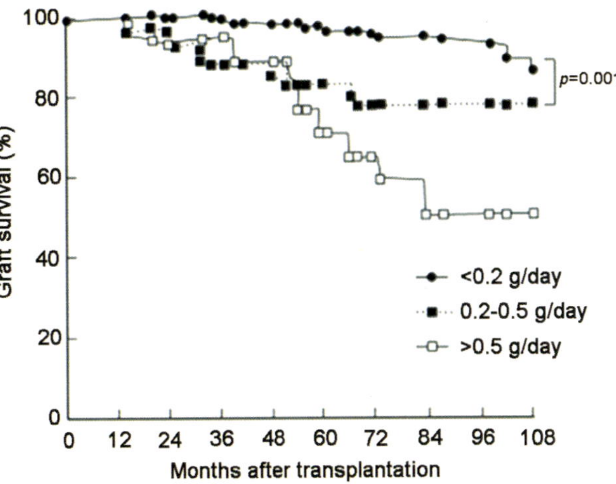

Figure 35.3: Proteinuria at 1 year post transplant and effect on subsequent graft survival

Approach to Proteinuria (Table 35.6)

Table 35.6: Approach to proteinuria

Timeline	
1st month post transplant	Assess proteinuria at least once in the 1st month If ESRD is due to FSGS measure proteinuria daily for 1st week; weekly for 4 weeks Screen proteinuria by PCR or ACR and confirm by 24 hours urine collection Consider renal biopsy if unexplained proteinuria > 1.5 gm or new onset proteinuria > 300 mg
2-12 months post transplant	Assess proteinuria at least once in 3 monthly If proteinuric, measure proteinuria every monthly for 12 months Screen proteinuria by PCR or ACR and confirm by 24 hours urine collection Consider renal biopsy if unexplained proteinuria >1.5 gm or new onset proteinuria > 300 mg
> 1 year post transplant	Assess proteinuria at least once yearly If proteinuric, measure proteinuria every 3 monthly Screen proteinuria by PCR or ACR and confirm by 24 hours urine collection Consider renal biopsy if unexplained proteinuria >1.5 gm or new onset proteinuria > 300 mg

Clin J Am Soc Nephrol 2011;6:1786-93.

PCR: Urine protein/creatinine ratio; ACR: Urine Albumin/creatinine ratio.

Treatment

Goals of proteinuria reduction include symptom management such as controlling oedema, prevention of proteinuria-related complications-hyperlipidemia and venous thrombosis, and delaying progression to end-stage renal disease. Treatment of post-transplant proteinuria is focussed on the: (1) Non specific treatments reduce proteinuria; (2) Specific treatment for the cause of proteinuria; and (3) Cardiovascular risk treatment. Proteinuria treatment, especially for low-grade proteinuria, is often limited to controlling blood pressure or using angiotensin-converting enzyme inhibitors (ACEi), which can reduce the concentration of proteins in urine.

Non-Specific Treatment of Kidney Transplant Proteinuria

(1) Control blood pressure (systolic blood pressure lower than 130 mm Hg); (2) Use ACEi and/or angiotensin II receptor blockers (ARB) at the highest tolerated dose, even if the patient does not have hypertension; (3) Control the lipid profile, preferably using statins; (4) Maintain an adequate BMI; (5) Reduce the amount of proteins in the diet; and (6) Stop smoking.

Blood Pressure Control

Blood pressure during the first year after transplantation has been associated with allograft survival independent of graft function. The KDIGO transplant guidelines recommend maintaining blood pressure at less than 130 mm Hg systolic and less than 80 mm Hg diastolic. They recommend treatment with any class of anti-hypertensive unless urine protein excretion is 1 g/day or greater; ACEi or ARB is suggested for these patients.

Blockade of the Renin-Angiotensin System: Blockade of the renin-angiotensin-aldosterone system (RAAS) with ACE I or ARB has become standard therapy for the treatment of proteinuria in non-transplant CKD. In patients with post-transplant proteinuria, treatment with inhibitors of the renin angiotensin-aldosterone system (RAAS) may reduce proteinuria, but there is no evidence from randomized studies that this strategy results in improved graft survival or better patient survival. Opelz *et al.*[8] found no association between ACEi or ARB use and graft survival in 17,209 kidney transplant recipients. ALLOGRAFT study using losartan or placebo within 4 to 8 weeks after transplantation did not show any change in the outcome between the two groups.

Pentoxifylline: Pentoxifylline is a nonspecific inhibitor of the enzyme 3′,5′-phosphodietsterase which has been shown to decrease proteinuria. Shu *et al.* assessed the efficacy of pentoxifylline for 6 months in renal transplant patients (n=17) with biopsy proven chronic allograft nephropathy. Patients had already been treated with an ACEi or an ARB for more than 1 year. Urine protein excretion improved significantly in 5 (30%) patients, remained stable in 9 (53%) and worsened in 3 (17%) by 3 months.

Vitamin D Analogues seems to have a beneficial anti-proteinuric effect through down regulating renin synthesis.

Diet, Reduced Salt Intake and Protein Restriction: Proteinuric patients should be advised to consume a diet with a moderate protein and low sodium content. Patients with chronic kidney disease, a sodium intake of not exceeding 1.5 g (70 mmol/day) is advocated. The recent data show that even a modest reduction in dietary sodium intake may be very beneficial in kidney patients. High dietary sodium is related to increased albuminuria. It also may decrease the anti-proteinuric benefits of RAS blockade.

Two randomized, controlled trials published in the 1990s evaluated the role of dietary protein restriction in reducing proteinuria in kidney transplant recipients. A significant reduction in albuminuria and proteinuria was seen with protein restriction of 0.55 or 0.70 g/kg per day. However, there are no data about impact of dietary protein restriction on long-term kidney function or allograft survival and overall nutritional status of renal transplant recipients (Table 35.7).

Rituximab Therapy

B cells induce T cell activation, mediate antibody-independent autoimmune damage, and express co-stimulatory molecules and cytokines, maintaining T cell activation in autoimmune diseases. Rituximab chimeric anti CD 20 antibody treatment leads to B cell depletion caused by B cell apoptosis, antibody-dependent cellular cytotoxicity or phagocytosis, suppressing interactions between B cells and T cells, which may prevent relapses in patients with nephrotic syndrome. Rituximab seems to act on podocytes by down regulation of sphingomyelin phosphodiesterase acid-like 3b (SMPDL-3b) protein and acid sphingomyelinase (ASMase). Usual dose is 375/m^2 given every 1-2 weeks interval for 2-6 doses. Combination of Plasmapheresis and Rituximab has shown to be better efficacy in some reports. Rituximab therapy showed high rate of therapeutic success (82%), histologic resolution (40%) and lack of significant effect of MN recurrence on graft survival. A response was seen

Table 35.7: Risk of recurrence, graft loss and preventive strategies in patients with Glomerulonephritis

Glomerulonephritis	**Clinically relevant* recurrent risk**	**Risk of graft loss due to recurrence 5–10 years after Tx**	**Prevention/Treatment strategies**
IgA nephropathy Occur immediately, diagnosis is made 3 years after Tx	13–46	2–16	Induction with ATG Plasmapheresis (PP) and sterioid pulses in case of crescentic IgA GN ACEI and/or ARB for patients with proteinuria ± renal impairment due to recurrent IgAN
FSGS **High risk of recurrence:** Young age, mesangial proliferation, a rapid progression to ESRD	20–50	13–20	Avoid well matched living donors Pre-emptive perioperative PP for 2 weeks PP + high dose CNI ± Rituximab for early recurrence Oral galactose to reduce circulating factor Chronic PP with or without cyclophosphamide or cyclosporine–relapse after initial course of PP Avoid omission of calcineurin inhibitors in sirolimus-based immunosuppressive regimen
MPGN type 1	20–25%	15%	No effective preventive or treatment measures
MPGN type 2	80–100	30%	Exclude secondary cause May benefit from Eculizumab
Membranous GN Recurrence 2nd/3rd year	10–30	10–15	No effective preventive or treatment measures exclude secondary causes
ANCA-associated glomerulonephritis	17	6–8	Defer transplant until the disease inactive Cyclophosphamide for recurrence Combine therapy with PP, cyclophosphamide ± I.V. immunoglobulin for recurrence with high titre of ANCA and cellular crescents in renal biopsies
SLE	2–9	2–4	Defer transplant until the disease inactive. Consider mycophenolate mofetil for recurrence

FSGS: Focal segmental glomerulosclerosis; MPGN: Membrano proliferative GN; SLE: Systemic lupus erythematosus.

in 81% of the pediatric cases reported in the literature for recurrence of nephrotic syndrome as compared to 50% of adult.[10]

Cardioprotection

Proteinuria and renal insufficiency causes this increased cardiac morbidity and mortality. The following measures should be included: control blood pressure (lower than 130 mm Hg); use statins maintaining an LDL-cholesterol level lower than 100 mg/dl (less than 80 mg/dl in high-risk patients); tight control of glycaemia in diabetic patients; stop smoking; use aspirin and use beta blockers. The only measure that is proven, based on prospective, controlled and randomised studies, is that using statins is effective in transplant patients.

Conclusion

Post transplant proteinuria is common and is associated with reduced patient and allograft survival. Ideal cut-off for pathological and significant proteinuria in the transplant population remains undefined as even small amount increases risk of failure. Studies correlating biopsy findings with proteinuria after transplantation have confirmed that transplant specific causes are more common. Treatment options remain limited, and there is much uncertainty in the value of proteinuria-reducing therapies to improve clinical outcomes, such as patient and graft survival.

Key Points

1. Post-transplant proteinuria is common and could be due to multiple causes.
2. Proteinuria even low grade (<500 mg/day) is sensitive indicator of reduced graft survival.
3. The reduction in survival of the graft with proteinuria is probably due to aetiology. Needs evaluation to find out the cause of damage/proteinuria.
4. To treat proteinuria–three aspects should be considered; the cause, its reduction with nonspecific measures and reduction of associated cardiovascular risk.

References

1. Knoll GA. Proteinuria in kidney transplant recipients: Prevalence, prognosis and evidence-based management. Am J Kidney Dis 2009;Dec;54(6):1131-44.
2. D'Cunha PT, Parasuraman R, Venkat KK. Rapid resolution of proteinuria of native kidney origin following live donor renal transplantation. Am J Transplant 2005;5:351-55.
3. Amer H1, Cosio FG. Significance and management of proteinuria in kidney transplant recipients J Am Soc Nephrol 2009 Dec;20(12):2490-92.
4. Sancho-Calabuig A, PallardóMateu LM, Avila Bernabeu AI, *et al.* Very low grade proteinuria at 3 months post transplantation is an earlier marker of graft survival. Transplant Proc 2009;41:2122-25.
5. Letavernier E, Pe'raldi MN, Pariente A, Morelon E, Legendre C. Proteinuria following a switch from calcineurin inhibitors to sirolimus. Transplantation 2005; 80:1198-1203.
6. Verhave J, Boucher A, Dandavino R, *et al.* The incidence, management and evolution of rapamycin-related side effects in kidney transplant recipients. Clin Transplant 2014;28:616-22.
7. Na Ree Kang, Jung Eun Lee, Wooseong Huh *et al.* Minimum proteinuria One Year after Transplant is a Risk Factor for Graft Survival in Kidney Transplantation. J Korean Med Sci 2009 Jan;24(Suppl 1):S129-34.
8. Opelz G, Zeier M, Laux G, *et al.* No improvement of patient or graft survival in transplant recipients treated with angiotensin-converting enzyme inhibitors or angiotensin II type 1 receptor blockers: A collaborative transplant study report. J Am Soc Nephrol 2006;17:3257-62.
9. Lam NN1, Tonelli M2, Lentine KL3, Hemmelgarn B2, Ye F4, Wen K4, Klarenbach S4. Albuminuria and post transplant chronic kidney disease stage predict transplant outcomes. Kidney Int 2017 Aug;92(2):470-78.
10. Kazumoto Iijima, Mayumi Sako, Kandai Nozu. Rituximab for nephrotic syndrome in children. Clin Exp Nephrol 2017;21:193-202.

CHAPTER

36 A Renal Transplant Patient with Progressive Graft Dysfunction Due to Chronic Allograft Injury

Vivek Kute

Professor, Department of Nephrology and Clinical Transplantation, Institute of Kidney Diseases and Research Center, Dr. HL Trivedi Institute of Transplantation Sciences [IKDRC-ITS], Ahmedabad

CASE

A 45-year-old male patient Mr ABC a known case of CKD-ESRD with basic disease of IgA Nephropathy diagnosed 5 years back, presently on maintenance hemodialysis 3 times per week since 8 months with blood group of B+ received a deceased donor organ with 1 out of 6 HLA match (A,B,DR). Patients Panel Reactive Antibody was 20%. Deceased donor was extended criteria donor with serum creatinine value of 2.1 mg/dl at the time of organ procurement and cause of brain death was road traffic accident. Cold ischemia time was 17 hours.

Patient underwent open right iliac fossa renal transplantation after obtaining negative lymphocyte and flow cross match.

Patient was induced with IV methyl prednisolone 500 mg per day for 3 days and thymoglobulin 2 mg/kg intraoperatively single dose. Patient's intraoperative and immediate post-operative course was uneventful with creatinine of 1.7 mg/dl achieved on day 5. After that patient's creatinine was stuck around 1.7 mg/dl and increased to 2.4 mg/dl on day 9. Ultrasound guided percutaneous allograft biopsy was done and was suggestive of Banff grade IB acute cellular rejection. Patient was treated with 3 doses of methyl prednisolone 500 mg each, after which patient creatinine was decreased to 1.4 mg/dl.

For next 12 months patient did well, after 12 months patient presented to transplant OPD with complaint of minimal pedal edema, decreased urine output. Patient's blood pressure was also on higher side. Patient was admitted and investigated. His serum creatinine was found to be 2.7 mg/dl and proteinuria of 1.5 gm/24 hours. After taking informed consent allograft biopsy was performed and this was suggestive of acute antibody mediated rejection with diffuse C4d staining. Patient was found to have donor specific antibody against anti-HLA B51 with titer of 5000 MFI and anti-HLA DQ7, DQ8 with titer of 10000 MFI. Patient was treated with 3 doses of methyl prednisolone, 5 total plasma exchanges, IV immunoglobulin 100 mg/kg for 5 doses and rituximab 200 mg. Patient's serum creatinine decreased from 2.7 mg/dl – 1.9 mg/dl.

Patient did well for next 8 months and again presented to transplant OPD with complaint of pedal edema and asymptomatic rise in creatinine of 2.3 mg/dl allograft biopsy was performed and was suggestive of chronic antibody mediated rejection with DSA anti-HLA B51 7000 MFI and and anti-HLA DQ7, DQ8 with titer of 8000 MFI.

What are the Next Treatment Options?

Chronic Graft Dysfunction Management Overview

Both immunological and non-immunological factors play a role in progressive graft dysfunction and loss over time. Use of the previous term "chronic allograft nephropathy" is now discouraged and histopathological diagnosis should always be sought. Chronic rejection implies an immune mediated process, but optimum treatment is unknown.[1]

Contributors to chronic allograft dysfunction are:[2]

Alloantigen dependent	Alloantigen independent
• Chronic T cell mediated rejection • Chronic B cell mediated rejection • HLA mismatches • Prior sensitization • Inadequate immunosuppression	• CNI toxicity • Delayed graft dysfunction • Prolonged cold ischemia • Reduced nephron number • Donor factors • Recurrent recipient disease • BK virus nephropathy

Assessment of Patient with Chronic Graft Dysfunction

The monitoring of the graft function over time is one of the fundamental roles of a transplant follow-up clinic. Most patients will be asymptomatic. Key investigations include:

Serum creatinine and eGFR: It is important to consider changes in these over time in a similar manner to native kidney CKD.

Therapeutic drug levels, especially calcineurin inhibitor (CNI) levels: These should be considered over time and in the context of an individual patient's context.

Urinalysis and urine protein/creatinine ratio (uPCR): Proteinuria is a marker of renal injury, as well as of progressive transplant dysfunction, and overall CV morbidity and mortality.

HLA antibody screen: Measure monthly for the first 3 months and then 3 monthly for 1 year, then annually. Cost of qualitative luminex donor specific antibody (DSA) is 2500-3000 and quantitative luminex DSA is 30000. Qualitaive testing can be performed first and if positive then quantitative testing for DSA can be performed and this is cost effective also.

CMV and BK virus screening by CMV DNA and BKV DNA PCR method.[3]

They should be performed at time of graft dysfunction especially after anti-rejection therapy and monitoring response to anti-viral therapy.

Some centers perform "protocol biopsies" regardless of the function, to assess overall graft health and individualize management especially immuno-suppression.

The interpretation of a transplant biopsy performed for chronic graft dysfunction is complex and requires careful clinical histological correlation.

Is there Need to Measure Transcript Levels in Biopsies?

Molecular Microscope Diagnostics System (MMDx) is new microarray biopsy service. It provides the probability of rejection so you can assess transplant care. MMDx is a central diagnostic system that uses a MyGeneChip™ Custom Microarray from Thermo Fisher Scientific to measure transcript levels in biopsies, apply algorithms and compare algorithm results to a set of reference biopsies. The system complements conventional biopsy processing to improve the assessment of rejection and injury in transplanted organs.

How to Manage Patient with Chronic Graft Dysfunction?

General Measure

1. **Hypertension**

   The rationale for controlling hypertension in transplant recipient is two-fold that is, to reduce CV risk and slow progressive GFR loss.

   KDIGO guidelines suggest a target BP of <130/80 mm Hg.

   Patient should be educated regarding the benefits of lifestyle interventions for BP control.

   ACE inhibitors and ARB's are most favored group of anti-hypertensive followed by calcium channel blockers.

   Every drug should be looked for drug-drug interactions with CNI.[4]

2. **Management of Cardiovascular Disease (CVD)**

   CVD is the most common cause of death with a functioning graft in renal transplant patients.

   Renal transplant is considered to be cardio-protective as compared to patients who continue on hemodialysis.

   Immune suppressive drugs can exacerbate the cardiovascular disease risk.[5]

3. **Dyslipidemia**

   Dyslipidemia often results in raised total cholesterol, LDL cholesterol, and triglycerides as well as increased levels of intermediate lipoproteins.

   ALERT is the only larger RCT of statin treatment in renal transplant recipients and demonstrated a significant reduction in non-fatal MI and cardiac death in the Fluvastatin group.

   Patients should be educated regarding the benefits of life style modification for lipid control.

   Avoid smoking.[6]

   Optimum blood sugar controls in diabetics and NODAT patients.

   Statins are metabolised by CYP3A4 which is inhibited by CNI particularly cyclosporin and it should always be kept in mind that this combination can result in increased side effects of statin as well as CNI toxicity.

4. **Maintain good fluid balance.**

5. **Avoid nephrotoxic agents.**

6. **Management of the CNI Toxicity.**

   The earliest functional change is vasoconstriction, but structural toxicity, with histological change in the arterioles, glomeruli, and tubules eventually supervenes. Some degree of damage is inevitable in all patients taking a CNI.

   CNI induced arteriolar changes including swelling of the medial smooth cells and associated occasional endothelial or smooth muscle cell necrosis. The mature lesion demonstrates PAS positive hyaline nodules in the media and adventitia of the afferent arteriole.

   Thrombotic microangiopathy (TMA) may also be present, and focal segmental glomerulosclerosis (FSGS) can occur in the glomeruli secondary to arteriolar injury.

   Interstitial fibrosis and tubular atrophy is considered nonspecific caused by nephron drop out.

CNI minimization.

Dose reduction to aim for a lower therapeutic level.

Complete withdrawal, usually with a switch to sirolimus.

Other agents, such as belatacept, may have a role in future.[7]

How to Manage Rejection?

Management of Antibody Mediated Rejection (AMR)

Acute antibody mediated rejection is caused due to either increase in preexisting donor specific antibody (DSA) or due to de novo DSA formation. It is managed as per based on duration of renal transplant and the stage of rejection. It can be classified as per following categories:

Hyper Acute AMR

This type of rejection occurs on table or within 48-72 hours of transplant. The intensity of hyper acute rejection is so severe that most of the times it has to be treated with immediate graft nephrectomy. In very rare instances, it can be suppressed with high dosages of methyl prednisolone.

Acute AMR

This is the most common detectable presentation of AMR.

It is mainly seen as late cause of rejection but can be present within three months of renal transplant. Treatment is dependent upon the duration of transplant.

DSA testing should be done at the start of treatment. AMR occurring within one year of renal transplant is treated using methyl prednisolone injectable (7-10 mg/kg, a max of 1000 mg) per day for three days with intravenous immunoglobulin (100 mg/kg) for five days. In addition to the above anti-rejection medications, it is advised to do plasmapheresis for max 6 sessions on alternate day, 1-1.5 times the plasma volume with albumin as replacement agent preferably. Depending on the peri tubular capillary (PTC) score, if positive, additional treatment with rituximab (100-500 mg) or Bortezomib 2 mg/kg (4-8 doses) at interval of 4 days is advised.

If AMR occurs after 1 year of transplant, treatment given is same as mentioned above except plasmapheresis is not done. Rituximab is still given if PTC score >0.

Subclinical AMR

As against the management of cell mediated rejection, subclinical rejections in case of AMR are treated in the same manner as clinical AMR.

Chronic Active AMR

Chronic active AMR on biopsy should be treated with a trial of injectable methyl prednisolone 10 mg/kg for 3 doses along with intravenous immunoglobulin (IVIg) 100 mg/kg for 5 doses. Monitoring of DSA should be done and if present significantly, it should be treated with rituximab or newer immunosuppressant like proteasome inhibitors bortezomib for decreasing production of DSA and therapeutic plasma exchange for removal of DSA.[8]

Newer Immunosuppressant in Management of AMR

All the newer medications are in phase 2/3 of clinical trials:

1. **IL6 receptor blocker – Tocilizumab**

   In 1 study of 75 patients with chronic active AMR with or without transplant glomerulopathy, 37 patients who had failed high-dose IVIg, rituximab, and plasmapheresis received monthly doses of tocilizumab for 6 to 18 months and were found to have good outcomes when compared with published results.

2. **Compliment factor 5 inhibitor – Eculizumab**

   Eculizumab is a humanized monoclonal IgG antibody that binds to complement protein C5, inhibiting its cleavage to C5a and C5b and blocking the generation of the terminal complement complex C5b-C9. In a phase II randomized, open-label, multicenter trial of eculizumab vs placebo as an add-on to SOC desensitization protocols in living kidney donor recipients (NCT01399593), the eculizumab group failed to achieve a statistically significant reduction in the primary composite endpoint (occurrence of biopsy-proven AMR, graft loss, patient death, or loss to follow-up at the end of the 9-week treatment period post-transplant) when compared with placebo (9.8% vs 15.7%, P =.554).

3. **Complement INH inhibitor – Berinert and Cinryze**

   C1-INH is a serine protease inhibitor that inactivates both C1r and C1s and has multiple effects. C1-INH regulates proteases in the classical and lectin complement pathways and has major effects on regulation of the coagulation cascade as well as vascular permeability and inflammation by kinins.

4. **IdeS–immunoglobulin destructive enzyme of streptococcus pyogens**

   These are immunoglobulins derived from streptococcus pyogens. They destroy the antibodies completely. But the antibodies tend to recur to the previous level in next 15 days.[9]

Management of Acute Cellular Rejection (ACR)

ACR is seen mainly in first three months after transplant. Management is based on the Banff grade on renal biopsy.

Borderline rejection: It is a low level of rejection so usually managed by up regulating the dosage of steroids and calcineurin inhibitors.

Grade 1A: Managed by injectable methylprednisolone (7-10 mg/kg) for three days.

Grade 1B, 2 and 3: Managed by injectable methylprednisolone (7-10 mg/kg) for three days along with rabbit anti thymocyte globulin (rATG) 1-3 mg/kg over three days and can be up titrated to 5-10 mg/kg of total dosage.

If no improvement as in decrease in serum creatinine by 10% by five days then repeat biopsy is advised.

Our center experience: We suggest that a cumulative thymoglobulin 6 mg/kg, Rituximab 500 mg and or 8 doses of bortezomib 1.3 mg/m^2 and 8 sessions of therapeutic plasma exchanges can be used for treating allograft immune injury. Excessive immunosuppression carries risk of infections and death with functioning graft due to infections. After anti-rejection therapy prophylaxis should be given for CMV, PCP and fungal infection.

The Failing Graft

It is very easy to forget CKD basics in a transplant patient with deteriorating graft function.

Always explain the situation to the patient, with appropriate psychological support.

Management of secondary complications of the decreasing GFR like anemia and CKD MBD.

Ongoing control of BP and CV risk.

Early discussion regarding future dialysis and possible re transplantation. The earlier this is undertaken, the greater chance the patient will be able to choose the most acceptable modality for them.

Immunosuppression should not be stopped abruptly, AZA/MMF are generally stopped first followed by slow steroid withdrawal and progressive reduction of CNI.

Slow weaning will help to prevent inflammation in a remnant graft which can make the patient feel quite unwell and provoke the development of anti-HLA antibodies that might be dangerous in future transplantation.

Removal of the graft to prevent HLA sensitization is controversial – the patient may still become sensitized to antigens present in the vascular stump.

Prevention of Chronic AMR with Kidney Exchange

KDIGO guidelines reported that HLA mis-match is independent risk factor for acute and chronic immune injury (universal agreement). The chronic antibody mediated immune injury is caused by DSA. Better HLA matching before transplant improve long-term kidney allograft survival.

HLA matching has been best prognostic marker for long-term graft survival based on multiple regressions.[10] Basu *et al.*[11] reported that significant benefits, better long-term survival and lower infections due to less potent immunosuppression in Indian environment can be achieved by providing better-matched donors for HLA mismatched compatible pairs through Kidney Paired Donation (KPD). We suggest that compatible donor-recipient pair with poor HLA matching can be offered for KPD to achieve better HLA matching.

References

1. Paul LC. Chronic allograft nephropathy: An update. Kidney Int 1999 Sep;56(3):783-93. Review. PubMed PMID: 10469349.
2. Joosten SA, van Kooten C, Sijpkens YW, de Fijter JW, Paul LC. The pathobiology of chronic allograft nephropathy: Immune-mediated damage and accelerated aging. Kidney Int. 2004 May;65(5):1556-59. Review. PubMed PMID: 15086891.
3. Grinyo JM, Saval N, Campistol JM; ICEBERG STUDY Group. Clinical assessment and determinants of chronic allograft nephropathy in maintenance renal transplant patients. Nephrol Dial Transplant 2011 Nov;26(11): 3750-55. doi:10.1093/ndt/gfr091. Epub 2011 Apr 7. PubMed PMID: 21474575.
4. Li C, Yang CW. The pathogenesis and treatment of chronic allograft nephropathy. Nat Rev Nephrol 2009 Sep;5(9): 513-19. doi: 10.1038/nrneph 2009;113. Epub 2009 Jul 28. Review. PubMed PMID: 19636333.
5. Afzali B, Taylor AL, Goldsmith DJ. What we CAN do about chronic allograft nephropathy: Role of immunosuppressive modulations. Kidney Int 2005 Dec;68(6):2429-43. Review. PubMed PMID:16316321.
6. Agarwal A, Prasad GV. Post-transplant dyslipidemia: Mechanisms, diagnosis and management. World J Transplant 2016 Mar 24;6(1):125-34. doi: 10.5500/wjt.v6.i1.125. Review. PubMed PMID: 27011910; PubMed Central PMCID: PMC4801788.
7. Birnbaum LM, Lipman M, Paraskevas S, Chaudhury P, Tchervenkov J, Baran D, Herrera-Gayol A, Cantarovich M. Management of chronic allograft nephropathy: Asystematic review. Clin J Am Soc Nephrol 2009 Apr;4(4):860-65. doi:10.2215/CJN.05271008. Epub 2009 Apr 1. Review. PubMed PMID:19339427.
8. Garces JC, Giusti S, Staffeld-Coit C, Bohorquez H, Cohen AJ, Loss GE. Antibody-Mediated Rejection: A Review. Ochsner J. 2017 Spring;17(1):46-55. PubMed PMID: 28331448; PubMed Central PMCID: PMC5349636.
9. Pouliquen E, Koenig A, Chen CC, Sicard A, Rabeyrin M, Morelon E, Dubois V,Thaunat O. Recent advances in renal transplantation: Antibody-mediated rejection takes center stage. F1000Prime Rep. 2015 May 12;7:51. doi: 10.12703/P7-51.eCollection 2015. Review. PubMed PMID: 26097724; PubMed Central PMCID:PMC4447042.
10. Ferrari P1, Cantwell L, Ta J, Woodroffe C, D'Orsogna L, Holdsworth R. Providing Better-Matched Donors for HLA Mismatched Compatible Pairs Through Kidney Paired Donation. Transplantation 2017 Mar;101(3):642-48. doi: 10.1097/TP.0000000000001196.
11. Basu G, Daniel D, Rajagopal A, Neelakantan N, John GT. A model for human leukocyte antigen-matched donor-swap transplantation in India. Transplantation 2008;85:687-92.

CHAPTER 37

A Post Renal Transplant Patient with Cytomegalovirus (CMV) Disease

Dipankar Bhowmik[1], Arun Kumar S[2]

[1] *Professor, Department of Nephrology, All India Institute of Medical Sciences, New Delhi*
[2] *Assistant Professor, Department of Nephrology, All India Institute of Medical Sciences, New Delhi*

CASE

A 49-year-old male patient who had received kidney transplantation 8 months earlier for end-stage renal disease due to type 2 diabetes mellitus was admitted to the hospital with severe fatigue, diarrhea and loss of appetite for 3 weeks duration. The donor was his brother-in-law (authorized donor) and was transplanted on anti-thymocyte globulin (ATG) induction. Current immunosuppressive regimen consisted of tacrolimus, mycophenolate mofetil (500 mg thrice/day) and low dose prednisolone (5 mg/day). The dose of tacrolimus was titrated to achieve trough whole blood level of 6 ng/ml. The patient and donor were CMV positive (IgG serology) pre-operatively and received CMV prophylaxis with valganciclovir for 3 months after transplantation.

Clinically, the patient had fever with mild hypotension (90/60 mm Hg) which resolved with fluid bolus. On clinical examination, the abdomen was tender without signs of peritonitis and no localization. The rest of the physical examination was unremarkable. During hospital admission, the patient had fever with loose stools and persistent nausea. The initial blood cell count was within normal range (WBC $5.2 \times 10^9/l$), and blood chemistry revealed mild renal dysfunction (creatinine 2.1 mg/dl) as well as slightly elevated liver enzymes. Stool examination for Salmonella, Shigella and Clostridium difficile, and parasitological examination came back negative. Initial CMV serology was positive for IgM, whereas the previous serology done pre-transplant had been negative. Concomitant CMV viral load was elevated to 1,620,000 IU/ml (Cobas Taqman, Roche). Trough levels of tacrolimus was 5.6 ng/ml. Fundus examination was normal without sign of retinitis. Upper gastrointestinal tract endoscopy showed erosive gastritis. Immunostaining of gastric biopsies revealed CMV nuclear inclusions, suggesting CMV gastritis.

Patient was well hydrated and renal-dosed intravenous ganciclovir was administered for 2 weeks. The dose of mycophenolate mofetil was reduced to 500 mg twice/day. Repeat CMV viral load became undetectable after 2 weeks and diarrhea also subsided. Oral valganciclovir was then added in lieu of ganciclovir. The patient made a complete clinical recovery and attained baseline serum creatinine of 1.3 mg/dl. He was discharged with maintenance prophylaxis dose valganciclovir therapy for a total duration of 3 months. Patient did not have any recurrence of CMV infection for up to one year on follow-up and is on regular follow-up at present.

Infections in Renal Transplantation

The outcomes after kidney transplantation has improved significantly over the years. However, with advances in immunosuppressive agents, infectious complications are still an important cause of morbidity and mortality in this population. The risk of infection depends on the 'net state' of immunosuppression in the post-transplant setting which in turn depends on the immunosuppressive agent used, donor as well as environmental factors. Immunomodulatory infectious agents such as cytomegalovirus (CMV) can cause disease and also predispose to other opportunistic infections. Plausible reports of transmission of infections through kidney transplants have been described for a number of agents, including CMV. These 'donor-derived' infections also constitute a significant risk for post-transplant infections.

Cytomegalovirus (CMV) Infection

CMV is a universal herpes virus that infects 70-100% of the general population. CMV remains a common infectious pathogen in renal transplant recipients and other immunocompromised hosts, either presenting with asymptomatic viremia or as a viral syndrome or a tissue-invasive disease. Unlike immunocompetent adults, where CMV infection has a self-limited course or a mononucleosis-like syndrome, renal transplant recipients often present with serious manifestations. Apart from its direct deleterious effects, CMV infection has also shown to compromise transplant outcomes by triggering graft rejection by its immunomodulatory effects and increases the risk for other opportunistic infections. Hence, a systematic approach is needed to prevent and treat CMV in this population.

Pathophysiology

CMV infection is nearly ubiquitous with serological studies in India detecting seropositivity in over 95% in the pre-transplant population. In the transplant population, CMV infection occurs due to reactivation of latent infection, transmission from the transplanted organ or following a primary infection in seronegative patients. After the initial infection, CMV remains in a latent state in the host resulting in 'persistent' infection. Myeloid lineage cells constitute an important reservoir and CMV DNA has been found in CD34+ myeloid progenitor cells and dendritic cells. Reactivation and viral replication typically occurs in immunocompromised states as after renal transplantation. This risk is increased in the first 6 months after transplantation as the maintenance immunosuppression is maintained at a higher level to avoid rejection. Drugs which suppress T-lymphocyte suppression like anti thymocyte globulin (ATG) increases the risk of reactivation multifold. As the viral replication increases, there is cell to cell spread of the virus and the endothelial cells are then infected. The polymorphonuclear leukocytes and mononuclear cells take up the virus and the pp65 matrix protein when they come into contact with the infected endothelial cell. These endothelial cells get detached and can plug smaller capillaries and spread infections to distant organs. The deleterious effects of CMV result from direct cytopathic effect of the virus on various organs. Active CMV infection has also been shown to cause complement activation and contribute to tissue injury.

What are the Risk Factors for CMV Infection?

The risk of CMV in transplanted patients varies according to the organ transplanted, type of transplantation, the serological status of donor and recipient, immunosuppressive drugs used and additional risk factors. The risk is highest with heart-lung transplantation followed by liver transplantation and least with renal transplantation. The greatest risk factor is serological 'mismatch' between the donor (D) and recipient (R). The highest risk is when the recipient is seronegative and the donor being seropositive (CMV D+/R-); CMV D+/R+ and CMV D-/R+ are of intermediate risk while CMV D-/R- transplantation is considered to be low risk. The other factor increasing the CMV risk is the 'net' immunosuppression. Use of lymphocyte depleting agents (ATG), high maintenance immunosuppression, HLA mismatch, acute rejection, advanced age of donor/recipient and genetic polymorphisms decide the risk of active CMV infection.

Time Line of CMV Infection

CMV disease mainly occurs between 30 and 90 days after transplantation and was considered to be rare after 180 days as the net immunosuppression is reduced after this time period. However, the onset is delayed when post transplant antiviral prophylaxis is given. 'Late' CMV infection is usually defined as occurring more than 1 year after transplantation. The reported incidence of late CMV infection has shown a rise with the use of regular prophylaxis after transplantation and also use of better diagnostic modalities. In a case series of 2489 renal transplant patients, it was seen that 77 patients (3.1%) developed late CMV infection and 15% of these infections were in D-/R- recipients. Primary infections leading to late-onset CMV disease remain rare and are limited to a few case reports with some reported even after 10 years after transplantation. Due to the paucity of available data, duration of secondary prophylaxis is unknown in this population.

Definitions

Understanding the difference between CMV infection and CMV disease is essential to plan therapy. The definitions have been given by the American Society of Transplantation and CMV Drug Development Forum. *CMV infection* is characterized by the evidence of viral replication which is detected by molecular methods or antigenemia assays regardless of symptoms. *CMV disease* is said to be present when there is evidence of CMV infection with symptoms attributed to it. CMV disease can present as a 'viral syndrome' characterized by fever, malaise with cytopenia and deranged liver function tests. 'Invasive' disease characterized by the presence of organ specific symptoms with viral cytopathic effects in the target organ. The various CMV associated 'clinical syndromes' include gastrointestinal disease (esophagitis, gastritis, enterocolitis), pneumonia, hepatitis, retinitis, myocarditis and CNS disease. The various modes of presentation of CMV infection are enlisted in Table 37.1.

It must also be kept in mind that CMV disease often co-exists with other bacterial, fungal and viral infections. Hence steps must be taken to diagnose co-existing infections.

How to Diagnose CMV Infection?

Prior to transplant, the CMV serostatus of the donor and recipient are significant predictors of the risk for CMV infection post transplant and also determine the need for prophylaxis/preemptive treatment. CMV specific IgG testing should be done in all patients. Both IgM and combined IgG and IgM are less useful for screening purposes. If the results are equivocal, the higher appropriate CMV risk staging has to be done.

Table 37.1: Various presentations of CMV disease

Type of disease	Clinical presentation	Diagnosis
Asymptomatic CMV viremia	Asymptomatic	Detection of CMV infection in blood
CMV syndrome	Febrile illness	CMV viremia and cytopenia
CMV gastrointestinal disease	Nausea, vomiting, loose stools, GI bleeding (Occult/Frank)	CMV in biopsy specimens ± CMV viremia
CMV hepatitis	Nausea, vomiting, icterus	Transaminitis ± hyperbilirubinemia with CMV in biopsy/blood
CMV pneumonia	Dyspnoea, cough, LRTI features	CMV in BAL/lung biopsy
Others–Less common CMV retinitis, cystitis, myocarditis, pancreatitis, encephalitis	Features suggestive of corresponding organ involvement	CMV viremia + detection of CMV in biopsy samples/body fluids

BAL: Bronchoalveolar lavage; CMV: Cytomegalovirus; GI: Gastrointestinal; LRTI: Lower respiratory tract infection.

Serology in general has a limited role after transplantation. Though studies have shown that seroconversion at 6 months after transplant in D+/R- individuals reduces the risk for late CMV disease, it is not a useful predictor of future CMV disease. Viral culture has a poor sensitivity and is not used outside research purposes. A sensitive method used earlier was 'pp65 antigenemia' wherein pp65 antigen is identified within the leukocyte cytoplasm by immunofluorescence. With the availability of multiple automated platforms, quantitative CMV DNA testing is the present gold standard for diagnosis of CMV infection. As per the WHO international standard, the results are calibrated and reported in IU/ml. CMV DNA is detected earlier and in higher quantities in whole blood and hence preferred over plasma samples. With the availability of highly sensitive assays, studies have shown that viral load values <147 IU/ml following therapy is predictive of a clinical response.

With regard to tissue invasive disease, the presence of CMV cytopathic changes or CMV by immunohistochemistry is the gold standard for diagnosis. Patients with gastrointestinal disease may have low DNAemia and remain undetectable and hence need tissue biopsy for diagnosis. Tissue Quantitative nucleic acid testing (QNAT) and viral cultures may be more specific and need more studies before recommendation.

CMV specific immune monitoring assays include the commercially available QuantiFERON-CMV assay (ELISA based IFN-gamma release assay for CD8 T cells) and the ELISpot assay (assess both CD4 and CD8 cells). They may be predictive of disease but further studies are required before clinical recommendation.

Prevention of CMV Infection

Having seen that CMV infection is common and destructive, preventive strategies are of paramount importance to improve clinical outcomes. Routine prevention is not recommended in seronegative individuals (D-/R-). In other classes of preventive strategies include either universal prophylaxis or preemptive therapy as detailed below (Table 37.2).

Universal prophylaxis involves giving antiviral agents in the post-transplant period for 3-6 months. Until now, valganciclovir has been the most effective drug used for prevention of CMV in the post-renal transplant setting. The dosing of valganciclovir is also different in different centers. In general to improve the tolerability and to reduce costs 'mini-dosing' with half the dose (450 mg/day) is done. The use of intravenous ganciclovir and foscarnet for this purpose has been hampered by considerable adverse effects. Other well studied prophylactic options include high-dose acyclovir, valaciclovir and intravenous immune globulin; all of which have low efficacy and not used routinely. This strategy increases the risk of late onset CMV disease. Regarding the duration of prophylaxis, the Improved Protection Against Cytomegalovirus in Transplantation

Table 37.2: Comparison between Prophylaxis vs. Preemptive therapy

	Prophylaxis	Preemptive therapy
CMV disease prevention	Effective	Effective
Late CMV disease	Possible	Less likely
Resistance	Uncommon	Uncommon (if weekly monitoring)
Drug toxicity	Can occur	Less common
Costs	Cost of drugs	Cost of diagnostics
Other advantages	Prevent other herpes viral infections (HSV,VZV)	–

CMV: Cytomegalo virus; HSV: Herpes simplex virus; VZV: Varicella zoster virus.

(IMPACT) study reported a reduced risk of CMV disease in D+/R- patients with 200 days of prophylaxis (21.3%) compared to those given 100 days of prophylaxis (36.8%). Seropositive recipients can receive shorter course (3 months) of prophylaxis.

Preemptive therapy needs periodic monitoring of blood CMV to identify early replication and initiating therapy at a pre-determined threshold to prevent the progression to CMV 'disease'. The definition of a suitable 'threshold' has been a topic of contention and varies with the sensitivity of the test used, the serological status and the institutional protocol. Though the risk of late onset disease is reduced in this approach the logistics and cost involved in repeated monitoring is of concern in resource limited settings. Also, whether the low-level viremia has a deleterious effect on the graft and overall patient outcomes is debatable.

There are four randomized controlled trials which compare both these strategies in renal transplantation. When universal prophylaxis was compared to weekly monitoring for the initial 4 months, there was no difference between the two strategies with regard to CMV disease or long-term graft survival irrespective of the recipient serological status (R+ or R-). However, if less frequent monitoring is done, the risk of CMV disease increases and the long-term graft survival is reduced. The need for active surveillance after prophylaxis is not supported by the data available at present and should be carried out only in symptomatic patients. The recommended approaches for CMV prevention is detailed below in Table 37.3.

Table 37.3: Recommended approach for CMV prevention

Serostatus	Risk level	Recommendation
D-/R-	Low	No prophylaxis; Monitor according to clinical symptom and need
D+/R+	Intermediate	3 months of prophylaxis or Preemptive therapy
D+/R-	High	6 months of prophylaxis or Preemptive therapy

CMV immune globulin was earlier used for prevention but in the era of antivirals, the limited effectiveness, cost and infusion related toxicity limits its role in the present time. Present interest has been towards newer antiviral drugs and vaccines. The studies have been predominantly done in hematopoietic stem cell transplant recipients where maribavir, brincidofovir and anti-CMV vaccine ASP0113 have been unsuccessful. Letermovir inhibits the viral terminase enzyme and has shown promise in this setting and is being evaluated in larger trials. CMV vaccines are in the early stages of clinical development and not available for routine clinical use. Adoptive T cell therapy with CMV specific T cells for resistant and refractory CMV infection has shown promise in this subset of patients.

Though there are no prospective trials for secondary prophylaxis to prevent recurrence of CMV infection following therapy, prophylaxis with valganciclovir is generally given for 3 months after resolution of CMV viremia.

What is Treatment of CMV Infection?

The landmark VICTOR study had shown equal efficacy for both oral valganciclovir and intravenous ganciclovir for both CMV syndrome and tissue-invasive disease. Ganciclovir is preferred for life threatening CMV disease. Whenever feasible valganciclovir is better on account of its oral administration and better adverse effect profile. Valganciclovir (900 mg twice a day) or intravenous ganciclovir (5 mg/kg twice a day) is the dose for patients with normal graft function. Dosing has to be calculated precisely based on body weight and eGFR to avoid under-dosing thereby causing treatment failure or resistance or overdosing which results in drug toxicity. The intensity of immunosuppression has to be reduced and the anti-proliferative agents (Azathioprine or MMF) have to be stopped in severe disease. Intensive therapy should be given for 14 – 21 days and CMV DNA should be re-assessed after intensive phase. In the presence of leukopenia, antiviral drugs should not be stopped but granulocyte colony stimulating factor has to be tried to avoid treatment failure or drug resistance. Once there is clinical response, ganciclovir can be substituted by oral valganciclovir. Weekly CMV DNA assessment should be done if feasible. Once negative or below lower limit of quantification (LLOQ), secondary prophylaxis can be given for 3 months. In patients intolerant to both these drugs, foscarnet is the second-line agent to be tried.

Drug resistance manifests as persistent or increasing viremia and/or symptomatic disease during antiviral therapy. Patients on strong immunosuppressive therapy, preemptive therapy (in comparison to universal prophylaxis) and prior cumulative exposure to either of the drugs for > 6 weeks are at risk for resistance. Any patient who fails to respond to therapy even after 6 weeks of therapy has to be evaluated in detail for the same. The most common cause is UL97 kinase gene mutations which affect drug phosphorylation needed for antiviral activity. The UL54 DNA polymerase gene mutations confer ganciclovir resistance with cross-resistance to cidofovir and foscarnet. The appropriate management of antiviral resistance is relatively unknown due to the limitations in diagnosis of the same. Optimisation of host factors with increased dose of ganciclovir (10 mg/kg twice a day) may suffice for lower levels of resistance due to UL97 mutations. Foscarnet is the second drug of choice but its use is limited by the toxicity profile. Some cases resistant to all the aforementioned agents may respond to cidofovir. Use of CMV Ig or CMV specific T cell infusion may be useful as add-on therapy. Salvage therapy with maribavir (UL 97 linase inhibitor) or letermovir (UL56 terminase inhibitor) may hold promise for the future.

A simple algorithm for management of CMV disease in post-transplant patients is given in Figure 37.1.

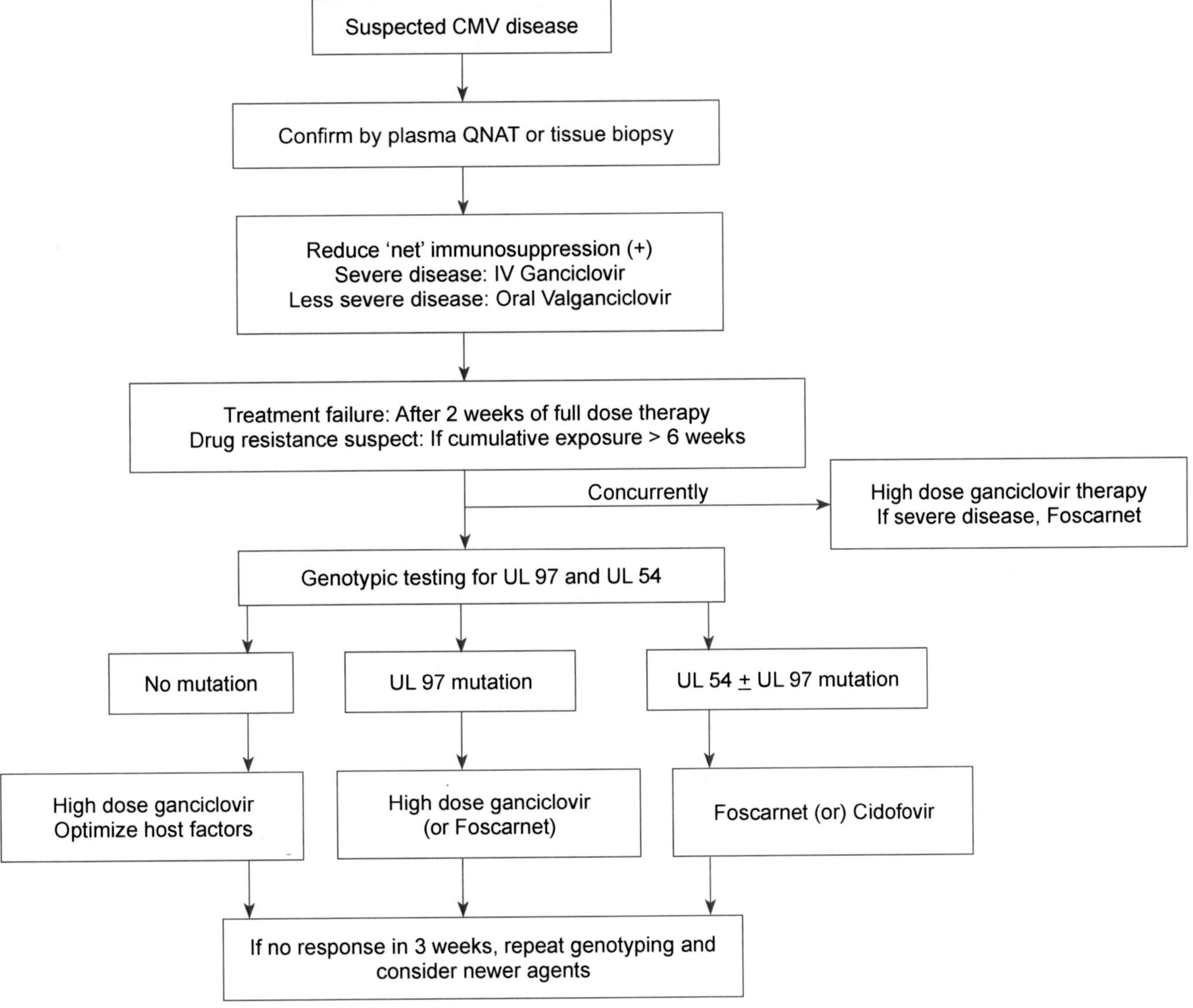

Figure 37.1: Management of CMV infection in post-transplant patients

Our patient presented with symptomatic CMV gastrointestinal invasive disease after prophylaxis and was confirmed by both QNAT and tissue biopsy specimens. He responded to ganciclovir therapy which was followed by valganciclovir prophylaxis as suggested. The serological status, use of strong immunosuppression (ATG) increased the risk of CMV at the end of prophylaxis period in our patient. In addition to antiviral agents, we had reduced the dose of the anti-proliferative agent (MMF) and hence reduced the 'net' immunosuppression. Hence, successful management of CMV disease is possible if suspected early and treated appropriately.

Conclusion

With an ever-increasing knowledge about CMV infection and advances in both diagnostics and therapeutics, management of CMV infection has become effective in the last decade. Nevertheless, there are some gaps in our knowledge with regard to the preventive strategy, threshold levels of viremia, secondary prophylaxis and resistant CMV infection. CMV infection is preventable and treatable and may not be the 'troll of transplantation' it was described as earlier.

Key Points

- Cytomegalovirus infection is common after renal transplant with 'direct' effects presenting as a viral syndrome or invasive disease and 'indirect' immunomodulatory effects increasing the risk of rejection and adverse graft outcomes.
- The initial post-transplant period poses the highest risk for symptomatic CMV infection/reactivation and depends on the 'net' immunosuppression of the patient.

Contd.

Contd.

- The risk varies according to the organ transplanted, the serological status of donor and recipient and immunosuppressive drugs used. D+/R- has the highest risk for CMV disease.
- Prompt diagnosis can be made by Quantitative CMV DNA testing and in tissue invasive disease from the tissue biopsy. Valganciclovir and intravenous ganciclovir are effective treatment options.
- Preventive strategies employing valganciclovir is effective and can either be part of a universal prophylaxis regimen or as a component of preemptive therapy.
- Emerging problem of drug resistance needs to be addressed and newer treatment options require further validation.

Suggested Reading

1. Kaminski H, Fishman JA. The Cell Biology of Cytomegalovirus: Implications for Transplantation. Am J Transplant 2016;16(8):2254-69.
2. Ljungman P, Boeckh M, Hirsch HH, *et al.* Definitions of Cytomegalovirus Infection and Disease in Transplant Patients for Use in Clinical Trials. Clin Infect Dis 2017;64(1):87-91.
3. Hayden RT, Sun Y, Tang L, *et al.* Progress in Quantitative Viral Load Testing: Variability and Impact of the WHO Quantitative International Standards. J Clin Microbiol 2017;55(2):423-30.
4. Fisher CE, Alexander J, Bhattacharya R, *et al.* Sensitivity of blood and tissue diagnostics for gastrointestinal cytomegalovirus disease in solid organ transplant recipients. Transpl Infect Dis 2016;18(3):372-80.
5. Humar A, Limaye AP, Blumberg EA, *et al.* Extended valganciclovir prophylaxis in D+/R- kidney transplant recipients is associated with long-term reduction in cytomegalovirus disease: Two-year results of the IMPACT study. Transplantation 2010;90(12):1427-31.
6. Witzke O, Hauser IA, Bartels M, *et al.* Valganciclovir prophylaxis versus preemptive therapy in cytomegalovirus-positive renal allograft recipients: 1 year results of a randomized clinical trial. Transplantation 2012;93(1):61-68.
7. Helantera I, Lautenschlager I, Koskinen P. The risk of cytomegalovirus recurrence after kidney transplantation. Transpl Int 2011;24(12):1170-78.
8. Kotton CN, Kumar D, Caliendo AM, *et al.* The Third International Consensus Guidelines on the Management of Cytomegalovirus in Solid Organ Transplantation 2018. 10.1097/TP.0000000000002191.
9. Asberg A, Humar A, Rollag H, *et al.* Lessons Learned From a Randomized Study of Oral Valganciclovir Versus Parenteral Ganciclovir Treatment of Cytomegalovirus Disease in Solid Organ Transplant Recipients: The VICTOR Trial. Clin Infect Dis 2016;62(9):1154-60.
10. Chou S. Approach to drug-resistant cytomegalovirus in transplant recipients. Curr Opin Infect Dis 2015a;28:293-99.

CHAPTER 38

A Renal Transplant Recipient with Recurrent Urinary Tract Infections and Graft Dysfunction

Raj Kanwar Yadav[1], Kishore Kumar Ariga[2], Sushma Yadav[3]

[1]Associate Professor, Department of Nephrology, AIIMS, New Delhi
[2]Senior Resident, Department of Nephrology, AIIMS, New Delhi
[3]Senior Resident, Department of Obst and Gynae, SHKM GMC, Nalhar

CASE

Mr B, 35-year-old male, case of autosomal dominant polycystic kidney disease (ADPKD) which was diagnosed 6 years before renal transplantation, when he was 29 years old and he had a progressive course to end stage renal disease. He also had bilateral renal calculi with hydronephrosis in the past for which bilateral stenting was done. He underwent live renal transplantation with wife as a donor, basiliximab induction and triple drug immunosuppression (Tacrolimus, Mycophenolate and Prednisolone). During workup for transplantation, he was diagnosed to have multiple urethral strictures for which endoscopic dilation was done before transplant. Immediate post-transplant, he had a lowest serum creatinine of 1.1 mg/dl. He developed symptoms of dysuria and fever on POD7 and urine showed pus cells and culture grew E. coli for which sensitive antibiotics were given for 2 weeks and cultures became negative. He developed new onset diabetes post-transplant (NODAT) which was treated with insulin. After 3 months of transplantation he was again admitted with fever and dysuria and urine culture grew klebsiella and he received IV antibiotics for 4 weeks and was discharged on antibiotic prophylaxis. Uroflowmetry was suggestive of obstructive pattern because of stricture urethra and endodilatation was done. After one month of discharge from hospital he was admitted again with graft pyelonephritis with graft dysfunction (Serum creatinine-2 mg/dl). He again grew klebsiella and IV antibiotics were given for 6 weeks. Retrograde urethrogram and Micturating urtherogram showed grade III reflux in the graft. He was advised clean intermittent catheterisation to be done regularly and was discharged with normal serum creatinine and antibiotic prophylaxis for urinary tract infection (UTI). He had 3 further episodes of breakthrough UTI with graft dysfunction even on antibiotic prophylaxis. PET-CT ruled out possibility of cyst infection in native kidneys. After treating his UTI with adequate antibiotics his serum creatinine settled around 2.0 mg/dl which is stable for last 8 months.

This case describes a patient with ADPKD, post renal transplant on immunosuppression with multiple risk factors for UTI (stricture urethra, NODAT, prior urological procedure, immunosuppression, cyst infection, renal stones in the native kidney) and graft pyelonephritis leading to persistent graft dysfunction because of recurrent UTI.

Urinary Tract Infections in Renal Transplant Recipients

Renal transplantation is the treatment of choice for end stage renal disease patients (ESRD). Immunosuppression and altered genitourinary tract anatomy places these patients at high risk of infections and complications. Bacterial infections are a major cause of morbidity and mortality post renal transplantation. Urinary tract infections (UTI) are the most common infectious complication after renal transplantation. Fungal and Mycobacterial UTI can also occur post renal transplantation. Asymptomatic bacteriuria (ASB) has the highest incidence followed by cystitis, allograft pyelonephritis and urosepsis. Emphysematous allograft pyelonephritis is very rare.

Prevalence

Solid organ recipients developed UTI in 4.4% of patients in one large series. Renal transplant recipients had highest incidence of UTI among solid organ recipients with an incidence of 0.45 episodes per 1000 days of transplant and a frequency of 7.3% (82% had cystitis and 18% had pyelonephritis).[1] Incidence of UTI varies between studies from 4% to 75% mainly because of different diagnostic criteria used to diagnose UTI, different follow-up time after transplantation and including patients with ASB.

Clinical Definitions in Renal Transplant Patients[2]

Symptomatic UTI: UTI are defined by $>10^5$ CFU/ml from the urine sample with accompanying symptoms such as dysuria, suprapubic, flank or allograft pain, fever, or chills.

Asymptomatic Bacteriuria (ASB)

- **In men:** A single, clean-catch voided urine specimen with one bacterial species isolated in a quantitative count ≥ 10^5 CFU/ml in the absence of symptoms or signs of UTI.
- **In women:** Two consecutive voided urine specimens with isolation of the same bacterial strain in quantitative counts ≥ 10^5 CFU/ml in the absence of symptoms or signs of UTI.
- If a urine sample is collected through catheterisation, a single urine specimen with isolation of a single bacterial species in a quantitative count ≥ 100 CFU/ml is enough to identify bacteriuria in women or men.

Uncomplicated UTI: Outgrowth of bacteria with >10^5 CFU/ml from a properly collected urine sample, where the patient has symptoms of dysuria, frequency and urgency. Urinary tract is functionally normal.

Complicated UTI: Outgrowth of bacteria with >10^5 CFU/ml from a properly collected urine sample, where the patient has symptoms of fever, allograft pain, chills, malaise or bacteraemia with same organism in urine and blood. UTI with functional or structural renal tract abnormalities is also complicated UTI.

Recurrent UTI: ≥3 episodes in 1 year (OR) ≥2 episodes in 6 months.

Risk Factors

Most of the episodes of UTI occur in the initial 6 months of transplantation. Many factors promote the onset of UTI in a renal allograft recipient as follows: (Table 38.1).

Table 38.1: Risk factors predisposing to UTI in transplant recipients

Type	Factors
Recipient	Female gender Advanced age Recurrent UTI prior to renal transplantation Diabetes mellitus Urinary tract abnormalities (reflux, bladder dysfunction, Neurogenic bladder, Enlarged prostate, hydronephrosis) Prior urological operations Prolonged length of dialysis Re-transplantation
Organ	Deceased donor Duplicated ureter
Transplantation	Foreign material (ureteral stent, bladder catheter) Immunosuppressive regimen: Mycophenolate, azathioprine, Anti Thymocyte Globulin Acute rejection CMV infection Graft dysfunction Instrumentation of the urinary tract >2 episodes of ASB after transplantation

Diagnosis

The clinical features of classical UTI may be masked in transplant recipients due to surgical denervation of ureter and kidney along with immunosuppression. The diagnosis of UTI should not be based alone on classical symptoms. Cystitis generally presents with frequency, urgency, dysuria, hematuria and suprapubic pain. Sepsis may be the first presentation of UTI. Suspect UTI in renal allograft patients with fever, raised WBC counts, abdominal or graft site pain, sepsis or asymptomatic graft dysfunction. Acute allograft pyelonephritis is diagnosed on both clinical findings such as fever, pyuria and/or tenderness, along with an outgrowth of a microorganism in the urine culture.

Microbiology

Gram negative bacterial organisms account for the majority of UTIs post-transplant. *Escherichia coli* is the most common bacterium associated with UTI among transplant recipients. Other causative organisms for UTI are: *Klebsiella pneumoniae, Pseudomonas aeruginosa, Proteus mirabilis, Morganella morganii, Enterococcus faecalis, Enterobacter species, Corynebacterium urealyticum* and *Candida species.*

Candida albicans is the main cause of fungal UTI. Diabetics are more predisposed for fungal UTI and it is difficult to treat. Patients with indwelling catheters usually have polymicrobial infections. Studies have demonstrated up to 70% resistance in Gram positive and Gram negative organisms for TMP-SMX.

Initial Evaluation of UTI

1. Clinical examination
   a. Look for temperature, blood pressure, tachycardia.
   b. Graft site, loin and supra pubic tenderness.
   c. Check for enlarged and tender prostate, scrotal examination and vaginal atrophy.
2. Urine dipstick evaluation
   a. Nitrates, leukocyte esterase, blood and protein.
3. Urine microscopy, culture and sensitivity pattern.
4. Ultrasound KUB
   a. Native kidney, graft and bladder evaluation.
   b. Post void residual urine volume estimation.
5. Review excessive immunosuppression and initiate antibiotics.

Causes and Evaluation of Recurrent UTI

1. Calculi in graft or native kidneys
   a. X-rays, CT KUB
2. Complex cysts of kidneys
   a. CECT KUB

3. Cyst infection in polycystic kidneys
   a. PET-CT
4. Bladder dysfunction and outflow obstruction
   a. Uroflowmetry
   b. Urodynamic studies
   c. Cystoscopy
5. Reflux
   a. Micturating cystourethrogram
6. Transplant ureteric obstruction
   a. Renal dynamic scan

Additional investigations with instrumentation carries the risk of further infection during the procedure. Early post-transplant infection should prompt culture of transport medium to detect donor derived infection. It is important to rule out BK virus and CMV infection patients with pyelonephritis. Graft rejection and UTI can coexist simultaneously and the only way to distinguish is by graft biopsy.

Management of UTI

Complicated UTI after transplant requires initiation of empirical antibiotics covering both gram positive and gram-negative organisms. Infections of lower UTI without signs and sepsis can be managed on an outpatient basis but hospitalisation is required for pyelonephritis with intravenous antibiotics. After the initial therapy, definitive therapy should be guided by culture sensitivity reports. Third generation cephalosporins and carbapenems are usually needed in cases of graft pyelonephritis with renal dysfunction. Eradication of organisms should be confirmed with negative urine culture results. Drug interactions with immunosuppressive agents should be reviewed when antibiotics are initiated in renal transplant patients. Erythromycin, Rifampicin and azoles increase the levels of Cyclosporine and Tacrolimus. Trimethoprim decreases the levels of cyclosporin when administered intravenously. Aminoglycosides and Amphotericin increase nephrotoxicity. Oral fluoroquinolones (ofloxacin, ciprofloxacin), co-trimoxazole and fosfomycin can be given orally on outpatient basis (Fig. 38.1).

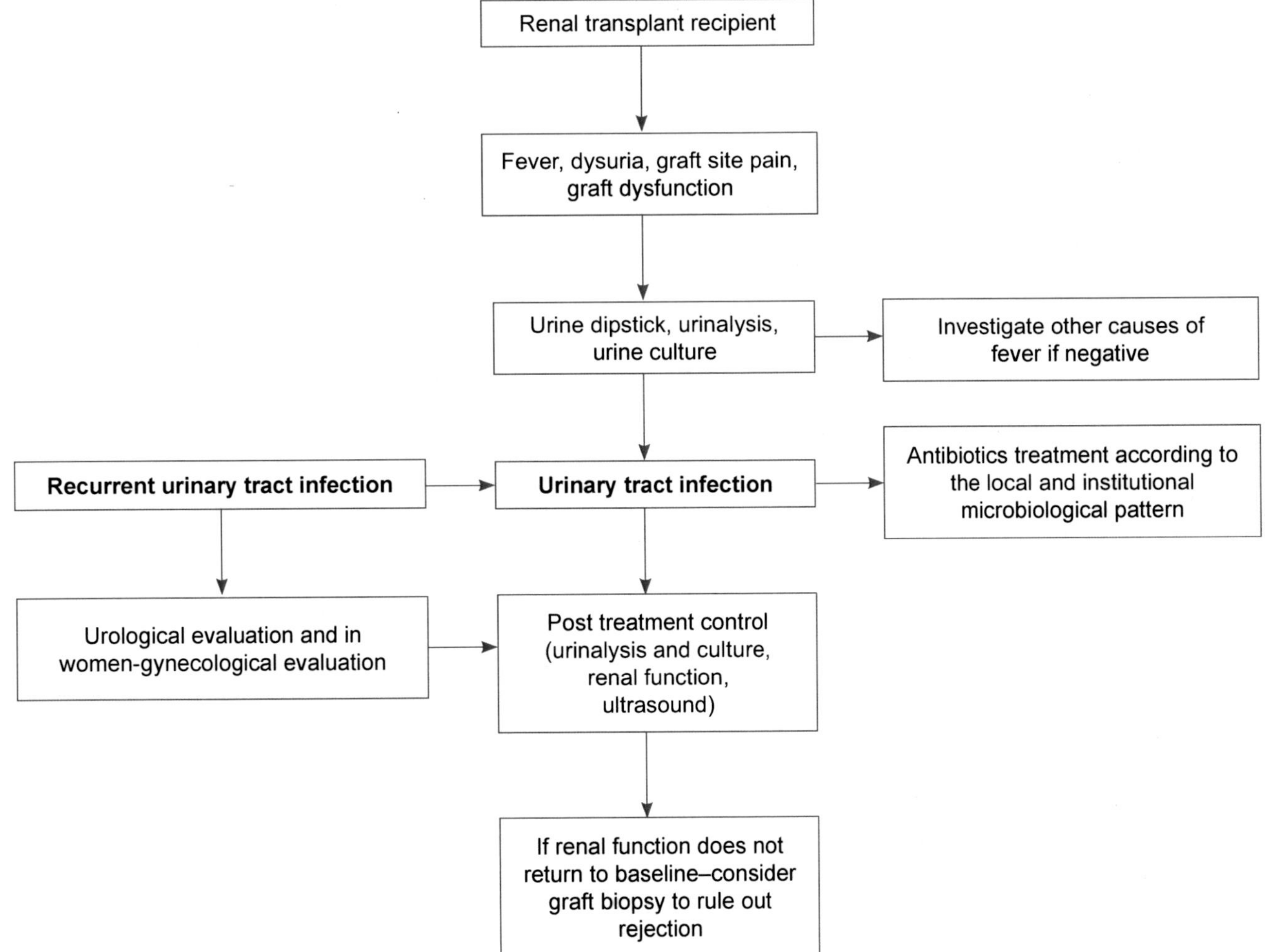

Figure 38.1: Algorithm for management of UTI in renal transplant recipients

Early (less than 6 months) uncomplicated UTIs needs to be treated for 10-14 days of antibiotics. Late uncomplicated UTIs can be treated with antibiotics for 5-7 days. Pyelonephritis and UTIs with systemic features require IV antibiotics for 2 weeks. Pyelonephritis may be associated with bacteremia, metastatic spread, impaired graft function and even death. Recurrent and relapsing UTIs should receive prolonged antibiotic course (4-6 weeks). Suspected foci of infection like stent should be identified and removed promptly.

Fungal UTI requires treatment with systemic antifungals like fluconazole or amphotericin B. Suggested fluconazole regimen for candida UTI is 200 mg stat followed by 100 mg once a day for a minimum 14 days. BK virus nephropathy requires decrease in immunosuppression as the mainstay of treatment.

Surgical management of UTI includes early removal of catheters and stents in the immediate post-transplant period, adequate drainage of urinary tract obstruction (percutaneous nephrostomy), detection and treatment of urinary tract calculi if present and drainage of infected cysts in native kidneys or nephrectomy.

Asymptomatic Bacteriuria–Is It Benign?

Incidence of asymptomatic bacteriuria (ASB) is reported variedly between studies ranging from 17 to 51%. Risk factors associated with ASB are female sex, delayed graft function, Foley's catheter use, glomerulonephritis as primary renal disease and re transplant. Persistent ASB is a risk factor for pyelonephritis. Renal scars may develop in patients with ASB. It can act as a local stimulus for immune reactivation in urinary tract and may be a risk factor for rejection. Increased levels of urinary IL-8 are reported in renal transplant recipients with ASB.

In a retrospective study of 189 transplant recipients followed over 3 years, 51% developed 298 episodes of ASB. Majority of episodes were within first year of transplant. Single episode of ASB was not associated with pyelonephritis, whereas 2–5 or more than 5 episodes of ASB were strongly associated with pyelonephritis. The incidence of pyelonephritis among recipients with ASB was 7.6 episodes per 100 patient years versus 1.07 episodes per 100 patient years among recipients without ASB.[3]

There are no clear recommendations for treatment of ASB. Many transplant physicians still, however, treat asymptomatic bacteriuria after transplantation. Reasons include the possibility that denervation of the kidney graft and the use of immunosuppressive medications mask the clinical features of UTI, and the fear that kidney transplant recipients may be at higher risk for developing severe infections. In a retrospective study, out of 334 episodes of ASB only 101 were treated with antibiotics. Despite the treatment 45 ASB episodes persisted with resistant organisms. Spontaneous clearance occurred in 59% of untreated patients.[4] In another retrospective study, the risk of developing symptomatic UTI was almost three times higher after the treatment of ASB in comparison to no treatment.

In a recent Cochrane review based on two studies, treating renal transplant recipients with asymptomatic bacteriuria had uncertain effects on preventing symptomatic UTI, and entailed uncertain risks for selecting resistant strains. Persistence of asymptomatic bacteriuria was high regardless of treatment and although the available data were limited, so far, there is no evidence to suggest antibiotic treatment of asymptomatic bacteriuria would improve patient and graft outcomes such as all-cause mortality, graft loss, acute rejection, hospitalisation for UTI or graft function.[5] Further studies are underway which may give us further information regarding this entity post-transplant.

Asymptomatic candiduria requires treatment with antifungals in renal transplant recipients as fungal UTIs have high rate of complications. In summary, frequent episodes of ASB are also associated with the development of UTIs such as allograft pyelonephritis. ASB itself does not impair renal allograft function but persistent ASB is associated with allograft pyelonephritis and acute rejection. Treatment of ASB does not seem to be very effective. Consider not treating ASB occurring more than 3 months after renal transplantation unless there is an increase in serum creatinine.

Outcomes of UTI

Effect of UTI on renal allograft function varies on the type of UTI whether the patient has cystitis vs pyelonephritis vs sepsis and recurrence. Few observational studies show that UTI does not impair the renal allograft function whereas graft pyelonephritis and septicemia have been shown to affect the graft function.

In a large single centre retrospective cohort study of 2469 renal transplant recipients 7% had recurrent UTI and 19% had non-recurrent UTI. Recurrent UTI had poor graft and patient survival compared to non-recurrent UTI and no UTI.[6]

Antimicrobial Prophylaxis

Perioperative prophylaxis with antibiotics is routinely recommended post transplant. Single dose of antibiotic (2nd or 3rd generation cephalosporin) before surgery and continuation in immediate post transplant period is practised to prevent surgical site and urinary tract infections. Most centres prescribe up to 6 months of antibiotic prophylaxis.

KDIGO guidelines for the care of kidney transplant recipients suggest that all recipients receive UTI prophylaxis with daily trimethoprim-sulfamethoxazole for at least 6 months after transplantation.[7] Co-trimoxazole administered also prevents the occurrence of pneumocystis infections. Use of cotrimoxazole for first 9 months after transplant was associated with significantly decreased number of bacterial infection, overall UTI and non-catheter UTI. Ciprofloxacin is also effective in prevention of UTI after kidney transplantation but patients who were treated with ciprofloxacin were at risk of Pneumocystis jiroveci pneumonia (PCP). So, Cotrimoxazole is preferred over ciprofloxacin for prevention of UTI in the first 6 months after transplantation. In patients allergic to Cotrimoxazole nitrofurantoin is the alternative that can be used.

In a systematic review on antibiotic prophylaxis for urinary tract infections in renal transplant recipients, prophylaxis lowered the risk of sepsis with bacteraemia and risk of bacteriuria (symptomatic and asymptomatic). All cause mortality and adverse events were not significantly different. Symptomatic UTI and pyelonephritis were not reported.[5]

BK Virus Nephropathy

BK virus is a ubiquitous, double stranded polyoma virus that replicates in the host nuclei. They cause clinical disease only in immunosuppressed host. It causes BK associated nephropathy, which is characterized by tubule interstitial disease, sometimes mimicking acute rejection. It can also cause ureteral strictures leading to obstructive disease. It usually occurs 2-4 months post transplant. The important risk factors for BK virus nephropathy are use of steroid pulses for rejection episode, use of anti thymocyte globulins, diabetes and older age.

Diagnosis of BK Virus Nephropathy

BK virus can be detected by DNA polymerase chain reaction both in blood and urine. Though the viruria appears earlier than viremia, the BK viremia is better predictor of nephropathy. A viral load of more than 10,000 copies is strongly associated with nephropathy. The urine examination may reveal "decoy cells", which have enlarged nuclei with a single basophilic intranuclear inclusion. The gold standard for diagnosis is graft biopsy, which shows tubule interstitial inflammation and intranuclear viral inclusions. These can be confirmed with immunohistochemistry.

Treatment of BK Virus Nephropathy

The mainstay of treatment is reduction of immuno-suppression; mostly stopping the mycophenolate and decreasing the dose of calcineurin inhibitors. Antiviral therapy with leflunamide or cidofovir has been used in conjunction with decrease in immunosuppression. Persistence of viremia is associated with progressive graft dysfunction and failure.

Key Points

- UTI is the most frequent infectious complication post-transplant with negative consequences for both patient and graft.
- Risk of UTI is multifactorial and depends on host, organism and anatomical factors.
- Mainstays of management are patient education, appropriate treatment of infective episodes, review of immunosuppressive therapy, and selective use of prophylactic antibiotics.
- Treatment of UTI should focus on narrow spectrum of antibiotics to prevent resistance.
- Treatment of ASB has uncertain effects on preventing symptomatic UTI but with risk of resistance emergence.

References

1. Vidal E, *et al.* Bacterial urinary tract infection after solid organ transplantation in the RESITRA cohort. Transpl. Infect. Dis. Off. J. Transplant. Soc 2012;14,595-603.
2. Hollyer I and Ison MG. The challenge of urinary tract infections in renal transplant recipients. Transpl. Infect. Dis. Off. J. Transplant. Soc 2018;20, e12828.
3. Fiorante S, *et al.* Systematic screening and treatment of asymptomatic bacteriuria in renal transplant recipients. Kidney Int 2010;78,774-81.
4. El Amari EB, *et al.* Outcome of treated and untreated asymptomatic bacteriuria in renal transplant recipients. Nephrol. Dial. Transplant. Off. Publ. Eur. Dial. Transpl. Assoc.-Eur. Ren. Assoc 2011;26,4109-14.
5. Coussement J, Scemla A, Abramowicz D, Nagler EV and Webster AC. Antibiotics for asymptomatic bacteriuria in kidney transplant recipients. Cochrane Database Syst. Rev. 2018;2,CD011357.
6. Britt NS, *et al.* Effects of recurrent urinary tract infections on graft and patient outcomes after kidney transplantation. Nephrol. Dial. Transplant. Off. Publ. Eur. Dial. Transpl. Assoc. - Eur. Ren. Assoc 2017;32,1758-66.
7. Kidney Disease: Improving Global Outcomes (KDIGO) Transplant Work Group. KDIGO clinical practice guideline for the care of kidney transplant recipients. Am. J. Transplant. Off. J. Am. Soc. Transplant. Am. Soc. Transpl. Surg 2009; 9 Suppl:3,S1-155.

CHAPTER

39

A Post Renal Transplant Recipient with Diarrhea

Ashish Nandwani[1], Arushi Nautiyal[2]

[1] *Consultant, Nephrology, Manipal Hospital, Dwarka, New Delhi*

[2] *Consultant, Nephrology, Jaipur Golden Hospital, Rohini, New Delhi*

CASE

A 30-year-old male with chronic kidney disease stage 5 underwent live renal transplant with his wife as donor. He was a 5/6 mismatch and received Anti-thymocyte globulin (ATG) as induction therapy with triple drug immunosuppression namely–tacrolimus, mycophenolate and prednisolone. He was treated for biopsy proven acute rejection 2 months after his transplant with pulse methyl prednisolone. At 3 months post transplant, he developed abdominal pain along with diarrhea along with low grade fever. His evaluation showed graft dysfunction with leucopenia. He was managed with IV hydration and broad spectrum antibiotics, however his diarrhea persisted. He underwent colonoscopy and biopsy was taken, which was suggestive of CMV colitis as cause of diarrhea. He was managed with IV Ganciclovir along with reduction in MMF doses. Patient responded to treatment with resolution of diarrhea and graft dysfunction.

Discussion

Renal transplants have helped patients with end stage renal disease attain better quality of life, as it allows freedom from dialysis and other complications associated with deranged renal functions. However long-term immunosuppression requirement in solid organ transplants are associated with increased risk of opportunistic infections, malignancies and drug related effects contributing adversely to overall wellbeing and mortality. Still renal transplant confer longer survival versus remaining on long-term dialysis and is thus the preferred mode of renal replacement therapy.

Gastrointestinal symptoms in the post transplant period are often under-reported by patients and not given due importance by treating physicians, though they can be associated with significant dimunition in quality of life. A higher than general population prevalence of inflammatory bowel syndrome associated with symptoms of anxiety and depression was reported in a Turkish cohort of renal transplant recipients.

Diarrhea is classified as per WHO as *acute watery* and *acute bloody* diarrhea which can last from hours to days; both can lead to dehydration, the latter also increases risk of developing sepsis. *Perisistent diarrhea* lasts 14 days or longer and can lead to malnutrition and dehydration. In a renal transplant recipient, the causes of diarrhea can vary from infective causes, medication induced, related to dietary intake, tumors or due to autoimmune conditions such as inflammatory bowel disease. Thus a variety of diagnostic tests are sometimes required to accurately ascertain the cause.

In the study by Bunnapradist *et al.*, post kidney transplant diarrhea was assessed in medicare beneficiaries enrolled in USRDS, cumulative incidence of diarrhea at 3 years post transplant was 22%, most cases were reported in the first year. Most cases had unspecified non-infectious etiology as cause of diarrhea.

Graft dysfunction can occur secondary to dehydration or altered drug levels of calcineurin inhibitors. Mycophenolate mofetil doses are often altered by treating physicians in absence of apparent infectious etiology of diarrhea, this can lead to increased risk of rejection and graft dysfunction. Tacrolimus exposure has been found to be increased in states of persistent diarrhea, this phenomenon has been ascribed to decrease of intestinal *P glycoprotein* which is involved in tacrolimus drug efflux, this can lead to several adverse effects including nephrotoxicity, necessitating monitoring of tacrolimus trough levels and dose modifications. *Chronic diarrhea* can cause development of malnutrition and weight loss, leading to morbidity and increased susceptibility to infections. Fat malabsorption in chronic diarrheal states can lead to excessive enteric oxalate absorption predisposing to renal oxalate crystal deposition, causing tubular injury and necrosis.

Lee *et al.*, looked at commensal flora in the gut in transplant recipients. They found altered flora and lesser commensals in patient with diarrhea in early post transplant period (3 months), however were unable to specify if diarrhea lead to alteration of gut microbiota or vice versa.

Causes of Diarrhea in a Renal Transplant Recipient

Infectious Causes

Gut related opportunistic infections are usually seen after the first month.

While enteric bacteria–E coli, salmonella spp., parasites such as giardia and viruses like rota virus are commonly responsible for causing diarrhea in the general as well as in transplant populations, organisms such as microsporidia, cryptosporidium and cytomegaloviruses are mostly reported in immunosuppressed patients.

The DIDACT study assessed diarrhea in renal transplant recipients presenting with severe diarrhea, it was able to detect a microbiological cause of diarrhea in 22 out of 108 patients, most commonly implicated organisms were bacteria followed by parasites, protozoans and then viruses. Coste *et al.*, studied techniques such as multiplex PCR versus standard cultures and assays for better detection of microbiological causes of diarrhea, they identified bacteria as most common pathogens followed by viruses and lastly parasites as assessed by both techniques.

Bacterial

The occurrence of *Clostridium difficile infection* (CDI) has been reported in various studies to range from 3-16% in renal transplant recipients, often in the first few months after transplant. It is typically related to antibiotic associated diarrhea and pseudomembranous colitis. It is diagnosed with presence of its toxin in stool, or by its endoscopic appearance of pseudomembrane. It can lead to development of abscesses, intestinal obstruction and fulminant colitis thus leading to morbidity and mortality rates between 2.3-8.5% in solid organ transplant recipients. *Risk factors* associated are age greater than 55 years, thymoglobulin use, recent hospital stay and length of stay and especially a recent use of antibiotics. Fluoroquinolones and cephalosporins have especially been linked to the very virulent strain BI/NAP1/027. The latest IDSA guidelines recommend oral Vancomycin or Fidaxomicin for 10 days even in non severe first episode, Metronidazole to be used if either of the two are unavailable. In recurrent episodes oral Vancomycin should be used as a tapered and pulsed regimen. Fecal microbiota transplantation (FMT) should be considered in case of multiple recurrences. Kelly *et al.* retrospectively assessed use of FMT in patients who were immunocompromised, 24% of the study population consisted of solid organ transplant recipients, use of FMT in recurrent CDI was seen to be associated with an overall cure rate of 89%.

Campylobacter jejuni enteritis commonly presents as acute self limiting diarrhea often associated with abdominal pain and fever in the general population, not necessitating treatment. It may also present with blood and mucus in feces resulting from colorectal inflammation. Severe colitis and even bacteremia are more commonly reported in the elderly or immunocompromised individuals, requiring antibiotic therapy. A zoonotic illness, chickens and poultry are a major source of infection along with unpasteurised milk. Amongst renal transplant diarrhea it has been detected in 4-10% cases by standard cultures and assays and upto 28% when detected by PCR. This organism is typically susceptible to Macrolides, Fluoroquinolones, Carbapenems and Aminoglycosides. Resistance to Fluoroquinolones is increasingly being detected, Azithromycin is often first line preferred drug.

Campylobacter spp along with enteropathogenic, enterotoxigenic strains of Escherichia coli are often implicated in traveller's diarrhea. Samonella spp, Shigella and other enteric pathogens such as Yersinia account for 2-3% cases of diarrhea.

Viruses

Cytomegalovirus (CMV) involving the gastrointestinal tract is its most common tissue invasive manifestation. It commonly presents as esophagitis, colitis with ulcerative lesions. The risk of CMV disease is greatest in patients with thymoglobulin induction and those with discordant CMV serologies, especially the D+/R- pair. Due to universal adoption of viral prophylaxis in high risk patients, a later onset of CMV disease has been seen which is reported to be upto 30% in D+/R- pair, occurring at a median of 61 days after stopping prophylaxis. Humar *et al.* were able to demonstrate a lower incidence of confirmed CMV disease in patients who were given prophylaxis for 200 days as opposed to 100 days upto 12 months post transplant. CMV GI disease is usually diagnosed by the identification of the virus in histopathology or its antigen by immunohistochemistry/ DNA hybridisation in tissue biopsies obtained upon endoscopic studies, as quantitative PCR detection in blood is often negative in CMV GI disease, however a study by Durand *et al.* revealed a differing sensitivity and specificity of PCR detection depending upon donor-recipient serologies pretransplant, a sensitivity of 100% was seen in D+/R- pair in liver and renal transplant recipients. Treatment requires IV Ganciclovir in severe disease followed by oral valganciclovir. Resistance to the first line drugs may necessitate use of drugs such as Foscarnet.

Norovirus infection is emerging as one of the leading causes of viral gastroenteritis. In immunocompetent persons it usually leads to a self limiting illness, however in immunocompromised individuals can often lead to chronic and relapsing diarrhea and its ensuing complications. In a retrospective analysis by Weil *et al.* who assessed renal transplant patients admitted for diarrhea, 16 out of 20 patients screened were positive for norovirus diarrhea, 94% of whom had chronic illness. These patients in comparison to bacterial or parasitic diarrheal infections had a greater weight loss at time of admission, prolonged course and a greater likelihood of requiring mycophenolate mofetil dose reduction. Most patients who were followed were also detected to have prolonged shedding of the virus. Renal dysfunction was also reported in several patients, with 81% developing acute kidney injury. The virus has also been known to evolve inside the host especially when associated with chronic infection, as evidenced by heterogenous strains detected in stool samples in such patients. Norovirus antigens and RNA can be detected in stools samples, quantitative PCR is the most commonly used measure. No antivirals for treatment or vaccines for prevention are presently available for Norovirus infections, though are in research stage. Thus hand and food hygiene remain the best modalities for prevention of infection. Change from calcineurin inhibitors to mammalian targets of rapamycin have been advocated perhaps due to an indirect antiviral activity. Antiviral activity has also been ascribed to nitazoxanide with studies detailing its ability to decrease duration of symptoms and help to clear the virus.These studies enrolled immunocompetent persons only, however case reports of its efficacy in immunocomporomised persons are also available mostly in bone marrow transplant recepients and recently a pediatric renal transplant recipient.

Adenovirus infections are generally more common in children, however, it has also been identified in adults associated with a 4.1% incidence. It also has a higher incidence in the first year post transplant, possibly related to higher immunosuppression during that period, induction therapy and absolute lymphocyte counts. Humar *et al.* summarised adenovirus infections in solid organ transplant recipients and identified gastrointestinal symptoms in 10% of their study population. Cidofovir can be used in severe infectious states.

Rotaviruses are also a common cause for diarrhea in general population and transplant recipients, though it is mostly associated with a self limiting illness.

Parasites

Parasitic infections of gastrointestinal tract in transplant recipients are usually associated with a low morbidity and are difficult to detect and diagnose as they are often asymptomatic. Intestinal *amebiasis* and *giardiasis* can present as diarrheal illness or unexplained eosinophilia, their course tends to resemble infections in immunocompetent persons.

However, opportunistic parasites such as Strongyloides, Microspsora, Cryptosporidium may lead to serious illness with reported fatal outcomes.

Strongyloides stercoralis is an endemic parasite in tropical areas. In a study at a tertiary centre in India, half of the patients in a study cohort diagnosed with strongyloides infection were immunocompromised. Eosinophilia is usually a common accompaniment, however use of corticosteroids leads to a blunting of this response, thus it is a poor marker in immunocompromised to assess for infection. Parasitic infection with strongyloides leads to autoinfection due to hatching of the eggs in the intestine of the host itself and blood invasion of larvae, which can lead to chronic or subclincal infections, serious illness is kept at bay by a person's immunity but is exaggerated in immunocompromised persons leading to syndrome of hyperinfection. It can present as disseminated disease in such patients leading to diarrhea, intestinal obstruction, pneumonia and even multiorgan failure due to massive proliferation of the larvae and organ invasion. Larvae detection in stool generally require multiple and fresh stool samples. Serology testing of IgM and IgG antibodies by ELISA are also useful especially with negative stool tests in patients with high suspicion. RT-PCR stool assays are useful in detecting active disease, though are not universally available. Diagnosis in disseminated illness is easier as large number of larvae can be dectected in stool or body fluids such as bronchoalveolar lavage, CSF. First line treatment is usually by ivermectin, alternative medication is albendazole. The duration of therapy in hyperinfection and disseminated states is usually till 2 weeks after persistent negative stool examination along with reduction of immunosuppression.

Cryptosporidium is a ubiquitous parasite, it infects the epithelial cells of the gastrointestinal tract, after being acquired through contaminated water or food. In immunocompromised persons it can lead to development of acute severe diarrhea or chronic/prolonged illness. In a tertiary centre in northern India, it was detected as a cause for diarrhea leading to hospitalisation in 28% post renal transplant recipients over an eleven- year period. This study also found the incidence of cryptosporidium diarrhea to be greater in persons on tacrolimus and MMF based immunosuppression, as opposed to cyclosporin and MMF regimen. Enterocyte infection by the parasite has been implicated in altered metabolism of tacrolimus by intestinal CYP3A4, leading to increased drug levels. The organism is usually identified by modified Ziehl-Nielsen staining in stool microscopy, serology by immunofluoresence or ELISA improves detection rates. Nitazoxanide is commonly used in treatment of cryptosporidial diarrhea, immunocompromised persons usually require longer duration of therapy, need for combination therapy in relapse cases with Azithromycin/fluoroquinolones or use of paromomycin have also been reported.

Microsporidioisis causing intestinal involvement and diarrhea has also been reported in solid organ transplant recipients. Most commonly implicated species being Enterocytozoon bieneusi which infects intestinal as well as biliary epithelia. Champion *et al.* described 10 renal transplant recipients with microsporidial diarrhea presenting as afebrile subacute diarrhea.

Diagnosis is by identification of spores in stool samples, which requires specialised techniques such as fluorescent marking of spore wall, PCR assays can also be utilised. Treatment has been most successful with reduction of immunosuppression, however Fumagilin, derived from Aspergillus fumigatus is a therapeutic option in patients in whom immunosuppression taper is not desirable. Use of this drug has been associated with cytopenias especially thrombocytopenia, it is also reported to cause decrease in trough levels of tacrolimus.

Drugs

Mycophenolate Mofetil

Mycophenolate mofetil is a commonly used drug in present day regimens, as its use has led to reductions in acute rejection rates and thus better graft survival, it also allows for dose reduction of calcineurin inhibitors. It has been commonly implicated in adverse gastrointestinal symptomatology in the post transplant period which often leads to dose reductions or discontinuation, increasing the risk of graft rejection. The GI symptoms associated with MMF are varied and can present as nausea, vomiting, diarrhea or even lead to malabsorption and weight loss. Selbst *et al.* studied the various histological changes in colonic biopsies in solid organ transplant patients on MMF presenting with diarrhea. They identified inflammatory bowel disease-like changes in 28%, graft-vs-host disease (GVHD)-like in 19%, colitis-like in 16% and ischemia like changes in 3%. It has also been implicated in causing duodenal villous atrophy. MMF induced GI toxicities are considered to be a result of mycophenolate acid, its active metabolite, it interferes with the de novo purine synthesis pathway affecting lymphocyte proliferation and also intestinal epithelial cell replication. MMF induced chronic diarrhea is also linked to increased risk of infection related diarrhea, especially norovirus. Reporting of GI symptoms has been found to be greater with higher dose use. Enteric coated Mycophenolate sodium (EC-MPS) was expected to ameliorate the gastrointestinal effects of MMF as local toxicity of MPA acyl metabolite has also been implicated in GI toxicity. EC-MPS delivers the drug in the small intestine and has been observed to achieve comparable peak concentrations to MMF. Although few open label trials have reported benefits in GI symptomatology after conversion, various randomised trials failed to show any significant difference. Gastrointestinal symptoms account for 20-39% of MMF dose changes as per few retrospective analyses, dose changes also lead to increased vulnerability of the graft, with almost two-fold increase in risk of rejections with >50% dose reduction. Thus all possible alternative causes should be excluded, non immunosuppressive drugs should be minimised before considering changes to MMF prescription.

Calcineurin Inhibitors (CNI)

Diarrhea has been associated with use of CNIs especially when in combination with MMF. Amongst them, tacrolimus has been more commonly implicated, as per Symphony trial, patients receiving low dose tacrolimus with MMF group had a greater incidence of diarrhea as compared to standard or low dose cyclosporine with MMF. Similar results were reported by Heller *et al.*, wherein within one year of renal transplantation, 31% of patients on tacrolimus developed diarrhea as opposed to 12% patients on cyclosporine. Cyclosporine reduces enterohepatic recirculation of MMF metabolites, whereas tacrolimus does not which leads to greater intestinal exposure and toxicity with the metabolites. Tacrolimus is also associated with increased intestinal motility by its interaction with motilin receptors in the gastrointestinal tract. Tacrolimus levels also increase in diarrheal states, thus leading to a vicious cycle. A subanalysis of the data of Symphony trial also reported higher tacrolimus levels prior to developing diarrhea. Though diarrhea with tacrolimus is usually mild and responsive to dosage reduction, rarely severe forms have been reported leading to malnutrition.

Mammalian Target of Rapamycin Inhibitors

The Symphony trial showed a greater frequency of diarrhea in patients on Sirolimus/MMF versus cyclosporine/MMF. The etiological mechanism is not understood yet. Its use is mostly associated with self limiting diarrhea.

Miscellaneous

Diarrhea in renal transplant recipient can also result from malabsorption syndromes such as *Celiac disease*, pre-existing or de novo *inflammatory bowel disease*, even *post transplant lymphoproliferative disorder* involving GI tract can present as chronic diarrhea. Such causes should always be considered and excluded in difficult diagnoses via serology, endoscopic evaluations and colonic biopsies. Use of non immunosuppressive medications such as proton pump inhibitors, antihypertensives, colchicine, antibiotics, iron supplements should also be minimised.

Diagnostic Evaluation of a Post Renal Transplant Diarrhea

Observations and interventions in the DIDACT study showed that discontinuing/minimising non immunosuppressive medication and appropriate management of infections allowed for no change in ongoing immunosuppression in 50% cases. Thus in evaluating chronic diarrhea in this population, non immunosuppressive drug prescription should be revised, standard stool cultures for bacteria, assessment for parasites–cyst and ova, CMV viremia should be first line investigations. Commercially available Multiplex PCRs can also be utilised as they allow for better detection of pathogenic organsims such as Campylobacter species, enteropathogenic and enterotoxigenic E. coli, Shigella species, Salmonella species, Yersinia, Clostridium difficile, Cryptosporidium, Enterocytozoon bieneusi, Enteric viruses (rotavirus, adenovirus, norovirus, and enterovirus). However these are not universally available and due to high sensitivity may detect non disease producing bacteria in stool samples such as eneteropathogenic E coli. Empirical antibiotics can be started in patients with febrile diarrhea, which are required long-term in small intestinal bacterial overgrowth syndrome mostly suspected with mixed culture growth. Endoscopic evaluations in DIDACT study did not provide significant contribution in diagnostic evaluation in majorty of its study population. However upper GI ensodcopies/colonoscopies should be undertaken in patients presenting with bloody diarrhea, significant weight loss, family history of inflammatory bowel disease as post transplant lymphoproliferative disorder, inflammatory bowel disease, CMV colitis are often diagnosed on such evaluations. If such history or suspicions are not present, they may be done if there is no resolution or recurrence of symptoms despite antimicrobial therapy or change of immunosupression. Tacrolimus and Sirolimus trough levels should be monitored and doses altered on their bases, as with tacrolimus high levels can lead to diarrhea as well as result from diarrheal states. MMF is most frequently modified in persistent diarrhea, an attempt to change to enteric coated MPS should be made, else dose reduced. If > 50% dose reduction is expected, a change to azathioprine can be considered as an alternate to MMF.

Diarrhea in a renal transplant recipient is often multifactorial and involve an interplay between degree of immunsuppression, drug related factors and infectious causes especially opportunistic infections. Other causes such as tumors, inflammatory bowel pathology should also be ruled out. Diarrhea in this population should be addressed before it leads to significant malabsorption or weight loss as it can increase morbidity and mortality.

Suggested Reading

1. Ponticelli C, Colombo D, Novara M, Basilisco G. Gastrointestinal symptoms impair quality of life in Italian renal transplant recipients but are under-recognized by physicians. Transpl Int 2010;23:1126-34.
2. Ekberg H, Kyllönen L, Madsen S, Grave G, Solbu D, Holdaas H. Clinicians Underestimate Gastrointestinal Symptoms and Overestimate Quality of Life in Renal Transplant Recipients: A Multinational Survey of Nephrologists. Transplantation 2007;84:1052-54.
3. Bunnapradist S, Neri L, Wong W, Lentine KL, Burroughs TE, Pinsky BW Incidence and Risk Factors for Diarrhea Following Kidney Transplantation and Association With Graft Loss and Mortality Am J Kidney Dis 2008;51:478-86.
4. Aulagnon F, Scemla A, DeWolf S, Legendre C, Zuber J. Diarrhea After Kidney Transplantation: A New Look at a Frequent Symptom. Transplantation 2014;98:806-16.
5. Shin HS, Chandraker A. Causes and management of postrenal transplant diarrhea: An underappreciated cause of transplant-associated morbidity. Curr Opin Nephrol Hypertens 2017;26.
6. Coste JF, Vuiblet V, Moustapha B, *et al.* Microbiological diagnosis of severe diarrhea in kidney transplant recipients by use of multiplex PCR assays. J Clin Microbiol 2013; 51:1841-49.
7. Maes B, Hadayab K, de Moore B, Cambierd P, Peeterse P, de Meesterf J. Results of the DIDACT Study. American Journal of Transplantation 2006;6:1466-72.
8. Fitzgerald C J, Whichard J and Nachamkin I. Diagnosis and antimicrobial susceptibility of Campylobacter species. In: Campylobacter, Nachamkin I, Szymanski CM, and Blaser MJ (Eds), ASM Press, Washington, DC 2008;227-43.
9. Arthurs SK, Eid AJ, Pedersen RA, Kremers WK, Cosio FG, Patel R. Delayed-Onset Primary Cytomegalovirus Disease and the Risk of Allograft Failure and Mortality after Kidney Transplantation. Clinical Infectious Diseases 2008;46: 840-46.
10. Jang EY, Park SY, Lee EJ, Song EH, Chong YP, Lee SO. Diagnostic performance of the cytomegalovirus (CMV) antigenemia assay in patients with CMV gastrointestinal disease. Clin Infect Dis 2009;48(12):e121-24.
11. Valar C, Keitel E, Dal Prá RL, Gnatta D, Santos AF *et al.* Parasitic Infection in Renal Transplant Recipients. Transplantation Proceedings 2007;39:460-62.
12. Bhadauria D, Goel A, Kaul A, Sharma RK, Gupta A, Ruhela V, Gupta A *et al.* Cryptosporidium infection after renal transplantation in an endemic area. Transpl Infect Dis 2015; 17:48-55.
13. Ciancio G, Miller J, Gonwa TA. Review of Major Clinical Trials with Mycophenolate Mofetil in Renal Transplantation. Transplantation 2005;80:S191-S200.
14. Weclawiak H, Ould-Mohamed A, Bournet B, Guilbeau-Frugier C, Fortenfant F, Muscari F *et al.* Duodenal villous atrophy: A cause of chronic diarrhea after solid-organ transplantation. Am J Transplant 2011;11(3):575-82.
15. Helderman JH, Goral S. Gastrointestinal complications of transplant immunosuppression. J Am Soc Nephrol 2002; 13:277.

CHAPTER

40 A Post Renal Transplant Patient with Post Transplant Diabetes Mellitus

Manish Jain[1], Abhishek Garg[2]

[1] Director, Medanta, The Medicity, Gurugram

[2] Consultant, Nephrology, Maharaja Agarsen Hospital, New Delhi

CASE

A 50-year-old male with chronic kidney disease (CKD)–basic disease being autosomal dominant polycystic kidney disease, underwent live renal transplant with his wife as donor. He was a 5/6 mismatch and received Anti-thymocyte globulin (ATG) as induction therapy with triple immunosuppression namely–tacrolimus, mycophenolate and prednisolone. He was treated for biopsy proven acute rejection 2 months after his transplant. He also gives history of hepatitis C infection which was treated after the transplant. At 6 months post transplant, he developed increased frequency of urination. His labs are creatinine-1.5 mg/dl, fasting blood sugar 94 mg/dl, 2 hours post prandial blood sugar–214 mg/dl and HbA1c 7.2. His family history is significant for presence of diabetes in his mother. This patient has developed post transplant diabetes mellitus (PTDM).

Discussion

Renal transplantation has now become standard of care for end stage renal disease (ESRD) and is associated with survival advantage as well as better quality of life as compared to patients on dialysis. Diabetes is an important complication following solid organ transplantation. It was first described in 1964 following liver transplant and was subsequently described in all solid organ transplants. Different studies have shown that development of PTDM increases the risk for long-term cardiovascular adverse events as compared with patients who do not develop diabetes post transplant. In addition, PTDM is accepted as a strong independent risk factor for global mortality and graft failure.

Over the years, different names like steroid induced diabetes, transplant associated hyperglycemia, new-onset diabetes after transplantation (NODAT) and post transplant diabetes mellitus (PTDM) have been used to describe diabetes developing after transplant. Until recently NODAT was the preferred name. However in 2014, the International Expert Panel consisting of transplant nephrologists, diabetologists, surgeons and clinical scientists recommended changing the terminology NODAT back to PTDM. These investigators also suggested excluding transient post transplant hyperglycemia from diagnosis of PTDM.

Historically different definitions have been used to diagnose post transplant diabetes mellitus (PTDM) which has resulted in wide variations in reported incidence in literature. To overcome this lack of standard definition, International Consensus Guidelines were set by panel of experts from fields of diabetes and transplant in 2003. They recommended that PTDM should be diagnosed based on definition of diabetes mellitus as described by World Health Organization (WHO) and American Diabetes Association (ADA) for general population (Table 40.1).

The incidence of PTDM in analysis of United States Renal Data System (USRDS) data was 16% at the end of 12 months. Recent studies in era of tacrolimus put incidence of PTDM to be around 20%. Studies from India have shown incidence of PTDM ranging from 16% to as high as 34%.

Risk Factors

Multiple risk factors have been identified for development of PTDM. Certain risk factors are not modifiable like patient age, ethnicity, genetic background, Autosomal dominant polycystic kidney disease (ADPKD) as a cause of CKD, pre-transplant impaired blood glucose tolerance and family history of diabetes.

Table 40.1: Current criteria as per ADA guidelines to diagnose PTDM
1. Symptoms of diabetes and Random Plasma Glucose > 200 mg/dl (11.1 mmol/l) or
2. Fasting Plasma Glucose (FBG) ≥126 mg/dl (7.0 mmol/l) or
3. Two-hour Post Glucose >200 mg/dl (11.1 mmol/l) during an Oral Glucose Tolerance Test (OGTT)

Amongst modifiable factors are obesity, metabolic syndrome, HLA antigen mismatch and drugs like steroids, Calcineurin inhibitors (CNI) which includes cyclosporine and tacrolimus.

Hepatitis C virus (HCV) infection and Cytomegalo virus infection (CMV) infection are considered as risk factors which can be potentially modified with timely treatment (Table 40.2).

Demographics

Age has been universally accepted as a significant risk factor for PTDM. Investigators from different parts of world have found that risk of PTDM is significantly higher in recipient who are in 5th decade of their life or higher. Studies done in India have also consistently shown age to be a significant risk factor for PTDM.

Male gender has been considered as risk factor for PTDM by some investigators but most of the studies have not been able to confirm this association.

ADPKD has been variably shown as a risk factor for PTDM but the underlying mechanisms associating PTDM and ADPKD are not yet known. A possible explanation is that some genes interfering with insulin secretion and hepatic gluconeogenesis are co transmitted with ADPKD gene mutations.

Obesity

Obesity is associated with peripheral insulin resistance which in turn may lead to increased chances of developing PTDM. Increasing BMI, especially >30 kg/m^2 increases the risk of PTDM significantly as was shown in analysis of both Organ Procurement and Transplantation Network (OPTN) and USRDS data.

Family History

A positive family history has been associated with high chances of developing PTDM in kidney allograft recipients. Interestingly as per Indian studies 50-60% of kidney allograft recipients who develop PTDM have a family history of diabetes. This makes it all the more important for us to be aware of family history of diabetes in our transplant patients.

Infections

Hepatits C has been shown to be a risk factor for PTDM. Exact mechanism by which hepatitis C increases risk of diabetes is not clear but both insulin resistance and islet cell damage are thought to play a role. However all these studies were done in an era when directly acting anti virals were not available. It remains to be seen if the risk for developing PTDM remains same with early and effective treatment of Hepatitis C with newer directly acting anti virals (DAA).

CMV infection has also been shown to increase the risk by two- to four-fold for developing PTDM. Most likely mechanism is apoptosis of beta cells of pancreas.

Hypomagnesemia

Earlier studies have shown conflicting results between serum magnesium levels and PTDM. However, a meta analysis done in 2016 confirmed the association between hypomagnesemia and PTDM. Further large studies are needed to confirm the risk associated with hypomagnesemia and effect of magnesium supplements.

Immunosuppression

Choice of induction agent is not universally accepted as a risk factor for PTDM. Only a few studies have shown that induction with Basiliximab is associated with higher chances of development of PTDM while most of the studies did not find any difference.

Glucocorticoids are perhaps the oldest immuno-suppressive agents in use. They are associated with

Table 40.2: Risk factors for PTDM

Modifiable	Non modifiable	Potentially modifiable
Obesity	Age	Hepatitis C
Steroids	Ethnicity and race	Cytomegalovirus infection
Calcineurin inhibitors	Family history	
	Impaired glycemia	
	ADPKD	
Transplant related	**Unrelated to transplant**	
Steroids	Age	
Calcineurin inhibitors	Ethnicity and race	
Cytomegalovirus infection	Family history	
	Impaired glycemia	
	Obesity	
	Hepatitis C	

hyperglycemia and risk of diabetes, both in normal as well as post transplant population. Predominant mechanism is by increased peripheral insulin resistance. Glucocorticoids impair insulin mediated glucose uptake by directly interfering with components of the insulin signalling cascade.

Even though steroid withdrawal has consistently shown to decrease the incidence of PTDM but this reduction has to be weighed against increased risk of Biopsy proven acute rejection which often necessitates use of intermittent high doses of steroids. Rejection episodes treated with steroid pulses have been shown to increase the risk of developing PTDM. So any attempt to reduce the risk of PTDM by alteration in immunosuppression must be weighed against the increased risk of rejection and its consequences.

Even though both cyclosporine and tacrolimus are associated with PTDM, tacrolimus has been observed to be more diabetogenic. CNIs impair the functioning of islet cells by inhibiting nuclear factor of activated T cells (NFAT) pathway. They also cause pancreatic islet cells damage in form cytoplasmic swelling and vacuolization (tacrolimus more than cyclosporine). A meta-analysis by Heisel *et al.* found that insulin-treated diabetes occurred in 9.8% of renal transplant recipients on tacrolimus versus 2.7% on cyclosporine. This increased risk of PTDM with tacrolimus was observed across liver, heart and lung transplant groups as well. In USRDS data, the unadjusted cumulative incidences of PTDM at 3, 12 and 36 months were 13.5%, 22.1% and 31.8%, respectively for patients receiving tacrolimus, compared with 7.8%, 14.2% and 21.9% kidney allograft recipients not receiving tacrolimus.

Efficacy Limiting Toxicity Elimination (ELITE) study also support this increased risk of PTDM with tacrolimus as compared to cyclosporine and sirolimus. Another study showed that number of tacrolimus trough levels >15 ng/ml in first month post transplant was significantly associated with increased risk of PTDM.

In contrast to the effects of calcineurin inhibitors, the use of azathioprine and Mycophenolate mofetil (MMF) is not associated with a higher risk of diabetes. In fact in one large study they were associated decreased risk of PTDM (Azathioprine – 16% lower risk and MMF – 22% lower risk). The reasons for these associations are not clear, but it is possible that the use of MMF or azathioprine allowed use of lower doses of calcineurin inhibitors which are more likely to cause PTDM.

Sirolimus has also been shown to be associated with increased risk of PTDM in kidney transplant recipients.

Patient and Graft Outcomes

PTDM has been associated with increased risk of major cardiovascular events, cardiovascular mortality and overall mortality in post renal transplant population. Rates of graft failure are also increased. However, association with death censored graft failure is heterogeneous, with most of studies reporting no association of PTDM with death censored graft failure. A possible explanation for association between PTDM and death censored graft survival found in few studies could be due to confounding factor of acute rejection.

Diabetes in general is accepted as a risk factor for infection in general population. Post transplant patients by virtue of being treated with immunosuppressive medications are at a higher risk for infections. Siraj *et al.* in retrospective analysis found infectious complications to be significantly higher in patients who developed PTDM as compared to those who did not have PTDM (52% vs 30%, p=0.036).

Management

In view of potential harmful effects of PTDM on long term patient and graft outcomes, it is imperative that PTDM be managed early and effectively. Lifestyle modifications in form of incorporation of healthy eating habits, regular exercise and weight loss in those who are overweight seems prudent at earliest sign of impaired glucose metabolism. Timely introduction of therapy in form of oral hypoglycemic drugs and insulin to adequately control PTDM appears to be a logical step. Role of newer agents like GLP-1 analogues and SGLT-2 inhibitors needs more scrutiny before they can be used in this specific subset of population. In order to achieve better control of PTDM, change of immunosuppression from more diabetogenic tacrolimus to less diabetogenic cyclosporine has been studied. The results however are mixed. Also any attempt to change immunosuprressive therapy has to be weighed against the chances of acute rejection.

Suggested Reading

1. Cosio FG, Kudva Y, Velde MVD, Larson TS, Textor SC, Griffin MD, *et al.* New onset hyperglycemia and diabetes are associated with increased cardiovascular risk after kidney transplantation. Kidney International 2005;67(6):2415-21.
2. Hjelmesæth J, Hartmann A, Leivestad T, Holdaas H, Sagedal S, Olstad M, *et al.* The impact of early-diagnosed new-onset post-transplantation diabetes mellitus on survival and major cardiac events. Kidney International 2006;69(3):588-95.
3. Sharif A, Hecking M, Vries APJD, Porrini E, Hornum M, Rasoul-Rockenschaub S, *et al.* Proceedings From an International Consensus Meeting on Post transplantation Diabetes Mellitus: Recommendations and Future Directions. American Journal of Transplantation 2014 Jun;14(9):1992-2000.
4. Davidson J, Wilkinson A, Dantal J, Dotta F, Haller H, Hernandez D, *et al.* New-Onset Diabetes After Transplantation: 2003 International Consensus Guidelines 1. Transplantation 2003;75 (Supplement).

5. Prakash J, Rathore SS, Singh TB, Choudhury TA, P, U. New onset diabetes after transplantation (NODAT): Analysis of pre-transplant risk factors in renal allograft recipients. Indian Journal of Transplantation 2012;6(3):77-82.
6. Lakshminarayana GR, Sheetal LG, Anil M, Rajesh R, George K, Unni VN. New Onset Diabetes after Renal Transplantation (NODAT): Prevalence, Risk Factors and Treatment. Journal of Medical Science and Clinical Research 2016;4(1):8969-75.
7. Bora G, Guleria S, Reddy V, Tandon N, Gupta N, Gupta S, *et al.* Risk Factors for the Development of New-Onset Diabetes Mellitus in a Living Related Renal Transplant Program. Transplantation Proceedings 2010;42(10): 4072-73.
8. Sanyal D, Das P, Gupta S, Bhattacharjee K. Evaluation of Pre-Transplant Risk Factors as Independent Predictors on the New Onset of Diabetes after Renal Transplants (NODAT). Journal of endocrinology and thyroid research 2017;2(1):1-4.
9. Kasiske BL, Snyder JJ, Gilbertson D, Matas AJ. Diabetes Mellitus After Kidney Transplantation in the United States. American Journal of Transplantation 2003;3(10):178-85.
10. Shah T, Kasravi A, Huang E, Hayashi R, Young B, Cho YW, *et al.* Risk Factors for Development of New-Onset Diabetes Mellitus After Kidney Transplantation 2006;82(12):1673-76.
11. Patel DD, Modi KP, Patel AK, Chaudhary V. New Onset of Diabetes Mellitus in Indian Renal Transplant Recipient–A Retrospective Study. International Journal of Pharmacy and Pharmaceutical Sciences 2015;7(11):228-32.
12. Santos L, Rodrigo E, Piñera C, Quintella E, Ruiz JC, Fernández-Fresnedo G, *et al.* New-onset Diabetes After Transplantation: Drug-Related Risk Factors. Transplantation Proceedings 2012;44(9):2585-87.
13. Matas AJ, Gillingham KJ, Humar A, Ibrahim HN, Payne WD, Gruessner RWG, *et al.* Posttransplant Diabetes Mellitus and Acute Rejection: Impact on Kidney Transplant Outcome. Transplantation 2008;85(3):338-43.
14. Siraj E, Abacan C, Chinnappa P, Wojtowicz J, Braun W. Risk Factors and Outcomes Associated with Posttransplant Diabetes Mellitus in Kidney Transplant Recipients. Transplantation Proceedings 2010;42(5):1685-89.

CHAPTER 41

A Post Renal Transplant Recipient with Post Transplant Lymphoproliferative Disorder

Aniket Hase[1], **Ashish Nandwani**[2]

[1] *Consultant, Nephrologist and Renal Transplant Physician, Jupiter Hospital, Thane, Maharashtra*

[2] *Consultant, Nephrologist and Renal Transplant Physician, Manipal Hospital, New Delhi*

CASE

A 32 years old female, underwent renal transplant for her end stage renal disease 2 years back. Her native kidney disease was reflux nephropathy. Donor was her husband (36 years old). She received induction with anti thymocyte globulin (ATG) 3 mg/kg. She was on triple drug immunosuppressants: Tacrolimus 1.5 mg twice a day, Mycophenolate 500 mg twice a day and prednisolone 5 mg once a day. Her HbsAg, HCV and HIV markers were negative. Her graft function was stable. Sr Creatinine varied between 1-1.3 mg/dl. Her tacrolimus trough level was 4.5 ng/ml. HLA had all six antigens mismatch, lymphocyte crossmatch was negative.

Two years post transplant patient presented with low grade fever mainly in evening, loss of appetite and loss of weight. She gave history of distention and pain in abdomen, and loose motions intermittently. There was no blood or mucus in stool. Diarrhea persisted despite of stopping mycophenolate. There was no history of cough, hemoptysis, no history of joint pains and bone pains. She was treated with metronidazole and doxycycline.

Physical examination revealed anemia, pulse was 110/min collapsing. Blood pressure was 150/70 in right upper limb in supine position. There was generalized wasting of muscles and edema. Abdominal examination showed hepatosplenomegaly with free fluid in abdomen. There was non tender lump in right iliac fossa separate from transplanted kidney. Cardiovascular system examination revealed normal heart sounds with ejection systolic murmur in left 2nd space. Respiratory system and nervous system were unremarkable.

Laboratory investigation revealed normocytic normochromic anemia with mild thrombocytopenia. Urine revealed proteinuria 600 mg/24 hours without active sediment. Sr. creatinine was 1.3 mg/dl. Sr. proteins were 6.8 g/dl and albumin 2.8 g/dl. Alkaline phosphatase was 500 IU, markedly raised LDH 1800 IU, ALT 20, AST 15 IU. Blood glucose was 80 mg/dl. X-ray chest showed mediastinal widening. CT chest showed mediastinal lymph node enlargement. CT abdomen showed hepatosplenomegaly with ileocecal mass and ascites. Transplant kidney was slightly enlarged. No dilatation of PCS. Para aortic lymph nodes were enlarged. PET CT showed metabolically active focus in chest and abdomen. CT guided biopsy of lymph node showed diffuse large B cell lymphoma. EBV DNA was positive with 220860 copies per ml. BKV blood and urine PCR was negative. Bone marrow examination was unremarkable. Patient's mycophenolate was stopped and dose of tacrolimus was reduced by 50%. Patient received cycle of CHOP and Rituximab. Before 2nd cycle she developed bilateral pneumonia and succumbed to septic shock and acute respiratory distress syndrome (ARDS).

Discussion

The renal transplant remains the best treatment modality for ESRD patient. The long-term risk of rejection vs infection and malignancy has been increasing. Lymphoproliferative malignancies are one of the most common malignancies in solid organ transplant recipient.

Incidence

This is the most serious and fatal complication of chronic administration of immunosuppressive drugs. The overall incidence of Post Transplant Lymphoproliferative Disorder (PTLD) is 0.6% to 1.5% of patients after kidney transplantation.[1] It is 30-50 times higher than general population. The incidence is highest in first year when recipients are receiving highest dose of immunosuppressant.[2]

Risk factors: The major risk factors implicated in pathogenesis of PTLD are the overall net immunosuppression and Epstein-Barr Virus (EBV) positivity. Patient who are EBV negative and receive grafts from EBV positive individuals are at highest risk of acquiring infection and PTLD. EBV is incorporated into B lymphocytes during primary infection. EBV infected B cells are thought to be normally "held in check" by cytotoxic T cells. This defense mechanism of immunosurveillance is lost because of T cell immunosuppression, promoting development of PTLD.[3] The other risk factors reported are advance age or pediatric age, HLA mismatch in unrelated donors, administration of antithymocyte globulin or anti CD3 antibody, pre-transplant malignancies and chronic graft versus host disease.

Classification

According to WHO classification three main types of PTLD have been described in transplant recipients.[4]

1. Early lesions characterized by polyclonal B cell proliferation with no evidence to suggest malignant transformation.
2. Polymorphic PTLD are polyclonal or monoclonal lymphoid infiltrate that demonstrate evidence of malignant transformation but do not meet all the criteria's for one of the B cell or T/NK cell lymphomas recognized in immunocompetent patient.
3. Monomorphic PTLD is characterized by monoclonal lymphoid proliferations that meet the criteria for one of the B cell or T/NK cell lymphomas. The most common subtype is diffuse large B cell lymphoma. Other types are Plasma cell myeloma and peripheral T cell lymphoma. Classical Hodgkin's lymphoma like PTLD is rarely reported in renal transplant recipients. More than 80% of post-transplant lymphomas are of B-cell origin; approximately 15% are T-cell lymphomas.

Clinical Presentation

The clinical presentation of PTLD is highly variable. The most common presentation of PTLD is fever, weight loss, malaise, fatigue and non-specific constitutional symptoms. The lymphadenopathy is common. The extra nodal involvement occurs in more than 2/3 of cases. It may involve allograft like heart, kidney, lung, bowel transplant and up to 10% to 15% of PTLD present with central nervous system involvement. EBV negative PTLD may present later (6.4 versus 1.5 years post transplantation) as compared to EBV positive PTLD and are much more virulent with median survival of 1 versus 37 months. EBV negative PTLD has been reported in up to 30%.[5] This clinical presentation can mimic tuberculosis, atypical mycobacterial infection and fungal infections.

Diagnosis

Diagnosis of PTLD is challenging task and requires high index of suspicion. Positive positron emission tomography favors and highly suggestive of PTLD. PET-CT also useful evaluating response to therapy. Gold standard remains biopsy and histopathology. CT abdomen, Chest and bone marrow is required for staging purposes.

Treatment

Early lesions are managed by reduction of immunosuppressants alone. Decreasing cyclosporine or tacrolimus by 50% and discontinuing azathioprine or mycophenolate mofetil is often recommended. Approximately 25%-50% of patients respond to reduction in immunosupprression alone.[6-8]

Polymorphic PTLD that express CD 20 can be managed by reduction of immunosupprression and Rituximab. In monomorphic PTLD, suggested treatment in addition to reduction of immunosuppression is rituximab and chemotherapy such as CHOP (cyclophosphamide, prednisolsone, doxorubicin, vincristine). CHOP with rituximab has overall response rate of 90%.[9] The role of antiviral therapy with acyclovir or gancyclovir has been controversial. Antiviral agents may be effective in patients with early or polymorphic disease, but there has been no clear benefit for antiviral therapy demonstrated in monomorphic disease in which transformed B lymphocytes do not have actively replicating EBV infection. Radiation Therapy modality is typically used to treat CNS disease.[10] A Case reports of successful autologous stem cell transplants in patients with chemotherapy-sensitive PTLD at relapse have been reported with preservation of graft function.[11]

Prognosis

The prognosis in PTLD varies with clonality, extent of disease. Published series suggest overall survival rates ranging between 25% and 30% Mortality with monomorphic PTLD has been reported to be as high as 80%. T-cell lymphomas have an extremely poor prognosis.[12]

Prevention

Limiting the levels of immunosuppression and avoiding OKT3 and ATG are important in preventing PTLD. Vaccination against EBV may provide protection against PTLD, particularly in EBV-naïve pediatric patients. Antiviral prophylaxis is another strategy that has been examined in a number of studies with variable results.[13]

References

1. Al-Mansour Z, Nelson BP and Evens AM. Post-transplant lymphoproliferative disease (PTLD): Risk factors, diagnosis and current treatment strategies. Current Hematologic Malignancy Reports 2013;8(3),173-83. doi:10.1007/s11899-013-0162-5.
2. Opelz G and Henderson R incidence of non-Hodgkin lymphoma in kidney and heart recipient Lancet 1993;342 (8886-87):154.
3. Gottschalks, Roosly CM and Heslop HE. Post transplant lymphoproliferative disorder Ann. Rev Med 2005;56:29-44.
4. Snerdlow SH, Campo E and Harris NL *et al.* World Health Organization classification of tumors of Haematopoietic and lymphoid tissues IARC press on 2008.
5. Leblond V, Davif Charlotte F *et al.* Post transplant lymphoproliferative disorder not dissociated with Epstein-Barr Virus: A distinct entity J clin Oncol 1998;16(6)2052-53.

6. Nalesnik MA. Clinical and pathological features of post-transplant lymphoproliferative disorders (PTLD). Springer Semin Immunopathol 1998;20:325-42.
7. Benkerrou M, Durandy A, Fischer A. Therapy for transplant-related lymphoproliferative diseases. Hematol Oncol Clin North Am 1993:7:467-75.
8. Starlz TE, Nalesnik MA, Porter KA *et al.* Reversibility of lymphomas and lymphoproliferative lesions developing under cyclosporine-steroid therapy. Lancet 1984;1:583-87.
9. Tsai DE, Hardy CL Tomsezewski JE *et al.* Reduction in immunosuppression as initial therapy for post transplant lymphoproliferative disorder: Analysis of prognostic variable and long-term follow of 42 adult patients. Transplantation 2001;171(8):1076.
10. Penn I, Porat G. Central nervous system lymphomas in organ allograft recipients. Transplantation 1995; 59:240-44.
11. Komrokji RS, Oliva JL, Z and M *et al.* Mini-BEAM and autologous hematopoietic stem-cell transplant for treatment of post transplant lymphoproliferative disorders. Am J Hematol 2005;79:211-15.
12. Savage P, Waxman J. Post transplant lymphoproliferative disease. Q J M 1997;90(8):497.
13. Hymes LC, Warshaw BL. Sirolimus in pediatric patients: Results in first 6 months. Pediatr Transplant 2005;9:520-22.

CHAPTER 42

Renal Histopathology–Clinicopathological Cases

Rajan Duggal

Associate Director, Head, Histopathology and Cytopathology, BLK Super Speciality Hospital, Pusa Road New Delhi

In this chapter we will discuss regarding the histopathological changes of common renal diseases.

CASE 1

Minimal Change Disease (MCD)

Clinical History:

25 years female with anasarca; Gross proteinuria; No hypertension; UPCR – 10.7gm/day; C3 and C4–Normal; Creatinine 0.4; ANA 1:40; Urine R/M–Protein 2+; RBCs–Nil.

Clinical Diagnosis:

Nephrotic syndrome? MCD ? FSGS ? MGN? Lupus.

Microscopy: Images 42.1 and 42.2

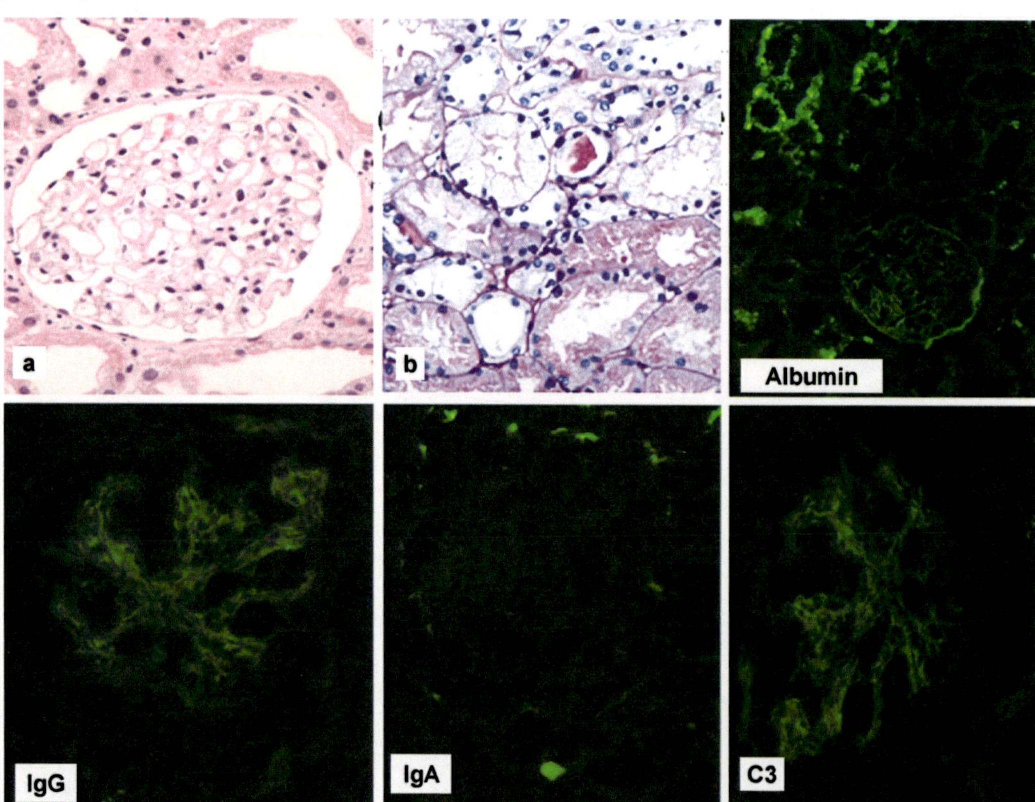

Figure 42.1: Kidney biopsy reveal normal glomerular morphology (a) No membrane thickening, mesangial/endocapillary/extracapillary proliferation seen. Tubules show cytoplasmic vacuolization (b) indicating significant proteinuria. Immunofluorescence is negative for all immunoglobulins and complement. Albumin stain highlight protein absorption droplets, however the glomeruli show negative staining

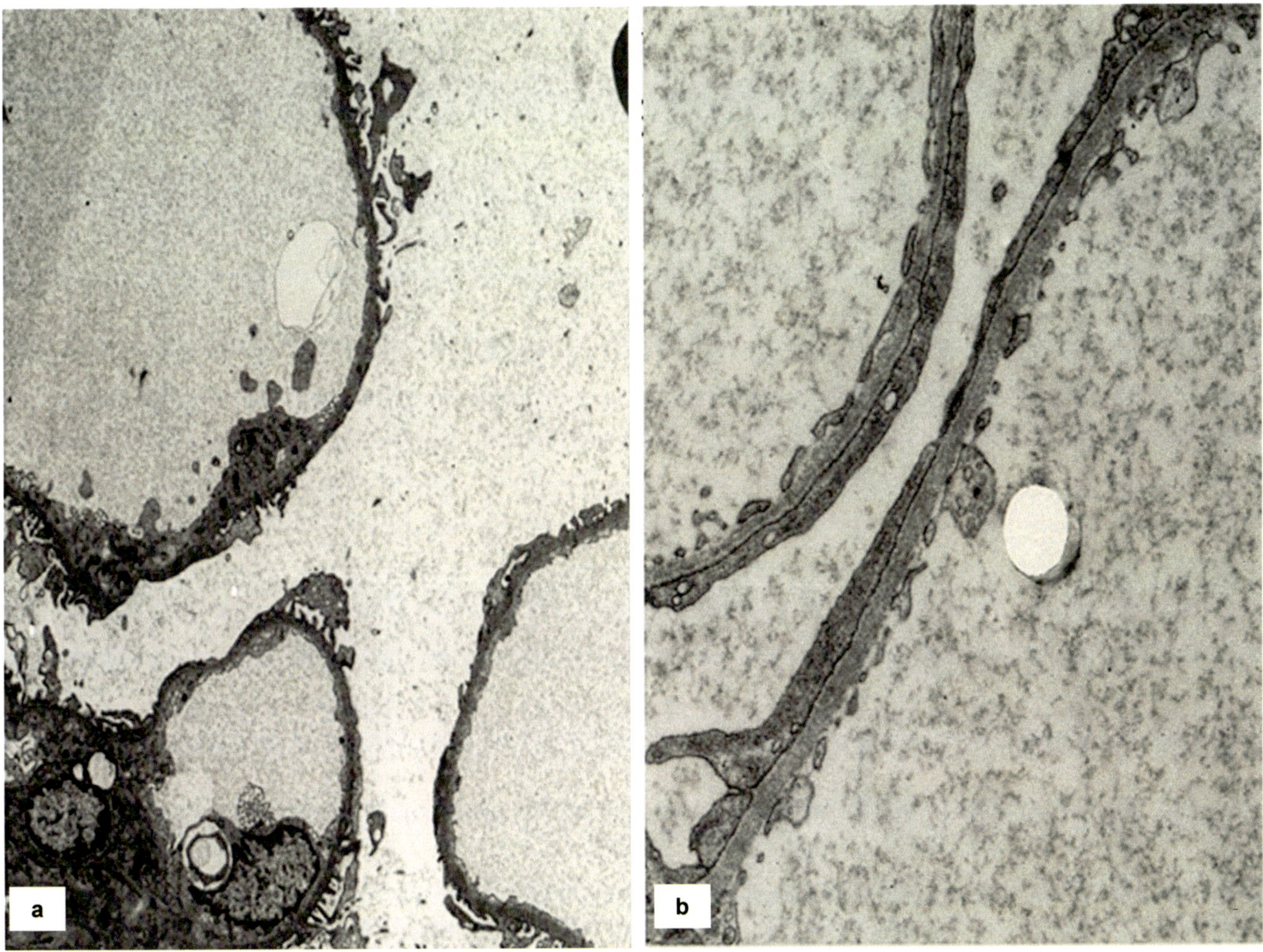

Figure 42.2: Electron microscopy show diffuse podocytic foot process effacement (a) Low magnification; (b) High magnification

CASE 2

Focal Segmental Glomerulosclerosis, Primary (FSGS)

Clinical History:

44 years female presented with bilateral pedal edema × 2 months duration. No other complaints. UPCR-18; Urine R/M: 3+ protein; RBC: 0-1; WBC: 0-1; Serum creatinine: 0.4.

Clinical Diagnosis:

? MCD ? FSGS.

Microscopy: Images 42.3 and 42.4

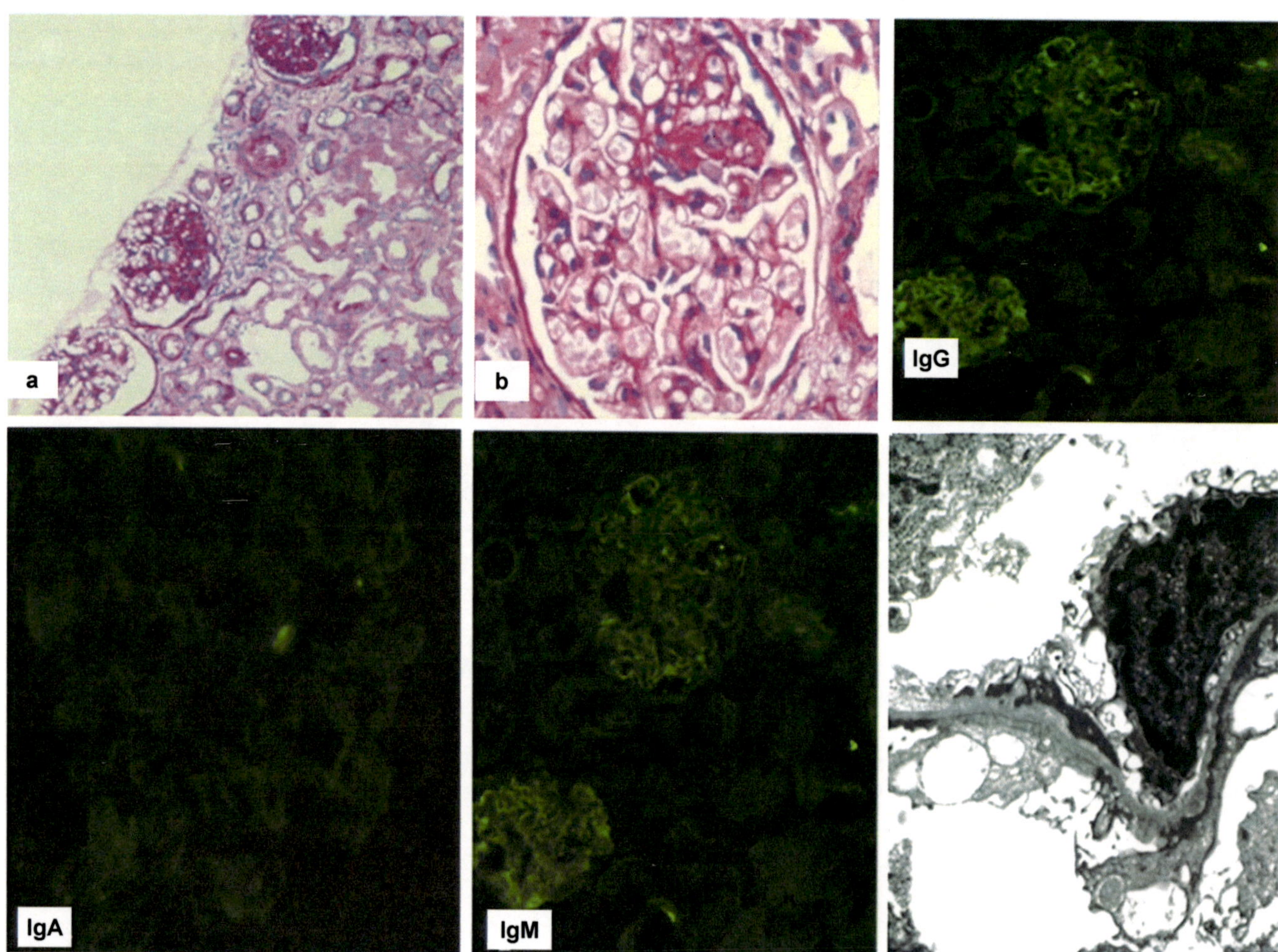

Figure 42.3: Low power magnification show 2 glomeruli with segmental sclerosis lesion (a). Higher magnification of the segmental sclerosis lesion (b). Immunofluorescence is negative for IgG, IgA, IgM. Electron microscopy show diffuse podocytic foot process effacement

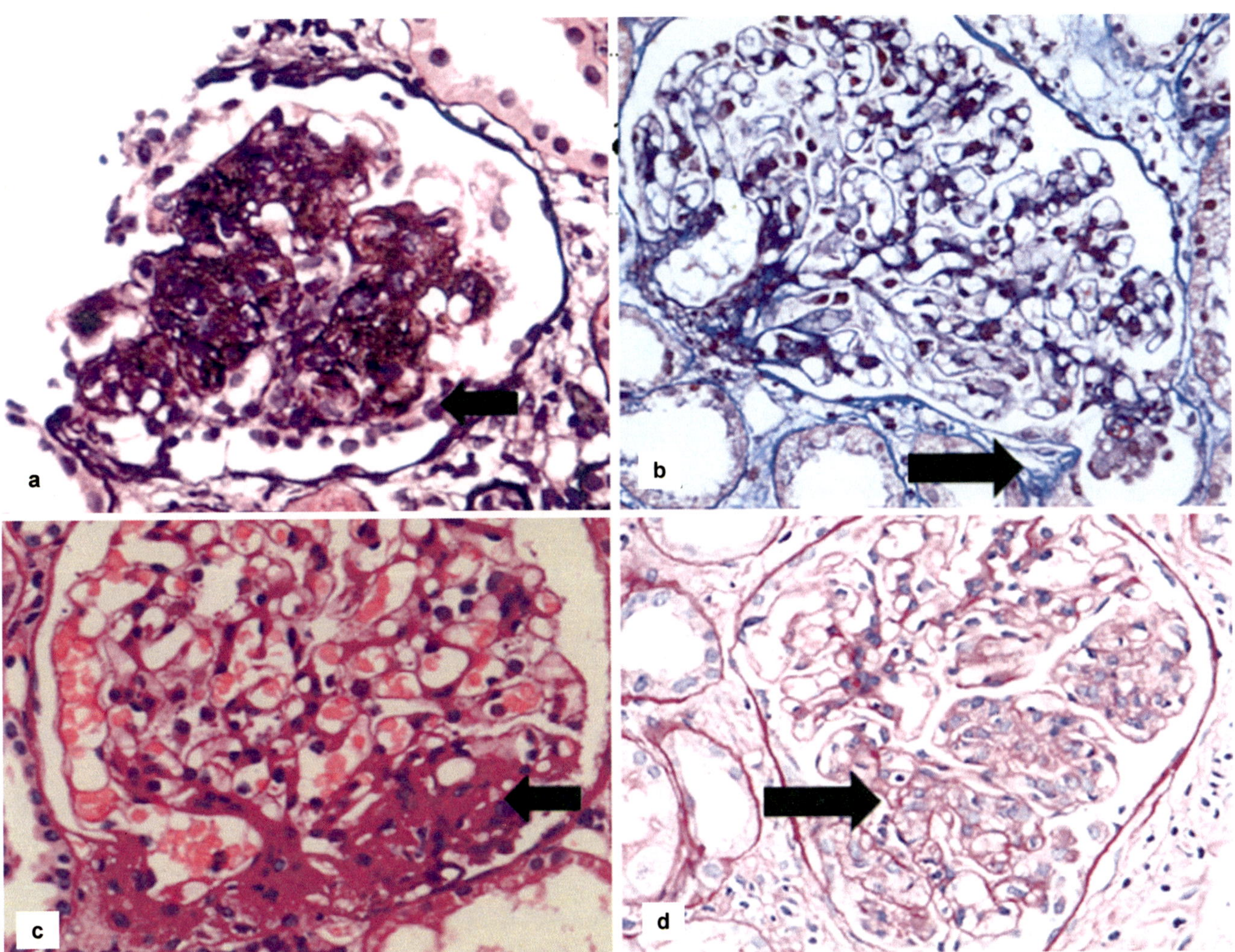

Figure 42.4: Photograph panel show morphologic variants of focal segmental glomerulosclerosis. Collapsing variant show global glomerular tuft collapse with proliferation of overlying podocytes (a). Tip variant of FSGS show segmental endocapillary foam cells projecting into the tubular pole (b). Perihilar FSGS show segmental sclerosis lesion near the hilar area (c). Cellular variant of FSGS show endocapillary cellularity. The endocapillary cells are composed of endothelial cells and foam cells (d)

CASE 3

Focal Segmental Glomerulosclerosis, Secondary (FSGS)

Clinical History:

48 years female with diabetes mellitus type 2 and hypertension × 15 years. Nephrotic range proteinuria history of hernia repair. Presently pedal edema and high BP. Presently Urine albumin creatinine ratio–11430.6 mg/gm protein; Creatinine–0.8; C3–Normal; Albumin–3.58.

Clinical Diagnosis:

?Diabetic Nephropathy?Hypertensive nephrosclerosis ?FSGS.

Microscopy: Image 42.5

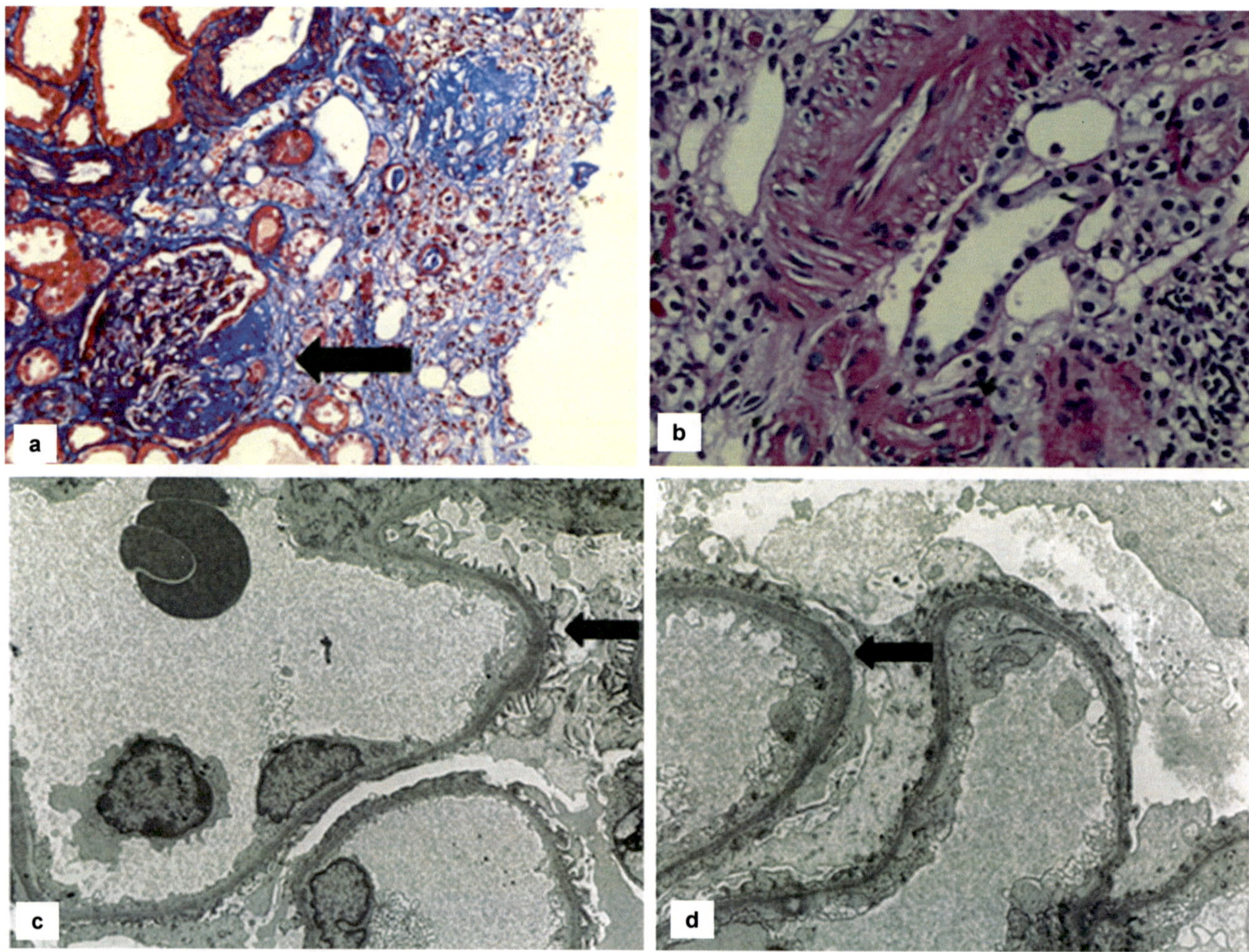

Figure 42.5: Low power magnification of Masson's trichrome stain show 1 globally sclerosed glomerulus alongwith 1 glomerulus with segmental sclerosis lesion (a). No mesangial matrix expansion or nodular glomerulosclerosis lesion seen thereby excluding possibility of advanved diabetic nephropathy. Majority of the blood vessels show moderate medial thickening with vascular hyalinosis indicating hypertensive nephrosclerosis with possibly secondary FSGS lesion (b). Immunofluorescence is negative for all immunoglobulins and complement (not shown). Electron microscopy show preserved podocytic foot processes in majority of the glomerular capillary loops (c). Few capillary loops show minimal subendothelial expansion with reactive endothelium and focal podocytic foot process effacement indicating secondary podocytopathy, possibly related to hypertension (d)

CASE 4

Alport's Disease

Clinical History:

44 years female with history of pedal edema-10 days. Family hisotry of kidney disease. Mother with ESRD on hemodialysis expired. Patient sister and brother both received kidney transplant. Brother at 18 years of age expired. Sons of both sisters history of proteinuria and microscopic hematuria.

Clinical Diagnosis:

? Familial FSGS ? Alport's disease.

Microscopy: Image 42.6

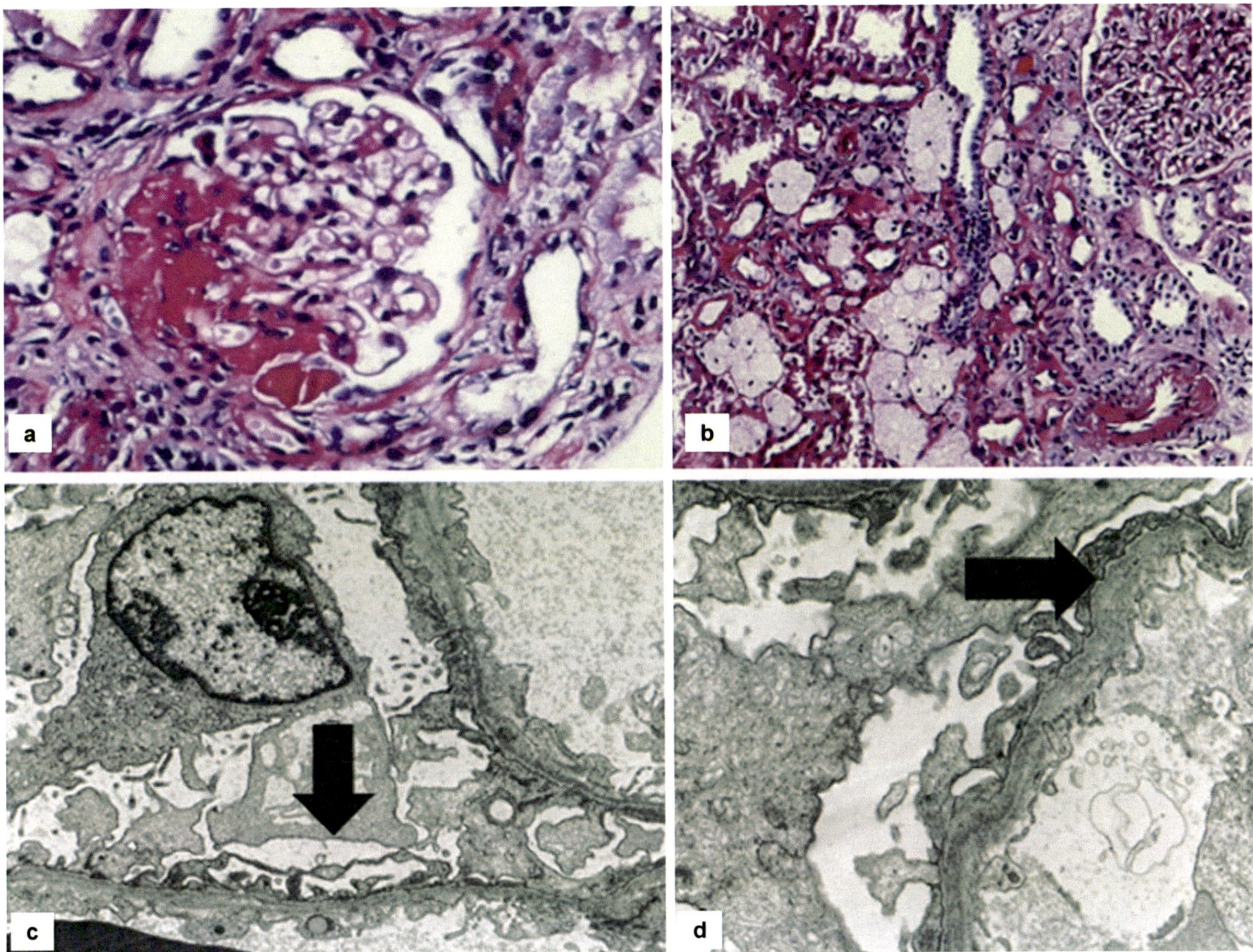

Figure 42.6: High power magnification of PAS stained section show 1 glomerulus with segmental sclerosis lesion (a). Numerous interstitial foam cells are seen (b). Electron microscopy show preserved podocytic foot processes as highlighted by arrow, thereby excluding possibility of primary podocytopathy (c). In addition, few capillary loops show fragmentation of lamina densa with baskey weave appearance (d)

CASE 5

C1q Nephropathy

Clinical History:

19 years old male presented with nephrotic range proteinuria. No active urine sediments, mild azotemia. No history of diabetes, hypertension and mixed connective disorder.

Clinical Diagnosis:

? MCD.

Microscopy: Image 42.7

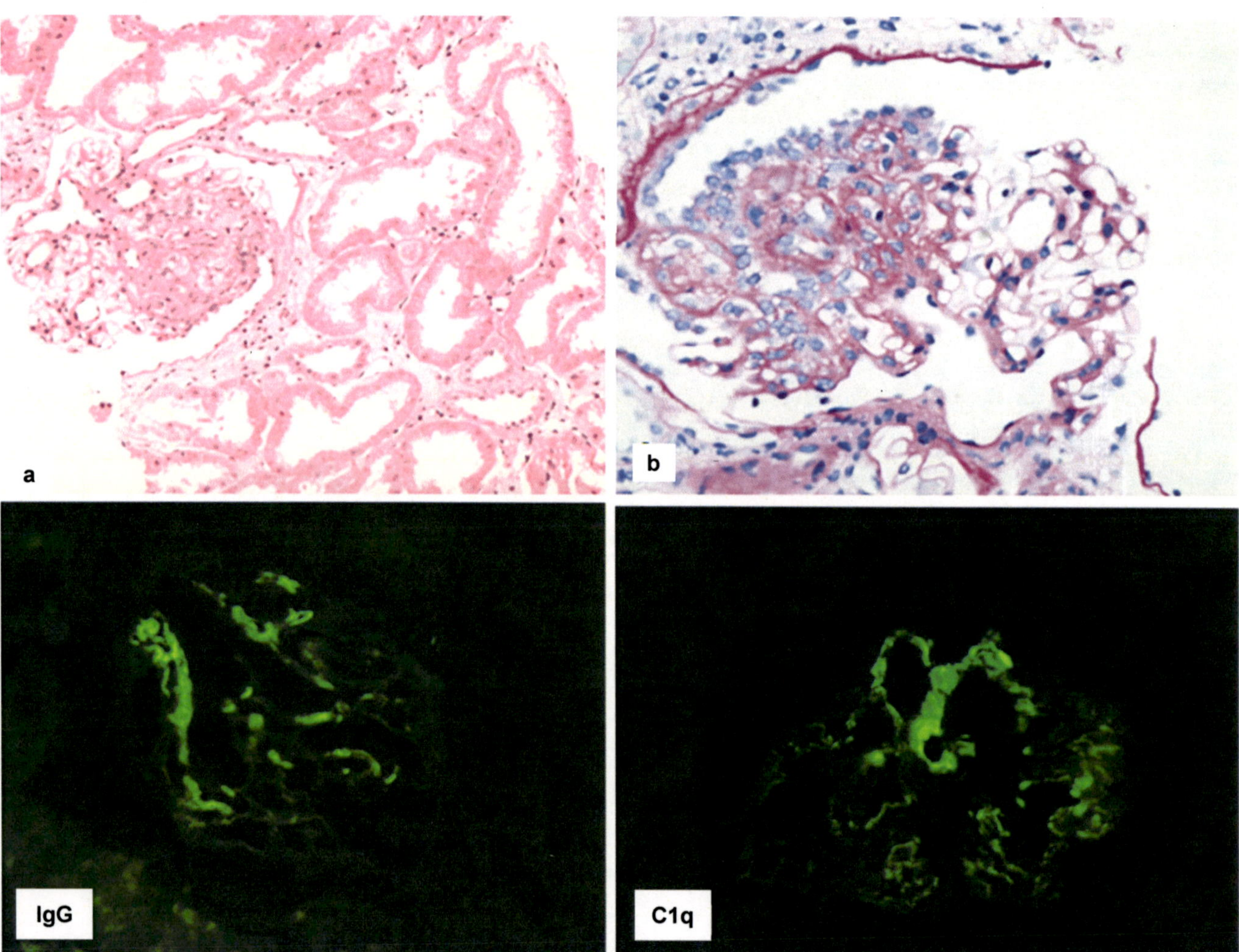

Figure 42.7: PAS stained section show 1 glomerulus with segmental sclerosis lesion (a) Low magnification; (b) High magnification. Immunofluorescence show mesangial deposits of IgG and C1q

Comment: C1Q nephropathy (C1qN) is an uncommon glomerular disease characterized by dominant or codominant (≥2+) mesangial staining for C1q, usually with immunoglobulins, in the absence of clinical or laboratory evidence of SLE. The overall biopsy prevalence of C1qN ranges from 0.2% to 9% but has been reported in up to 16.3% of children with treatment-resistant nephrotic syndrome. C1qN is mostly diagnosed in children and young adults but may occur at any age. Pediatric C1qN cases with MCD features typically respond well to steroids but may have a higher incidence of frequent relapses. Most of the reported cases with FSGS like morphology were treated with steroids and had generally poor response, not unlike primary FSGS.

CASE 6

Membranous Glomerulopathy, Primary (MGN)

Clinical History:

47 years male hypertension since 5 years on Irbesartan. No diabetes mellitus. Nephrotic range proteinuria detected during evaluation for mild facial puffiness and lower limb swelling on and off. No rashes/joint pains/decrease in urine output. Normal serum creatinine. Urine R/M: Proteins 3+; UPCR: 4 gm; Complements: Normal.

Clinical Diagnosis:

Nephrotic syndrome ? MGN ? FSGS

Microscopy: Image 42.8

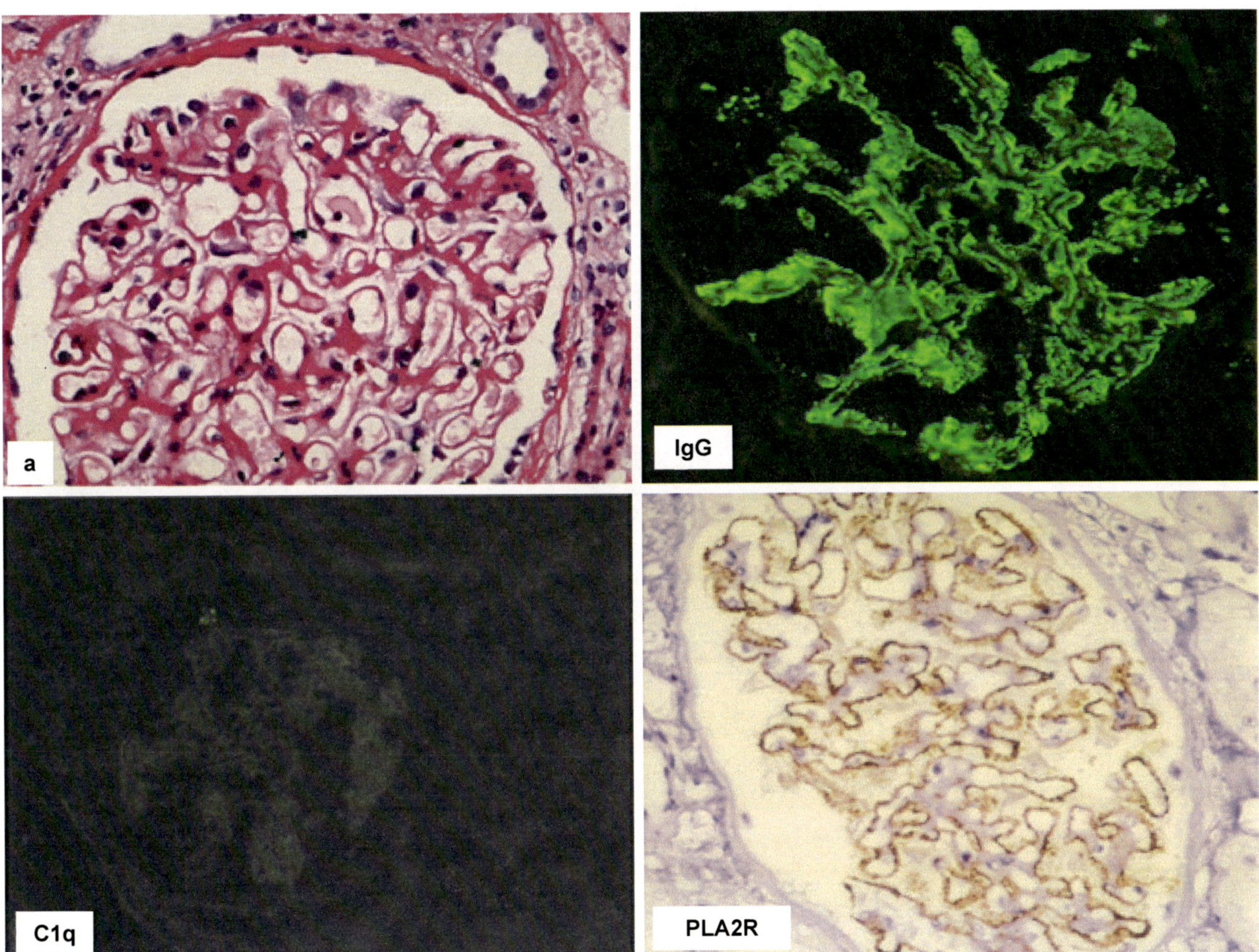

Figure 42.8: PAS stained section show moderate thickening of the glomerular capillary wall (a). Immunofluorescence show granular deposition of IgG along capillary loops without C1q staining. In addition, PLA2R immunohistochemistry show granular staining along capillary loops indicating PLA2R associated primary MGN

CASE 7

Membranous Glomerulopathy, Secondary (MGN)

Clinical History:

17 years old female presented with significant proteinuria. History of hypothyroidism, dyslipedemia and ANA postivity. ? Nephrotic syndrome.

Microscopy: Image 42.9

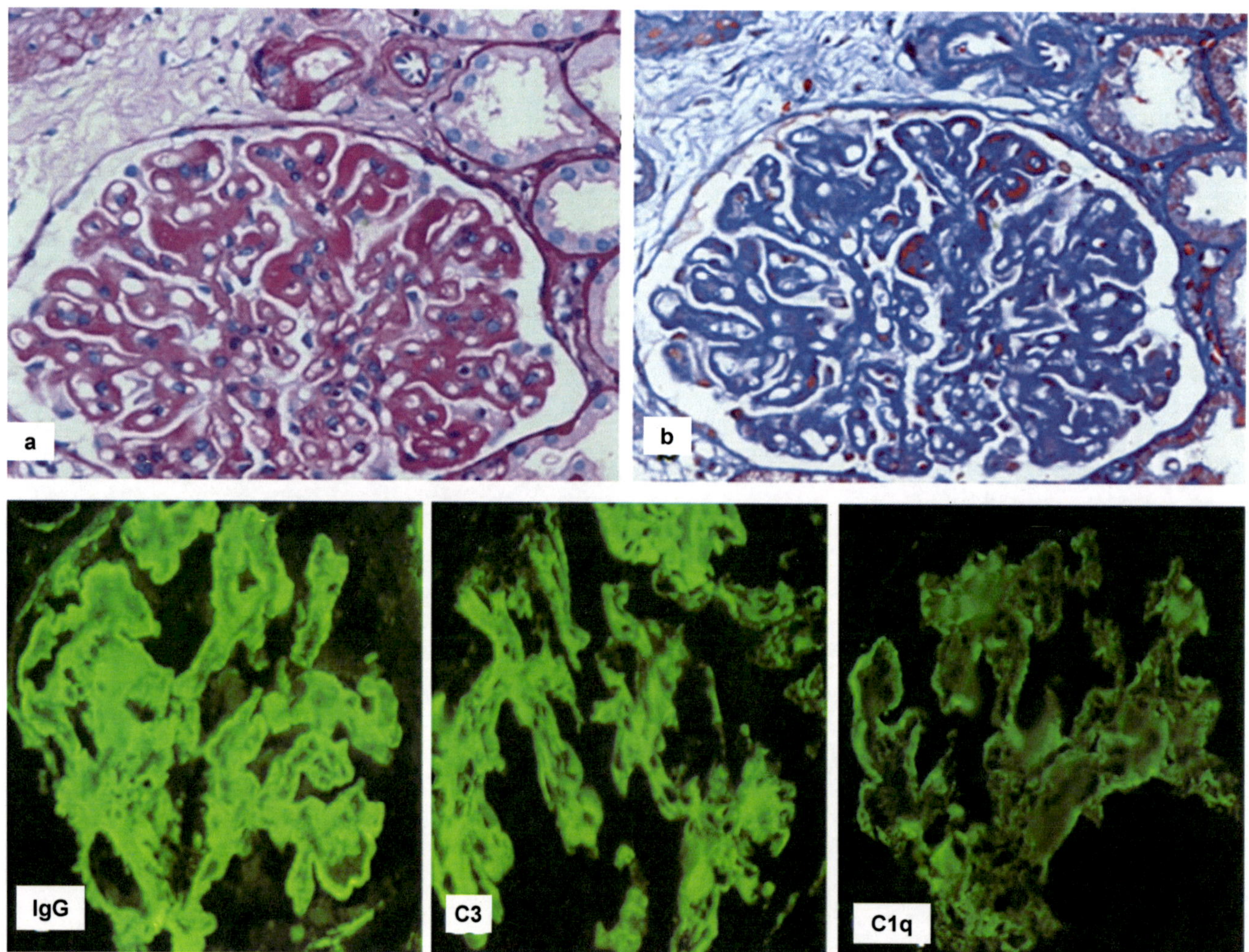

Figure 42.9: PAS stained section show moderate to severe thickening of the glomerular capillary wall (a). Masson's trichrome stain show few fuschinophilic red colored deposits along capillary wall (b). Immunofluorescence show granular deposition of IgG, C3 and C1q along capillary loops indicating secondary MGN (possibly Class V Lupus Nephritis)

CASE 8

IgA Nephropathy (IgAN)

Clinical History:

41 years male with proteinuria and microscopic hematuria. History of synpharyngitic hematuria? IgA nephropathy.

Microscopy: Images 42.10 and 42.11

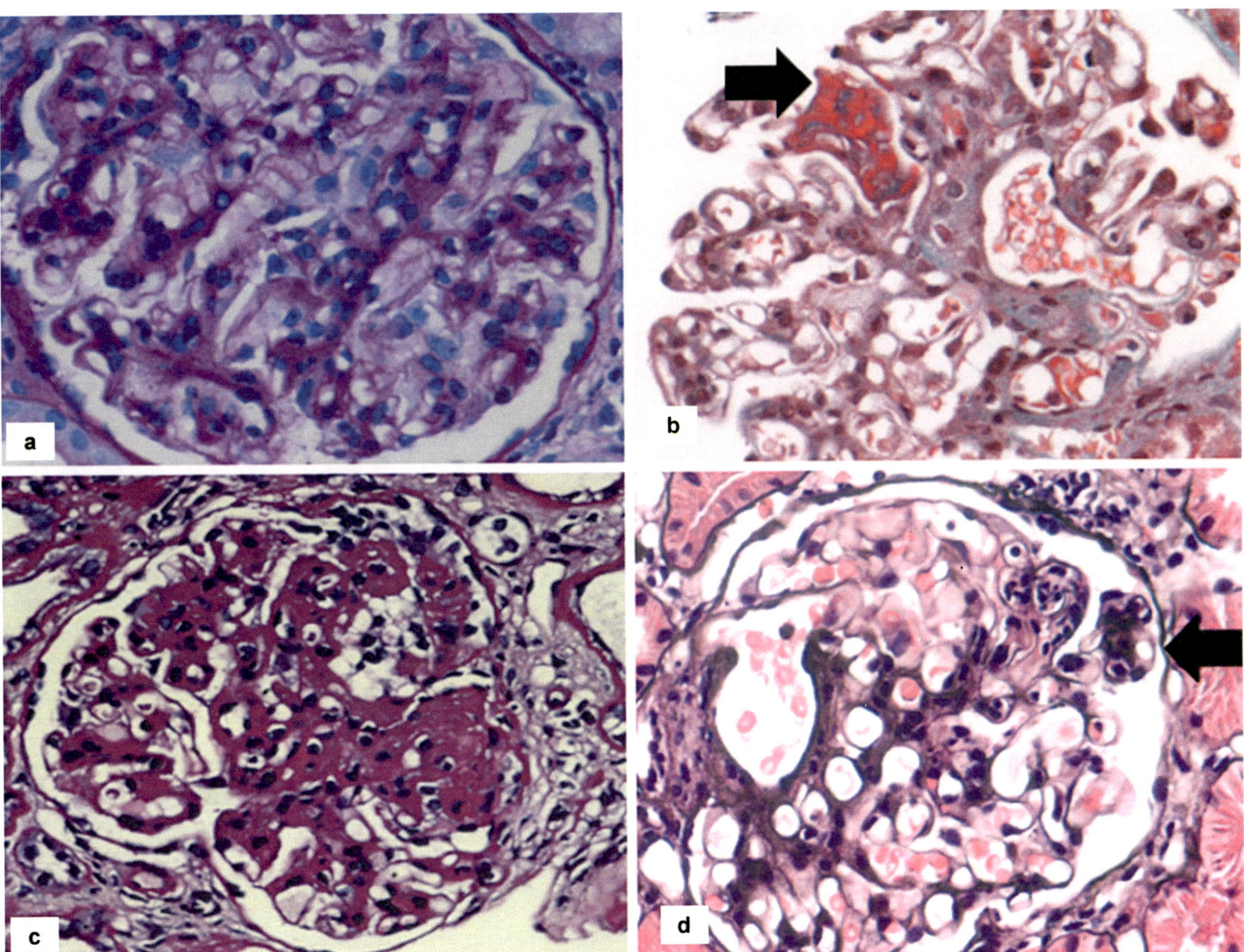

Figure 42.10: Photomicrograph panel show variable glomerular morphology in form of mesangial hypercellularity (a), segmental necrotizing lesion (b), segmental sclerosis lesion (c) and segmental endocapillary hypercellularity (d)

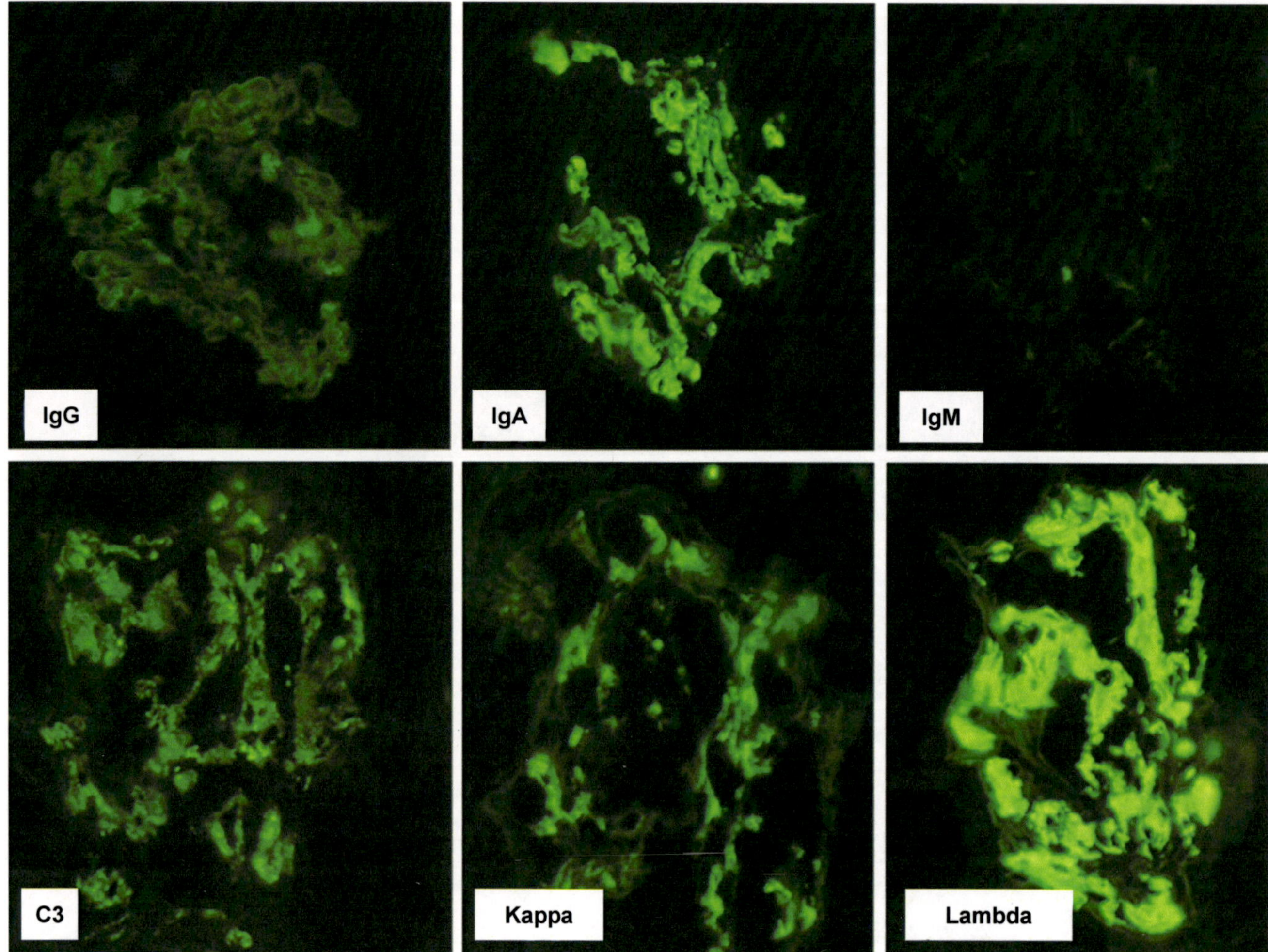

Figure 42.11: Immunofluorescence studies show dominant IgA deposits with more significant lambda staining than kappa

CASE 9

Lupus Nephritis

Clinical History:

29 years old female known case of SLE with renal impairment and proteinuria. Urine R/M: Protein 4+; WBC 0-2; 24 hours urine protein 2469 mg; serum creatinine 1.6 mg/dl; ANA+ve; dsDNA+ve.

Microscopy: Images 42.12 and 42.13

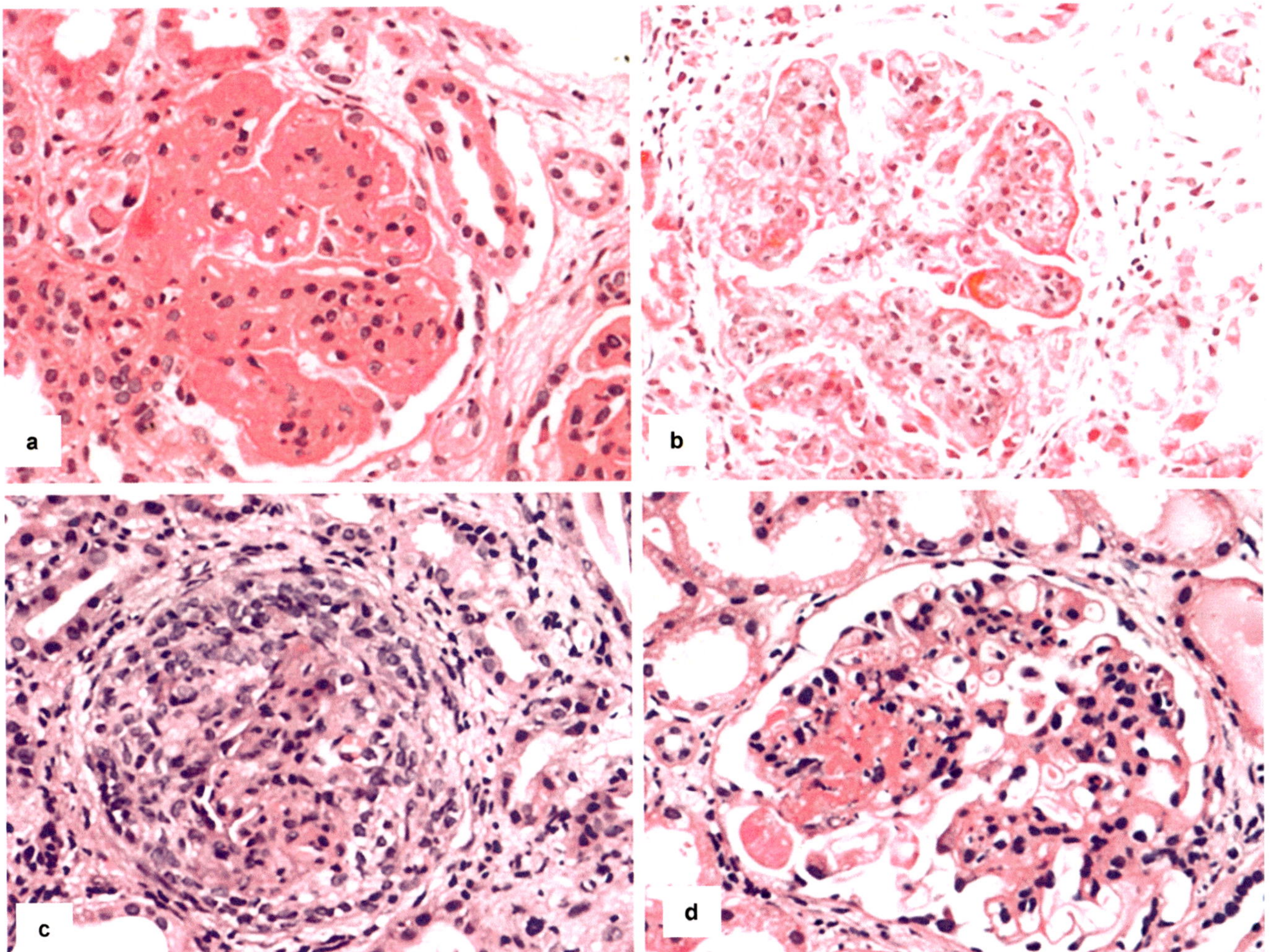

Figure 42.12: Photomicrograph panel show variable glomerular morphology in form of thickening of the glomerular capillary wall (a), lobular accentuation with fuschinophilic wire-loop like deposits with endocapillary proliferation (b), global circumferential cellular crescent (c) and segmental necrotizing lesion (d)

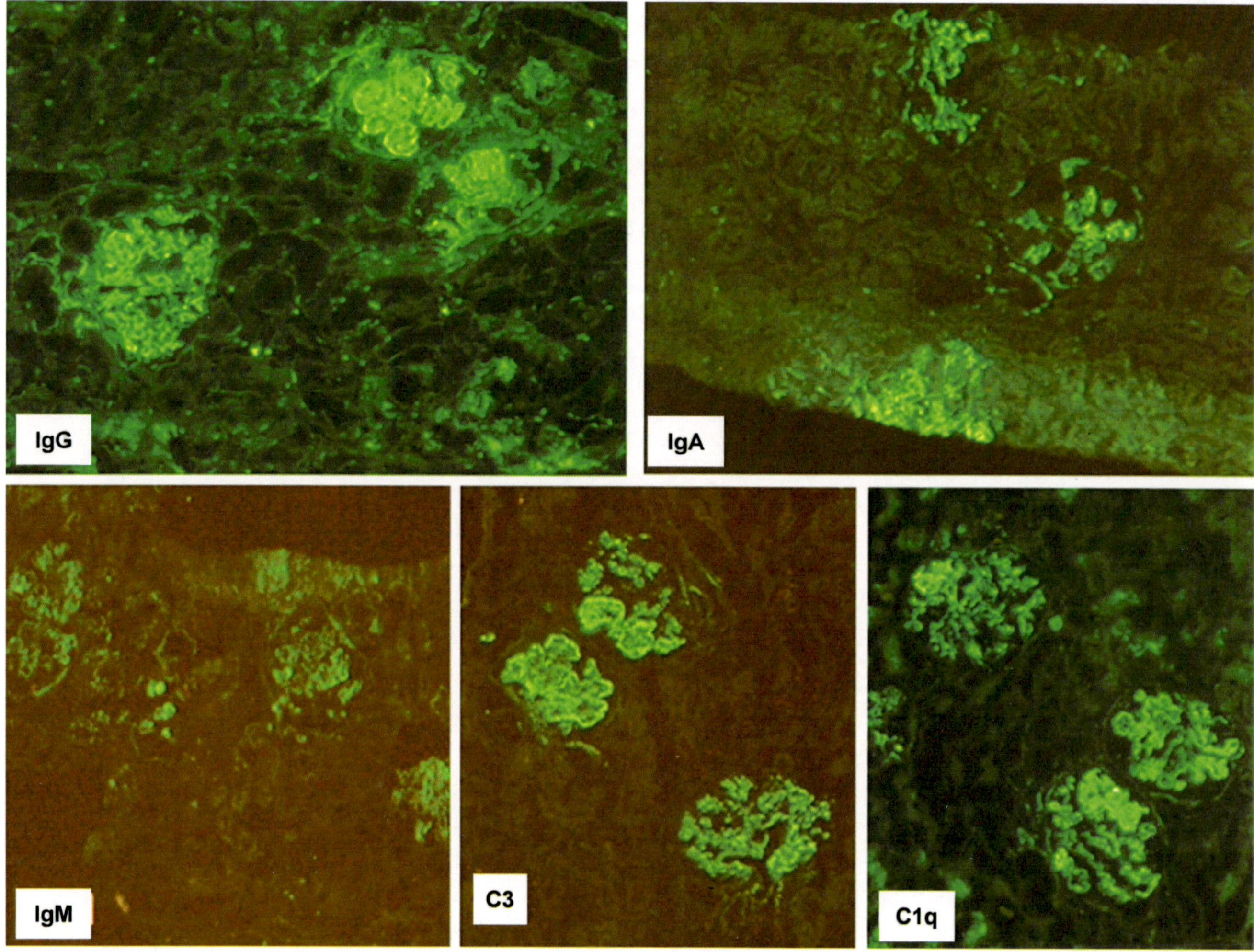

Figure 42.13: Immunofluorescence studies show full house immunofluorescence pattern with IgG, IgA,IgM, C3 and C1q staining

CASE 10

Post-Infectious Glomerulonephritis (PIGN)

Clinical History:

9 years male, had sore throat 13 days ago. Puffiness of face × 5 days. Serum creatinine at presentation is 13 mg/dl. No hypertension on presentation. Urine R/M: RBCs 20-25; Granular casts. Oliguria+; UPCR: 3.3 gm; C3: <16.9 (low); C4: Normal. Required hemodialysis. RPGN ? post-streptococcal with crescents.

Microscopy: Image 42.14

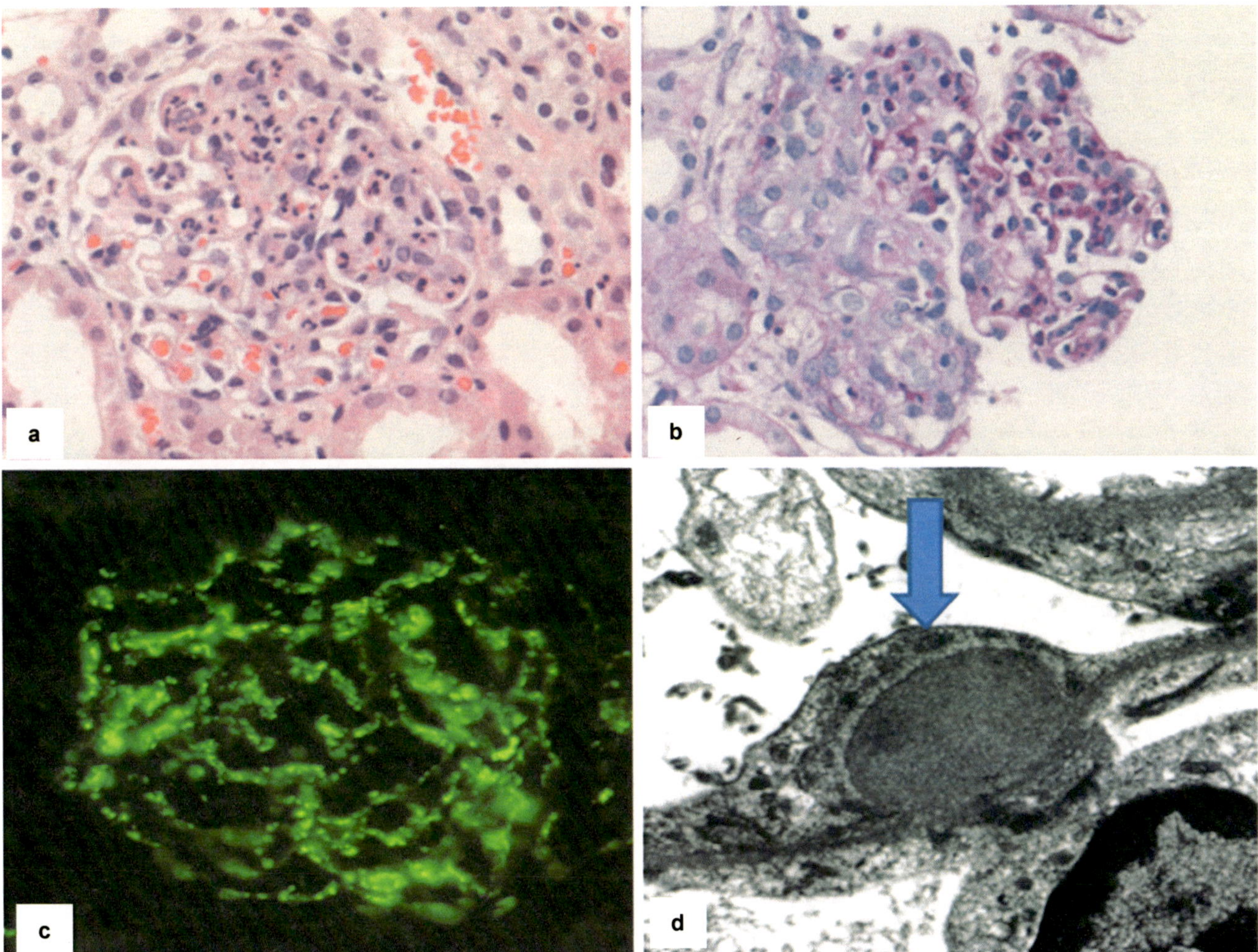

Figure 42.14: Photomicrograph panel show diffuse endocapillary proliferation rich in neutrophils (a). 1 glomerulus show segmental cellular crescent (b). Immunofluorescence show C3 deposits along capillary loops and mesangium in a dotted pattern (c). Electron microscopy show presence of subepithelial hump (d)

CASE 11

Membranoproliferative Glomerulonephritis, Immune-Complex Mediated (MPGN)

Clinical History:

70 years male recently diagnosed DM, HTN × 1 month ago. Presented with fluid overload and rise in serum creatinine from 1.5 to 2.0 mg/dl. UPCR–2.24; Microscopic hematuria; ANA and ANCA–Negative; C3–Low; C4–Normal.

Microscopy: Image 42.15

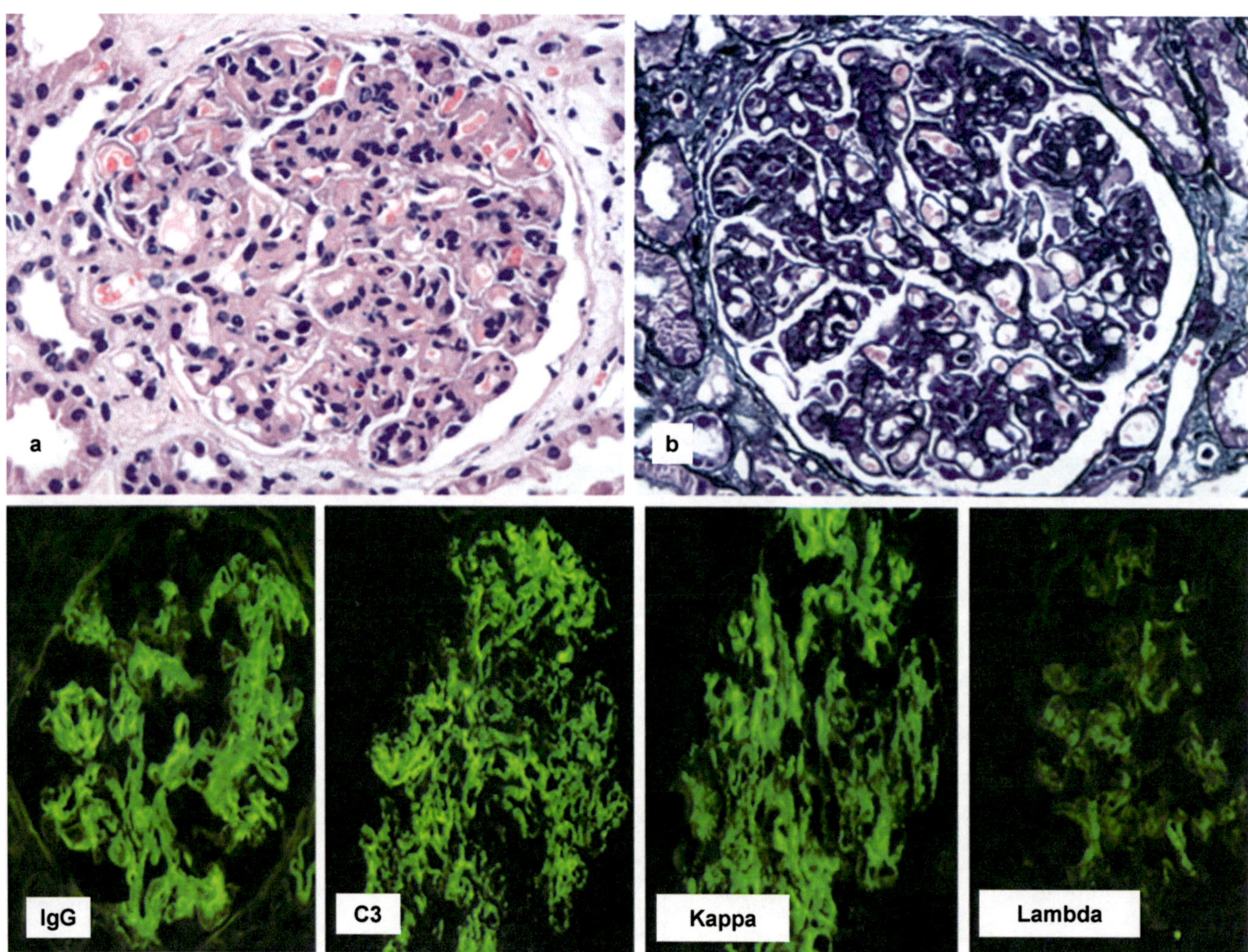

Figure 42.15: Photomicrograph panel show lobular accentuation with diffuse endocapillary proliferation rich in lymphocytes and neutrophils (a). Silver stain show segmental duplication of peripheral capillary wall with endocapillary proliferation (b). Immunofluorescence show granular IgG and C3 deposits along capillary loops and mesangium. Kappa and Lambda show no light chain restriction

CASE 12

Membranoproliferative Glomerulonephritis with Dysproteinemia

Clinical History:

46 years male hypothyroidism, hypertension. DM controlled on oral hypoglycemic agents. Anasarca+; Significant NSAIDs intake with decreased output. Urine R/M: 4+proteinuria; Creatinine 4.28mg/dl.

Microscopy: Image 42.16

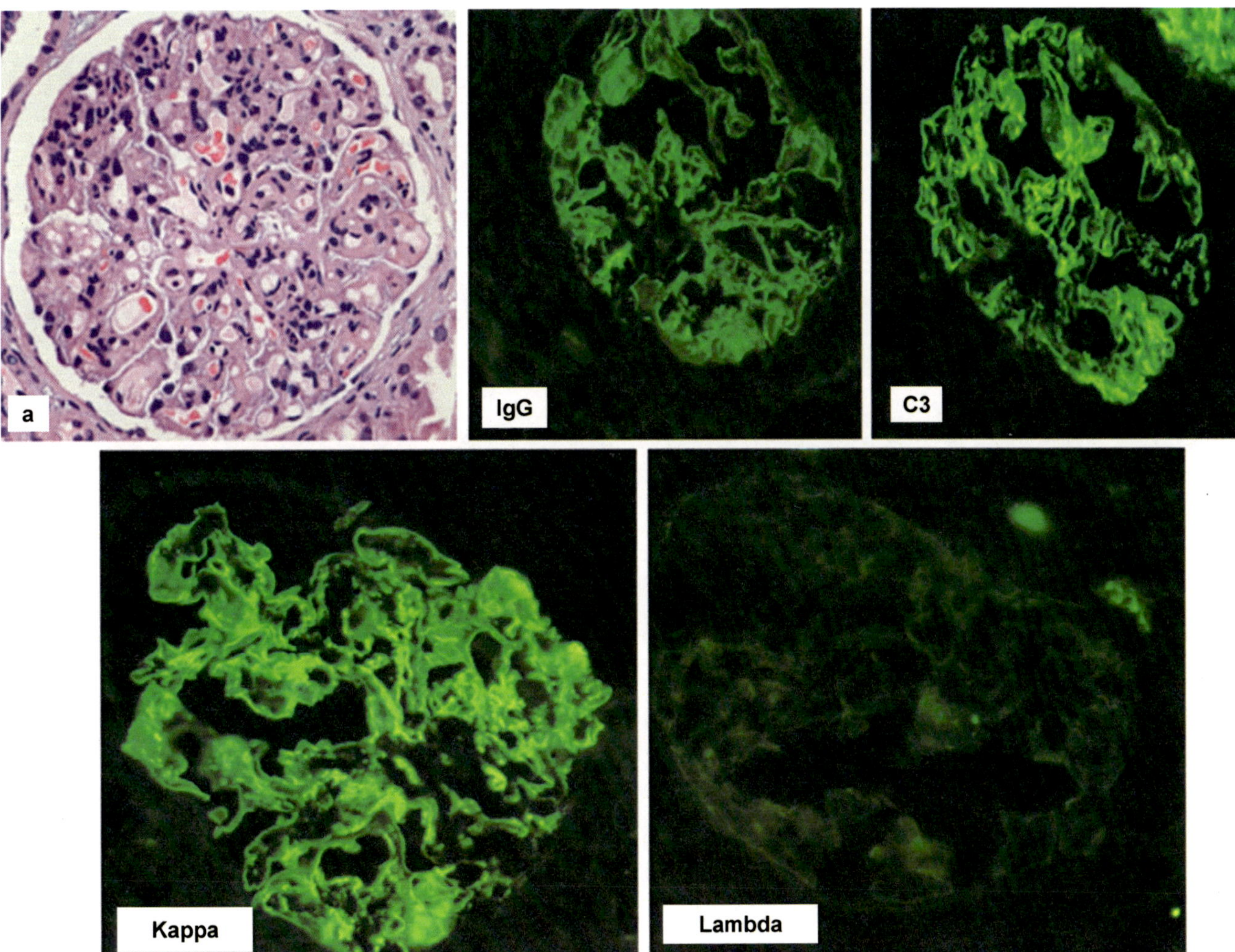

Figure 42.16: Photomicrograph panel show lobular accentuation with diffuse endocapillary proliferation rich in lymphocytes and neutrophils (a). Immunofluorescence show granular IgG and C3 deposits along capillary loops and mesangium. Kappa show 3+ staining and Lambda is negative, thereby indicating kappa light chain restriction

CASE 13

C3 Glomerulopathy (Includes C3 Glomerulonephritis and Dense Deposit Disease)

C3 Glomerulonephritis:

Clinical History:

15 years male with proteinuria and low C3. No history of infection.

Microscopy: Image 42.17

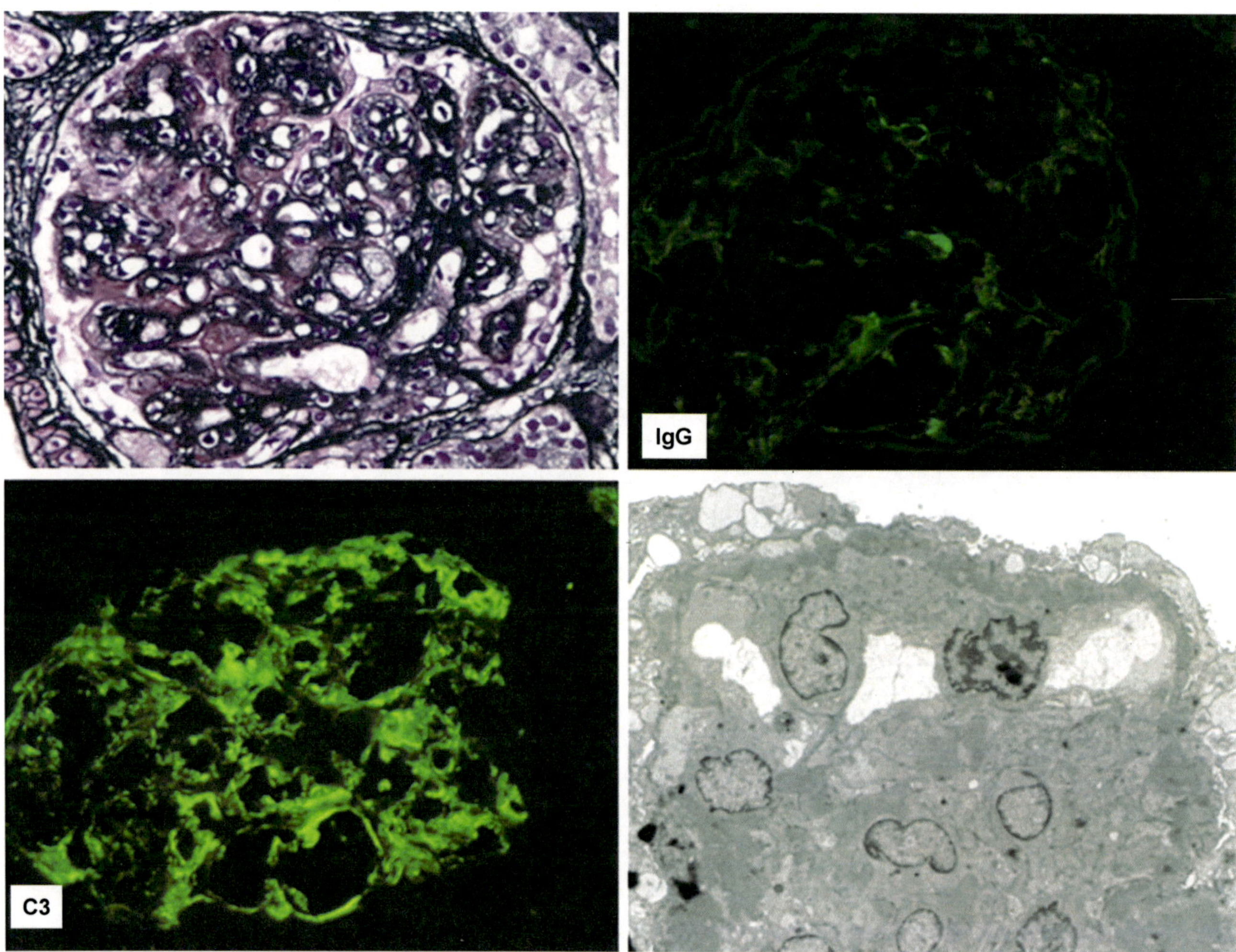

Figure 42.17: Photomicrograph panel show lobular accentuation with diffuse endocapillary proliferation rich in lymphocytes. In addition, there is non-uniform thickening of the glomerular capillary wall with extensive duplication. Immunofluorescence show dominant coarse C3 deposits along capillary loops and mesangium. Electron microscopy show presence of electron dense deposits in the subendothelial and mesangial location consistent with C3 glomerulonephritis

Dense Deposit Disease

Clinical History:

16 years male with nephrotic syndrome.

Microscopy: Image 42.18

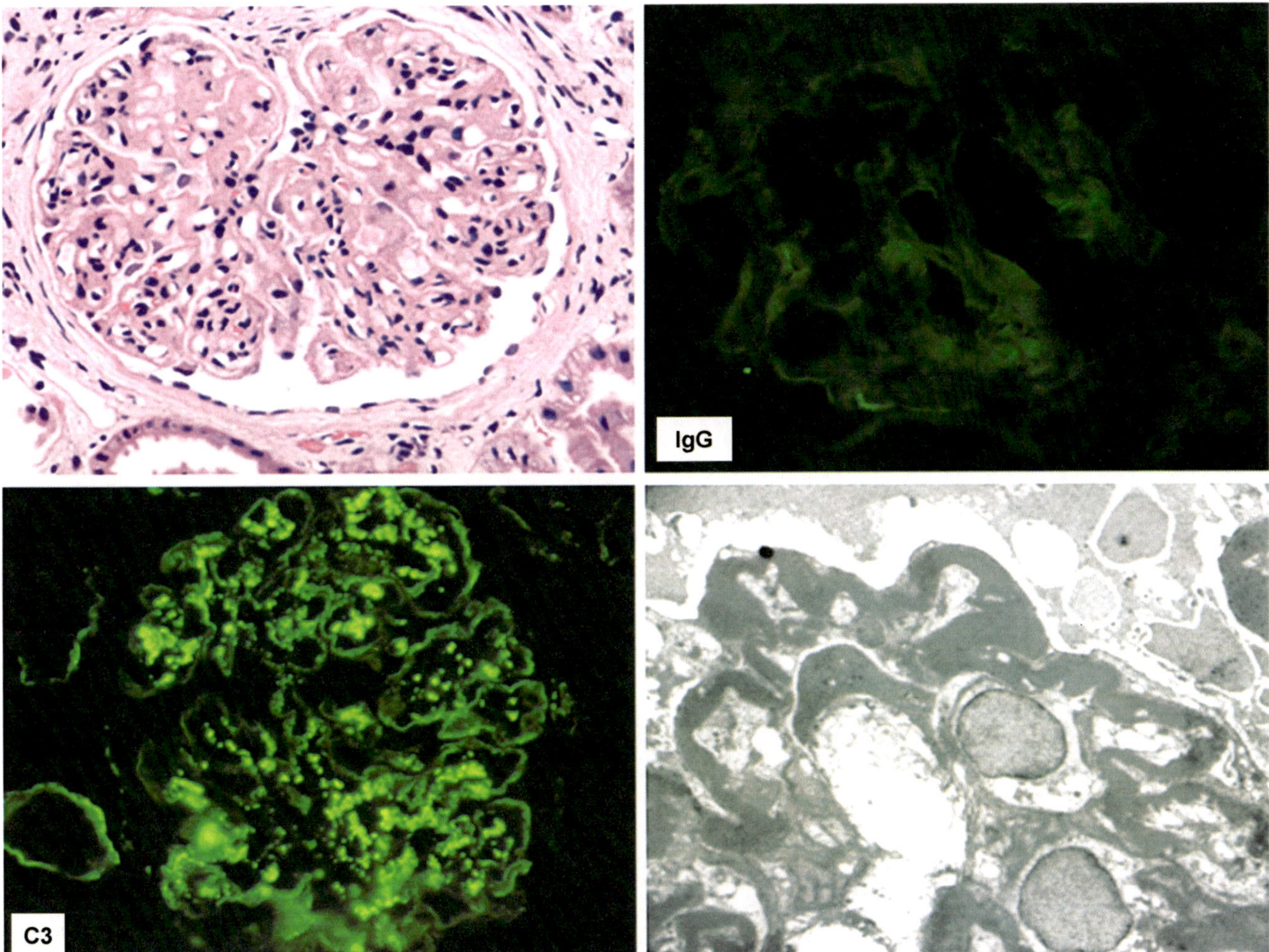

Figure 42.18: Photomicrograph panel show lobular accentuation with diffuse endocapillary proliferation rich in lymphocytes. In addition, there is non-uniform thickening of the glomerular capillary wall with extensive duplication. Immunofluorescence show dominant coarse C3 deposits along capillary loops and mesangium. Mesangial rings are seen. Electron microscopy show presence of dense osmiophilic intramembranous deposits consistent with dense deposit disease

CASE 14

Crescentic Glomerulonephritis

Includes Pauci-Immune Crescentic GN; Anti-GBM Glomerulonephritis; Immune-Complex Mediated GN

Pauci-Immune Crescentic GN

Clinical History:

62 years female known case of hypertension × 1 year alongwith AKI (S. Creatinine increased to 9.2 from 2.5). History of hematuria × 1 month. Urine R/M: Dysmorphic RBC.

Microscopy: Image 42.19

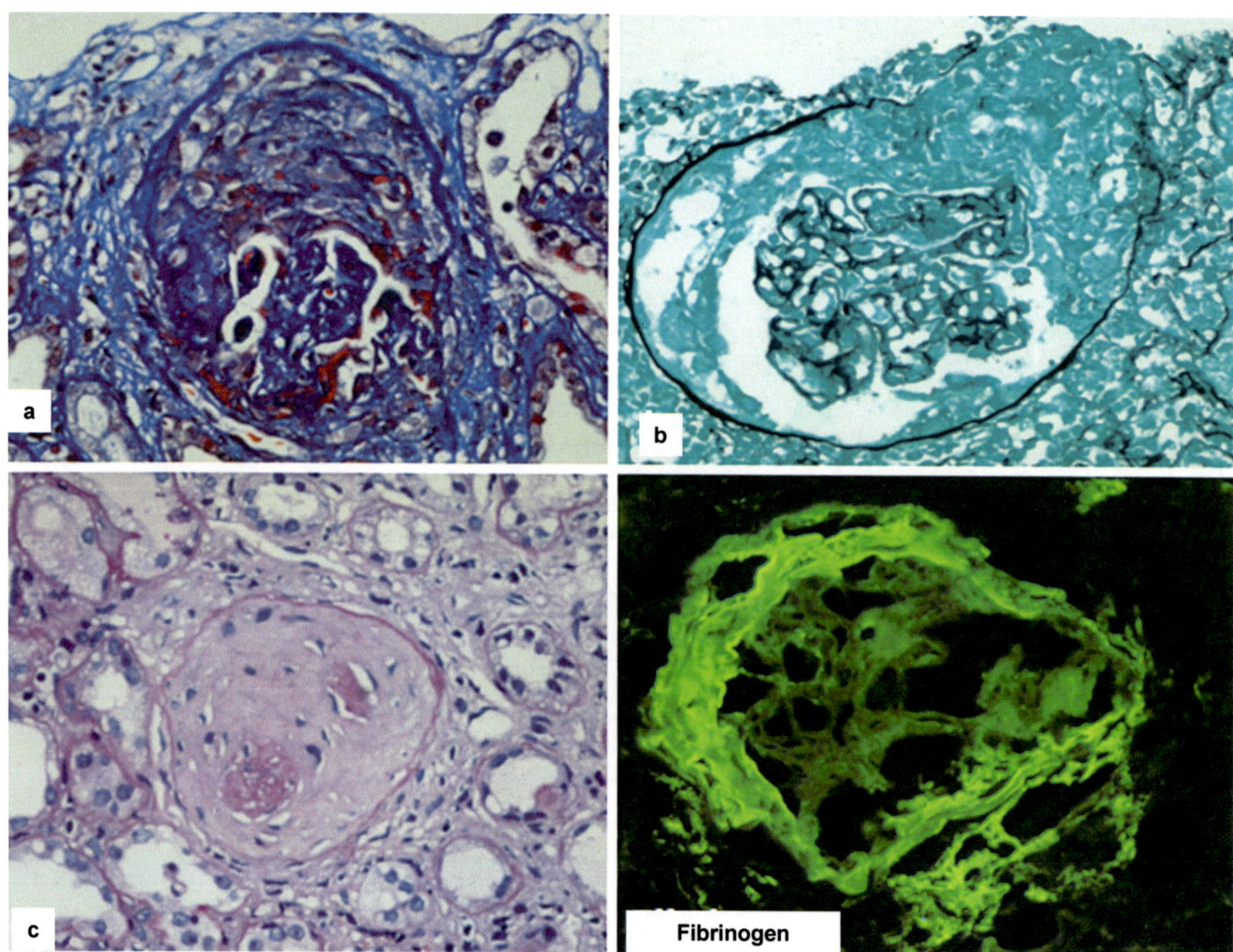

Figure 42.19: Photomicrograph panel show varying age of crescents. Cellular crescents are seen in (a, b) and fibrous crescent is seen in (c). In addition, there is evidence of segmental necrosis evident as fushinophilic deposits (a). Fibrinogen immunofluorescence highlight the crescent

Anti-GBM Crescentic GN

Clinical History:

68 years male non-diabetic, non-HTN. Advanced renal failure on hemodialysis. Active sediments. Proteinuria–580 mg/day.

Microscopy: Image 42.20

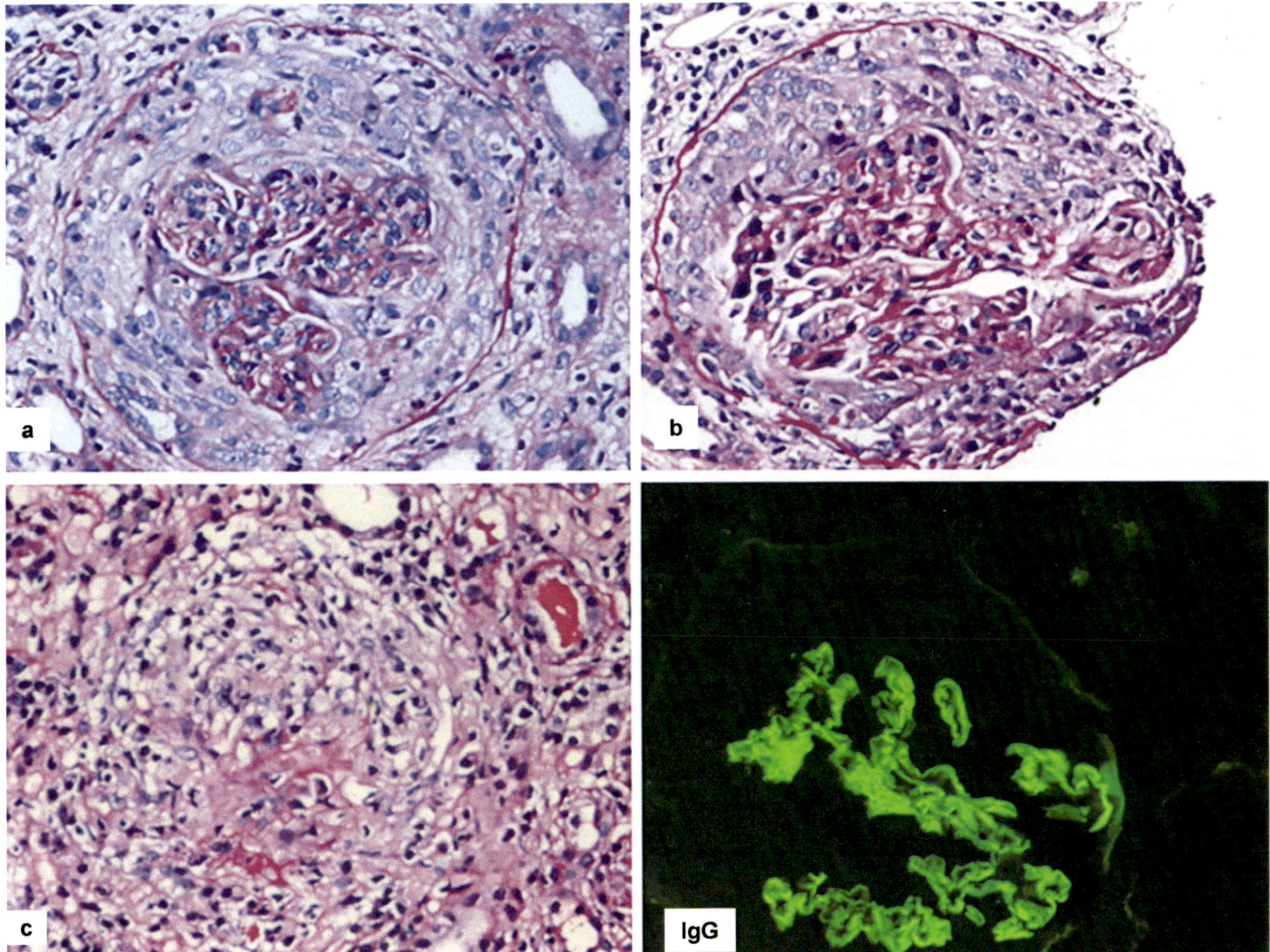

Figure 42.20: Photomicrograph panel show global circumferential cellular crescents of the same age (a, b, c). In addition, there is evidence of glomerulitis highlighted by rupture of Bowmann's capsule (c). IgG immunofluorescence show linear staining along glomerular capillary wall

Immune-Complex Mediated Crescentic GN

Clinical History:

52 years female with proteinuria under evaluation. HTN+; Bilateral lower limb swelling. UPCR–2 gm/day; Creatinine–2.9 mg/dl.

Microscopy: Image 42.21

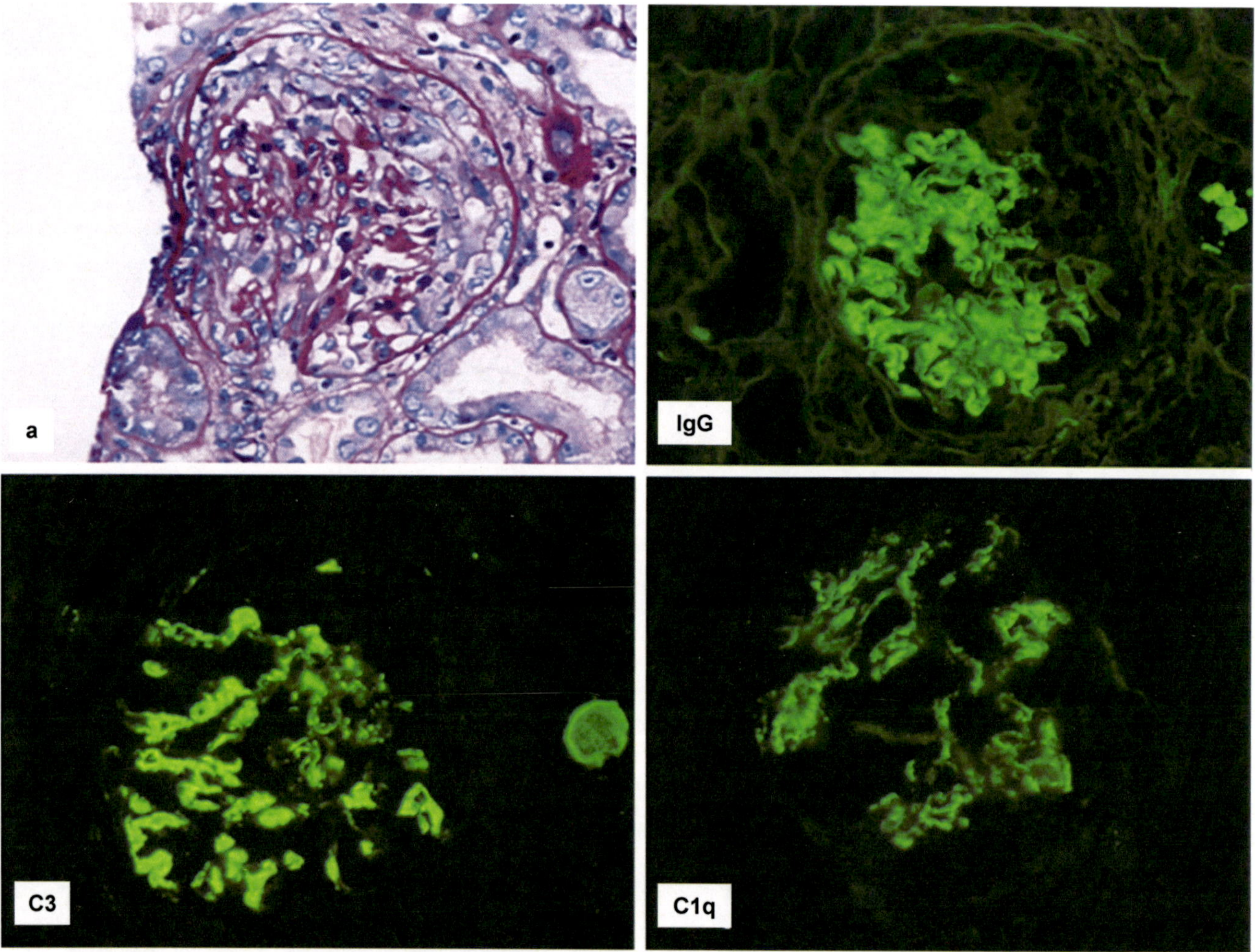

Figure 42.21: Photomicrograph panel show global circumferential cellular crescent. The underlying glomerular tuft show mild mesangial matrix expansion with minimal thickening of the glomerular capillary wall (a). Immunofluorescence show granular deposits of IgG, C3 alongwith minimal C1q consistent with immune-complex deposits

CASE 15

Diabetic Nephropathy Class III

Clinical History:

42 years male with Type 2 DM for 12 years. Presented with heavy proteinuria. UPCR–15.0 g/day. Serum Creatinine –1.2. No retinopathy. ? Diabetic nephropathy ? Associated MGN.

Microscopy: Image 42.22

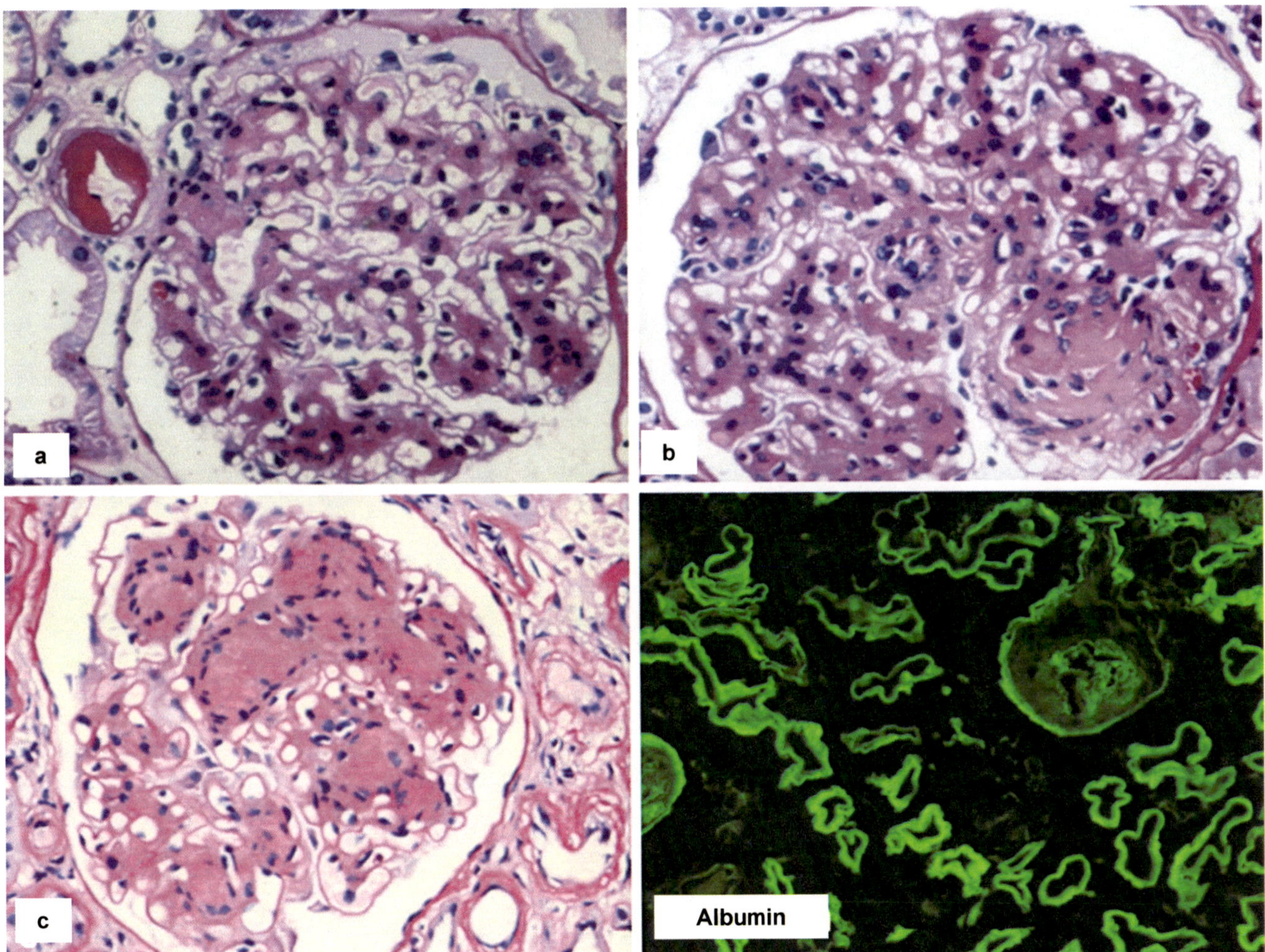

Figure 42.22: Photomicrograph panel show thickening of the glomerular capillary wall with moderate mesangial matrix expansion (a). Few glomeruli show classical PAS positive Kimmelsteil-Wilson lesion (b, c). Immunofluorescence show 2+ albumin staining along tubular basement membrane

CASE 16

Amyloidosis, Secondary

Clinical History:

48 years female known case of HTN × 1 year. Right hip Koch's received ATT × 1 year history of chronic NSAID intake. Pedal edema +; UPCR–9.6 gm; Creatinine is 1.5 mg/dl; ANCA ++ (pANCA) Nephrotic syndrome. ? Amyloidosis (Secondary) ? MGN ? MCD.

Microscopy: Image 42.23

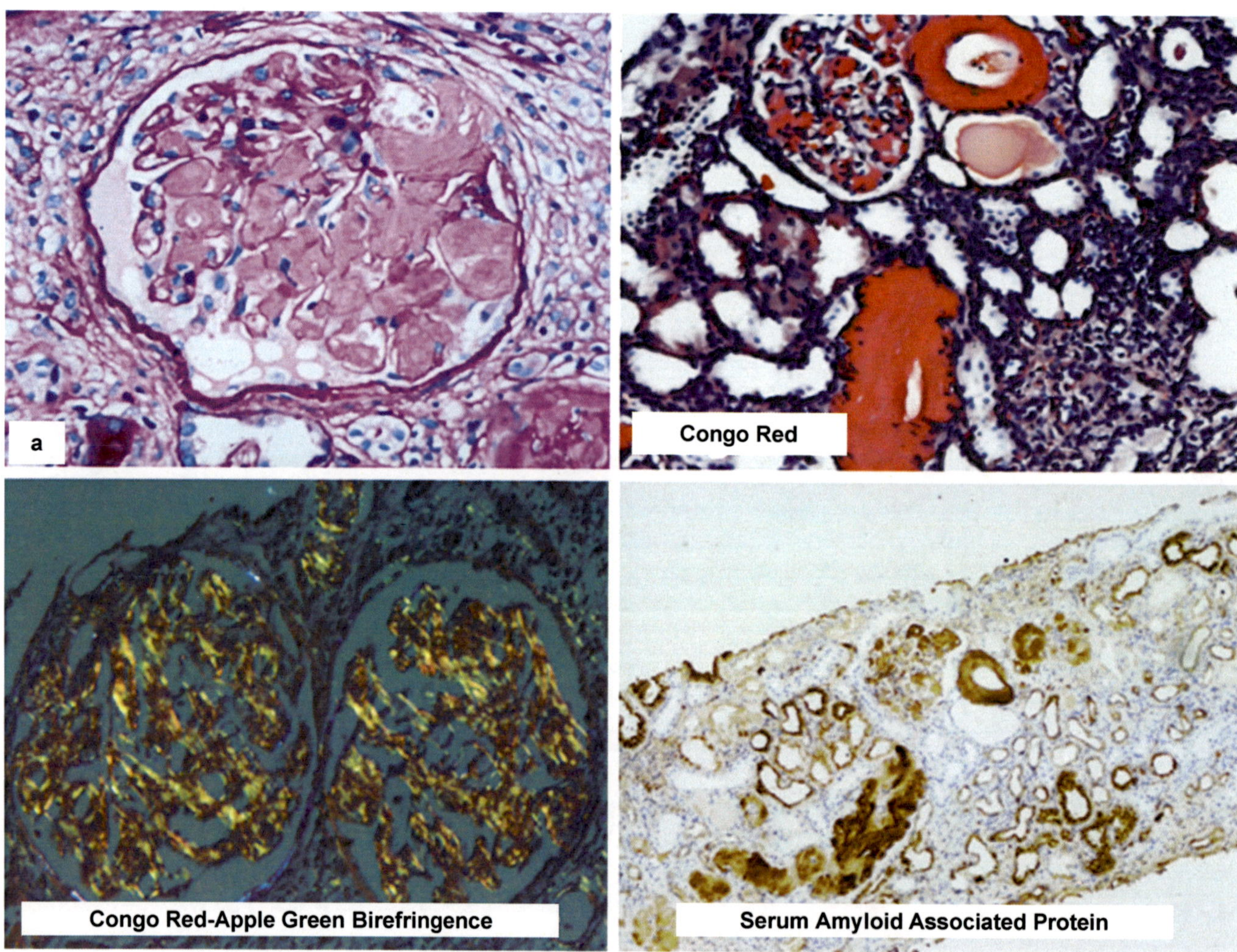

Figure 42.23: Photomicrograph panel show moderate mesangial matrix expansion by deposition of PAS negative amorphous material (a). Congo Red stain show congophilic deposits which reveal apple-green birefringence under polarized microscopy consistent with amyloid deposition (b, c). Serum amyloid associated protein is diffusely positive indicating post-inflammatory secondary amyloidosis. Kappa lambda immunofluorescence show no light chain restriction (not shown)

CASE 17

Amyloidosis, Primary

Clinical History:

55 years male with adult onset nephrotic syndrome, swelling over the body since 1 months. 4+ albuminuria.

Microscopy: Image 42.24

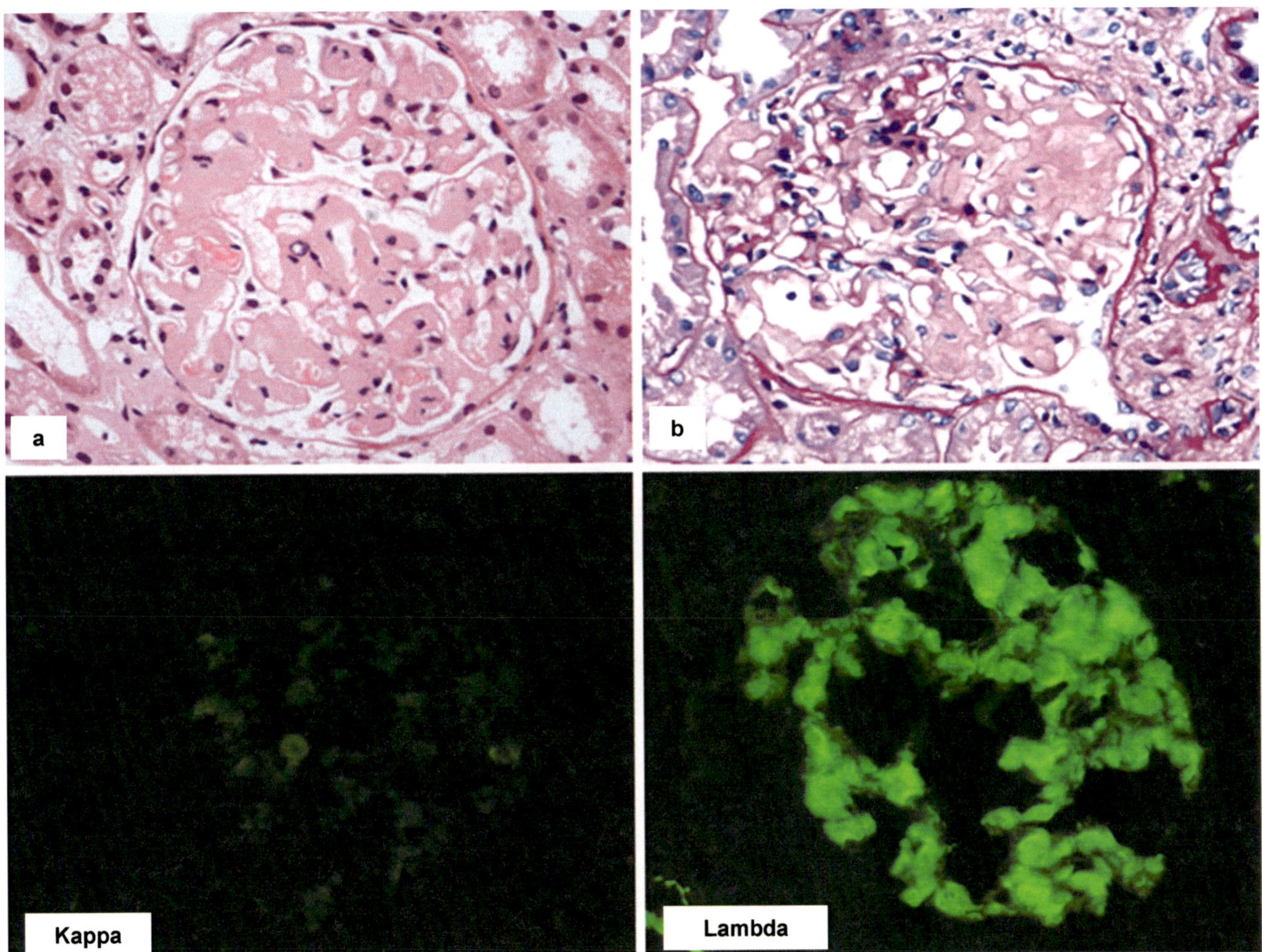

Figure 42.24: Photomicrograph panel show moderate mesangial matrix expansion by deposition of extracellular amorphous material (a). The deposition is PAS negative consistent with amyloid deposition (b). Kappa Lambda immunofluorescence show lambda light chain restriction indicating primary amyloidosis

CASE 18

Acute Tubulointerstitial Nephritis

Clinical History:

37 years male presented with vomiting. Bilateral flank pain with fever × 7 days. History of renal calculi 7 years back. Baseline creatinine is normal 1 year back. History of ingestion of diclofenac. BP–150/100. Not on any antihypertensive; Serum creatinine is 14 mg/dl; Urine R/M: Protein 1+.

Clinical Diagnosis:

?AKI ? AIN ? RPGN.

Microscopy: Image 42.25

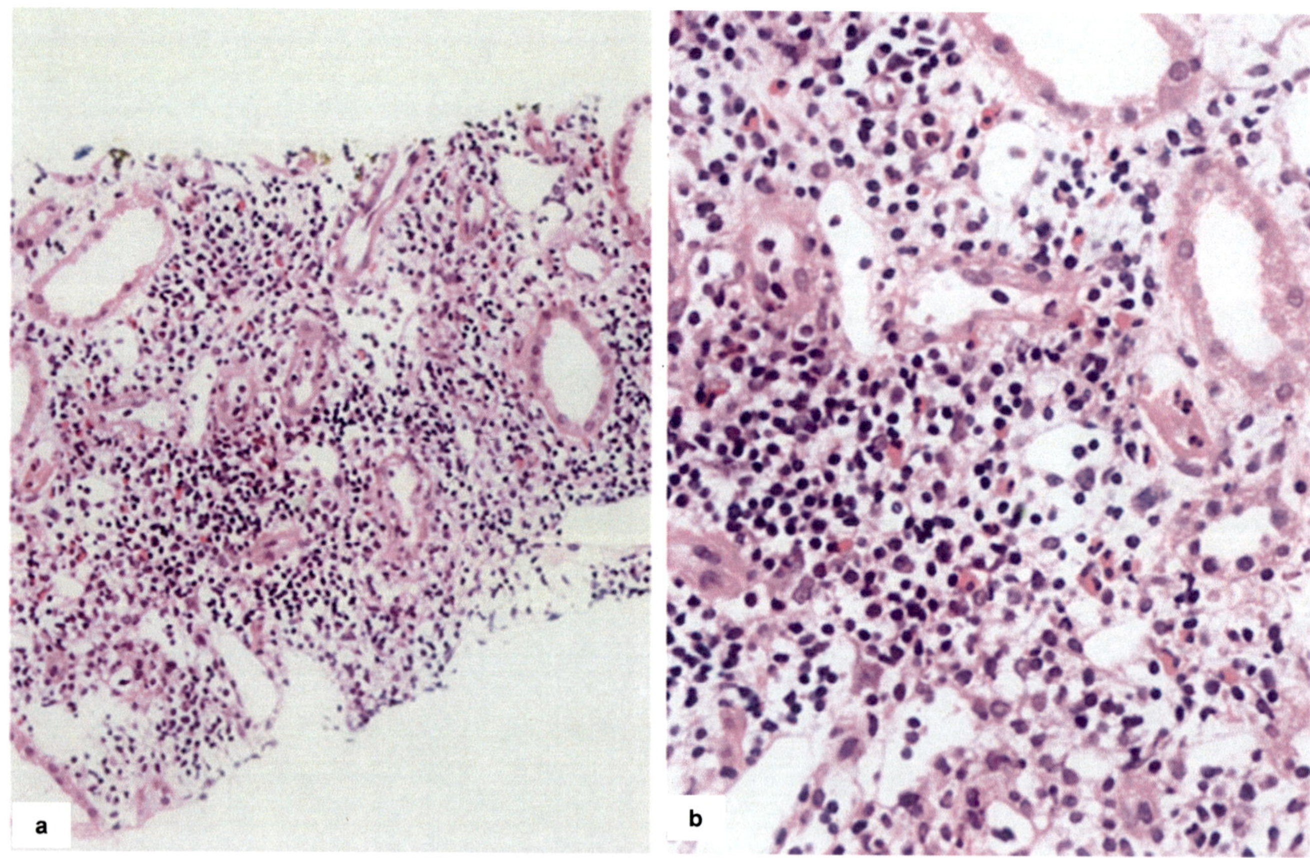

Figure 42.25: Hematoxylin and Eosin stained section show dominant pathology in the tubulointerstitial compartment in form of acute tubular injury alongwith moderate interstitial inflammation and interstitial edema. The interstitial infiltrate is composed of lymphocytes alongwith few scattered plasma cells and eosinophils

CASE 19

Myoglobin Cast Nephropathy

Clinical History:

20 years old male presented with acute kidney injury. History of rock climbing after taking alcohol followed by severe pain in legs, cola colored urine, oligoanuric. Serum creatinine 7 mg/dl, urine albumin 2+, SGOT–3233/SGPT–1536

Clinical Diagnosis:

? AKI? Myoglobinuria induced tubular injury.

Microscopy: Image 42.26

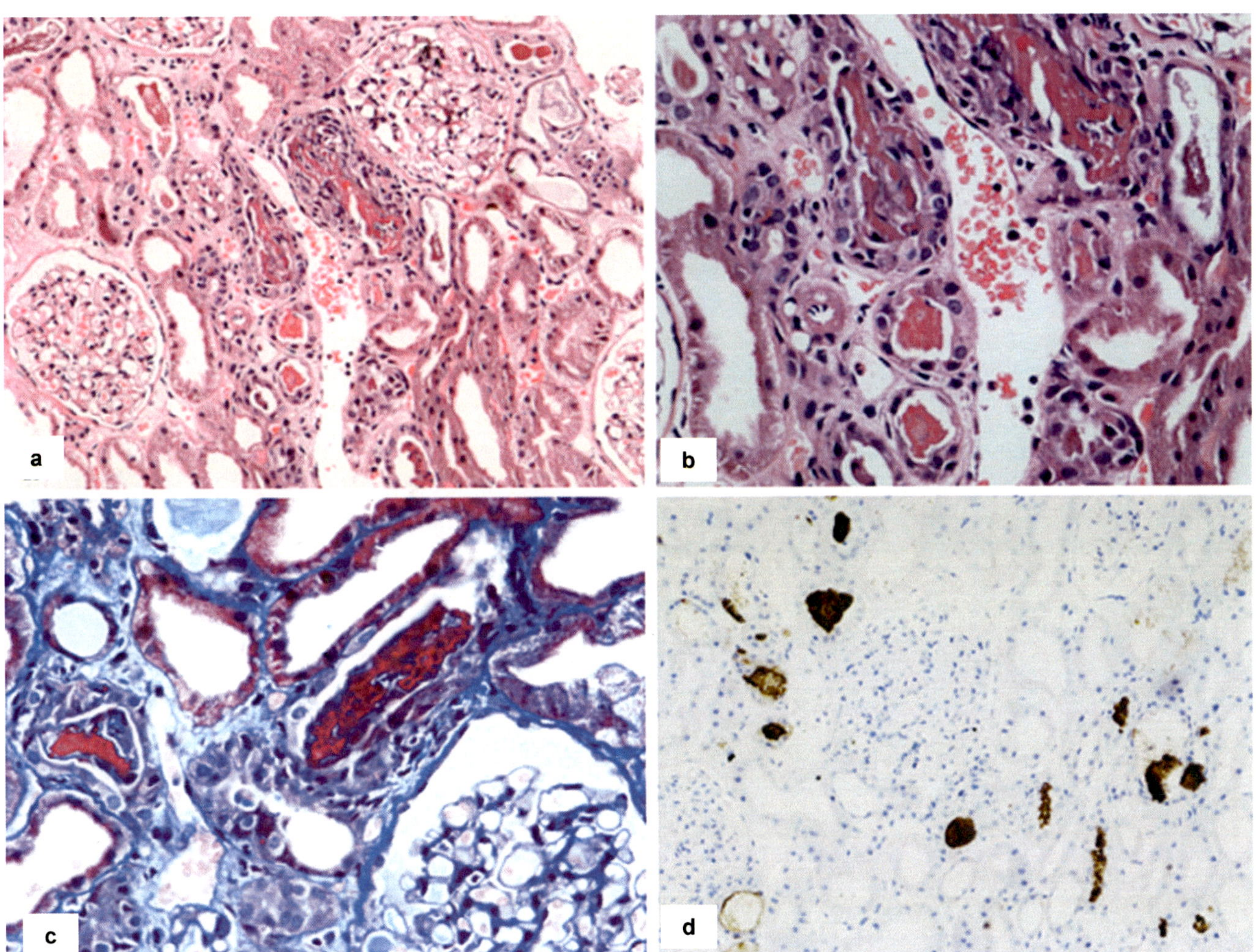

Figure 42.26: Hematoxylin and Eosin stained section show brick red cast tubular casts with beaded appearance (Low magnification in (a); Higher magnification in (b). Masson's trichrome stain highlight red colored tubular casts (c). Myoglobin immunohistochemistry confirm tubular casts (d)

Comment: Myoglobin deposition in tubular casts may result from trauma, increased muscle activity (such as severe exercise or seizure), exogenous toxins or medications (alcohol, illegal substances, cyclosporine, statins), hereditary myopathy, myositis, hypokalemia, hypophosphatemia or hyperosmolarity.

CASE 20

Light Chain Cast Nephropathy

Clinical History:

70 years male with deranged renal function. History of lower limb swelling × 3 months and generalized weakness for 1 month. Nondiabetic Nonhypertensive. Serum creatinine is 4.5 mg/dl. Urine R/M: Albumin ++; Pus cells 2-4/hpf; RBCs 3-5/hpf. No casts.

Clinical Diagnosis:

AKI? cause.

Microscopy: Image 42.27

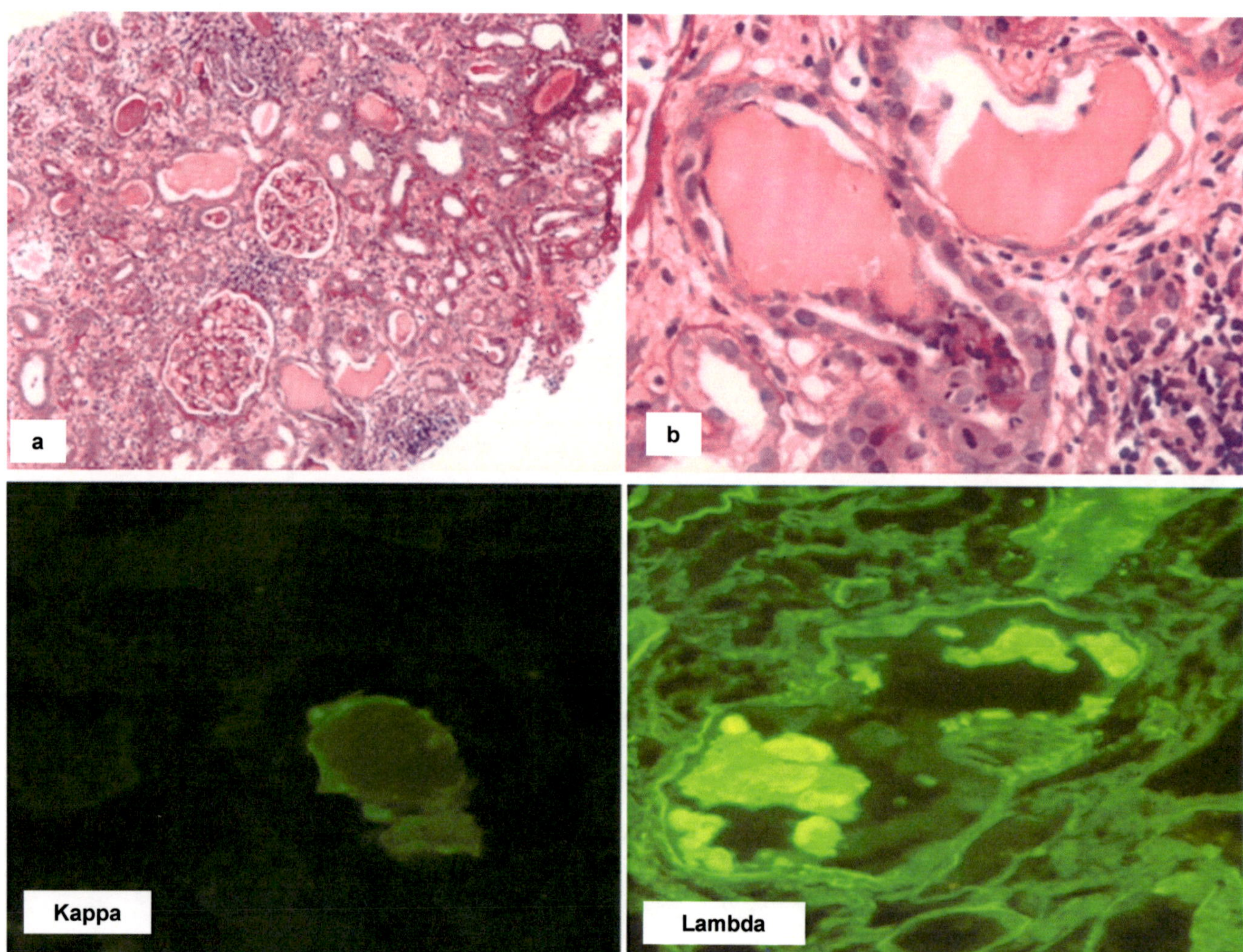

Figure 42.27: PAS stained section show presence of PAS negative tubular casts (a). High power magnification show PAS negative fractured casts with surrounding tubular epithelial reaction (b). Immunofluorescence studies show 3+ lambda staining in atypical tubular casts. The tubular casts show no kappa light chain staining, thereby indicating lambda light chain restriction. In addition, 2+ staining is seen along tubular basement membrane for lambda light chain and no staining is seen for kappa indicating early lambda light chain deposition disease

CHAPTER 43

Renal Transplant Pathology–Clinicopathological Cases

Rajan Duggal

Associate Director, Head, Histopathology and Cytopathology, BLK Super Speciality Hospital Pusa Road, New Delhi

Transplant Rejection

Overview of Banff Meetings

Till early 1990s, renal transplant rejection was classically classified into following broad categories:

1. **Hyperacute rejection:** Defined as immediate rejection of the renal graft within minutes to hours due to presence of preformed antibodies.
2. **Acute rejection:** Defined as rejection occurring after 5-7 days due to activated T-cells.
3. **Accelerated acute rejection:** Defined as an aggressive episode of rejection occurring within 5 days due to formation of antibodies in a presensitized patient.
4. **Chronic rejection:** Defined as slow progressive graft dysfunction starting after 3 months.

There was significant heterogeneity among pathologist in characterization of renal allograft biopsies. Hence, it was felt that standardization of renal allograft biopsy was necessary to guide therapy and to help establish an objective end-point in clinical trials. Hence, a group of pathologists, nephrologists, and transplant surgeons met in Banff Canada from 2-4 August, 1991, to formulate a schema for nomenclature and classification of renal allograft pathology. The schema underwent considerable revision over the next couple years through follow-up meetings and correspondence including circulation of slides and finally published in March 1993. Thereafter, the Banff group has been meeting at regular intervals. So far there have been a total of 14 Banff conferences.

Banff 1997 meeting constitutes a landmark document in the field of renal transplant pathology. It was developed using the 1st Banff schema and the CCTT (cooperative clinical trials in transplantation) modifications. The important changes introduced include:

Adequacy of renal transplant biopsy specimen: Two cores of tissue with cortex containing ≥ 10 glomeruli and atleast 2 arteries, and section thickness 3-4 μm.

Banff Diagnostic Categories

Category 1	Normal biopsy or non-specific changes
Category 2	Antibody-mediated changes
Category 3	Suspicious (borderline) for acute T cell-mediated rejection
Category 4	T cell-mediated rejection
Category 5	Interstitial fibrosis and tubular atrophy
Category 6	Other non-rejection changes

Hyperacute rejection in the 1st Banff was renamed as antibody-mediated rejection (ABMR), which included two subcategories: (A) Hyperacute rejection, and (B) Accelerated acute rejection. The diagnosis of acute accelerated rejection was based on positive repeat cross match.

Acute/active rejection: The grades of acute rejection were changed to type/grade.

Type (Grade) I: Tubulointerstitial inflammation only.

IA: Interstitial inflammation moderate-severe (i2,i3) and/or tubulitis moderate (t2).

IB: Tubulitis severe (t3).

Type (Grade) II: Intimal arteritis/Endothelitis.

IIA: Intimal arteritis mild-moderate (v1).

IIB: Intimal arteritis severe (v2).

Type (Grade) III: Transmural arteritis and/or fibrinoid necrosis (v3).

This classification of acute rejection still holds good, although it is now placed under acute T-cell mediated rejection.

Banff 2001 meeting recognized that antibodies play an important role in causing rejection. C4d staining of the peritubular capillaries was accepted as the marker of antibody-mediated rejection.

Banff 2005 meeting major revisions include:

- Change in the basic classification of rejection from acute and chronic to its pathophysiologic basis which is T-cell mediated rejection and antibody mediated rejection, either of which could be acute or chronic.
- Elimination of term chronic allograft nephropathy (CAN) by interstitial fibrosis and tubular atrophy (IFTA).

Banff 2007 meeting significant updates included:

- C4d staining of peritubular capillaries was graded: C4d0–Negative, C4d1–minimal 1-10%, C4d2–focal 10-50% and C4d3–diffuse >50%.
- Peritubular capillaritis was graded.

Banff 2009 meeting significant updates included:

- Six Banff working groups aiming at addressing unmet needs in transplantation pathology were established (isolated v lesion; fibrosis scoring; polyoma virus nephropathy staging; glomerular lesion scoring; molecular pathology; quality assurance).

Banff 2011 conference focused on refining diagnostic criteria for antibody-mediated rejection. The major outcome was acknowledgement of C4d negative ABMR. A new Banff working group was created to define diagnostic criteria for ABMR in kidneys independent of C4d.

Criteria for acute antibody-mediated rejection in renal allografts include 3 cardinal features:

1. Morphologic evidence of acute tissue injury, such as: (a) acute tubular injury; (b) neutrophils and/or mononuclear cells in peritubular capillaries and/or glomeruli, and/or capillary thrombosis; or (c) intimal arteritis/fibrinoid necrosis/intramural or transmural inflammation in arteries.
2. Immunopathologic evidence for antibody action, such as: (a) C4d and/or (rarely) immunoglobulin in peritubular capillaries; or (b) immunoglobulin and complement in arterial fibrinoid necrosis.
3. Serologic evidence of circulating antibodies to donor HLA or other anti-donor endothelial antigens.

Banff 2013 conference: The key outcome of this conference was defining criteria for diagnosis of C4d-negative ABMR and 3 new Banff working groups were initiated.

Acute/active ABMR; all three features must be present for diagnosis:

1. Histologic evidence of acute tissue injury, including one or more of the following:
    - Microvascular inflammation (g>0 and/or ptc>0).
    - Intimal or transmural arteritis (v>0).
    - Acute thrombotic microangiopathy, in the absence of any other cause.
    - Acute tubular injury, in the absence of any other apparent cause.
2. Evidence of current/recent antibody interaction with vascular endothelium, including at least one of the following:
    - Linear C4d staining in peritubular capillaries (C4d2 or C4d3 by IF on frozen sections, or C4d>0 by IHC on paraffin sections).
    - At least moderate microvascular inflammation (g+ptc ≥2).
    - Increased expression of gene transcripts in the biopsy tissue indicative of endothelial injury, if thoroughly validated.
3. Serologic evidence of donor-specific antibodies (DSAs) (HLA or other antigens).

Chronic, active ABMR; all three features must be present for diagnosis:

1. Morphologic evidence of chronic tissue injury, including one or more of the following:
    - Transplant glomerulopathy (TG) (cg>0), if no evidence of chronic thrombotic microangiopathy.
    - Severe peritubular capillary basement membrane multilayering (requires EM).
    - Arterial intimal fibrosis of new onset, excluding other causes.
2. Evidence of current/recent antibody interaction with vascular endothelium, including at least one of the following:
    - Linear C4d staining in peritubular capillaries (C4d2 or C4d3 by IF on frozen sections, or C4d>0 by IHC on paraffin sections).
    - At least moderate microvascular inflammation (g+ptc ≥2).
    - Increased expression of gene transcripts in the biopsy tissue indicative of endothelial injury, if thoroughly validated.
3. Serologic evidence of DSAs (HLA or other antigens).

C4d staining without evidence of rejection; all three features must be present for diagnosis:

1. Linear C4d staining in peritubular capillaries (C4d2 or C4d3 by IF on frozen sections, or C4d>0 by IHC on paraffin sections).
2. g=0, ptc=0, cg=0 (by light microscopy and by EM if available), v=; no TMA, no peritubular capillary basement membrane multilayering, no acute tubular injury (in the absence of another apparent cause for this).
3. No acute cell-mediated rejection (Banff 97 type 1A or greater) or borderline changes.

Banff 2015 meeting: The main aims of this conference were to review the clinical impact of 2013 changes related to the new diagnostic criteria for antibody-mediated rejection and to identify the next set of challenges in transplant diagnostics. In addition, prospects for introducing molecular diagnostics into the Banff classification was the main focus.

Banff 2017 conference focused on 2 areas: Clinical implications of inflammation in areas of interstitial fibrosis and tubular atrophy (i-IFTA) and its relationship to T cell-mediated rejection (TCMR), and the continued evolution of molecular diagnostics, particularly in the diagnosis of ABMR.

Banff 2019 meeting significant updates include:

- Clarifications and refinements to the criteria for chronic active (CA) T cell-mediated rejection (TCMR), borderline and antibody-mediated rejection (ABMR).
- Sessions on ABMR focused on biopsies showing microvascular inflammation in the absence of C4d staining or detectable donor-specific antibodies; the potential value of molecular diagnostics in such case.
- The capabilities of artificial intelligence and the potential for use of machine learning algorithms in diagnosis and personalized therapeutics in solid organ transplantation.

Drug Toxicity

Histologic changes of calcineurin toxicity in various renal compartments:

Tubular compartment: Single cell necrosis; Isometric vacuolization; Microcalcifications.

Vascular compartment: Smooth muscle swelling/ vacuolization; Single myocyte necrosis; medial and/ or adventitial hyaline deposits; fibrin thrombi or mucointimal edema suggesting vascular thrombotic microangiopathy (TMA).

Glomerular compartment: Fibrin thrombi (acute TMA) to glomerular capillary wall duplication (chronic TMA).

Infections

Many infections can affect immunosuppressed renal allograft recipients either as systemic or organ limited disease. Some infections, such as polyomavirus nephropathy (PVN) is restricted to kidney transplant. Other rare infections include CMV and Adenovirus infection.

PVN is defined morphologically and pathologists play a crucial role in patient management. A diagnosis requires histologic evidence of an intrarenal, productive polyomavirus infection in the medulla and /or cortex. Polyomavirus replication can be identified by light microscopy and the presence of intranuclear viral inclusion bodies or in early disease stages lacking inclusions also solely by IHC or alternatively by in situ hybridization. Thus, a definitive diagnosis of PVN is not established by laboratory tests, such as level of viremia, but rather requires a renal biopsy. The common histologic changes seen in PVN are presence of intranuclear viral inclusion bodies in epithelial cells and virally induced tubular epithelial cell injury and lysis.

CASE 1

Acute Cellular Rejection, Banff Type IA

Clinical History:

Post-renal transplant POD 13 days. No induction. Baseline creatinine is 1.4 mg/dl. Rise in serum creatinine to 2.0 mg/dl ? rejection ? ATN ? CNI toxicity.

Microscopy: Image 43.1

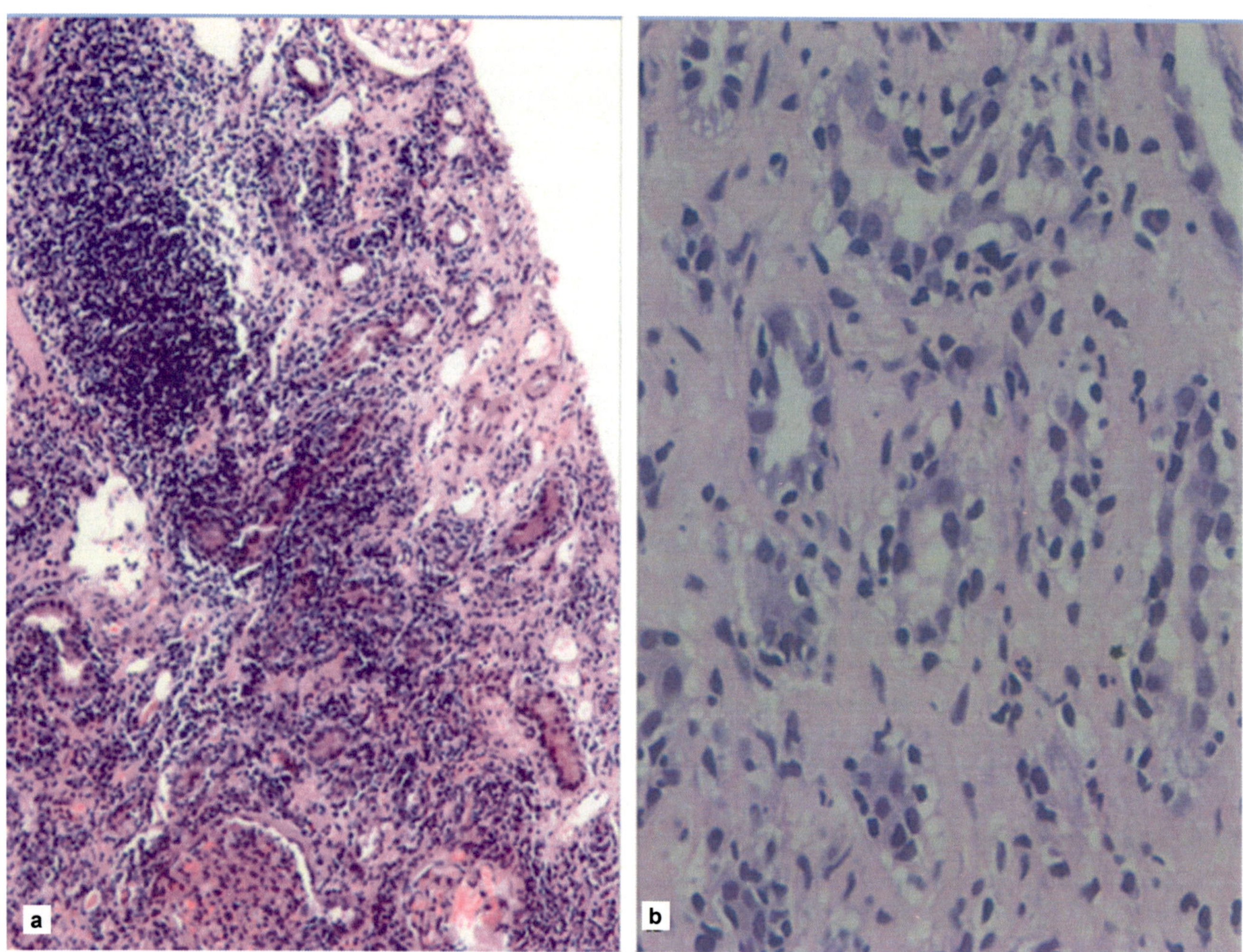

Figure 43.1: Allograft renal biopsy reveal moderate interstitial inflammation occupying 35-40% of the sampled renal cortex (a). Moderate tubulitis is seen in (b). C4d staining is negative (not shown)

Features are consistent with Acute Cellular Rejection, Banff IA.

Banff Score: g0 mm0 cg0 t2 ct0 i2 ci0 v0 cv0 ah0 ptc0. C4d0.

CASE 2

Acute Antibody Mediated Rejection

Clinical History:

32 years male post renal transplant (POD4 days). Allograft dysfunction with progressively falling platelets and hemoglobin. Basiliximab induction.

Microscopy: Image 43.2

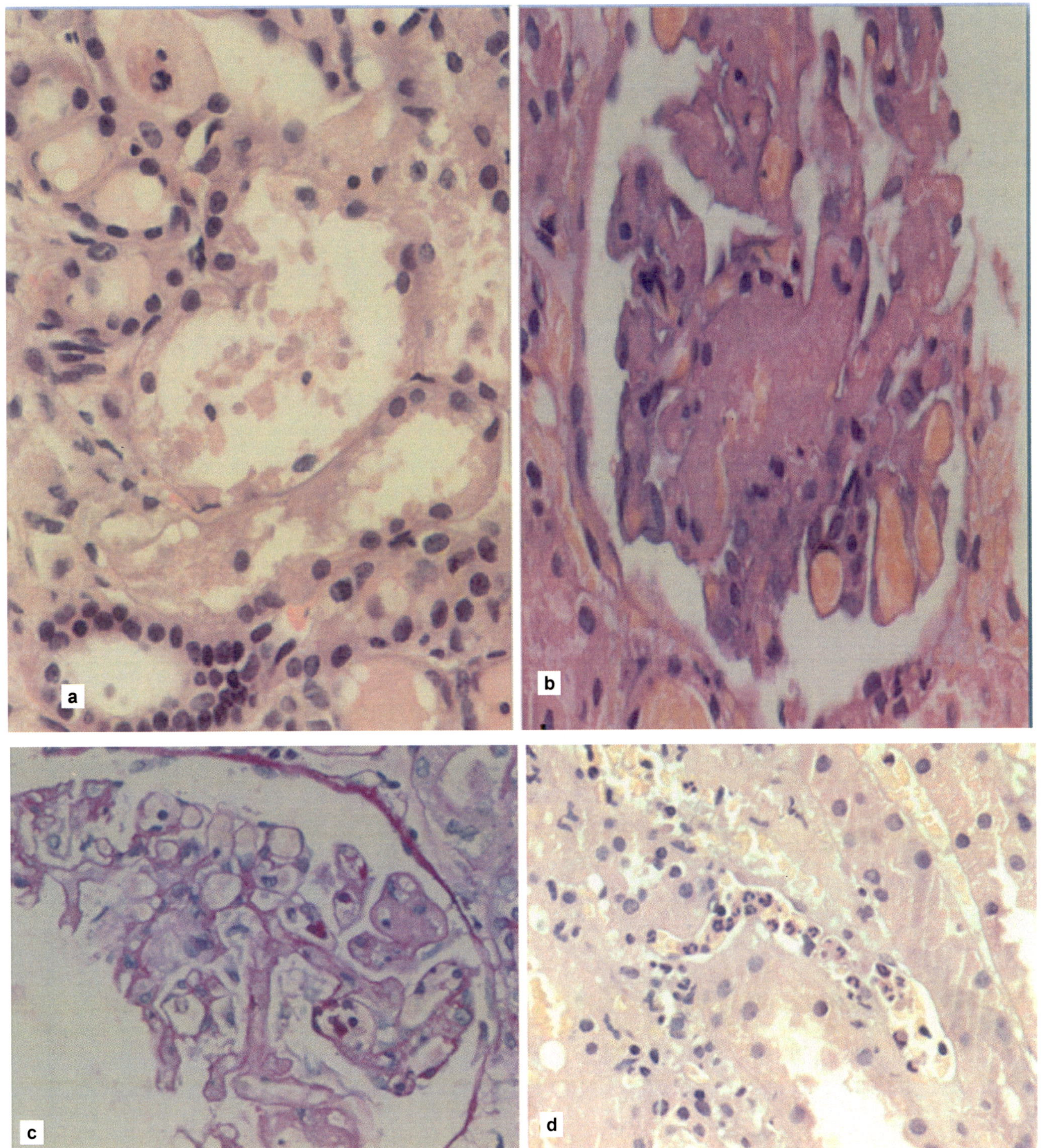

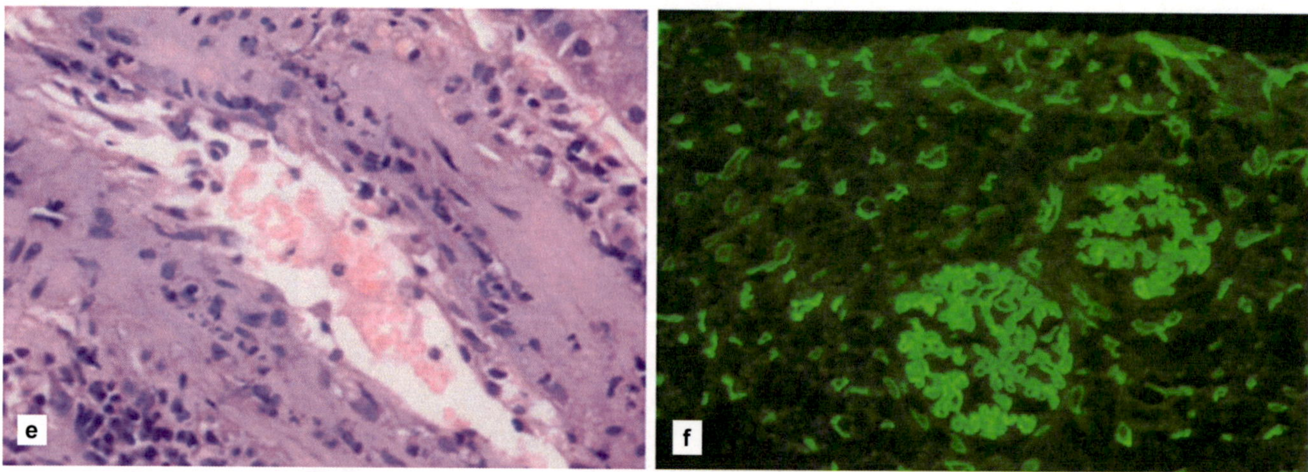

Figure 43.2: Allograft renal biopsy reveal diffuse acute tubular injury (a). Glomeruli show fibrin thrombi in capillary loops indicating acute glomerular thrombotic microangiopathy (b). Moderate microvascular inflammation seen in form of neutrophilic glomerulitis and peritubular capillaritis (c, d). Vessel show evidence of transmural inflammation along with necrosis consistent with type III vascular rejection/severe vascular rejection (e). C4d immunofluorescence show diffuse staining in peritubular capillaries (f)

Features are consistent with Acute Antibody Mediated Rejection.

Banff Score: g2 mm0 cg0 t0 ct0 i0 ci0 v3 cv0 ah0 ptc3. C4d3.

CASE 3

Chronic Antibody Mediated Rejection

Clinical History:

24 years male post renal transplant in 2010. Serum creatinine was 1.7 mg/dl in February 2017. Recent rise in serum creatinine to 3.6 mg/dl with chronic diarrhea. UPCR-3.0.

Microscopy: Image 43.3

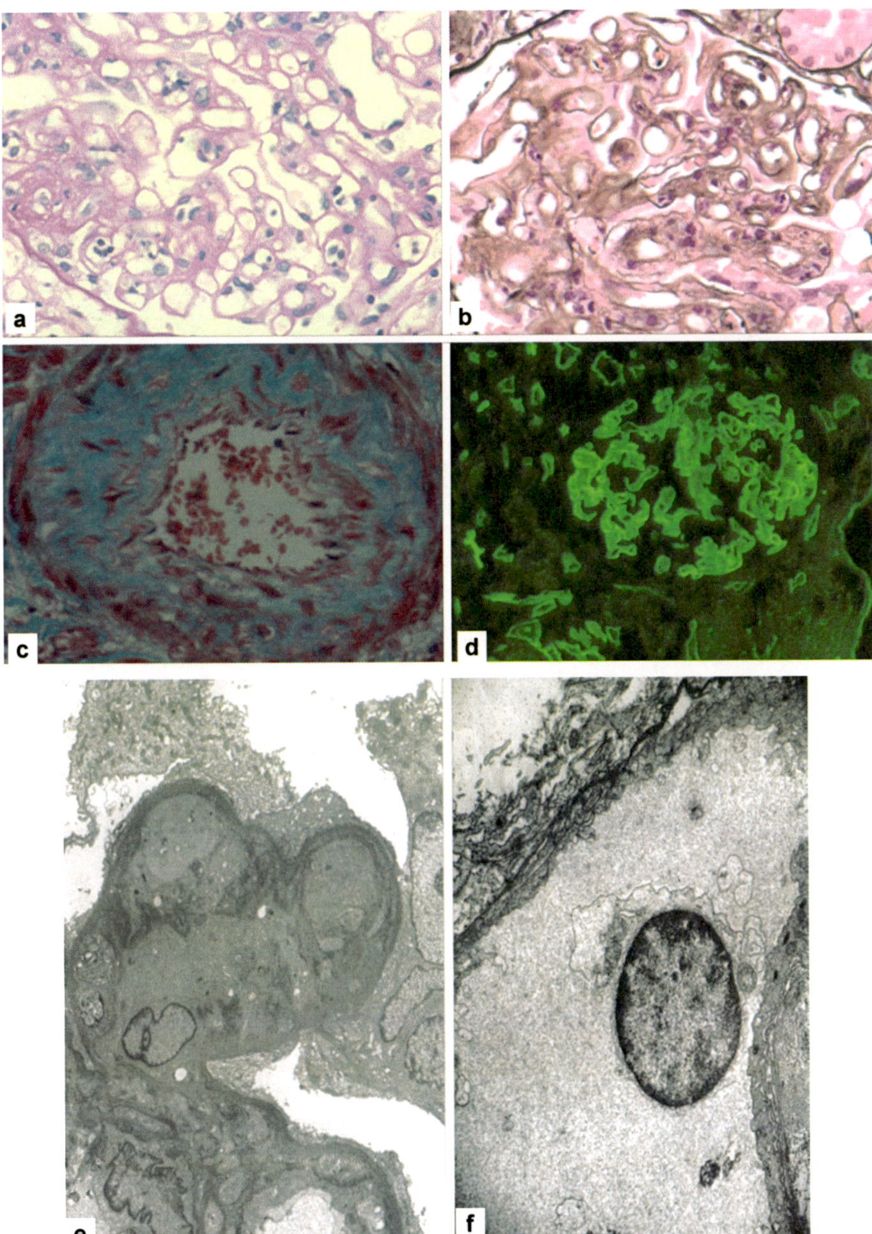

Figure 43.3: Allograft renal biopsy reveal mild thickening of the glomerular capillary wall with extensive duplication and minimal glomerulitis indicating advanced transplant glomerulopathy (a, b–PAS and Silver stain). Vessel show evidence of intimal sclerosis indicating transplant arteriopathy/chronic vascular rejection (c). C4d immunofluorescence show diffuse staining in peritubular capillaries (d). Ultrastructural examination show glomerular capillary wall multilamellation along with peritubular capillary basement membrane multilayering (e, f)

Features are consistent with Chronic Antibody Mediated Rejection.

Banff Score: g1 mm0 cg3 t0 ct1 i0 ci1 v0 cv2 ah0 ptc1. C4d3.

CASE 4

BKV Nephropathy

Clinical History:

28 years male post renal transplant (POD 8 months). Creeping creatinine 1.62—1.94—1.94—2.64 mg/dl.

Microscopy: Image 43.4

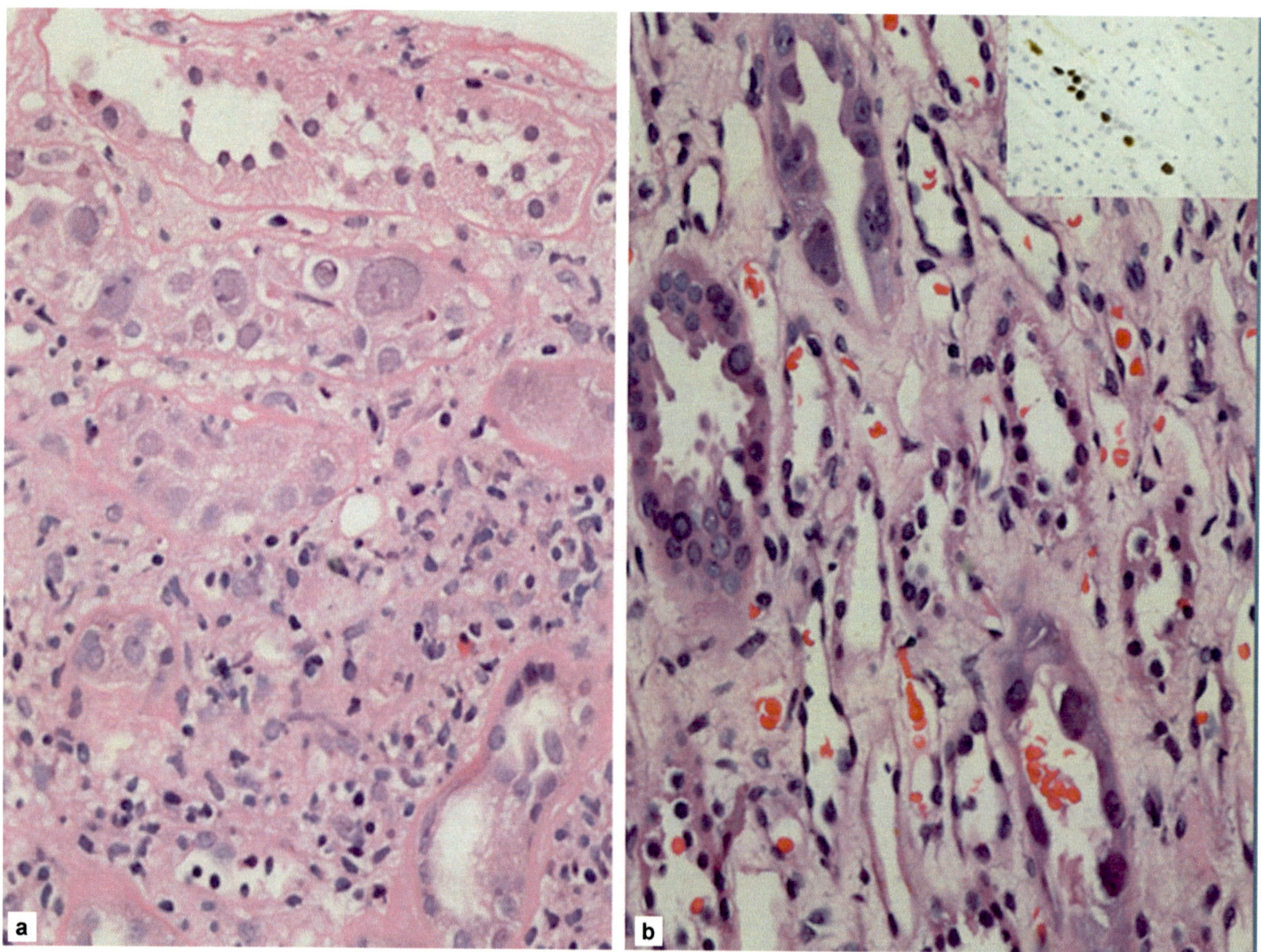

Figure 43.4: Allograft renal biopsy reveal presence of mild interstitial inflammation with evidence of mild tubulitis. In addition, few cortical and medullary tubules show evidence of nuclear enlargement with evidence of smudging and nuclear clearing (a, b). Inset show positive SV-40 stain in the nucleomegalic tubular epithelial cells. No tubular atrophy or interstitial fibrosis is seen (not shown)

Features are consistent with Polyoma virus nephropathy.

Banff Score: g0 mm0 cg0 t1 ct0 i1 ci0 v0 cv0 ah0 ptc0. C4d0.

CHAPTER

Application of Nuclear Medicine in Nephrology

Manas Sahoo[1], Rashmi Kavindram[2]

[1] *Consultant, Department of Nuclear Medicine, Medanta, The Medicity, Gurugram*

[2] *Consultant, Department of Nuclear Medicine, Medanta, The Medicity, Gurugram*

Clinical Indications for Genitourinary Scintigraphy

- Blood flow abnormalities.
- Function quantification:
  - Differential function.
  - Glomerular filtration rate, effective renal plasma flow.
- Mass vs. column of Bertin.
- Obstruction: Uteropelvic junction, ureteral.
- Pyelonephritis.
- Renal failure: Acute and chronic.
- Renovascular hypertension/renal artery stenosis.
- Renal vein thrombosis.
- Surgical complications.
- Transplant rejection.
- Transplant anastomosis assessment.
- Trauma.
- Vesicoureteral reflux.
- **Volume quantification:** Bladder residual volume.

^{99M}Tc-DMSA Scintigraphy

Dimercaptosuccinic acid is one of the most common renal cortical agent with about 40% concentrating in the cortex predominantly in the proximal tubules in the pars recta.[1-3]

Common Indications

- Detection of focal renal parenchymal abnormalities (cortical scar).
- Detection of renal sequelae, 6 months after acute infection.
- Accurate differential function.
- Detection of acute pyelonephritis.
- Detection of associated abnormalities: Abnormal duplex kidney, small kidney, dysplastic tissue, horseshoe kidney.
- Detection of ectopic kidney.
- Confirmation of non-functional multicystic kidney.

Contraindications

- Pregnancy.

Dose

- **Child:** 50 µCi/kg (minimum dose of 600 µCi).
- **Adult:** 5 mCi (185 MBq).

Procedure

- No diet restriction and fasting needed.
- Patient should be well hydrated.
- Radiopharmaceutical is injected intravenously. Image at 2 hours after injection. Patient should void prior to scan.

Radiation Burden

- Approximately 1 mSv/examination.[4-5]

Illustrations (Figs. 44.1 to 44.4)

Radionuclide Cystography (Direct and Indirect)

Vesicoureteral Reflux

Untreated reflux and infection are associated with subsequent renal damage, scarring, hypertension, and chronic renal failure.[6-8] Vesicoureteral reflux (VUR) occurs in approximately 1% to 2% of the pediatric population. In patients with acute pyelonephritis, VUR is present in approximately 40% of patients. In untreated patients, VUR is responsible for 5% to 40% of end-stage renal disease in patients under 16 years of age and 5% to 20% of adults younger than 50 years of age.

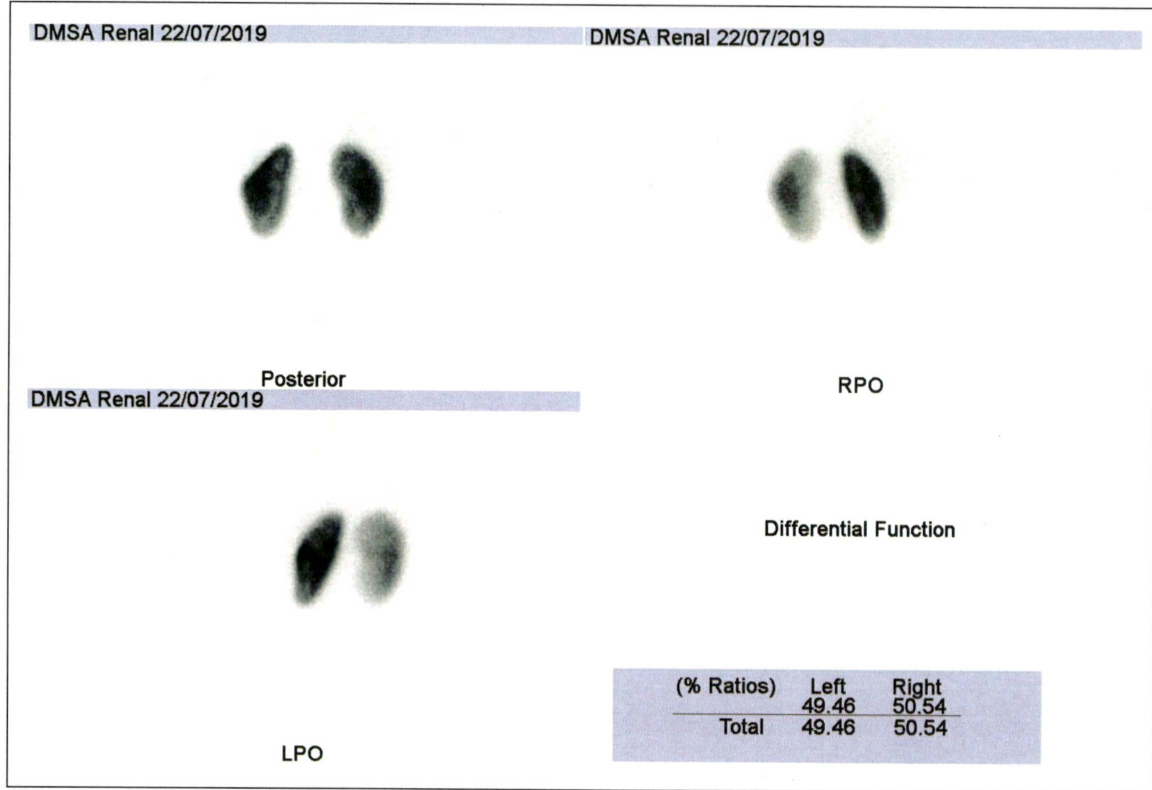

Figure 44.1: Bilateral normal functioning kidneys showing homogenous tracer uptake and no cortical scarring. Differential function is also calculated. Oblique views are acquired for better delineation of outlines

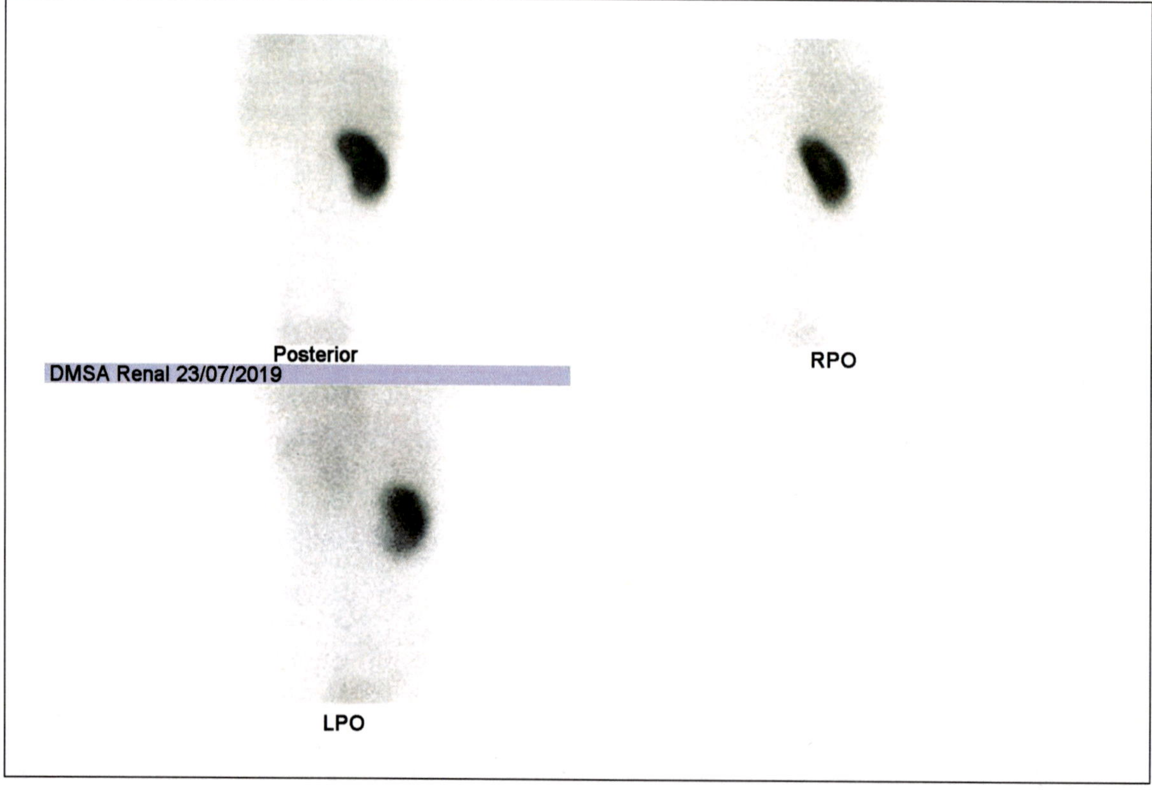

Figure 44.2: Left kidney is not seen with no significant tracer in left renal fossa – non functioning/non visualized kidney. Right kidney shows normal homogenous radiotracer uptake with well delineated outline

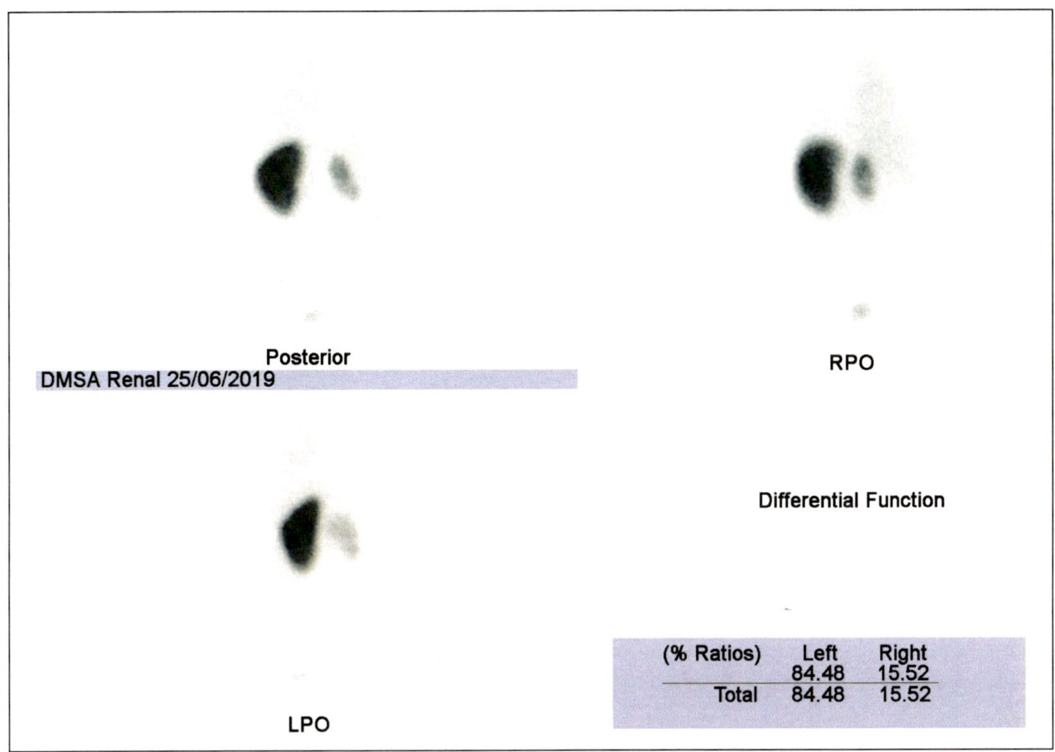

Figure 44.3: Left kidney shows normal homogenous radiotracer uptake with well delineated outline. Right kidney is small in size and shows reduced tracer uptake with ill defined outlines–representing poorly functioning scarred small right kidney

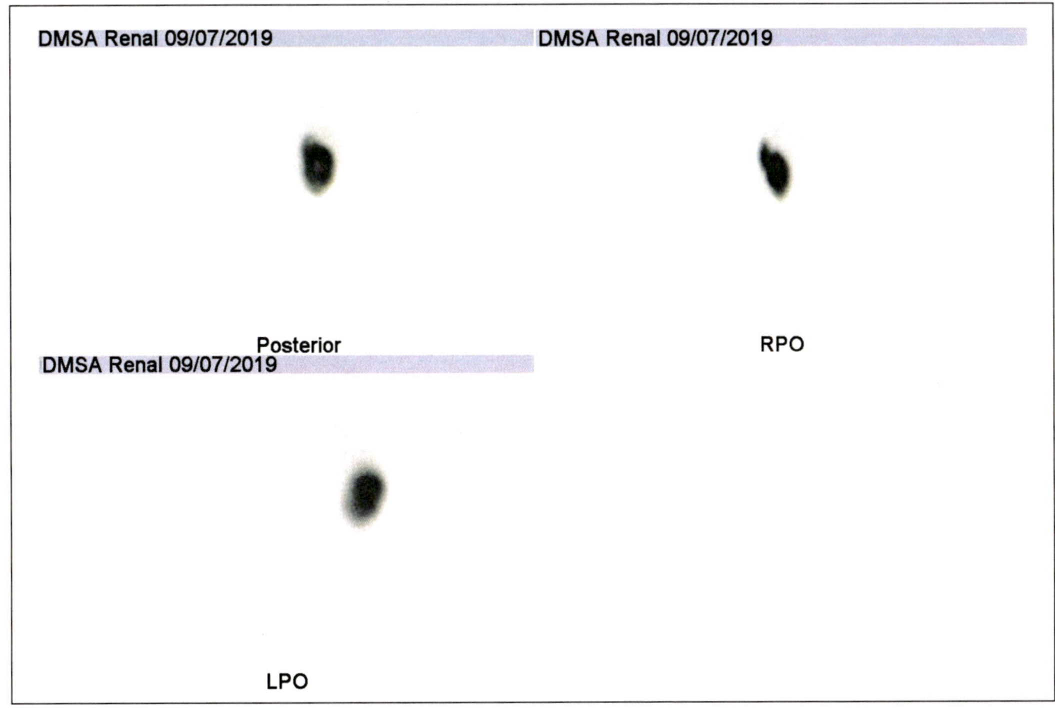

Figure 44.4: Left kidney is not seen with no significant tracer in left renal fossa–non functioning/non visualized kidney. Right kidney shows normal homogenous tracer uptake with cortical irregularity in the upper pole suggesting of cortical scarring

Advantages Over Micturating Cystourethrogram (MCU)

- Minimal radiation burden.
- Indirect radionuclide cystogram (IRC) offers the possibility of detecting VUR without a bladder catheterization and allows micturition to be studied under physiological conditions.[9-11]

Indications

- Detection of VUR in children after UTI (in boys the first catheter cystogram should be an MCU to visualize the urethra).
- Follow-up of children with known VUR during prophylactic antibiotic/bacteriostatic treatment.

- Assessment of the results of endoscopic or surgical treatment.
- Screening of siblings of children/parents with proven VUR.
- Detection and follow-up of VUR in children who are toilet trained (IRC). Assessment of the effect of the full and empty bladder on the drainage of the dilated upper tracts.[12-14]
- DRC can be also used for the detection of VUR in renal transplant recipients and for serial evaluation of bladder dysfunction (e.g., neurogenic bladder) for reflux.

Contraindications

- There are no contraindications. However children should not be catheterized during the active phase of UTI.
- In the presence of low lying or pelvic kidney VUR may be missed if a dilated lower ureter is being investigated.

Procedure

DRC Radiopharmaceutical

- Tc-99m Sulphur colloid, DTPA, MAG3, TcO4.

Dose

- 20-40 MBq for 500 ml saline; or
- 20 MBq for direct instillation technique.

Children are catheterized under aseptic conditions using a small size catheter. ^{99m}Tc radiotracer is mixed in 500 ml sterile isotonic saline warmed to body temperature and slowly fill the bladder under hydrostatic pressure. Filling of the bladder to capacity should take some 10 minutes.

When bladder capacity is reached, or when the child shows urge to void or when there is cessation of flow from the bottle in a nonvoiding patient the filling is stopped and the child is allowed to void.

The volume used should not markedly exceed the formula for bladder volume:

$$\text{Age} \times 30 + 30 \text{ cc} = (\text{Age in years} + 1) \times 30 \text{ cc.}$$

Radiation Burden

- Effective dose is approximately 0.048 mSv per 20 MBq of ^{99m}Tc (Fig. 44.5).

Glomerular Filtration Rate (GFR) Determination By Blood Sampling

Renal clearance of a substance can occur by two processes: glomerular filtration or tubular secretion. Of these processes, GFR is probably the most representative parameter of renal function. It is relatively constant under standard conditions, and, as opposed to tubular secretion, is independent of the urine flow.[15-18]

Indications

- Evaluation and follow-up of renal function in chronic glomerulopathies and diabetes mellitus.

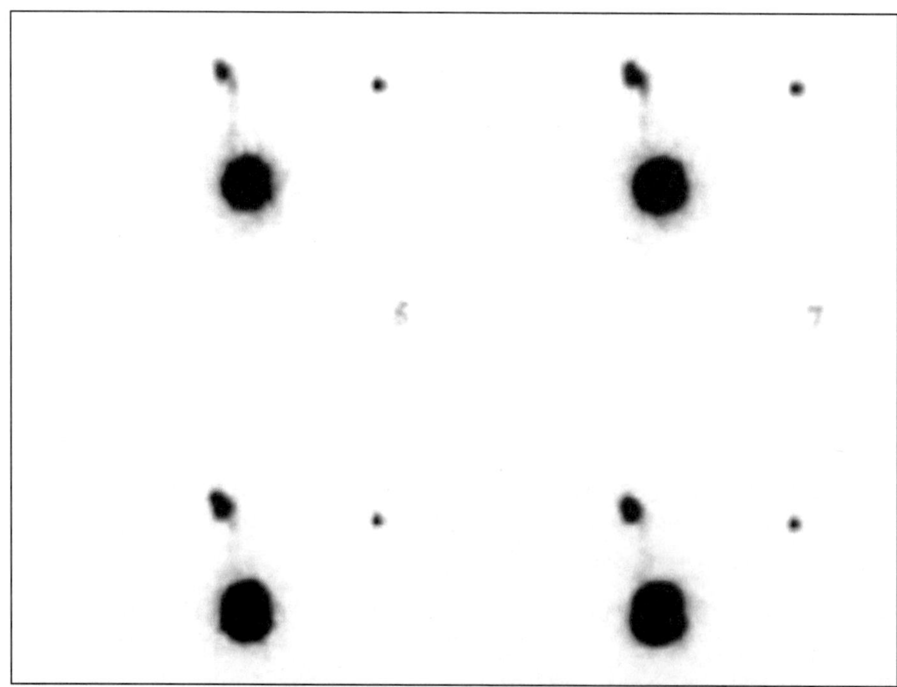

Figure 44.5: Upward tracking of tracer is noted on the right side upto the level of pelvis–suggesting of high grade reflux

- Evaluation and follow-up of renal side effects of chemotherapy or nephrotoxic drugs such as cyclosporin and antibiotics.
- Estimation of the single kidney GFR, in conditions such as unilateral or bilateral hydronephrosis, urinary tract infections with or without associated vesico-ureteral reflux, small kidney, single kidney, duplex kidney, urethral valves, pre- and post-operative follow-up.
- GFR determination can be considered each time renal impairment is suspected, even while plasma creatinine is in the normal range.

Contraindications

There are no contraindications.

Radionuclide

- Chromium-51 (51Cr); or
- Technetium-99m (99mTc).

Pharmaceutical

- Ethylene diamine tetraacetic acid (EDTA).
- Diethylene triamine pentaacetic acid (DTPA).

  Two methods are used:
- Slope-intercept method.
- Distribution volume method.

DTPA Dynamic Renal Scintigraphy

Agents for Glomerular Filtration Rate:

Tc-99m DTPA

Agents for Effective Renal Plasma Flow:

Tc-99m mercaptoacetyltriglycine (MAG3) and EC (ethylenedicysteine).

Standard renography allows estimation of two aspects of renal function.

The first aspect is renal clearance, i.e., the extraction of a tracer from the blood. DRF estimation is best undertaken approximately between one and two minutes after tracer injection.

The second function, which can be assessed by renography is the excretion, or disappearance, of the tracer from the kidney. This disappearance can simply be estimated by inspecting the renogram curve: An early peak followed by a rapidly descending phase is typical for normal excretion. An important delay in excretion is characterized by a continuously ascending curve. Several techniques have been proposed for quantifying the transit of tracer through the kidney.

Following intravenous injection, normal peak cortical uptake occurs by 3 to 4 minutes. By 5 minutes, the collecting system is seen; the bladder is typically visualized by 10 to 15 minutes. The T½ peak, or the time it takes for half of the maximal cortical activity to clear, is normally 15 to 20 minutes for Tc-99m DTPA.[19,20]

Normal Renogram

1. Initial blood flow (30-60 seconds).
2. Cortical uptake phase (normally 1-3 minutes).
3. Clearance phase representing cortical excretion and collecting system clearance.

Controversy exists in four areas, these are hydration of the child, bladder status/bladder catheterization, assessment of drainage post furosemide and the interpretation of impaired drainage.[21]

Hydration of the Child: The child should be adequately hydrated for both the standard and diuretic renogram.

Bladder Status and Effect of Gravity: In the presence of a full bladder, drainage from the kidney may be delayed, even in the normal kidney resulting in a flat renal curve.

Assessment of Drainage Post Furosemide: Assessment of drainage is controversial. The shape of the washout curve has been proposed to assess drainage. The classical method of analysis of the post diuretic curve is to assess the slope of this curve; however, the determination of this slope is not straightforward and many variants have been proposed, each resulting in a different slope value. Analysis of the post furosemide curve on its own is inadequate since important physiological variables are not taken into account; these include the function of the kidney, bladder status, and the effect of gravity and the volume of the renal pelvis.

The Interpretation of Impaired Drainage: Good drainage is easy to define, since the images, curves and numerical data all reveal little tracer in the kidney and collecting system at the end of the study. However, when drainage is reduced then there is little agreement as to what constitutes impaired drainage.

Mechanism of Uptake for Renal Scintigraphy Imaging Agents

- Clearance by glomerular filtration of DTPA is 100%.
- Clearance by tubular section of MAG3 is 100%.

Thus tubular tracers have greater extraction than the glomerular agent resulting in a lower background activity and a higher kidney to background ratio. For these reasons the tubular agents are preferred to 99m Tc-DTPA for estimation of DRF particularly in infants, for diuretic renography and indirect cystography. 99mTc-DTPA may be useful following renal transplantation when both blood flow as well as formal glomerular filtration rate (GFR) estimation (with blood sample analysis) is required.

Common Indications

- All uropathies, which require evaluation of individual renal function at diagnosis and during the different phases of surgical or conservative treatment and evaluation of the drainage function. Examples include dilatation immaterial of the cause (e.g., Pelvi-Ureteric and Vesico-Ureteric dilatation), bladder dysfunction, complicated duplex kidney, post trauma, asymmetrical renal function and reflux nephropathy.
- When dilatation of the collecting system exists, the standard renogram should be complemented by a diuretic renogram.
- Preceding Indirect Radionuclide Cystography (IRC).
- Evaluation of sustained systemic hypertension. If reno-vascular disease is suspected then captopril provocation may be used.
- Renal trauma.
- Follow-up of renal transplantation. Here the dose of tracer is increased and a rapid acquisition is required.

Contraindications

There are no contraindications. However, there are limitations: in the presence of poor renal function, accurate estimation of DRF and/or drainage may not be possible. In the presence of marked hydronephrosis, the interpretation of poor drainage is difficult since this could be due to either "partial hold-up" or simply because of the reservoir effect of the dilated system. In the presence of calculus obstruction, a renogram may be undertaken but no furosemide should be administered.

Dose Schedule

Minimum doses are: 99mTc-MAG3 = 15 MBq. 99mTc-DTPA = 20 MBq (for children).

Adult: 3-5 mCi (93-185 MBq).

Radiation Burden: The effective dose for an adult with normal renal function is 0.007 mSv/MBq.

Diuretic Administration (Furosemide) Dose: 1 mg/kg with a maximum dose of 20 mg for children, adults is 0.5 mg/kg.

Timing of Administration: There are three variations:

F + 20 - Furosemide is injected 20 minutes after the injection of tracer.

F – 15 - Furosemide is injected 15 minutes prior to the tracer – mostly used for post pyelopasty patient.

F – 0 - Furosemide is injected at the beginning of the study – most widely used method and the standard in pediatric population.

Diuretic Graphs

Illustrations (Figs. 44.6 to 44.8)

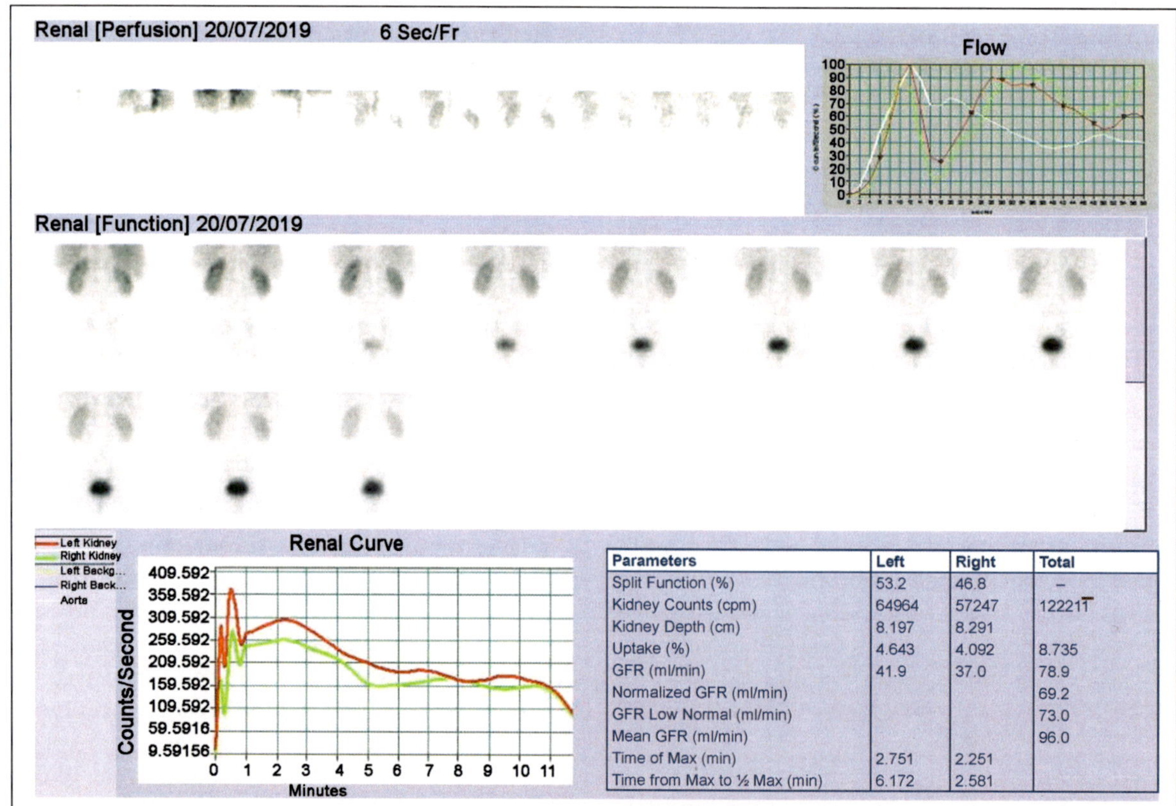

Figure 44.6: Bilateral kidneys show normal perfusion, cortical tracer uptake and subsequent drainage. Renogram curve shows normal pattern

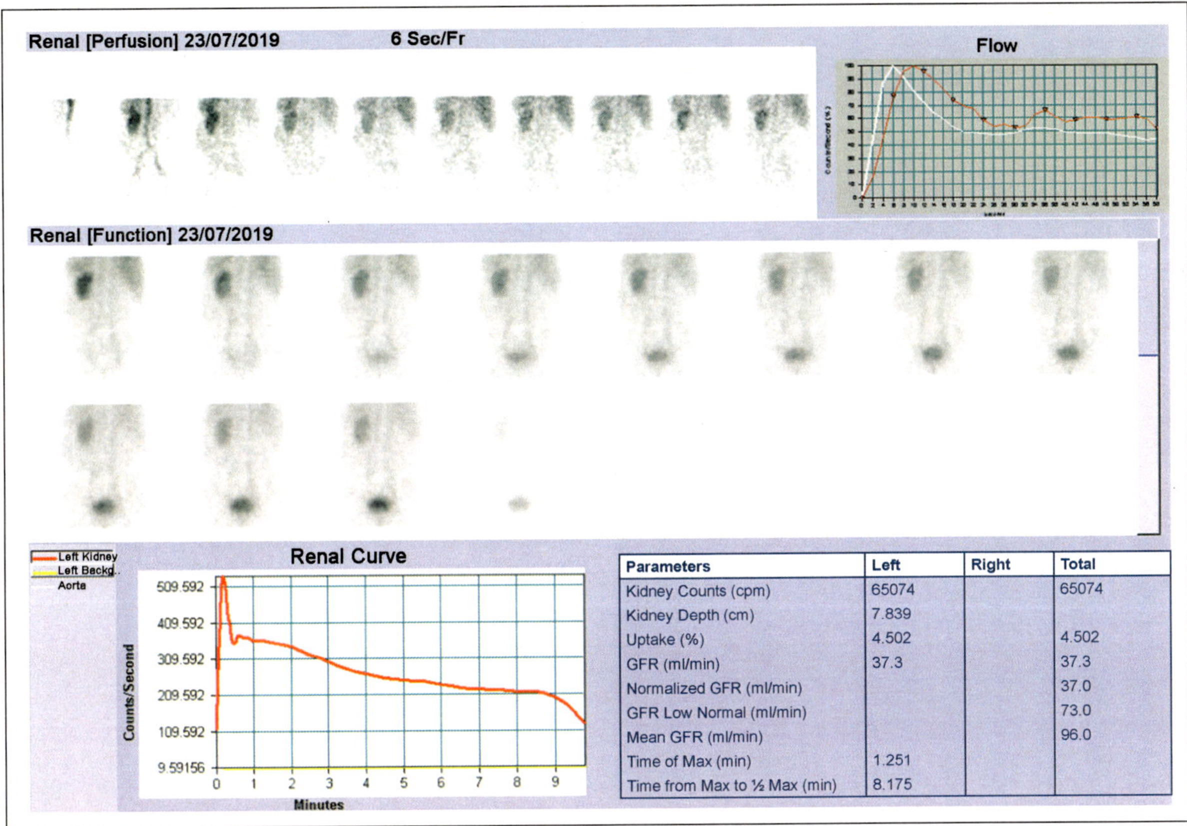

Parameters	Left	Right	Total
Kidney Counts (cpm)	65074		65074
Kidney Depth (cm)	7.839		
Uptake (%)	4.502		4.502
GFR (ml/min)	37.3		37.3
Normalized GFR (ml/min)			37.0
GFR Low Normal (ml/min)			73.0
Mean GFR (ml/min)			96.0
Time of Max (min)	1.251		
Time from Max to ½ Max (min)	8.175		

Figure 44.7: Left kidney shows normal perfusion, cortical tracer uptake and subsequent drainage. Right kidney shows no significant tracer uptake–non functioning right kidney

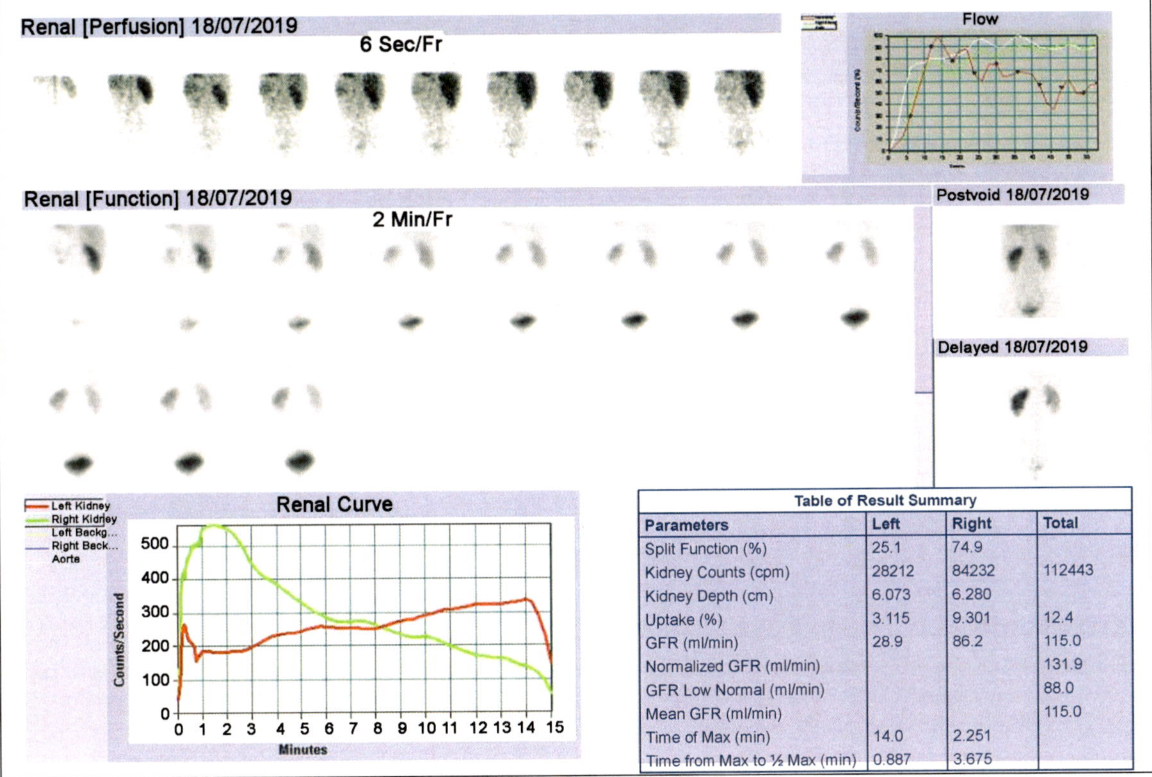

Table of Result Summary

Parameters	Left	Right	Total
Split Function (%)	25.1	74.9	
Kidney Counts (cpm)	28212	84232	112443
Kidney Depth (cm)	6.073	6.280	
Uptake (%)	3.115	9.301	12.4
GFR (ml/min)	28.9	86.2	115.0
Normalized GFR (ml/min)			131.9
GFR Low Normal (ml/min)			88.0
Mean GFR (ml/min)			115.0
Time of Max (min)	14.0	2.251	
Time from Max to ½ Max (min)	0.887	3.675	

Figure 44.8: Left kidney shows poor perfusion and cortical tracer uptake with no significant tracer clearance in delayed images–PUJO. Right kidney shows normal perfusion, cortical tracer uptake and subsequent drainage. Renogram curve confirms the same

Captopril Challenge Renography[22-23]

Useful for moderate-to-high risk of renovascular hypertension.

Patients need to be well hydrated before testing. Patients should drink only water and should not eat a solid meal within 4 hours of the study.

Short-acting ACEIs, such as captopril, should be withheld for 3 d before the study. Longer acting ACEIs should be withheld for 5-7 days.

Pathophysiology

Because of reduced renal plasma flow, filtration pressure and GFR fall. Increased renin and resulting angiotensin II produces vasoconstriction of the efferent glomerular arterioles, raising glomerular pressure and maintaining GFR. Captopril blocks the normal compensatory mechanism and GFR falls.

Interpretation: If the glomerular agent Tc-99m DTPA is used, the ACE inhibitor–induced drop in GFR pattern overall drop in function seen as slower uptake and a lower peak.

Looking at degree of change from baseline is critical with Tc-99m DTPA, and the greater the change, the higher the probability that RAS is causing significant RVH. A 10% decrease in relative function (differential function or split renal function) or a decrease in absolute function (GFR) greater than 10% is considered high probability. A change of 5-9% is intermediate or borderline.

If the protocol has been properly followed, sensitivity and specificity of ACE inhibitor renography is reportedly 90% and 95%, respectively. However, the sensitivity and specificity are lower in patients with elevated creatinine. The kidney must function well enough to actually show a change in function when ACE inhibitors are given. Therefore, a small shrunken kidney or one with poor baseline function can be difficult to interpret.

A normal ACE inhibitor study should be read as "low probability" of renin-dependent RVH. This means the post test chance of RVH is less than 10%. An "indeterminate" reading can be used for patients with very poor renal function or when an abnormal-appearing kidney does not change between baseline and ACE inhibitor examinations. When function markedly worsens on the ACE inhibitor challenge compared to the baseline study, the study is "high probability", with a greater than 90% chance of RVH. These patients are highly likely to improve with angioplasty or surgery.

Renal Transplant Evaluation

A baseline scan is a prerequisite for better understanding and differentiating ATN from other causes[24] (Table 44.1).

Surgical complications like urinoma/urinary leak can also be identified.

Table 44.1: Comparison between ATN and acute rejection

Disease	Baseline scan	Follow-up scan	Perfusion	Renal transit time
Acute rejection	Normal	Worsens	↓	↑
Vasomotor nephropathy (acute tubular necrosis)	Abnormal	Improves	Normal	↑

References

1. Mandell GA, Eggli DF, Gilday DL *et al.* Society of Nuclear Medicine procedure guideline for renal cortical scintigraphy in children. Society of Nuclear Medicine Procedure Guidelines Manual August 2003;195-98.
2. Piepsz A, Blaufox MD, Gordon I, *et al.* Consensus on renal cortical scintigraphy in children with urinary tract infection. Semin Nucl Med 1999;2;160-74.
3. Bjorgvinsson E, Majd M, Eggli KD. Diagnosis of acute pyelonephritis in children: Comparison of sonography and Tc-99m DMSA scintigraphy. Am J Roentgenol 1991; 157:539-43.
4. Smith T, Evans K, Lythgoe MF *et al.* Radiation dosimetry of Tc-99m DMSA in children. J Nucl Med 1996;37:1336-42.
5. Smith T, Gordon I, Kelly JP. Comparison of radiation dose from intravenous urography and Tc-99m DMSA scintigraphy in children. Br J Radiol 1998;71:314-19.
6. Rothwell DL, Constable AR, Albrecht M. Radionuclide cystography in the investigation of vesico-ureteric reflux in children. Lancet 1977;1:1072-75.
7. Maizels M, Weiss S, Conway JJ, Firlit CF. The cystometric nuclear cystogram. J Urol 1979 Feb;121(2):203-05.
8. Nasrallah PF, Conway JJ, King LR, Belman AB, Weiss S. The quantitative nuclear cystogram: An aid in determining the spontaneous resolution of vesicoureteral reflux. Trans Am Assoc Genitourin Surg 1978;70:52-55.
9. Treves ST, Zurakowski D, Bauer SB, Mitchell KD, Nichols DP. Functional bladder capacity measured during radionuclide cystography in children. Radiology 1996; Jan; 198(1):269-72.
10. Godley ML, Ransley PG, Parkhouse HF, Gordon I, Evans K, Peters AM. Quantitation of vesico-ureteral reflux by radionuclide cystography and urodynamics. Pediatr Nephrol 1990 Sep;4(5):485-90.
11. Van der Vis Melsen MJE, Baert RJM, Rajnherc JR. Scintigraphic assessment of lower urinary tract function in children with and without outflow obstruction. Br J Urol 1989;64:263-69.
12. Carlsen O, Lukman B, Nathan E. Indirect radionuclide renocystography for determination of vesico-ureteral reflux in children. Eur J Nucl Med 1986;12(4):205-10.

13. Rizzoni G, Perale R, Bui F, Pitter M, Pavanello L, Boscolo R, Passerini Glazel G, Macri C. Radionuclide voiding cystography in intrarenal reflux detection. Ann Radiol Paris 1986;29(3-4):415-20.

14. Nielsen JB, Jensen FT, Jorgensen TM, Charles P, Djurhuus JC. The diagnosis of vesico-ureteral reflux. Radiologic and nuclear medicine methods. Scand J Urol Nephrol 1985; 19(2):109-12.

15. Guignard JP, Torrado A, Feldman H, *et al.* Assessment of glomerular filtration rate in children. Helv Paediat Acta 1980;35:437-47.

16. Haenggi MH, Pelet J, Guignard JP. Estimation du debit de filtration glomérulaire par la formule DFG = KxT/Pcr. Arch Pédiatr 1999;6:165-72.

17. Cockcroft DW, Gault MH. Prediction of creatinine clearance from serum creatinine. Nephron 1976;16: 31-41.

18. Waller DG, Fleming JS, Ramsay B, *et al.* The accuracy of creatinine clearance with and without urine collection as a measure of glomerular filtration rate. Postgraduate Med J 1991;67:42-46.

19. Blaufox MD, Aurell M, Bubeck B, Fommei E, Piepsz A, Russell C, *et al.* Report of the Radionuclides in Nephrourology Committee on renal clearance. J Nucl Med 1996;37:1883-90.

20. O'Reilly P, Aurell M, Britton K, Kletter K, Rosenthal L, Testa T. Consensus on diuresis renography for investigating the dilated upper urinary tract. Radionuclides in Nephrourology Group. Consensus Committee on Diuresis Renography. J Nucl Med 1996;37:1872-76.

21. Upsdell SM, Leeson SM, Brooman PJ, O'Reilly PH. Diuretic induced urinary flow rates at varying clearances and their relevance to the performance and interpretation of diuresis renography. Br J Urol 1988;61:14-18.

22. Taylor Jr A, Nally J, Aurell M, Blaufox D, Dondi M, Dubovsky E, *et al.* Consensus report on ACE inhibitor renography for detecting renovascular hypertension. Radionuclides in Nephrourology Group. Consensus Group on ACEI Renography. J Nucl Med 1996;37:1876-82.

23. Prigent A, Cosgriff P, Gates GF, Granderus G, Fine EJ, Itoh K, *et al.* Consensus report on quality control of quantitative measurements of renal function obtained from renogram: International Consensus Committee from the Scientific Committee of Radionuclides in Nephrourology. Semin Nucl Med 1999;29:146-59.

24. Dubovsky EV, Russell CD, Bischof-Delaloye A, Bubeck B, Chaiwatanarat T, Hilson AJ, *et al.* Report of the Radionuclides in Nephrourology Committee for evaluation of transplanted kidney (review of techniques). Semin Nucl Med 1999;29:175-88.

CHAPTER 45

Uroflowmetry and Urodynamics

Mayank Bharti[1], Ramniwas Yadav[2], Varun Mittal[3]

[1] *Consultant, Uro-Oncology and Robotic Surgery, Fortis Memorial Research Institute, Gurugram*
[2] *Senior Fellow, Minimal Invasive Urology, Medanta, The Medicity, Gurugram*
[3] *Senior Consultant, Uro-Oncology and Robotic Surgery, Fortis Memorial Research Institute, Gurugram*

Introduction

The lower tract is composed of the urinary bladder, bladder outlet and urethra. Together they form a functional unit to store and empty the urine. Normally in storage phase, as the bladder is filled with urine, a sensation of filling is perceived at a certain moment and subsequently a strong desire to void is felt. Normally no uncomfortable sensation as urgency, pain or discomfort is perceived and there is no urinary leakage. Competence of the outlet and urethra and accommodation of the bladder make it possible to store urine at a low stable pressure throughout. Lower storage pressure insures adequate drainage of urine flow from the upper tract. The normal voiding phase is characterized by the voluntary initiation of micturition followed by forceful and continuous flow with no residual urine. Coordinated relaxation of pelvic floor and external urethral sphincter with simultaneous detrusor contraction contribute to the efficient emptying of urinary bladder. Urine flow can be intentionally interrupted by voluntary contraction of urethral sphincter and pelvic floor. Nervous control mechanisms via central and peripheral as well as somatic and autonomic, integrate all these functions. Aberrations at any level can lead to different symptoms and this helps us to diagnose the probable cause of dysfunction which is helpful to tailor treatment. Two broad types of lower urinary tract dysfunction including storage and voiding needs to be distinguished.

Urodynamic Study

Urodynamic investigation is a functional assessment of the lower urinary tract to provide objective explanation to symptoms of the lower and upper urinary tracts. Urodynamic studies comprise a series of tests. The appropriate test needs to be selected and the information provided is useful in establishing etiology and help to select the most appropriate intervention.[1] Urodynamic study should be performed and reported in accordance with the standards of the International Continence Society (ICS).[2]

The aim of this chapter is to provide basics of urodynamics study for practitioners dealing these cases regularly. Two most important and commonly performed studies in clinical practice are uroflowmetry with residual urine measurement and inflow cystometry with pressure flow studies.[3]

Uroflowmetry

Urine flow studies are the simplest of urodynamic techniques, because they are noninvasive and the necessary equipment is simple and relatively inexpensive.

Definitions

- Urine flow may be described in terms of flow rate and flow pattern, and may be continuous or intermittent.
- The basic information necessary in interpreting the flow trace includes the volume voided, the environment in which the patient passed urine and the pateint position, that is lying, sitting or standing
- Flow rate is the volume of fluid expelled via the urethra per unit time and is expressed in ml/s.
- Qmax is the maximum measured value of the flow rate.
- Voided volume (VV) is the total volume expelled via the urethra.
- Flow time is the time over which measurable flow occurs.
- Average flow rate (Qave) is voided volume divided by flow time.
- Time to maximum flow is the elapsed time from onset of flow to maximum flow (Fig. 45.1).[4]

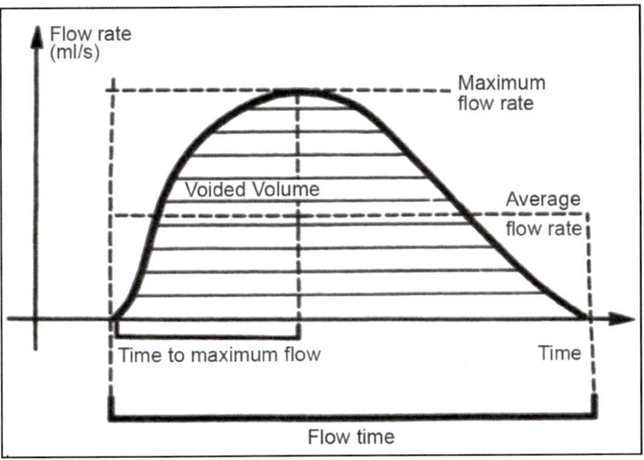

Figure 45.1: Graphic representation to understand various definitions in uroflowmetry

Method

- Make familiar with the equipment.
- Need 2 to 3 hours to perform the study and get the results.
- Adequate fluid intake to be ensured.
- Ask patient to hold the urine till full capacity.
- Flow room should be lighted well, clean with door closed so that patient passes urine in privacy.
- After passing measure post void urine volume with ultrasonography (USG), also called as bladder scan
- Ideally flow should be repeated 2 to 3 times but if voided volume is adequate then even once is sufficient.

Equipment

The available uroflowmeters use several different principles, as follows:

1. **Weight transducer flowmeter** involves weighing the urine voided, thereby measuring the volume of urine voided. It also calculates the urine flow rate by differentiation with respect to time.
2. **Rotating-disc flowmeter** has a spinning disc on which the urine falls. The disc is kept rotating at the same speed, in spite of changes in the urine flow rate; the weight of the urine tends to slow the rotation of the disc. The differing power needed to keep disc rotation constant is proportional to the urine flow rate. It is also possible to "weigh" urine by measuring the hydrostatic pressure exerted by a column of urine.
3. **Capacitance method:** Capacitance changes when quantity of fluid between the capacitor plates changes. Capacitor turns pressure into flow rates (Fig. 45.2).[5]

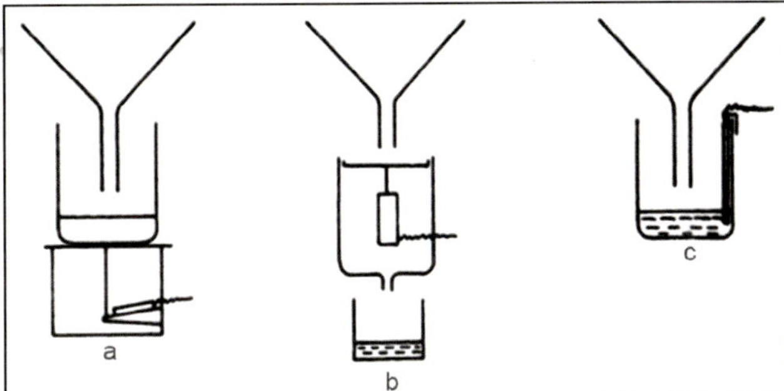

Figure 45.2: Line diagram to represent different types of urine flowmeters using (a) weight transducer, (b) spinning disc and (c) capacitance methods

Most commercially available flowmeters have acceptable accuracy. As flowmeter accuracy is limited flow rate should be expressed to the nearest whole milliliter (15 ml/s rather than 14.8 ml/s). The rapid changes in flow can be eliminated by using a sliding average. This process smooths the trace to remove positive and negative spikes.Volumes should be rounded to the nearest 10 ml. Results should be expressed as Maximum Flow Rate/voided Volume/Residual Volume (e.g., 10 ml/s/230 ml/20 ml).

Normal Flow Pattern

Flow curve has a "bell" shape (Fig. 45.3). Maximum flow is reached in the first 30% of any trace and within 5 seconds from the start of flow. The average flow is half the maximum flow value, (Q avg= ½ the Qmax).[5]

Factors Affecting Flow Rate

1. **Voided volume:** The flow rate varies according to volume voided and different traces can look quite different in the same unobstructed individual voiding different volumes. Although the traces look superficially different, they all have similar first and final phases. The final phase of a normal flow trace shows a rapid fall from high flow, together with a sharp cutoff at the termination of flow. Detrusor muscle when stretched achieves an optimal performance, but if stretched further it becomes inefficient. At more than 400 ml, the efficiency of the detrusor begins to decrease and Qmax is lower. Urine flow rate is highly dependent on the volume voided. Flow rates are highest and most predictable in the volume range between 200-400 ml. Through this range the maximum flow tends to be constant.The normal flow curve is bell-shaped but its appearance will differ quite markedly according to the volume of urine voided. Maximum flow is normally reached within 3s to 10s from the onset of micturition.
2. **Paper speed:** Appearance of trace also depends on paper speed of the recorder. If this is very slow then flow will appear as a vertical line and elongated in case it is faster. A paper speed of 0.25 cm/s is practical and allows easy interpretation.

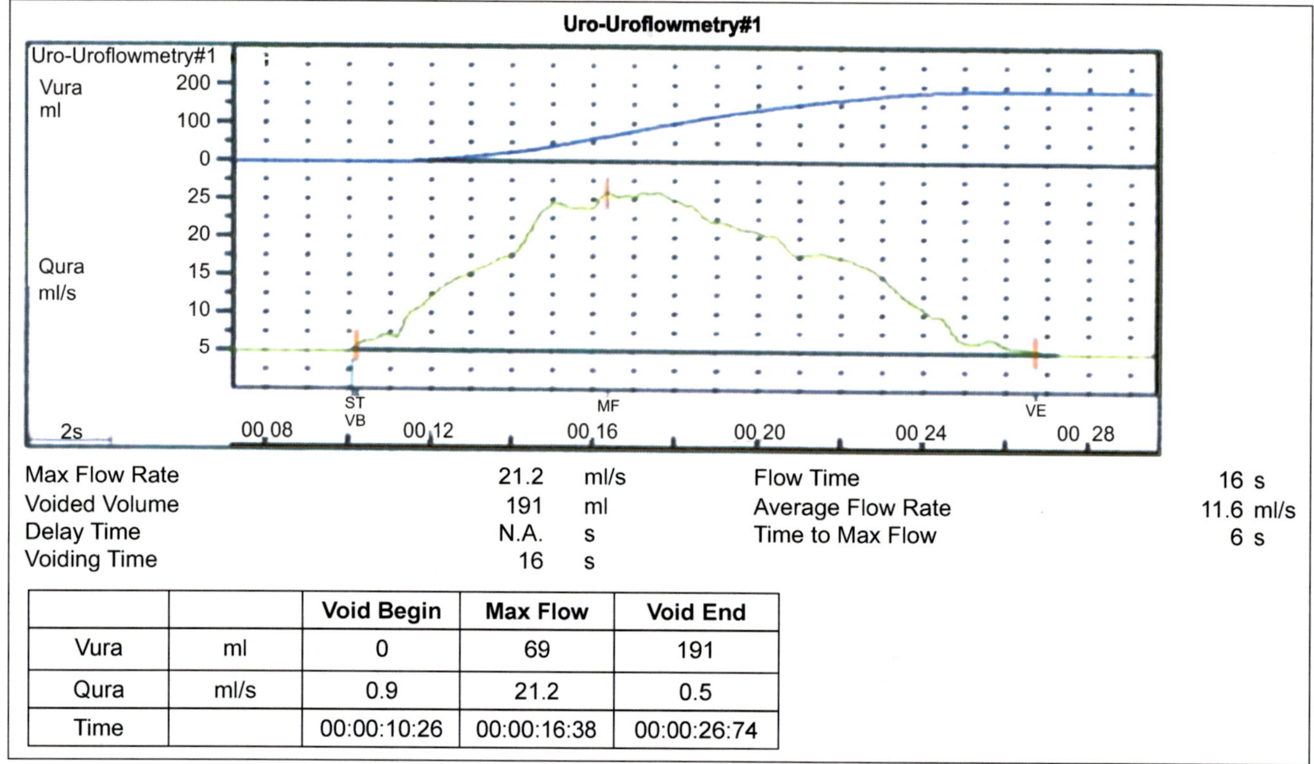

		Void Begin	Max Flow	Void End
Vura	ml	0	69	191
Qura	ml/s	0.9	21.2	0.5
Time		00:00:10:26	00:00:16:38	00:00:26:74

Figure 45.3: A representative normal uroflowmetry trace

3. **Age and sex:** Young men-Qmax greater than 15 to 20 ml/sec is considered as normal and <10 ml/sec as abnormal. These numbers decline with age by 1 to 2 ml/sec per 5 years resulting in a maximum flow of 5.5 ml/sec at 80 years. Normal woman Qmax is more than 30 ml/sec, the flow curve is bell shaped as in men, and the flow time is shorter. Maximum flow in women does not seem to be dependent upon age.
4. **Intermittent flow:** Flow time must be measured carefully, as the time intervals between flow episodes are disregarded. Voiding time is the total duration of micturition, including the interruptions. Where flow is continuous, voiding time is equal to flow time. The area beneath the curve or curves represents the volume voided (Fig. 45.4).[6]

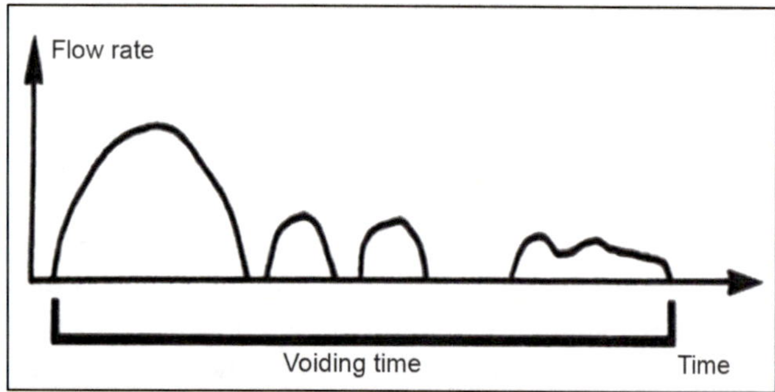

Figure 45.4: Intermittent flow trace representing the total voiding time

Abnormal Flow Patterns

1. **Bladder Outlet Obstruction:** Flow curves in obstructed patients are characterized by a low maximum and reduced average flow, with the average flow greater than half the maximum flow rate. Maximum flow is usually obtained relatively quickly (3-10 secs), but the flow rate then decreases slowly. In outlet obstruction the flow rate is expected to be continuous, although it may end in a terminal dribble. Obstruction may be "compressive", for example in benign prostatic obstruction, or "constrictive" as in a urethral stricture. The two types of obstruction give different types of trace.

- **Compressive obstruction:**
  - First third of the flow trace may appear relatively normal.
  - Qmax is reduced.
  - Latter part of trace usually is elongated into a pronounced "tail" of reducing flow rate.
  - Maximum flow is established soon after onset of voiding.
  - Flow is continuous or terminal dribble.
  - Qavg>> ½ Qmax.
  - Commonly noted in cases if benign prostatic hyperplasia (BPH), primary bladder neck obstruction (Fig. 45.5).
- **Constrictive" obstruction/stricture urethra**
  - Box pattern/"plateau"-shaped trace (Fig. 45.6).
  - No change in flow rate.
  - Qmax = Qavg.

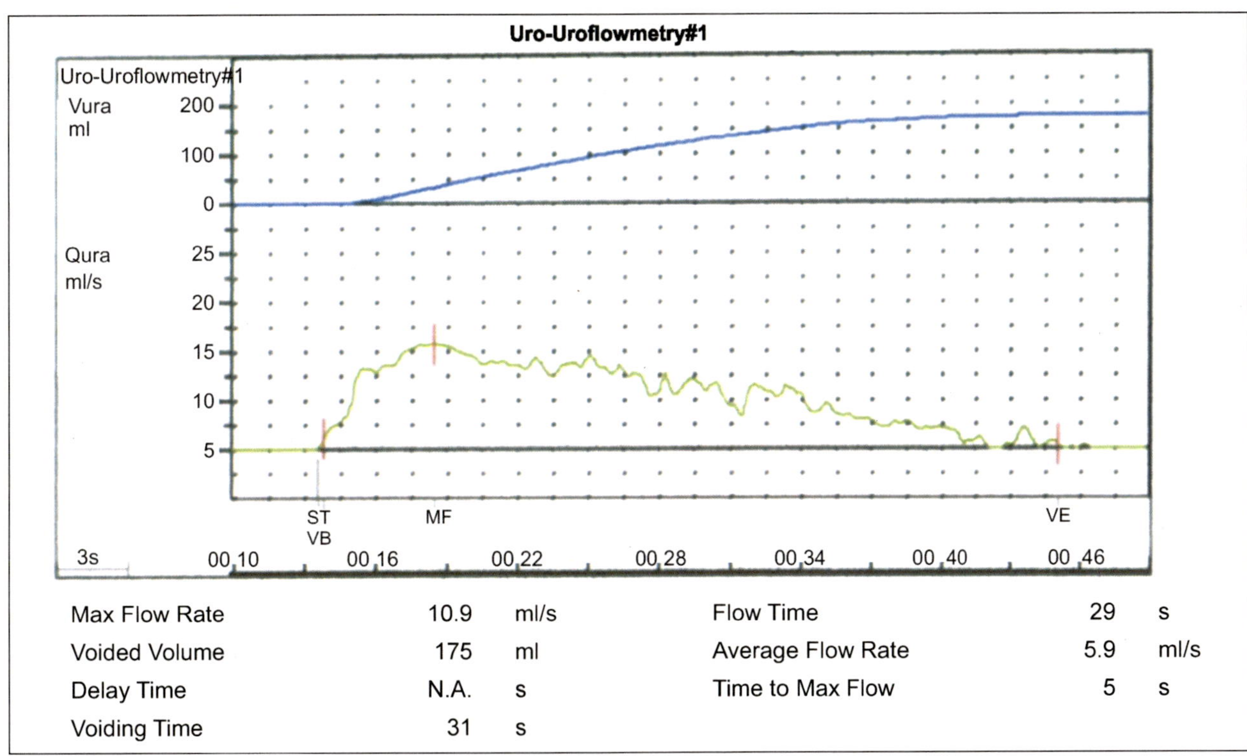

Figure 45.5: Uroflowmetry trace in a patient with benign prostatic hyperplasia leading to outlet obstruction

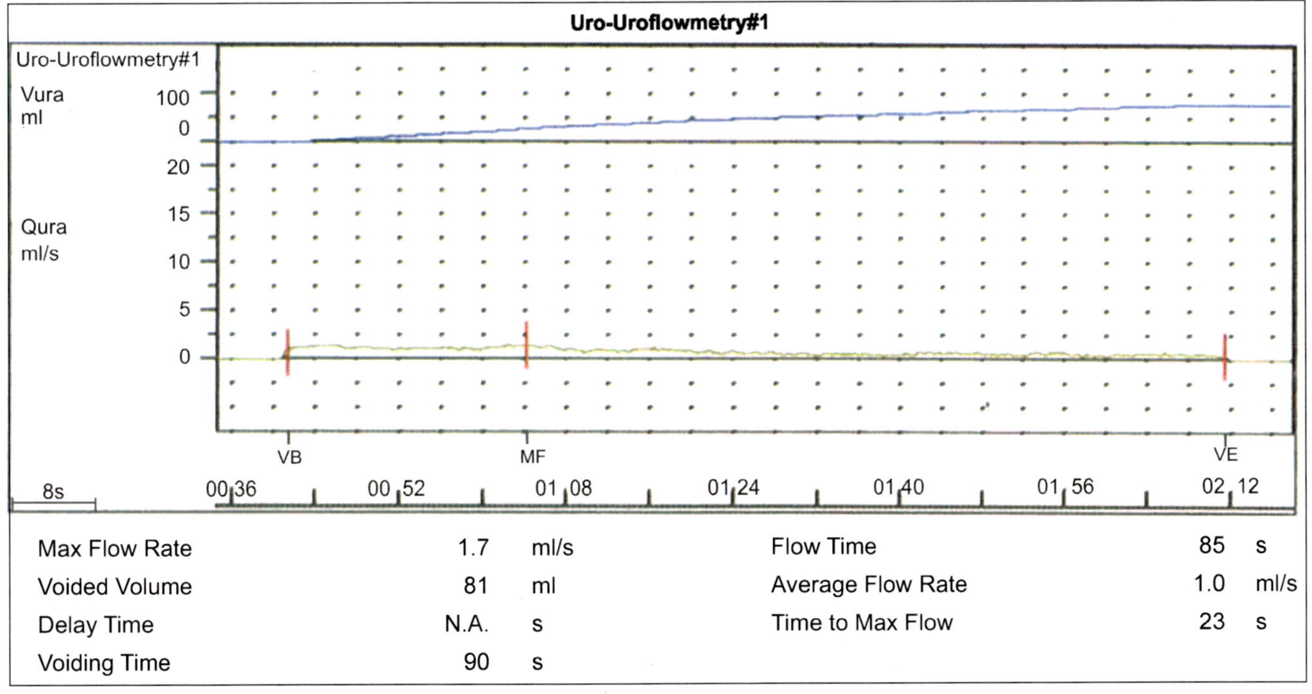

Figure 45.6: Uroflowmetry trace in a patient with stricture urethra

2. **Detrusor Underactivity:** Symmetrical trace with a low maximum flow rate is seen. The characteristic in detrusor underactivity is that the time to reach maximum flow is very variable and the maximum flow may occur in the second half of the trace/near the middle of the voiding time. Pressure flow study necessary to confirm as it may represent simply bladder outlet obstruction.

3. **Interrupted Flow Patterns:** Some patients are in the habit of using, their diaphragmatic and abdominal muscles to increase urine flow. Straining makes the flow trace irregular/discontinuous. With straining the changes in flow tend to be relatively slow and the stream is usually continuous. In general the flow increases as the patient strains, although this is not

the case in men with bladder outlet obstruction. The situation often needs further elucidation by a pressure-flow study (Fig. 45.7). Sometimes in case of underactive detrusor flow is completely dependent on abdominal straining and flow peaks and touches baseline (Fig. 45.8).[6]

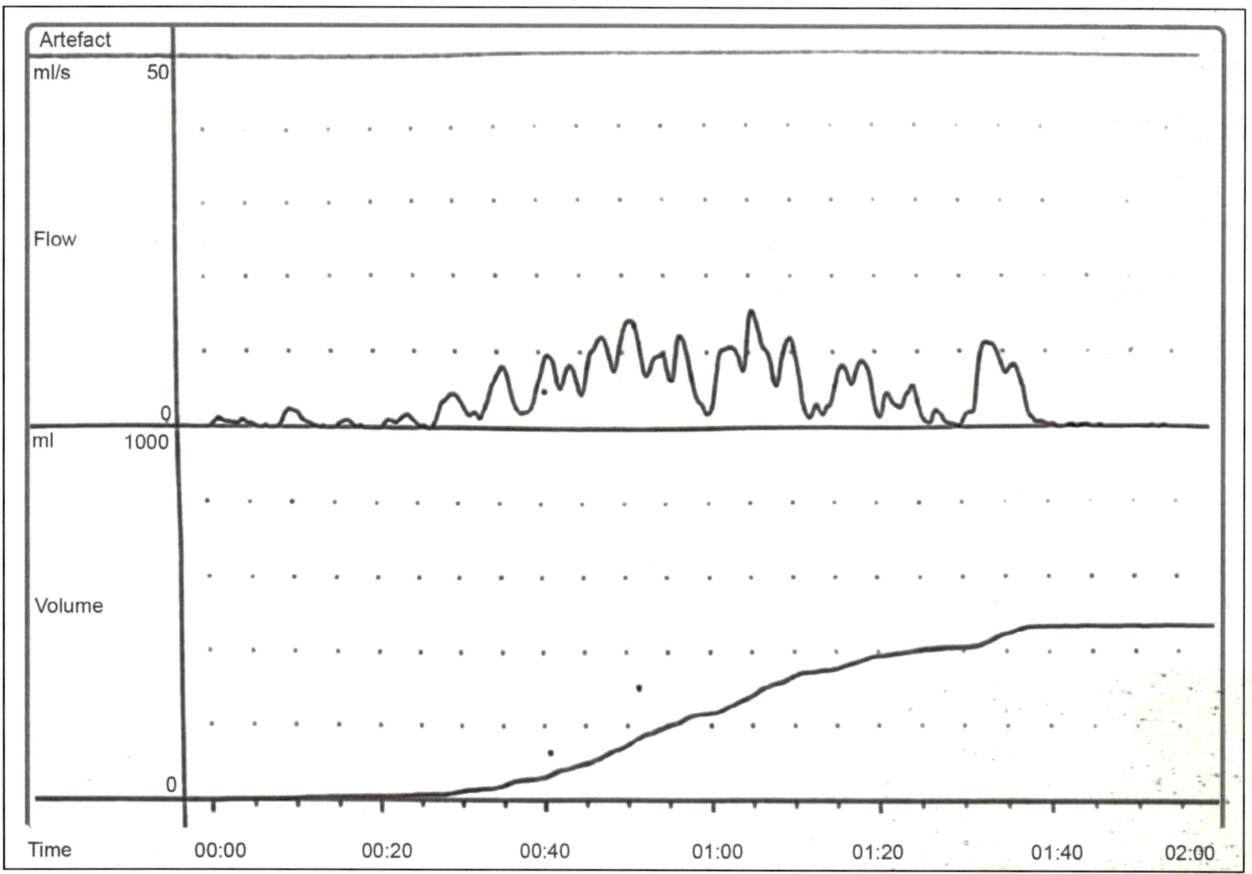

Figure 45.7: Uroflowmetry trace representing intermittent flow due to abdominal straining

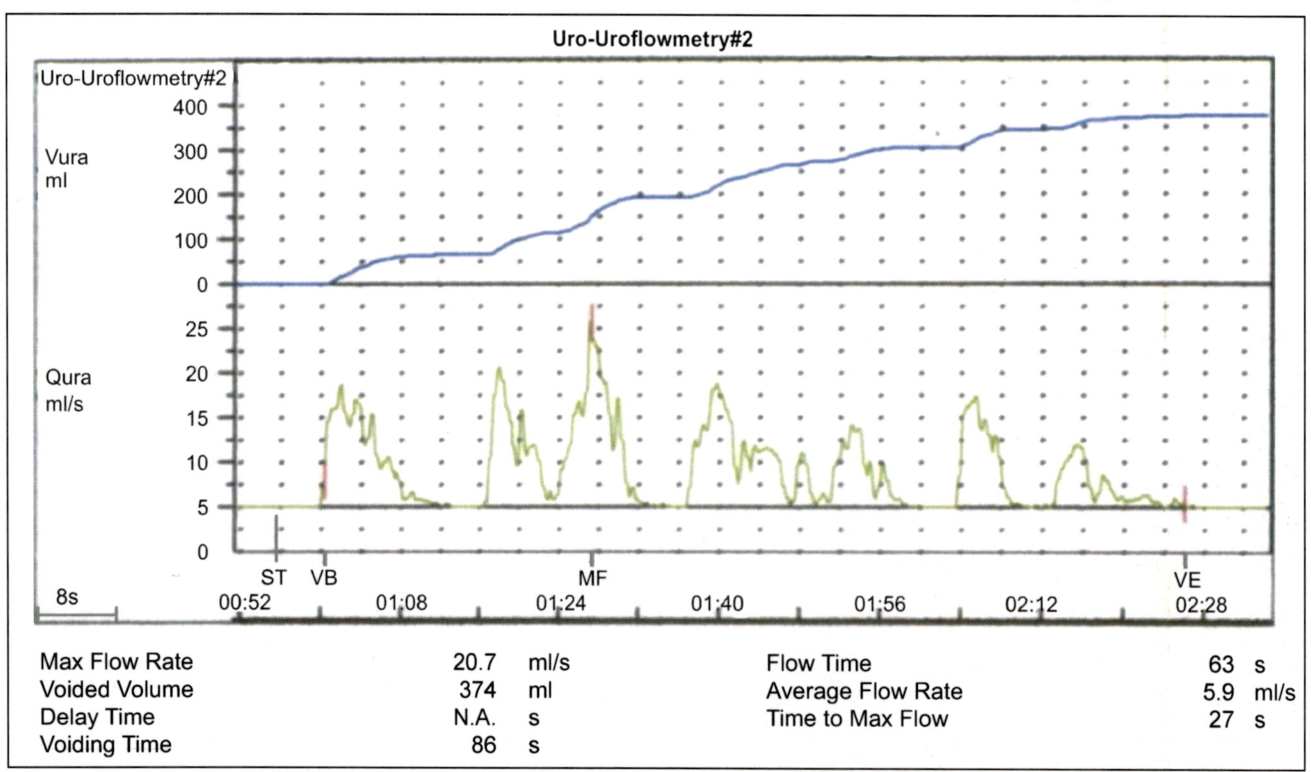

Max Flow Rate	20.7	ml/s	Flow Time	63	s
Voided Volume	374	ml	Average Flow Rate	5.9	ml/s
Delay Time	N.A.	s	Time to Max Flow	27	s
Voiding Time	86	s			

Figure 45.8: Interrupted flow with abdominal straining in case of detruxor underactivity

Recording of Post Void Residual Urine (PVRU)

On bladder scan the urinary bladder measurements are taken in all three dimensions, two in coronal and one in sagittal planes and product of all three is multiplied with factor 0.7, [{D1 × D2 × D3} × 0.7 = PVRU in ml]. Interobserver error is bound to happen.[7]

I. D1 – Fundus to neck in sagittal plane.

II. D2 – Anterior to posterior wall.

III. D3 – Coronal plane–right side to left side.

Cystometry

Role of Uroflowmetry is limited as mentioned above sometimes the trace is not representative of the actual clinical problem. There is no information about the storage phase. It can't diagnose between outlet obstruction and detrusor underactivity. Cystometry is the method of choice to study the storage and voiding phases of micturition and help further in correct understanding of the pathophysiology and aids in management.[3,6]

Indications of Cystometry

- Patients with persistent LUTS despite presumed appropriate therapy.
- Patients with LUTS who have both obstructive and marked instability symptoms.
- Patients with obstructive LUTS and neurologic disease.
- Younger men and women with LUTS.
- Patients with incontinence.
- All neurologically impaired patients who have neurogenic bladder dysfunction.
- Patients with neurologic disorders and those with a mismatch between symptoms and clinical findings.
- Children with persistent diurnal enuresis.
- Children with spinal dysraphism.
- Children with daytime urgency and urge incontinence.[8]

Method

- Patient informed in detail about the procedure–method, time taken (1-2 hours) and costs involved etc.
- Ensure there should be no active urinary tract infection.
- Informed written consent taken.
- Ensure rectum is empty or if constipated oral laxatives/enema given the night before study.
- Patient made familiar with urodynamic room and equipment.
- Patient voids and comes for the study.
- Study conducted with aseptic precautions.
- One shot of intravenous broad spectrum antibiotic is given 30 minutes before procedure.
- Patient placed in supine position.
- Paint and drape the patient.
- In neurologically normal patient empty the bladder using appropriate catheter (K90).
- In neurologically abnormal patient procedure done with residual urine.[9]

External Strain Gauge/Pressure Transducer

- Mounted on a stand and connected to patients' vesical and rectal catheter by Pressure monitoring (PM) line.
- Pressure wave bends a thin metal diaphragm in strain gauge and converts it into electrical discharge which is transmitted to computer (Fig. 45.9).

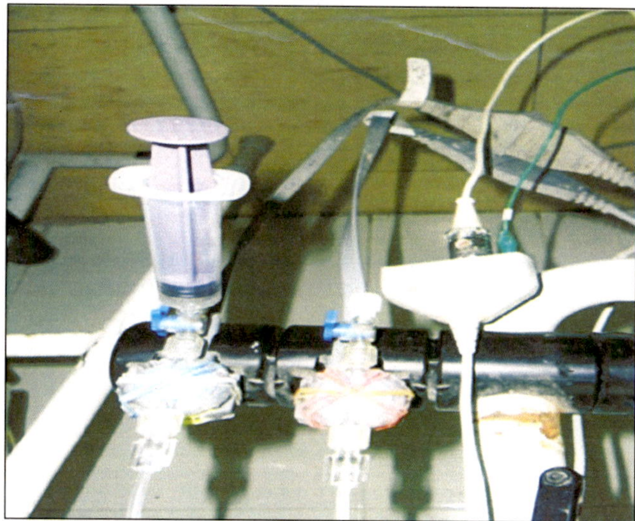

Figure 45.9: Stand with vesical and rectal catheter PM line attached to transducers

Catheters

- 7 Fr triple lumen catheter used to measure vesical pressure (Fig. 45.10).
- Rectal catheter–14-16 Fr Foley with filled bulb.
- Local anesthesia does not interfere with the recording of pressure.

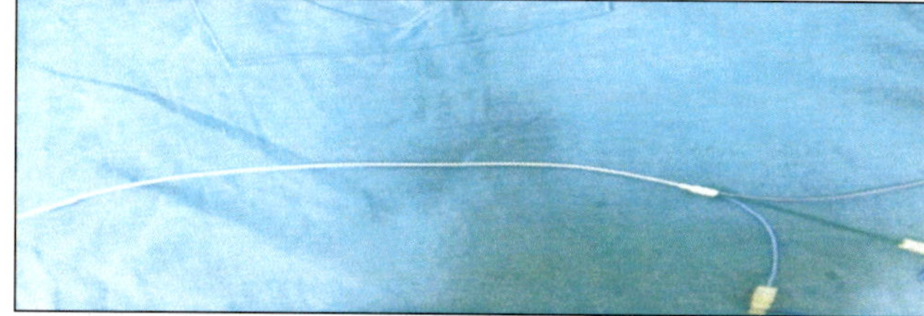

Figure 45.10: Triple lumen 7 Fr Urodynamic catheter

Placement of Vesical Catheters

- Triple lumen catheter is put per urethrally or through suprapubic route (Fig. 45.11).

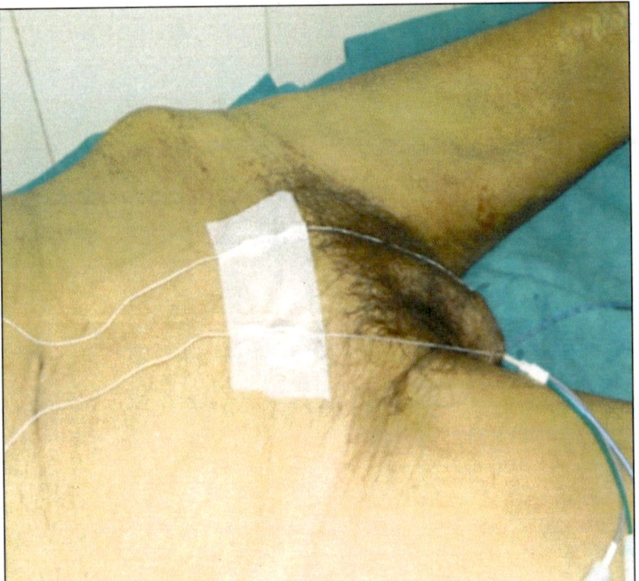

Figure 45.11: Triple lumen urodynamic catheter fixed on abdominal wall

- For Vesical Pressure (PVES) measurement catheter placed per urethrally till the box junction and then fixed to abdominal wall using thread so that it does not get displaced during filling or voiding phase.
- One lumen is for filling, second one for measuring vesical pressure (connected to pressure transducer by PM line), and third one for measuring urethral pressure. Urethral pressure is not measured routinely.

Placement of Rectal Catheter

- Measures pressure surrounding the bladder (Fig. 45.12).
- Rectal/vaginal/intraperitoneal/stomach/pre-peritoneal space used depending upon the situation.
- 14 Fr Foley's placed in rectum with 10 cc balloon inflation. Rectum pressure is transmitted by PM line into pressure transducer which covert it into electrical form.
- Catheter is taped to thigh.

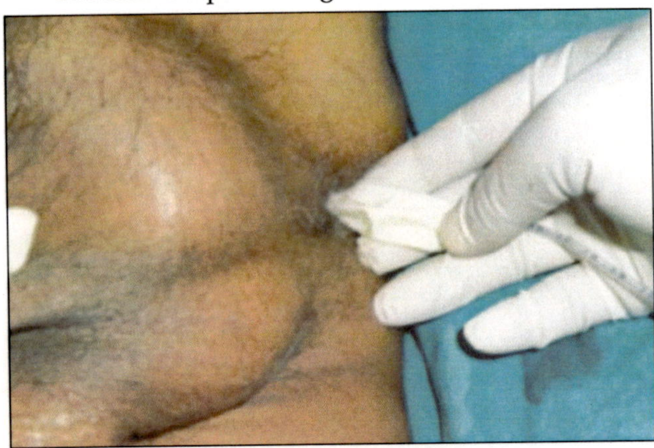

Figure 45.12: Rectal catheter being introduced

Placement of Electromyographic (EMG) Needle (For measuring Sphincteric Activity)

- **Men:** 50- to 75-mm-long needle is used. The needle is placed through the perineum, advancing toward the apex of the prostate under guidance from a finger in the rectum.
- **Women:** Needle is placed lateral to urethral meatus and advanced parallel to the urethra a distance of about 1 to 2 cm (Fig. 45.13).[10]

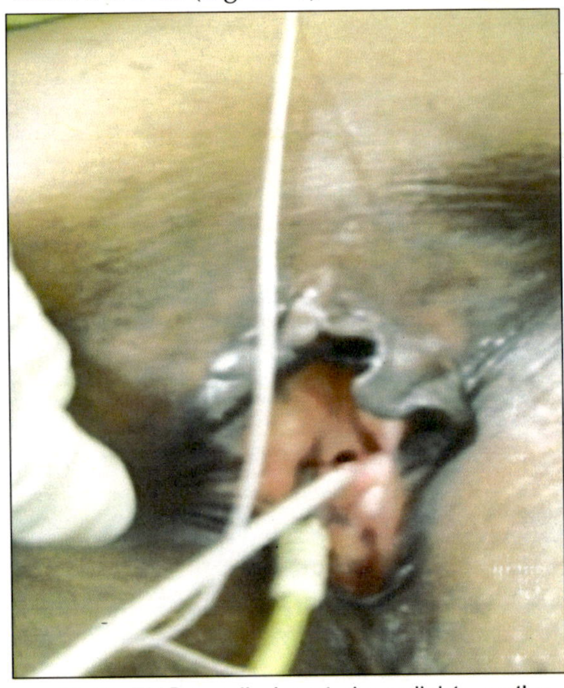

Figure 45.13: EMG needle inserted parallel to urethra in a female patient

Position

- With all the catheters and needle electrode strapped in situ patient sits on urodynamic chair comfortably (Fig. 45.14).
- Patient who is severely disabled need to do in supine position–pressure transducer position is readjusted to the pressure reference level.

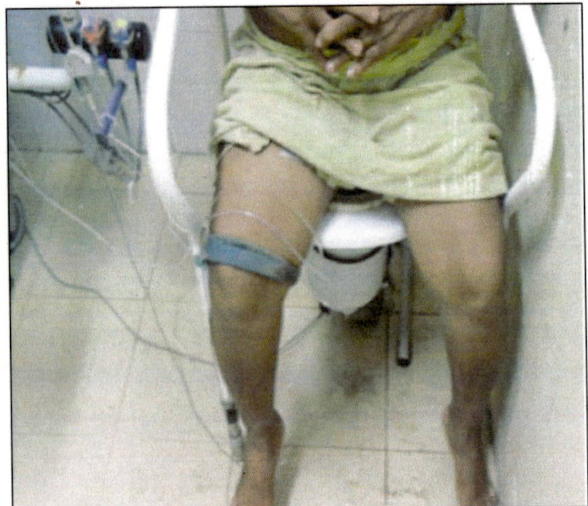

Figure 45.14: Patient positioned on a urodynamic chair

Media Used

- Water, saline both mimic urine and are used for filling bladder.

Temperature of Fluid

- Room temp: Around 22 to 24°C.
- Using fluid at body temperature is more physiologic.
- Cold fluid (<20°C) not used as it stimulates detrusor contraction at lower volumes.

Filling Rate

- Ideal filling rate= rate of urine production= BW(kg)/4.
- ICS formerly defined three categories of filling rate:
  - **Slow-fill Cystometry:** Up to 10 ml/min (physiological filling rate).
  - **Medium-fill Cystometry:** 10 - 100 ml/min.
  - **Fast-fill Cystometry:** >100 ml/min.
- Often the filling rate chosen will be a compromise between these two extremes, and a convenient rate, which does not prolong the test unduly, is 50 ml/min to 60 ml/min.
- In children and patients with neurological abnormalities and in particular patients with detrusor over activity secondary to spinal trauma, the bladder should be filled very slowly (<10 ml/min) because faster flow rates may produce artefactual low compliance.

What to Do About Residual Urine?

- Prior to catheterization the patient is asked to empty the bladder as fully as possible.
- If the patient self-catheterizes, then the patient is asked to do this before urodynamics commences and to empty the bladder and measure PVRU.

Procedure

- Setting zero level.
- Instruct the patient to inform the physician when first sensation, normal desire, strong desire, urgency is felt and cough command is given.
- Patient asked to withhold as much amount of urine as possible.
- Patient is asked not to void unless told to so.
- Before filling cough test is performed to ensure catheters are in place and are recording properly.
- Bladder is filled using sterile water or normal saline at a physiological rate.
- Various sensations are documented along with note of any urine leak or artefacts.
- **Quality control:** The patient is asked to cough every minute during filling and after voiding to ensure that the catheters have not become displaced during micturition.
- When the patient feels strong desire to void (Maximum cystometric capacity) then filling is stopped and voiding phase is begun.
- Patient voids in privacy and voids to completion.
- At the end of test cough test again performed to ensure that catheters were not displaced during voiding.
- Print of the graph is taken and analyzed (Fig. 45.15).[8,9]

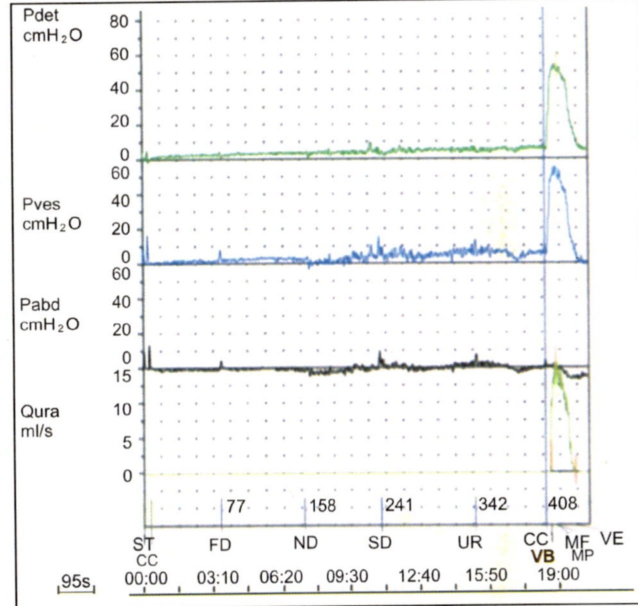

Figure 45.15: Cystometry trace representative of normal storage and voiding phase

Interpretation of Filling Phase

During filling following factors are assessed:

I. Bladder sensation.
II. Detrusor activity.
III. Bladder compliance.
IV. Urethral function.
V. Bladder capacity.

1. **Sensation:** First sensation of filling (FSF) happens at 50% of cystometric capacity. Normal desire to void occurs at 75% of cystometric capacity but voiding can be delayed if necessary. Strong desire to void (SDV) occurs at 90% of cystometric capacity. If less than above – means patient is having urgency. Look for any urine leakage simultaneously and if present means urge incontinence is also present and it usually associated with Detrusor Overactivity. Pain is always abnormal.

Abnormal Sensations

- **Hypersensitivity (urgency):** Early first sensation

(<100 ml), persists and increases, and limiting cystometric capacity to < 250 ml.

- **Reduced:** Late first sensation, normal and strong desire to void or urgency never occurs.
- **Absent:** Seen in spinal cord trauma, meningomyelocele.

2. **Detrusor Activity:** During bladder filling this can be either normal or increased (overactivity).The normal detrusor remains quiescent during filling and detrusor overactivity (DO) does not occur under any circumstances. During filling, detrusor pressure tends to remain near zero due to distensibility of bladder. Detrusor pressure (Pdet) = Vesical pressure (Pves) – Abdominal Pressure (Pabd) (if Pdet = 0 then Pves = Pabd). Detrusor overactivity exists when, during the filling phase, there are involuntary detrusor contractions. The overactive detrusor may be asymptomatic, and its presence does not necessarily imply a neurological disorder (Fig. 45.16). Neurogenic detrusor overactivity (NDO) or detrusor hyper-reflexia is a result of disturbance of the nervous control mechanisms and must be confirmed by objective evidence of a neurological disorder. Idiopathic detrusor overactivity or detrusor instability can be secondary to bladder infection, bladder outlet obstruction (BOO) due to various causes including benign prostatic hyperplasia/bladder neck contracture, bladder tumor or stones. There is no value for detrusor overactivity. In the past, these were documented as "unstable" only when they exceeded 15 cm H_2O. However, recently ICS has determined that there is no lower limit for the amplitude and that any contraction during the study resulting in the patient's sensation of the need to void is labelled as detrusor overactivity.

3. **Bladder Compliance:** In normal bladder function, intravesical pressure should change little from empty to full. Bladder compliance describes the relationship between change in bladder volume and bladder pressure ($\Delta v/\Delta p$).In the normal bladder with a capacity of 400 ml the change in pressure from empty to full should be <10 cm H_2O, giving a figure for normal compliance of >40 ml/cm of water. Normally compliance ranges from 40-120 cm of water. Bladder compliance is dependent on the rate of bladder filling, on bladder function, and on the neurological state of the patient. It is essential to determine whether or not low compliance is due to fast filling. When there is evidence of low compliance with a gradual increase in Pves, then bladder filling should stop for at least two minutes. If the intravesical pressure falls, then the reduced compliance was, at least in part, due to filling too fast. Once the pressure has stabilised then filling should be restarted, but at a significantly slower rate. If initial filling was at 50 ml/min then it should be reduced to 10 ml/min. Normal compliance is 40-120 cm H_2O. Impaired compliance is < 20 cm H_2O. Normal detrusor pressure during voiding is 40-60 cm H_2O in males and more than 80 cm H_2O indicated BOO.

4. **Urethral Function:** During the storage phase the urethral closure mechanism function is either normal or incompetent. The normal urethral closure mechanism maintains a positive urethral closure

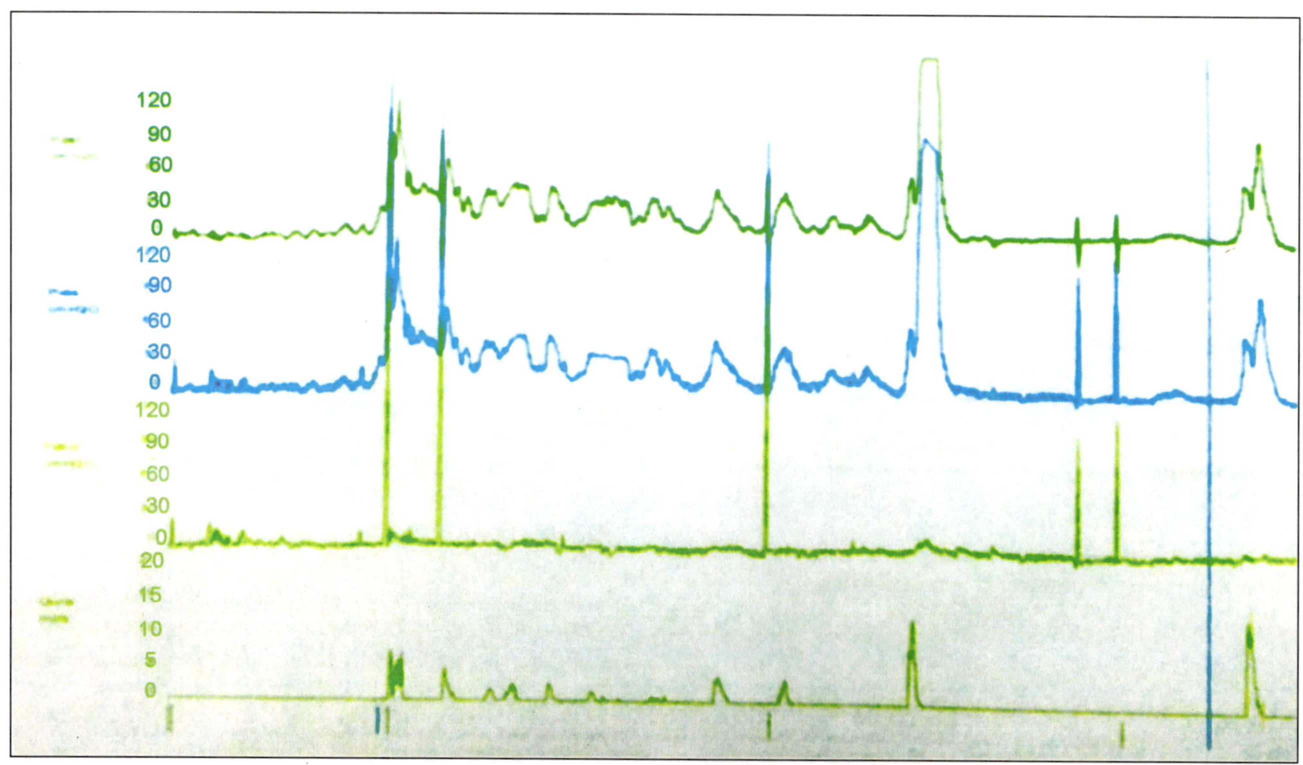

Figure 45.16: Detrusor overactivity with leak (urge incontinence)

pressure during filling, even in the presence of increased abdominal pressure. Incompetent urethral closure mechanism is one which allows leakage of urine in the absence of a detrusor contraction. Leakage may occur during coughing whenever intravesical pressure exceeds intraurethral pressure called as *urodynamic stress incontinence (USI)* or when there is an involuntary fall in urethral pressure called as *inappropriate urethral relaxation incontinence.*[10]

5. **Bladder Capacity:** In describing bladder capacity the ICS has recommended a few terms. *Cystometric capacity* is the bladder volume at the end of the filling cystometrogram, when the patient has a normal desire to void and "permission to void" has been given. Cystometric capacity is volume voided plus any residual urine. *Maximum cystometric capacity (MCC)* is the volume at which the patient feels that he or she can no longer delay micturition. *Maximum anesthetic bladder capacity* is the volume to which the bladder can be filled under either deep general or spinal anesthetic and may often be very different from the *maximum cystometric capacity, particularly in conditions such as DO or bladder hypersensitivity.*[10]

Interpretation of Voiding Phase

Detrusor activity and urethral (outlet) function should be defined separately. Detrusor activity is classified as follows:

- **Normal:** Detrusor contracts to empty the bladder with a normal flow rate.
- **Underactive:** Either the detrusor contraction is unable to empty the bladder or the bladder empties at a lower than normal speed.
- **Hypocontractile/Unsustained:** No effective detrusor contraction to produce urine flow. Whatever flow is there is mainly because of abdominal effort (Fig. 45.17).
- **Acontractile:** No measured detrusor pressure change occurs during voiding and whatever flow is there is mainly because of abdominal effort.[11]

Urethral (Outlet) Function During Voiding

- During voiding the urethra may be either normal or obstructive. A normal urethra is relaxed throughout voiding. An obstructive urethra is most commonly due to mechanical obstruction. If there is a mechanical obstruction, such as an enlarged prostate, then sphincter relaxation is likely to be normal. Urethral obstruction leads to increased voiding pressures (Fig. 45.18). In mechanical obstruction, the voiding pressures are constantly on higher side, whereas in case of urethral overactivity the voiding pressures may fluctuate as in detrusor-sphincter dyssynergia. Electromyography is needed to evaluate sphincter function. Females normally voids at low pressure

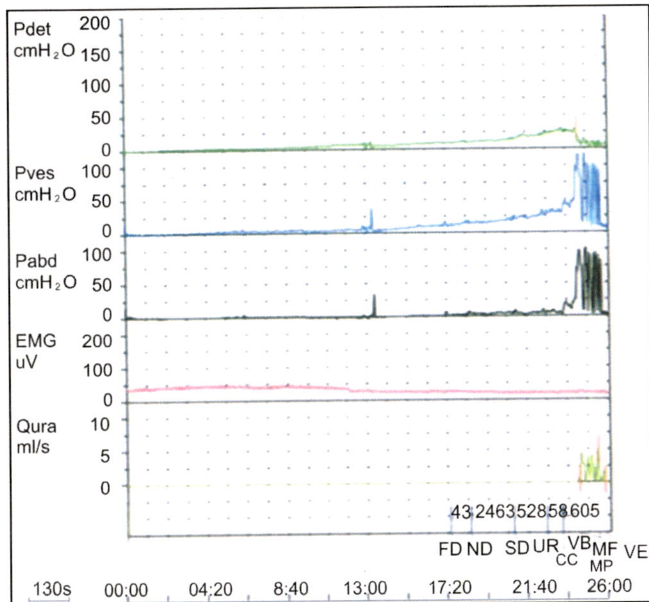

Figure 45.17: Cystometry representing hypocontractile/unsustained detrusor contraction

(Pdet < 30 cm H_2O) and Qmax of 30 ml/s. In females, Pdet of > 25 cm H_2O and Qmax of <12 ml/s is suggestive of bladder outlet obstruction.[12]

- Urethral obstruction due to urethral overactivity is characterised by the urethra contracting during voiding or the urethra failing to relax.
- **Urethral overactivity** can be classified as:
  - **Detrusor-sphincter dyssynergia (DSD):** Seen in patients with neurological disease and most classically in higher level (cervical) spinal cord injury. It is characterised by phasic contractions of the intrinsic urethral striated muscle during detrusor contraction (increased sphincteric pressure during voiding). This produces a very high voiding pressure and an interrupted flow.
  - **Dysfunctional voiding (DFV):** Produces the same urodynamic pattern as DSD but occurs in a different group of patients and has a different cause. DFV occurs, most characteristically, in children who are neurologically normal, the interrupted flow in these children is due to pelvic floor overactivity rather than to intrinsic striated muscle as in DSD. Most of the children have associated chronic constipation as well.[11,13]
- **Nonrelaxing urethral sphincter** obstruction is observed in meningomyelocele patients. There is a failure of urethral relaxation rather than urethral contractions during attempted micturition. The urethra opens except for the area of the striated muscle sphincter, at pelvic floor level. This condition produces a continuous obstruction with reduced flow rates. These patients often suffer from stress urine incontinence owing to sphincter incompetence during filling.[13]

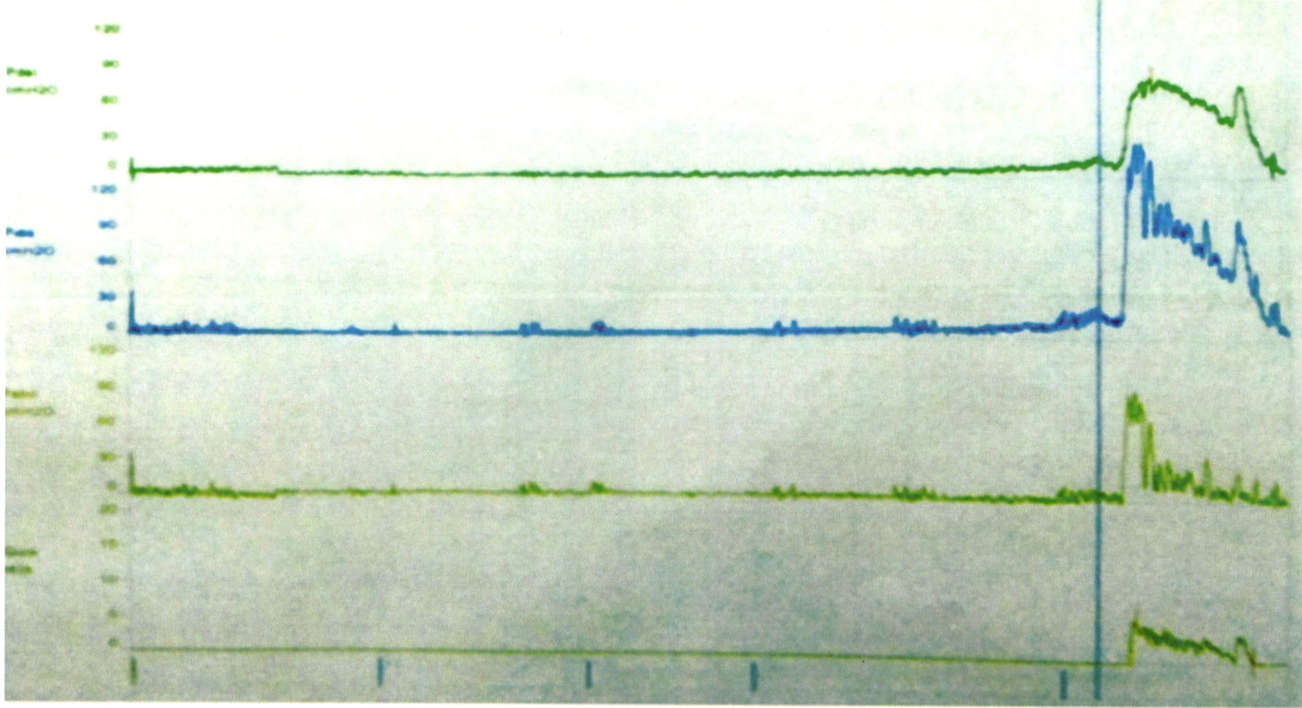

Figure 45.18: Cystometry representing normal storage phase with high voiding detrusor pressures and poor flow of urine suggestive of mechanical obstruction (bladder outlet obstruction)

Urodynamic Bladder Parameters

1. **Abrams Griffiths equation/ Bladder outlet obstruction index (BOOI):** BOOI= Pdet at Qmax– 2 (Qmax). Obstruction can be objectively defined with BOOI as follows:
   - Obstructed > 40.
   - Unobstructed < 20.
   - Equivocal if BOOI is 20-40.
2. **Slope of Schafer's lines, also known as the bladder contractility index (BCI):** BCI = Pdet at Qmax+ 5 (Qmax). It is interpreted as follows:
   a. Strong contractility if BCI >150.
   b. Normal contractility a BCI of 100-150.
   c. Weak contractility a BCI of less than 100.
3. **Leak point pressures:**
   a. **Detrusor leak point pressure (DLPP):** Defined as lowest detrusor pressure at which urine leakage occurs in the absence of a detrusor contraction. It was coined by McGuire for evaluating patients with low bladder compliance secondary to myelodysplasia. The urethral meatus is observed for leakage while bladder pressure is measured. When urine leakage is noted, the Pdet at that instant is recorded as the DLPP. Those with DLPP > 40 cm H_2O were at significantly higher risk for upper tract deterioration. The DLPP does not determine the etiology.
   b. **Valsalva leak point pressure (VLPP) or Abdominal leak point pressure (ALPP):** It is the intravesical pressure at which urine leakage occurs due to increased abdominal pressure in the absence of detrusor contraction. In a normal person detrusor pressure forces the urethral sphincter open whereas abdominal pressure cannot force a normally positioned and closed urethra. Leakage can be caused by abdominal pressure only when urethra is abnormal.
      i. **Method:** Bladder is filled to a capacity of 150-200 ml. Patient is asked to perform Valsalva maneuver until he/she leaks.The lowest pressure at which leak occurs is the VLPP.If no leak occurs the patient ask to cough.If no leak then repeat at 300 ml and then at cystometric capacity.
      ii. **Interpretation:** There is no normal value of ALPP.
         1. VLPP < 60 cm H_2O = Intrinsic Sphincter Deficiency (ISD).
         2. 60-90 cm H_2O = Urethral hypermobility with ISD.
         3. > 90 cm H_2O = Urethral hypermobility.
         4. >150 cm H_2O = Urethra is unlikely the cause of patients incontinence.

The ALPP measures the sphincter response to increased abdominal pressure. The lower the ALPP, "weaker" is the sphincter. The DLPP measures the bladder response to urethral or outlet resistance. The higher the resistance, higher is the DLPP, which is potentially dangerous to the upper tracts. The therapeutic aim is to keep ALPP high and DLPP low.[14,15]

The present chapter provides the basics of clinical urodynamics which can be applied to both adult and pediatric patients and also in both male and female patients. Further details and procedures including video urodynamics and pressure profilometry are beyond the scope of this chapter.

References

1. Homma Y, Batista J, Bauer S, Griffiths D, Hilton P, Kramer G, Lose G, Rosier PF. Urodynamics. Incontinence 2002; 317-72.
2. Abrams P, Blaivas JG, Stanton SL *et al*. Standardisation of terminology of lower urinary tract function. Neurourol Urodyn 1988;7:403.
3. Nitti VW. Pressure flow urodynamic studies: The gold standard for diagnosing bladder outlet obstruction. Reviews in urology 2005;7(Suppl 6):S14.
4. Nørgaard JP, Van Gool JD, Hjälmås K, Djurhuus JC, Hellström AL. Standardization and definitions in lower urinary tract dysfunction in children. British Journal of Urology 1998 May;81:1-6.
5. Lavelle JP, Phelan MW, Teahan S, Chancellor MB. Office Urodynamics. In Office Urology, Humana Press, Totowa, NJ 2001;407-16.
6. Rosier PF, Schaefer W, Lose G, Goldman HB, Guralnick M, Eustice S, Dickinson T, Hashim H. International continence society good urodynamic practices and terms 2016: Urodynamics, uroflowmetry, cystometry, and pressure-flow study. Neurourology and urodynamics. 2017 Jun;36(5):1243-60.
7. Schäfer W, Abrams P, Liao L, Mattiasson A, Pesce F, Spangberg A, Sterling AM, Zinner NR, Kerrebroeck PV. Good urodynamic practices: Uroflowmetry, filling cystometry, and pressure-flow studies. Neurourology and Urodynamics: Official Journal of the International Continence Society 2002;21(3):261-74.
8. Brucker BM, Nitti VW. Urodynamic Studies: Types and Indications. In Rapid and Practical Interpretation of Urodynamics, Springer, New York, NY 2015;3-25.
9. Abrams P. Urodynamics. London: Springer 2006 Jul 2.
10. Parsons M, Cardozo L. The classification of urinary incontinence. Reviews in Gynaecological Practice 2003 Aug 1;3(2):57-64.
11. Vignoli G. Urodynamics: A quick pocket guide. Springer 2016 Oct 6.
12. Okorocha I, Cumming G, Gould I. Female urodynamics and lower urinary tract infection. BJU international 2002 Jun;89(9):863-67.
13. Borawski KM. The EMG. In Practical Urodynamics for the Clinician, Springer, Cham 2016;77-87.
14. Peterson AC, Fraser MO, editors. Practical urodynamics for the clinician. Springer 2015 Nov 12.
15. Firoozi F, editor. Interpretation of Basic and Advanced Urodynamics. Springer 2016 Dec 20.

CHAPTER

Renal Imaging

Rajiv Yadav[1], Jammaludin[2]

[1] *Director and Head, Urologic Oncology and Robotic Surgery, Fortis Memorial Research Institute Gurugram*

[2] *Fellow, Urology, Medanta, The Medicity, Gurugram*

Renal Imaging is one of the important investigations to evaluate the patient with kidney and urinary tract disorders. Being retroperitoneal in location, kidneys are usually not accessible on physical examination, unless it is markedly enlarged in size due to cystic diseases or mass lesions. In such situations, imaging becomes necessary to know the size, shape, position and other information. The most frequently used imaging modalities are summarized in Table 46.1.

Table 46.1: Commonly used renal imaging modalities
Ultrasonography (USG) including Colour Doppler
Computed Tomography (CT)
Magnetic Resonance Imaging (MRI)
Voiding Cystourethrography (VCUG)
Retrograde or Ante Grade Pyelography
Intravenous Urography (IVU)
Renal Angiography
Nuclear Medicine Studies

Recommended Imaging Modalities for Kidney Diseases

The American College of Radiology (ACR) Appropriateness Criteria® are evidence-based guidelines to assist physicians in making the most appropriate imaging or treatment decision for a specific clinical condition. The recommended imaging modalities for kidney disease are summarized in Table 46.2.

The kidneys are paired retroperitoneal organs that lie at the level of the T12 to L3 vertebral bodies. Due to the right lobe of the liver, the right kidney usually lies slightly lower than the left kidney. In adults, the normal kidney is 9.0-12.0 cm in length, 3-5 cm wide, 3 cm in anteroposterior thickness. The left kidney is usually slightly larger than the right. Kidney length should not be less than three vertebral body lengths, and no more than four vertebral body lengths.

Table 46.2: The American College of Radiology–Appropriateness criteria® for kidney diseases

Kidney Disease	Imaging of Choice
Acute Onset Flank Pain–Urolithiasis	CT Abdomen and pelvis without contrast
Acute Pyelonephritis	CT Abdomen and pelvis without and with contrast
Proteinuria	USG Kidneys
Hematuria	USG Kidneys and bladder, CT
Renal Mass	CT Abdomen with or without contrast, MRI
Acute Kidney Injury/Chronic Kidney Disease	USG Kidneys and bladder
Renal Transplant Dysfunction	USG Transplant kidney
Reno Vascular Hypertension	MR Angiography without or with contrast CT Angiography with contrast
Renal Artery/Vein Thrombosis	CT with contrast
Lower Urinary Tract Infection	X-ray/CT cystography

On ultrasound in normal kidney, cortex is less echogenic than the liver, medullary pyramids are slightly less echogenic than the cortex. Cortex thickness equals or is more than 6 mm, if the pyramids are difficult to differentiate, the parenchymal thickness can be measured instead and should be 15-20 mm. Central renal sinus, consisting of the calyces, renal pelvis and fat, is more echogenic than the cortex. Normal ureters are generally not well seen on ultrasound. Bladder and prostate should be evaluated with full bladder.

Radiologic Atlas: Some of the clinically common conditions diagnosed radiologically are depicted in the atlas (Figs. 46.1-46.20).

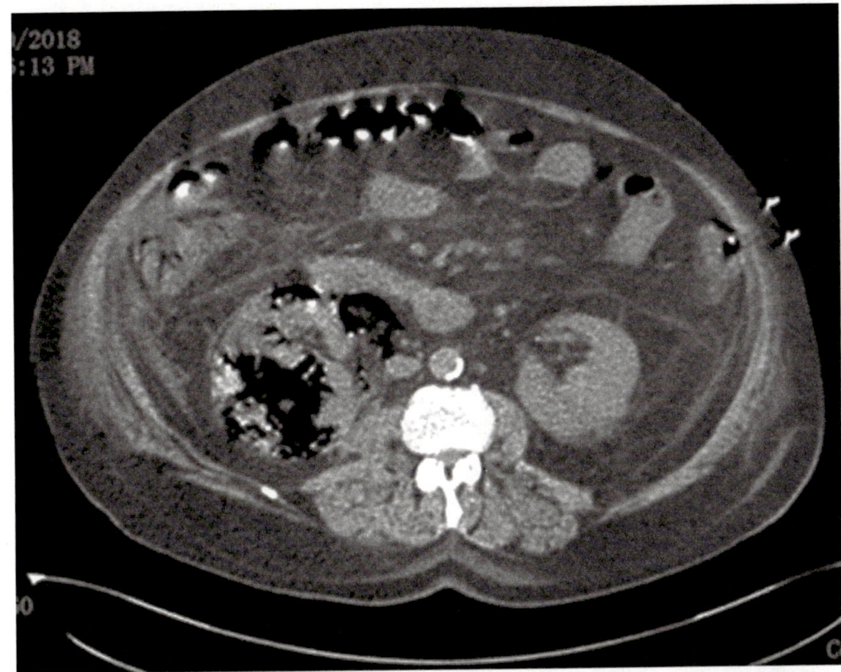

Figure 46.1A: CT scan axial view showing gas inside the right renal parenchyma, peri- and paranephric space–Emphysematous pyelonephritis

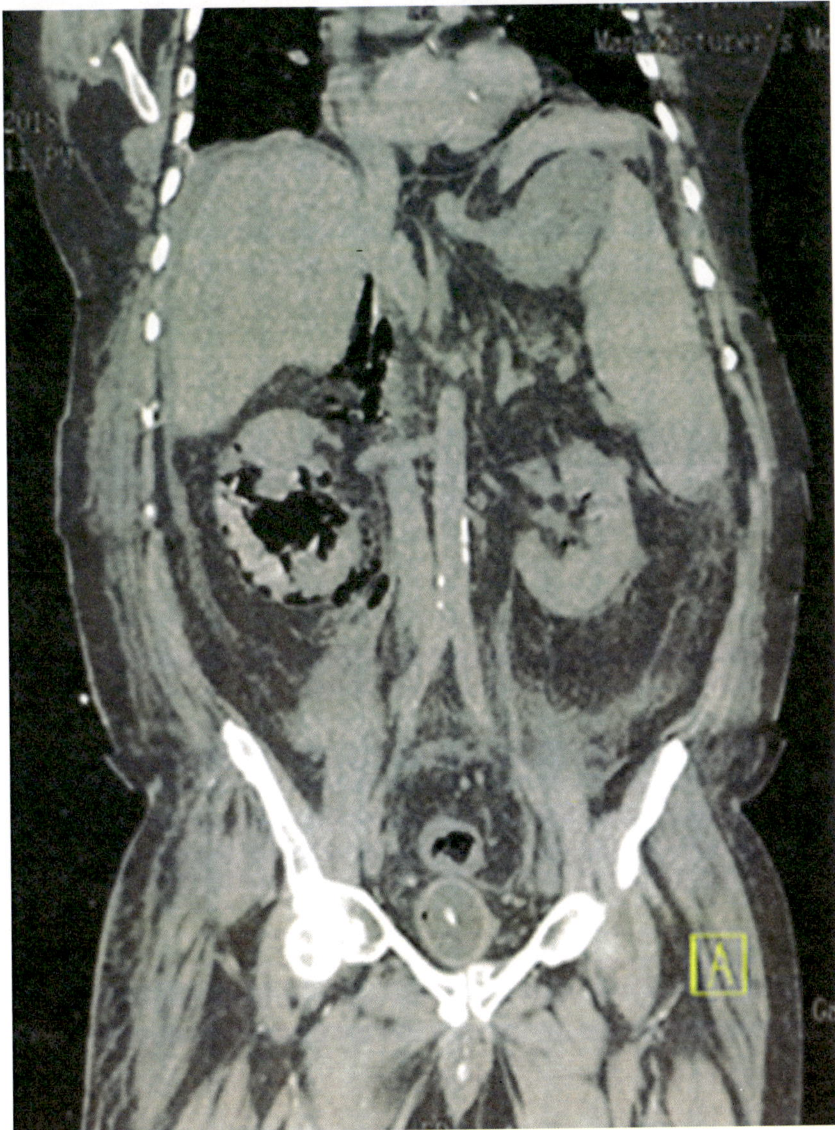

Figure 46.1B: CT scan coronal view showing gas inside the right renal parenchyma, peri- and paranephric space–Emphysematous pyelonephritis

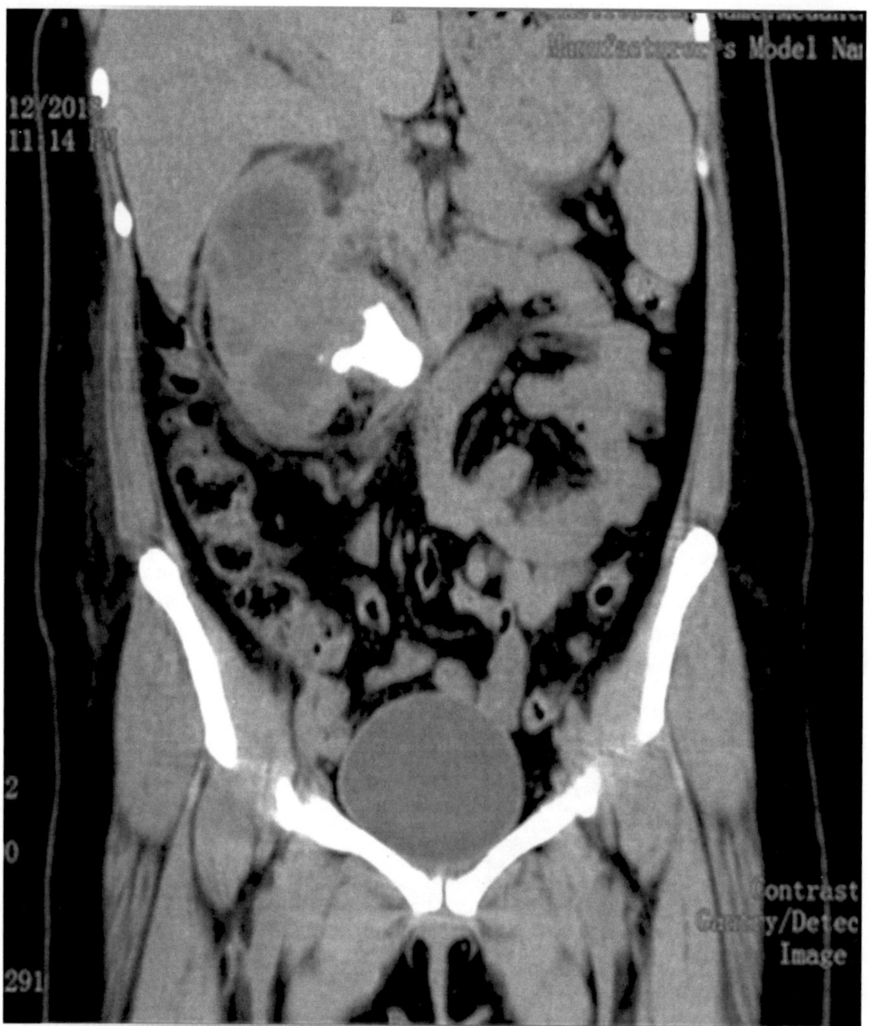

Figure 46.2: CT scan coronal view showing large stone in right renal pelvis with multiple focal hypodense lesion suggestive of pyonephrosis

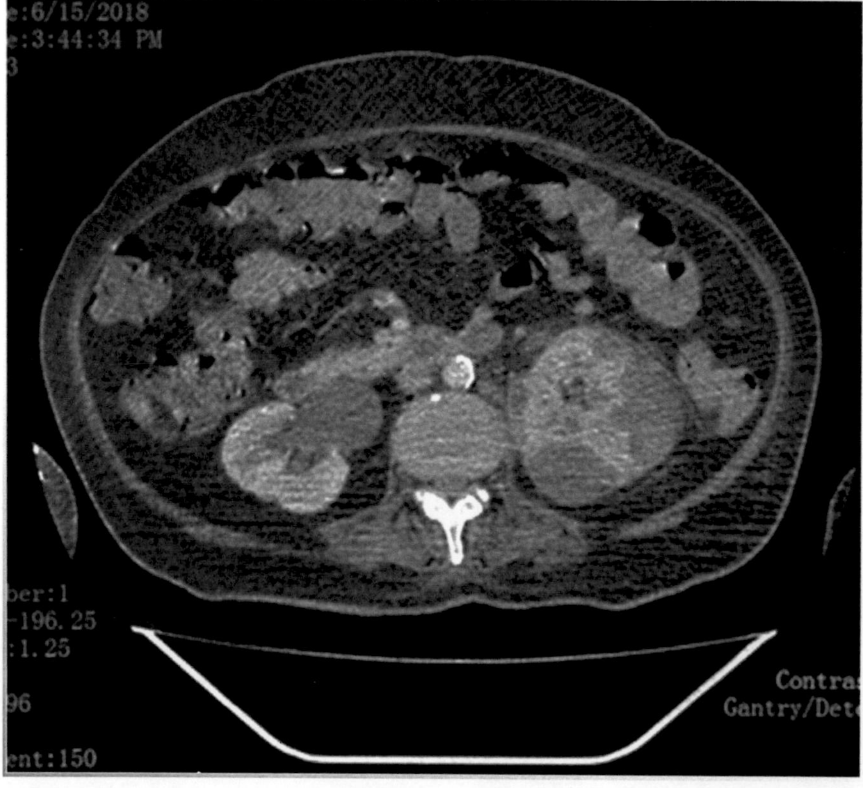

Figure 46.3: CT scan axial view showing enlarged left kidney with multiple focal hypodense lesion suggestive of pyonephrosis

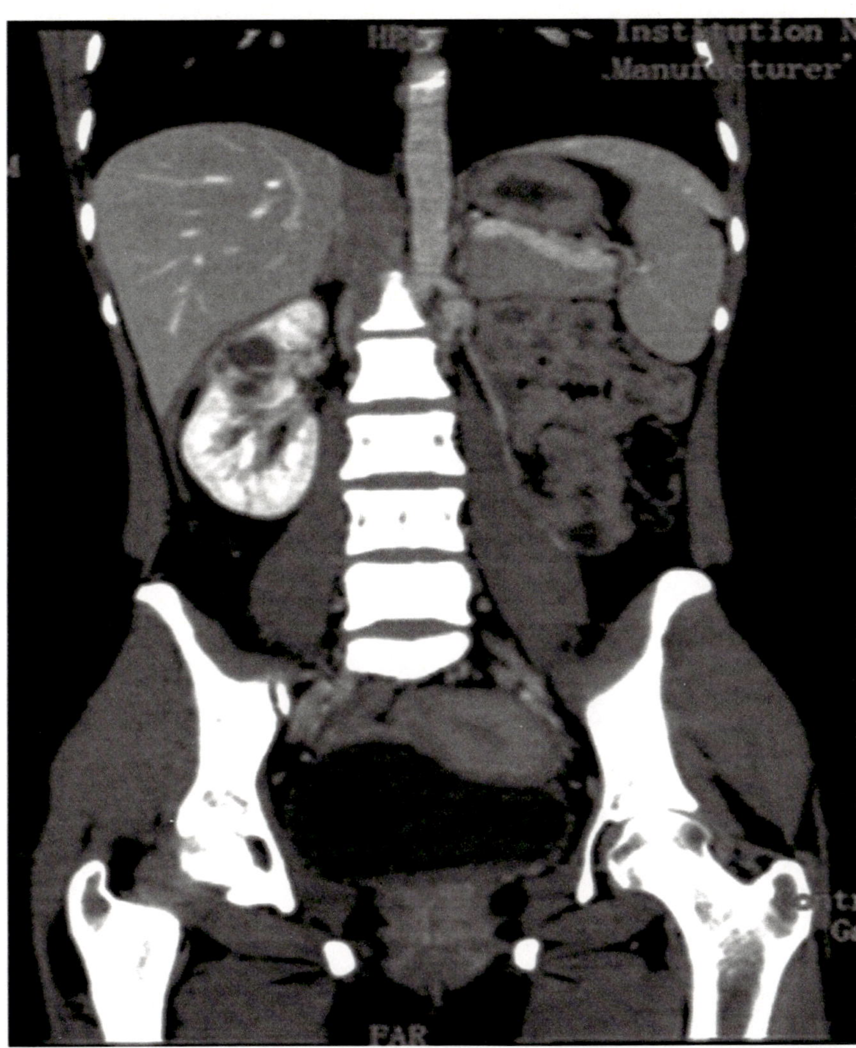

Figure 46.4: CT scan coronal view showing thick walled cystic lesion seen in the anterior cortex of the mid pole of the right kidney with enhancing septae suggestive of renal abscess

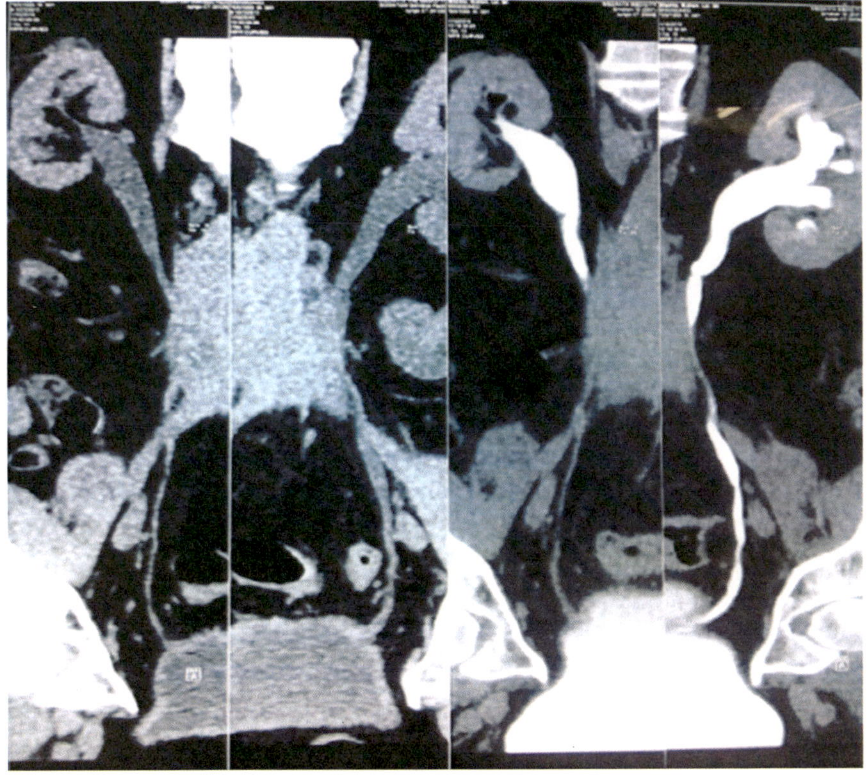

Figure 46.5: CT urography coronal view showing medial deviation of bilateral ureter and retroperitoneal concentric periaortic mass suggestive of retroperitoneal fibrosis

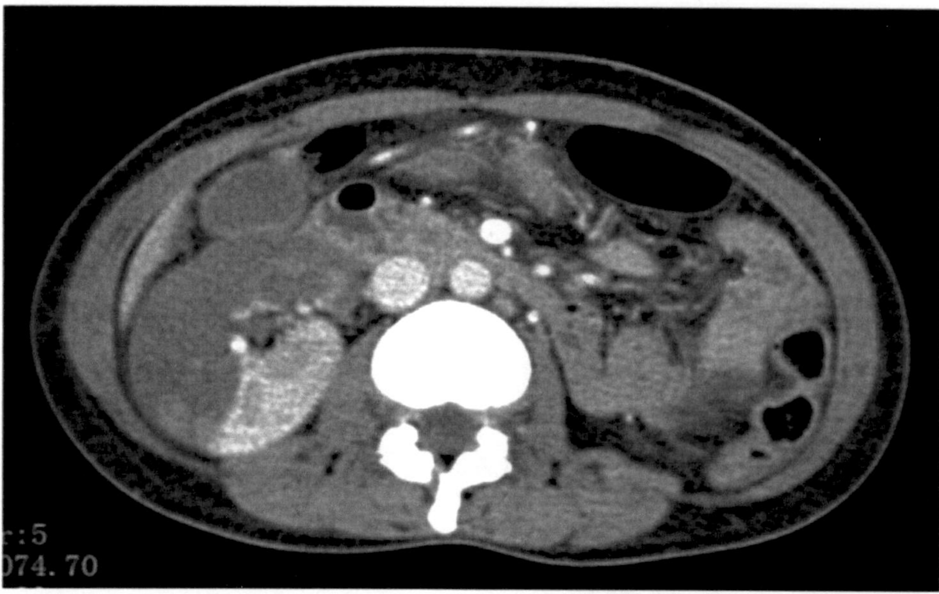

Figure 46.6: CT scan axial view showing enlarged right kidney with multiple wedge-shaped hypodense areas suggestive of infarcts

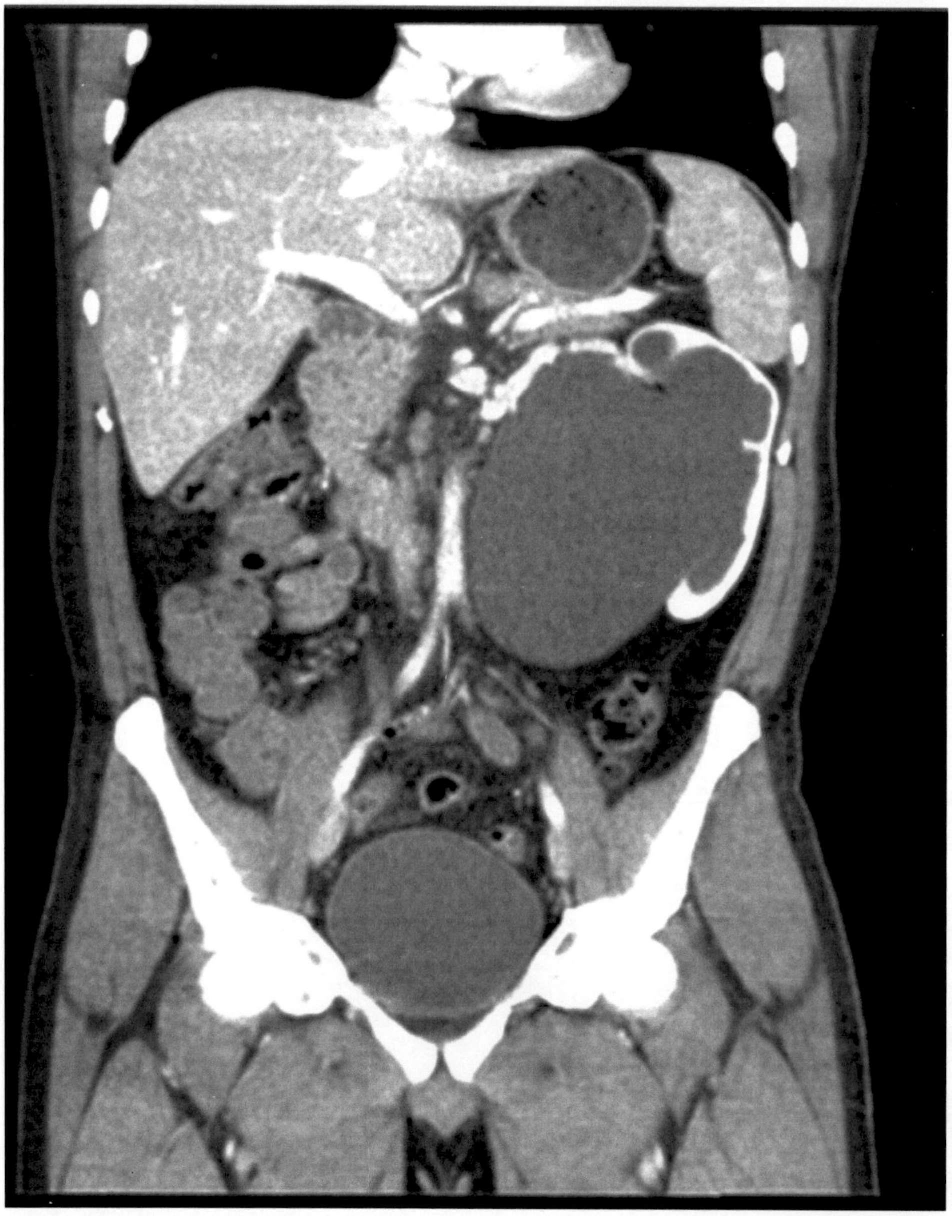

Figure 46.7: CT urography coronal view showing left PUJ obstruction with gross hydronephrosis and thinning of renal parenchyma

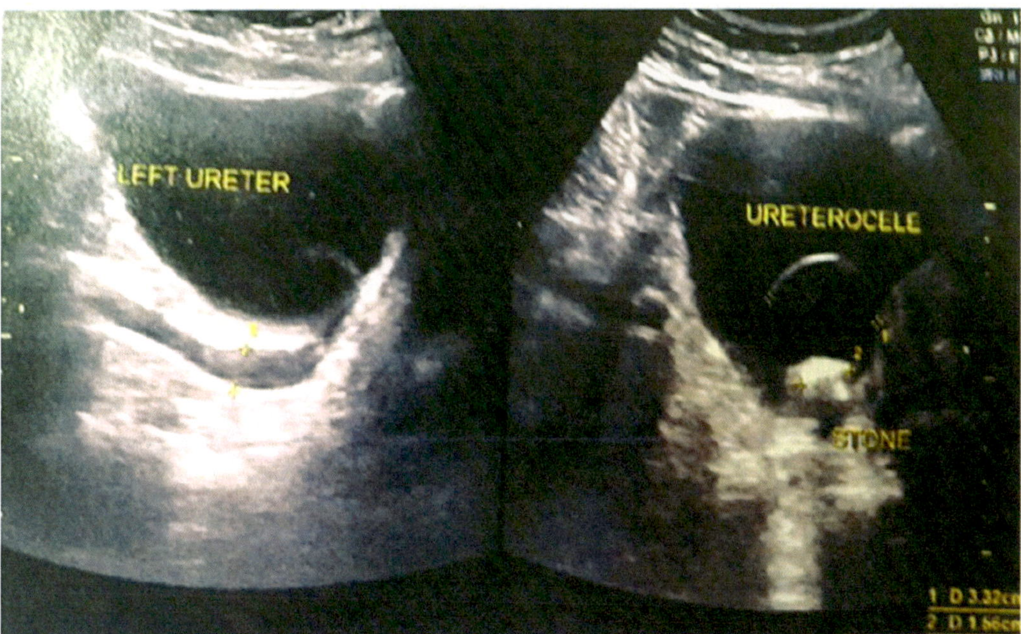

Figure 46.8: USG KUB findings revealed a thin-walled, cystic dilatation within the bladder with echogenic content that not extending beyond its wall as suggestive of ureterocele with calculus

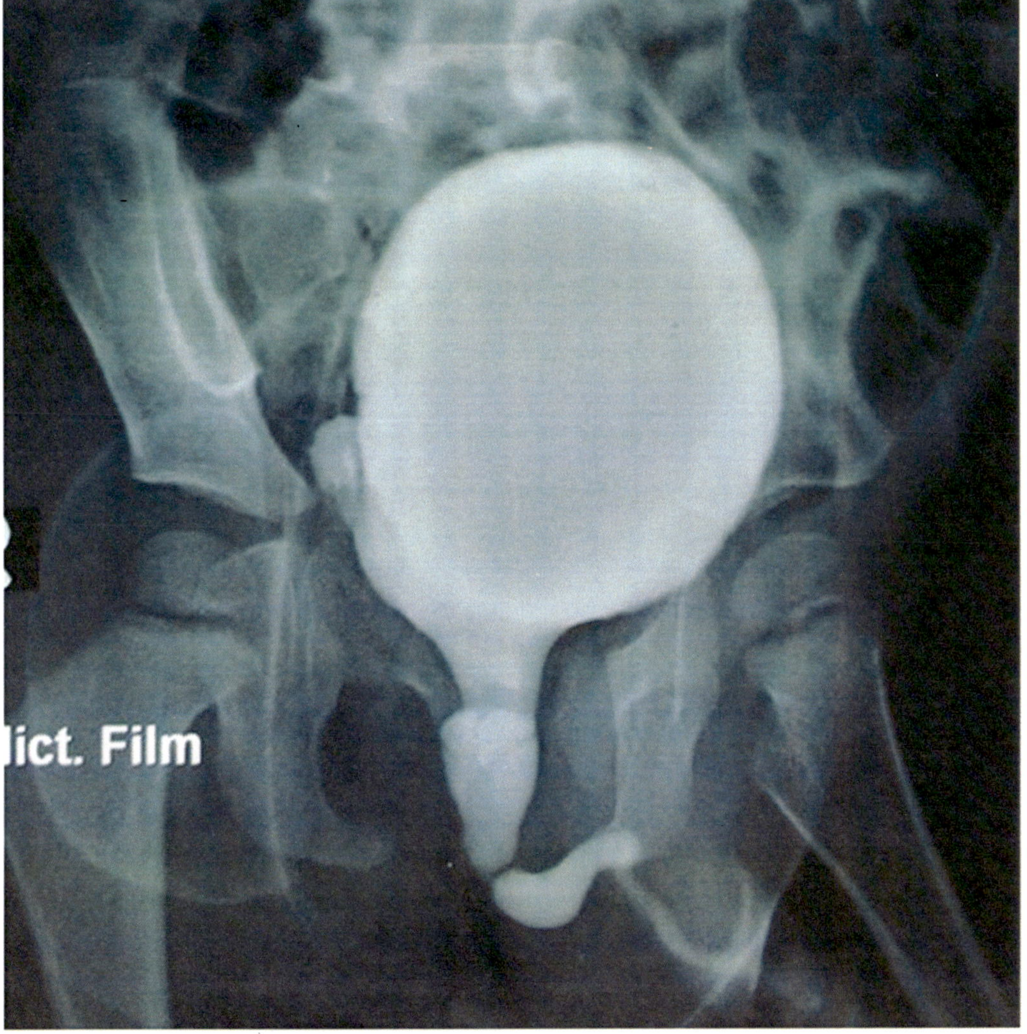

Figure 46.9: Micturating cystourethrogram–posterior urethral valve

- Bladder smooth walled with diverticula at right posterolateral surface.
- Posterior urethra dilated with filling defect at bulbo-membranous junction.
- Anterior urethra normal.

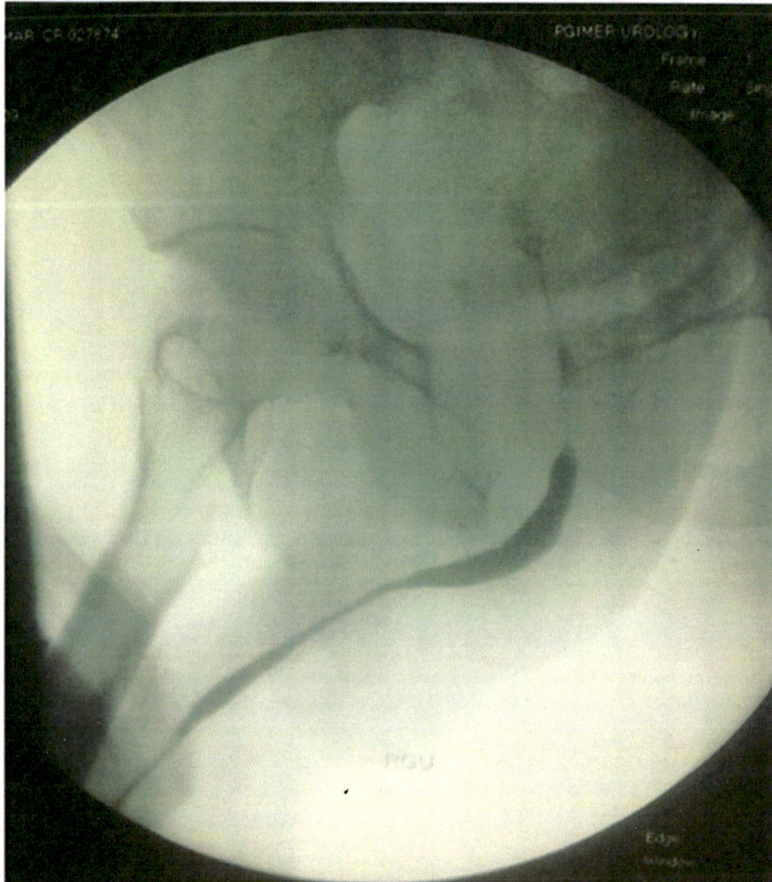

Figure 46.10: Retrograde urethrogram revealed 5 cm irregular stricture involving distal bulbar and proximal penile urethra

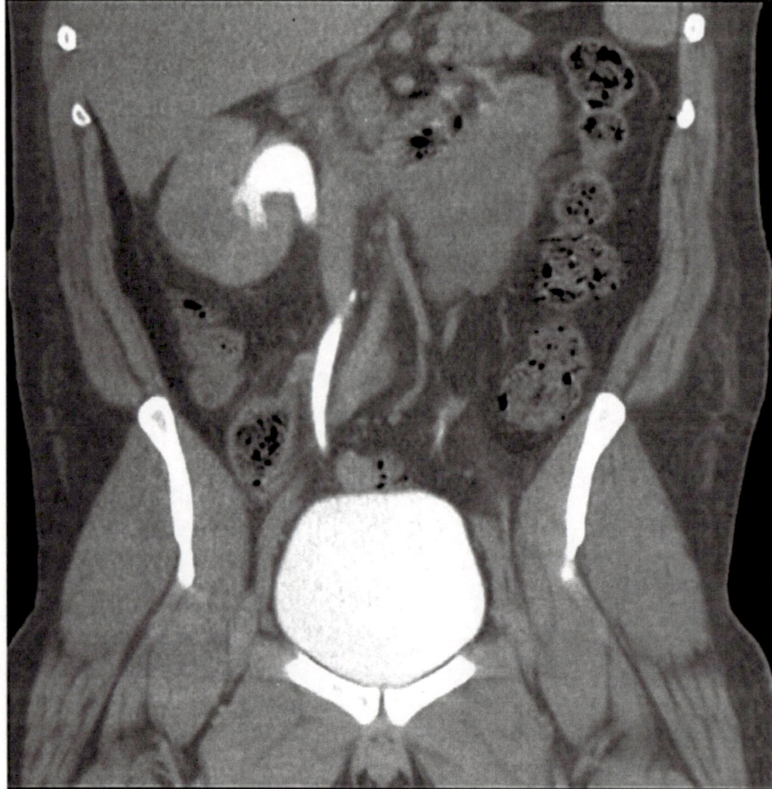

Figure 46.11: CT urography coronal view showing right hydroureteronephrosis with medial displacement of right ureter at mid ureter level–Retrocaval ureter

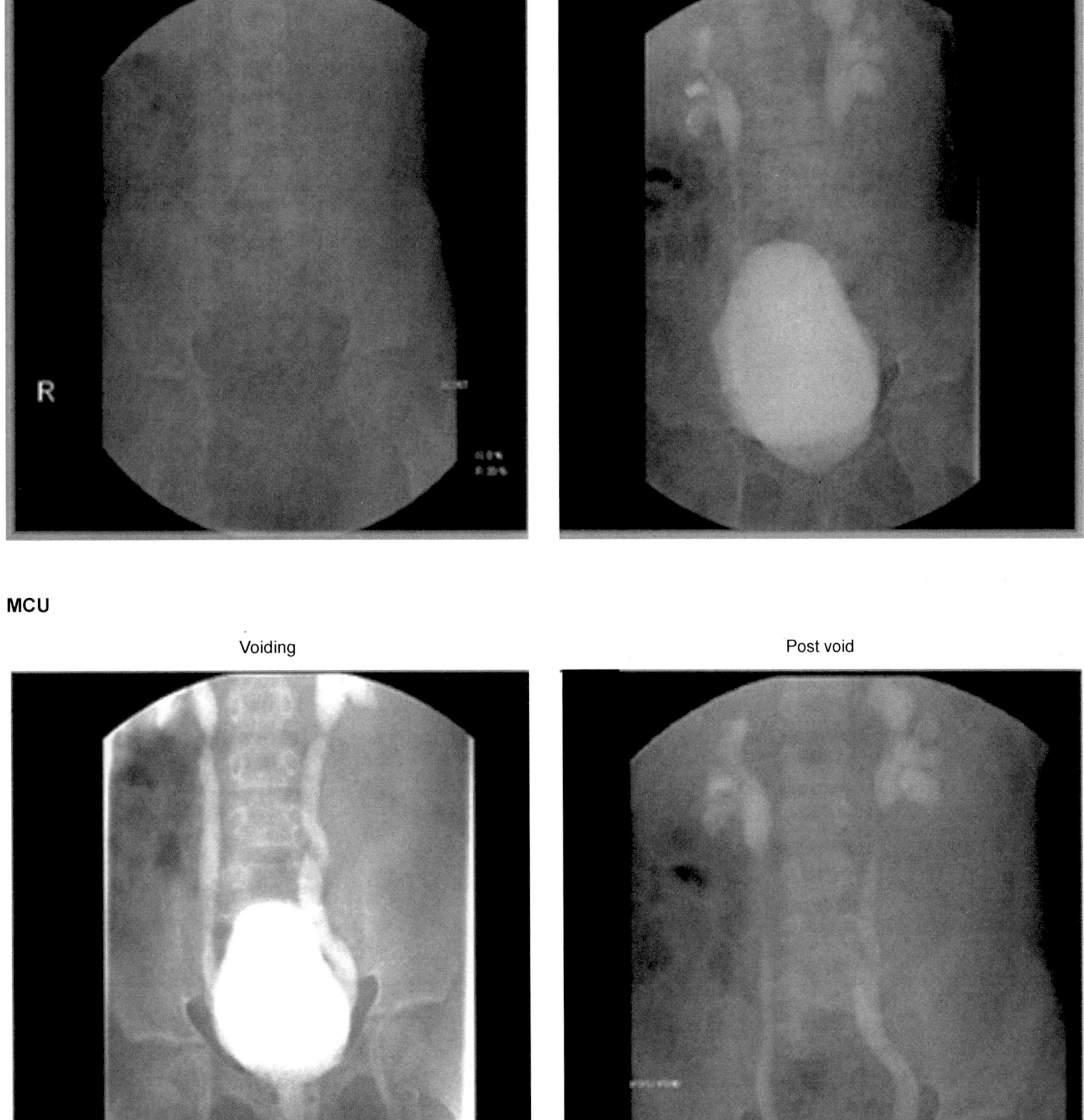

Figure 46.12: Micturating cystourethrogram–Vesicoureteric

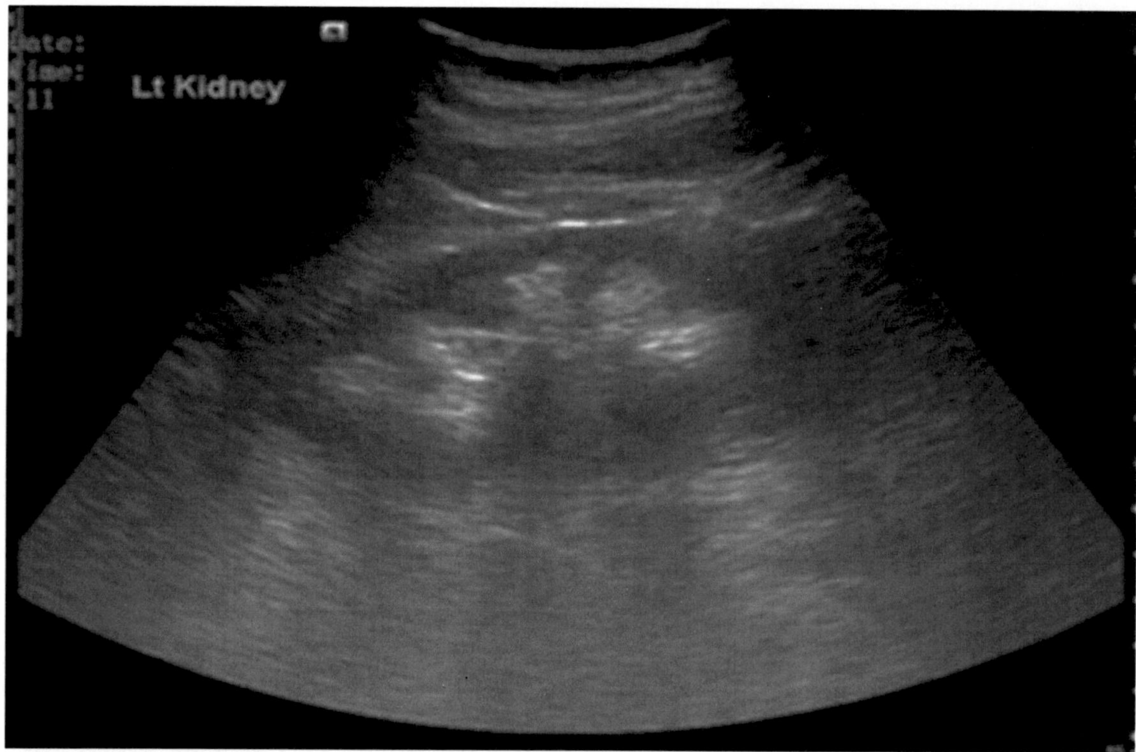

Figure 46.13A: USG showing Hyperechogenicity in medullary region bilateral kidney–Medullary calcinosis

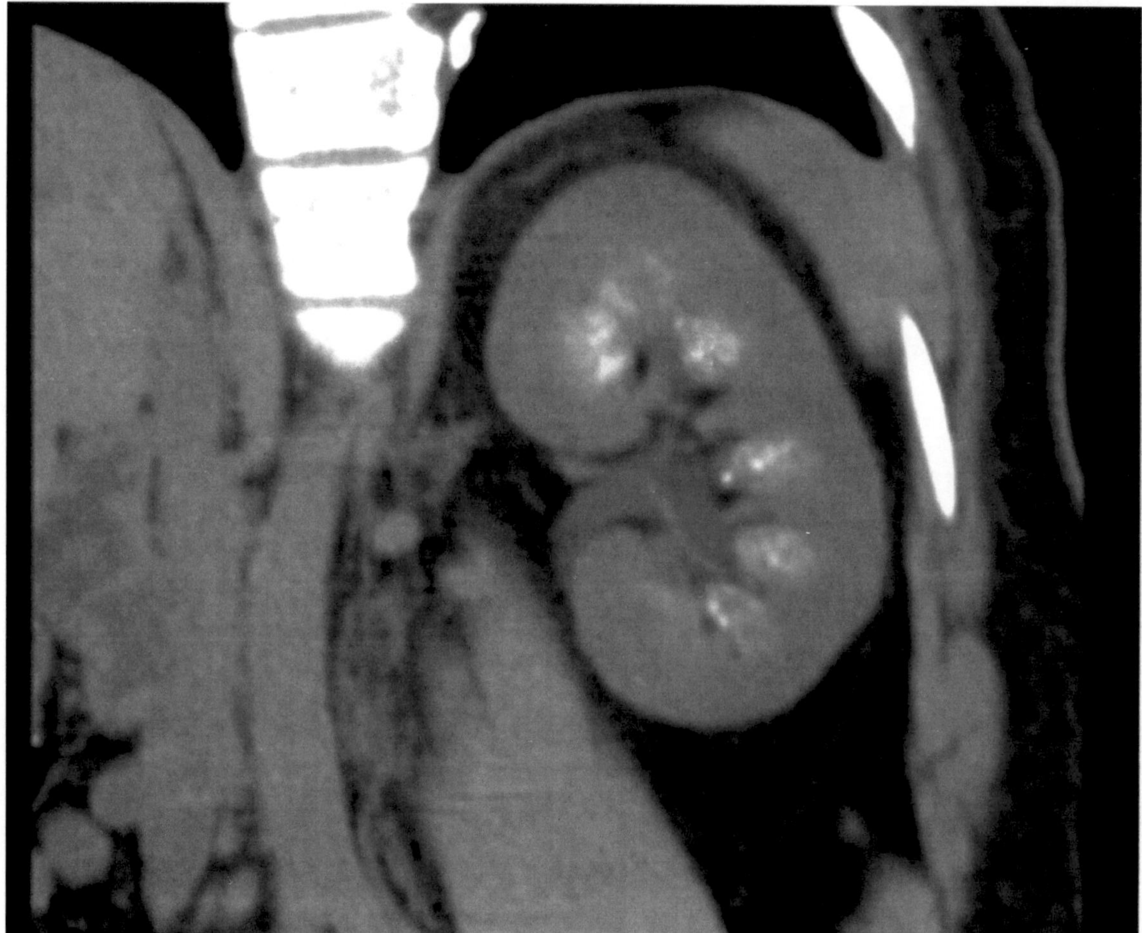

Figure 46.13B: NCCT coronal view showing medullary pyramids show striated hyperdensity giving brush border appearance–Medullary calcinosis

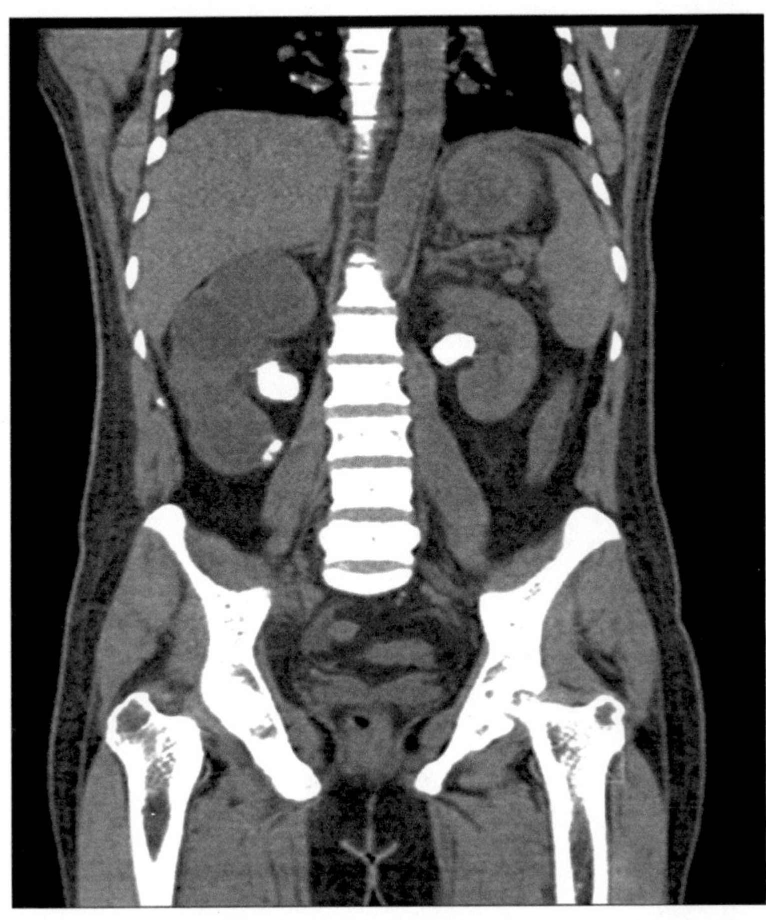

Figure 46.14: CT scan coronal view showing bilateral renal pelvis stone with right gross HDN and thinning of renal parenchyma

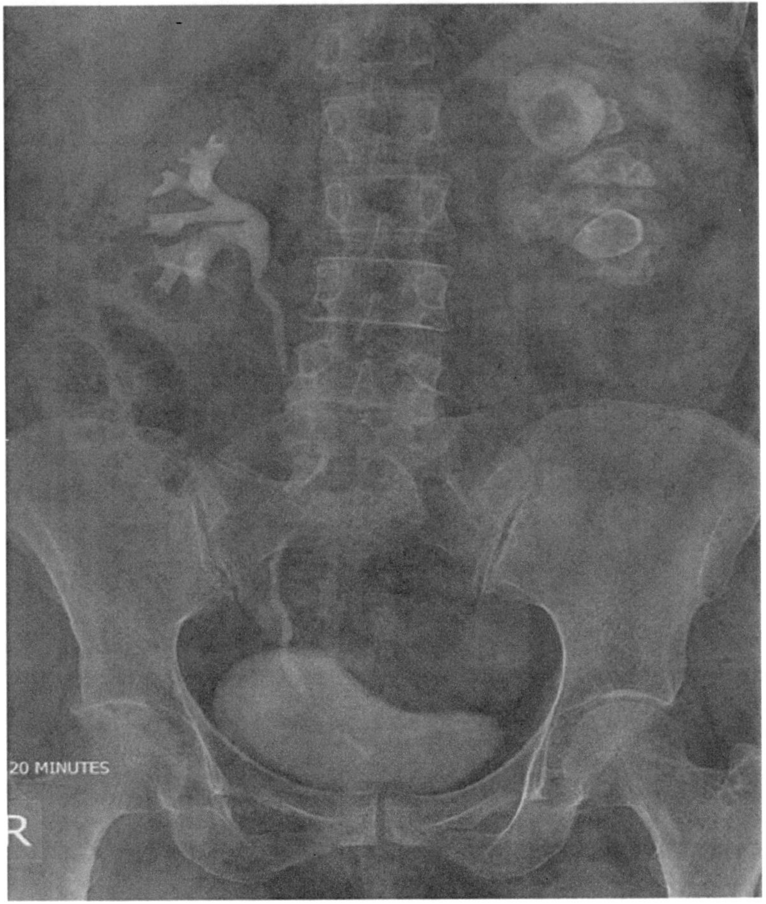

Figure 46.15: Intravenous urography (IVU) Multiple radiopaque stones (staghorn) visible in left kidney. Right pelvicalyceal system normal

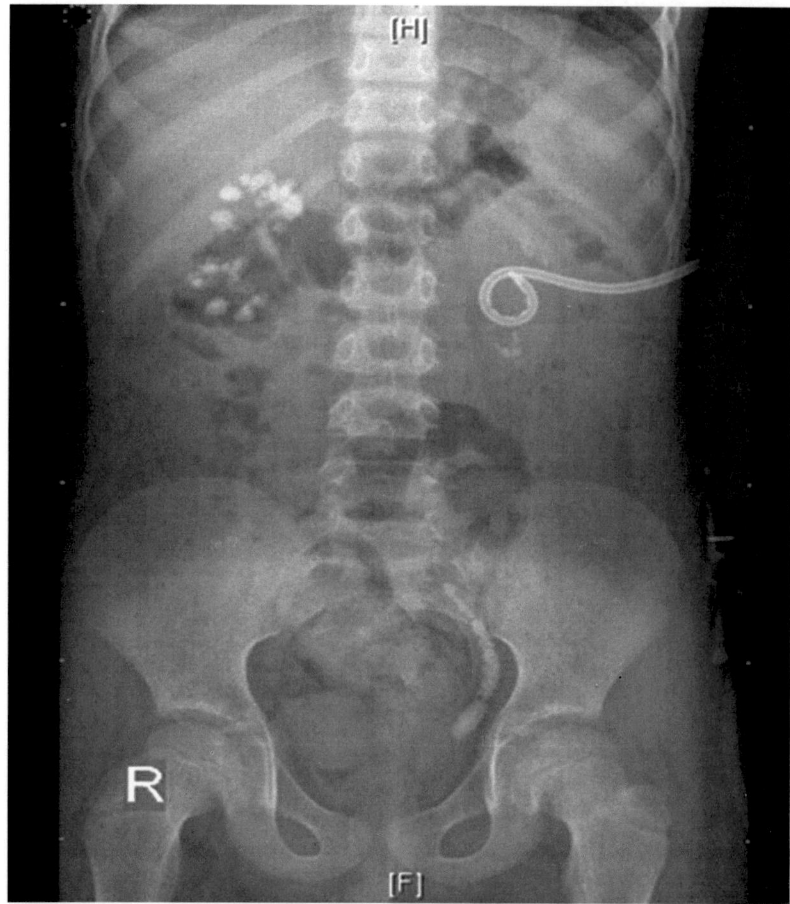

Figure 46.16: X-Ray KUB–*Bilateral multiple radiopaque stones suggestive of oxalate stones Left percutaneous nephrostomy tube in situ

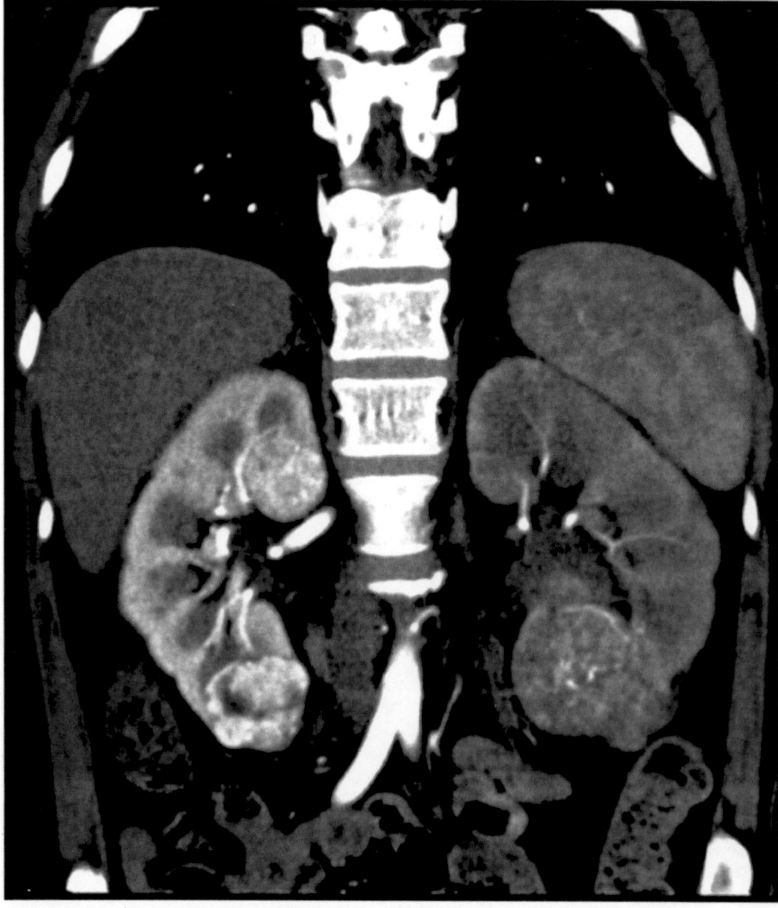

Figure 46.17: Coronal CT demonstrating heterogeneously enhancing mass at right upper and left lower pole

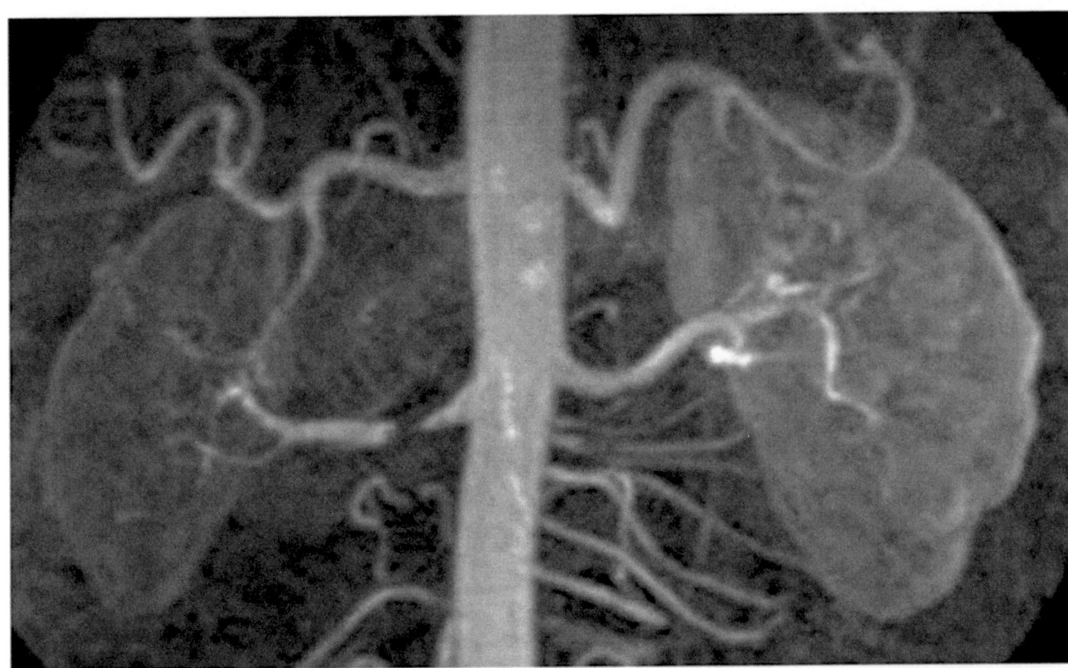

Figure 46.18: Renal angiogram showing right renal artery stenosis

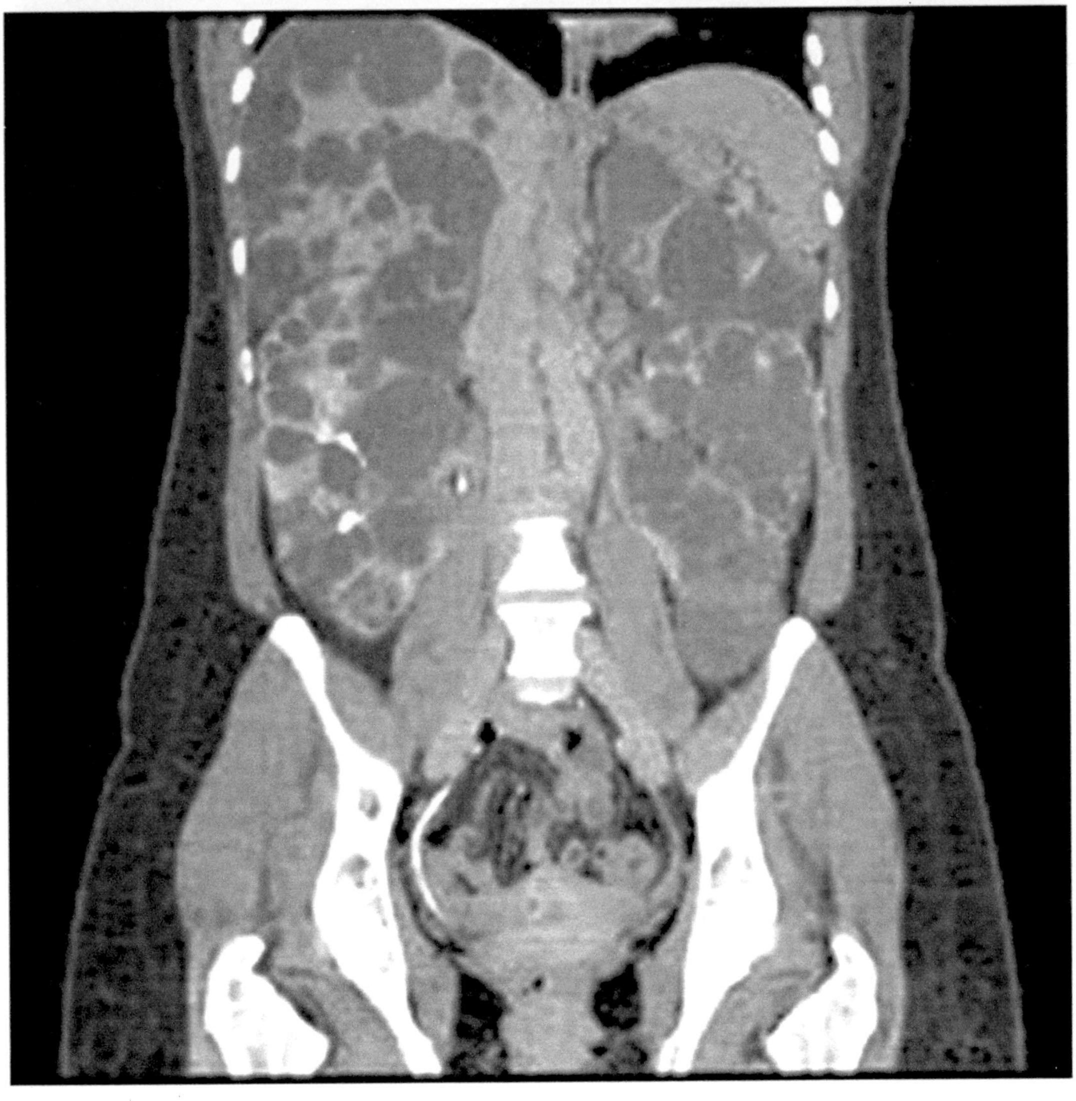

Figure 46.19: CT scan showing bilateral polycystic kidney disease

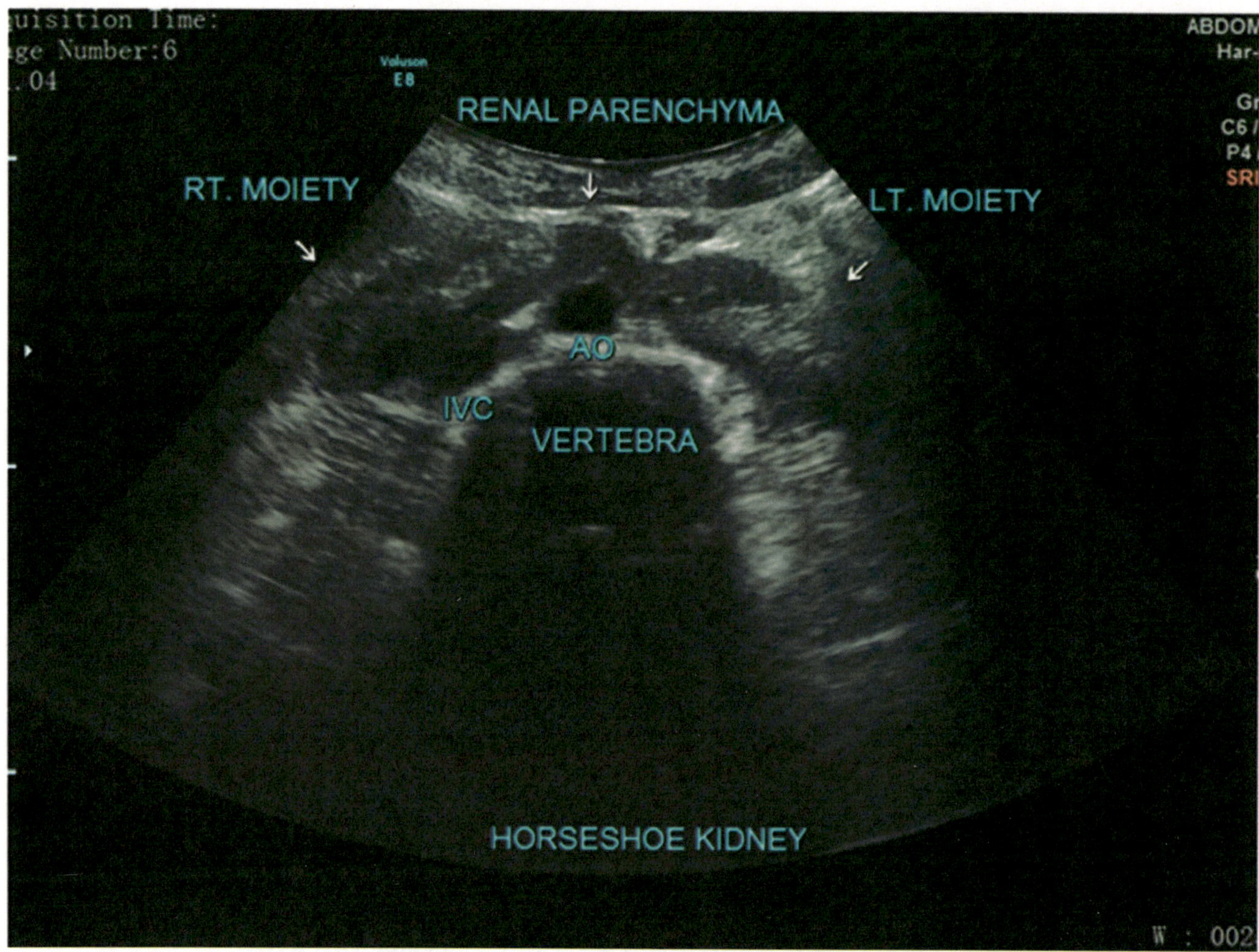

Figure 46.20: USG showing horseshoe kidney

Suggested Reading

1. American College of Radiology. Appropriateness criteria. Available at: http://www.acr.org/ac

CHAPTER

47

Retinal Abnormalities in Renal Diseases

Mayank Bansal

Consultant, Ophthalmologist and Vitreo-Retinal Surgeon in Delhi and Fortis Memorial Research Institute Gurugram

Retinal abnormalities are commonly seen in patients with renal diseases due to diabetes mellitus and hypertension. It is important to recognize them as they are helpful in diagnosis and overall management of patient. Following cases will be discussed in this chapter.

CASES

1. Diabetic Retinopathy.
2. Hypertensive Retinopathy.
3. Autoimmune Nephropathies–Wegener.
4. Other Syndromes–Bardt Beidel Syndrome.

CASE 1

Patient with sudden onset vision loss right eye, persisting for 1 year and a gradual vision loss in left eye. Known type 2 Diabetes, for 15 years, on treatment, poor sugar control. On general physical examination, he had a puffy face, pedal edema, and amputated left big toe. On ophthalmic examination, right eye vision was counting fingers at 3 meters (3/60), and left eye counting fingers at 6 meters (6/60). Right eye fundus examination revealed a Diabetic Vitreous Hemorrhage and Tractional Retinal Detachment (TRD) involving macula (Fig. 47.1a). Left eye fundus exam showed Proliferative Diabetic Retinopathy (PDR) with Diabetic Macular Edema (DME) (Fig. 47.1b).

Ophthalmic Investigations were performed. Optical Coherence Tomography (OCT), was done. An OCT scan of normal macula, is shown in Figure 47.2(a). The left eye image of our patient is given in Figure 47.2(b), showing a retinal thickening at the macula, DME. Right eye OCT image could not be captured due to vitreous hemorrhage.

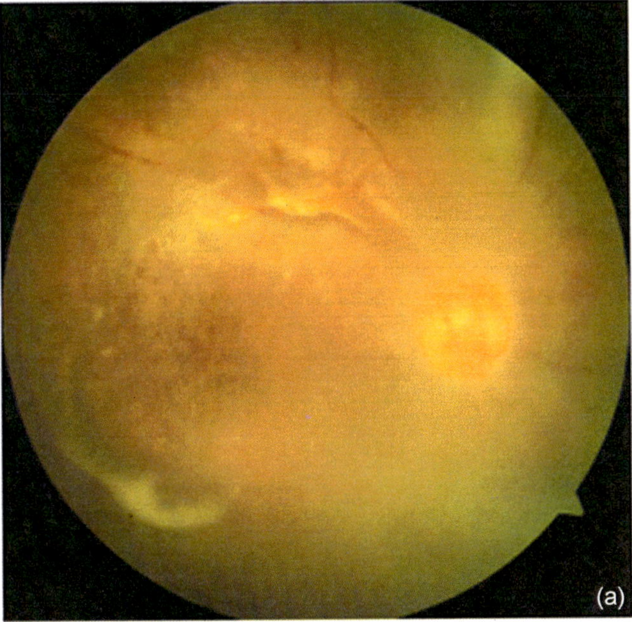

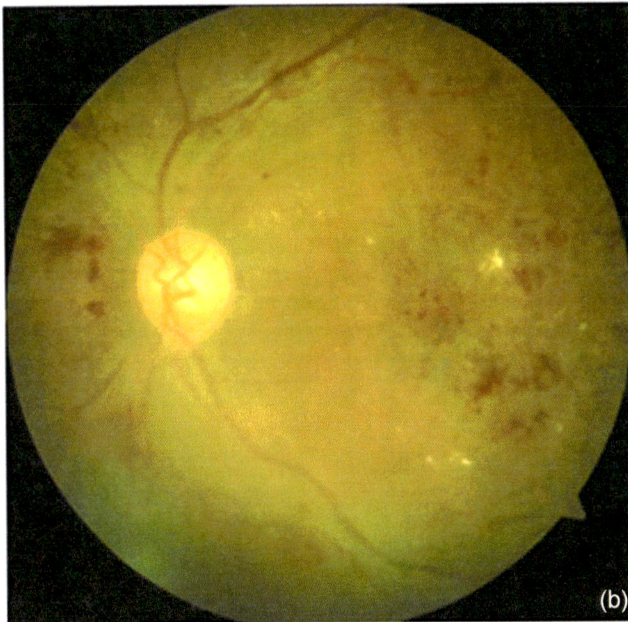

Figure 47.1: (a) Right eye fundus picture showing diabetic vitreous hemorrhage and tractional retinal detachment (TRD) involving macula (b) Left eye fundus picture showing proliferative diabetic retinopathy with diabetic macular edema

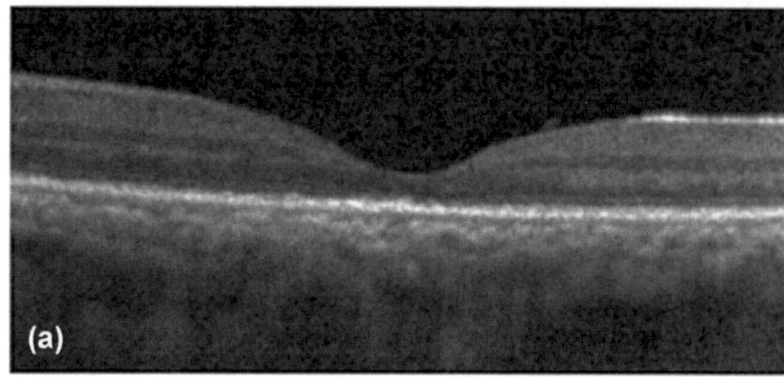

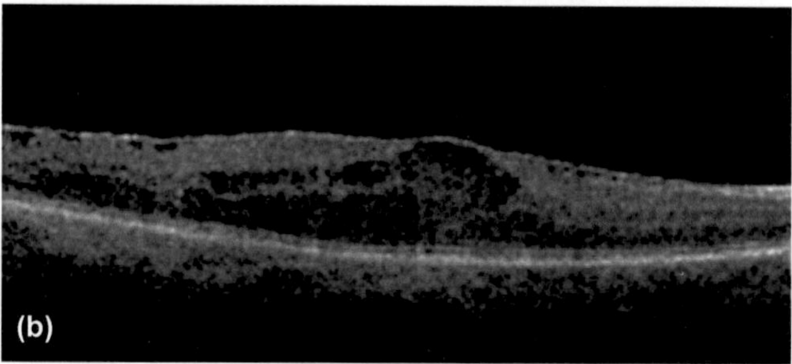

Figure 47.2: (a) OCT scan of normal macula, showing the foveal dip (b) OCT scan of our patient, left eye, showing hypo-reflective, intra-retinal fluid spaces, with a hyper-reflective membrane at the vitreo-retinal interface, the epiretinal membrane (ERM). Unlike the normal macula OCT scan, the foveal dip is lost

Fundus fluorescein angiography (FFA) was done, using 3 ml of 20% sodium fluorescein dye. The FFA image findings are shown in Figures 47.3(a) and (b).

Before further ophthalmic management, it was important to treat the patient and not just the eye. Systemic investigations, blood sugar profile, kidney function tests, lipid profile were done.

After systemic control of blood sugars, the right eye was operated for 25 gauge 3 port, *pars plana vitrectomy, endo-laser retinal photocoagulation* under local anesthesia. Post-vitrectomy the vision improved from 3/60 to 6/12 parts (on Snellen visual acuity chart) at 3 months follow-up. The pre- and post-operative fundus picture is shown in Figure 47.4.

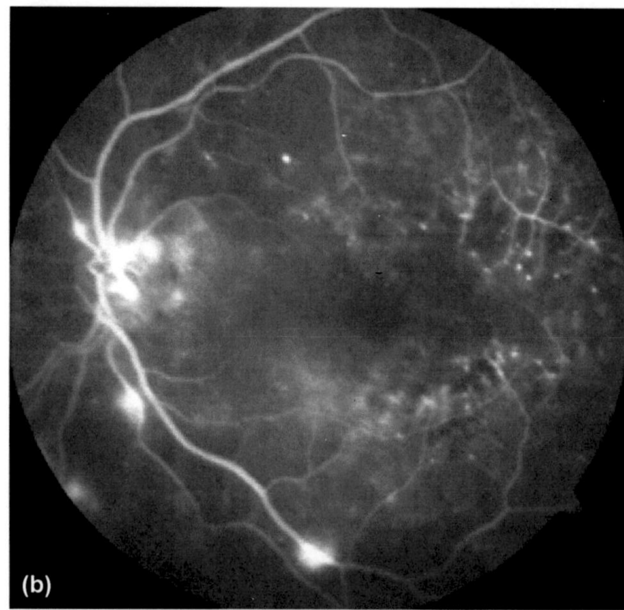

Figure 47.3: (a) Right eye fundus fluorescein angiography (FFA) image, in venous phase, showing an area of hyperfluorescence, corresponding to neo-vascularization on optic disc (NVD) and retinal neo-vascularization elsewhere (NVE) along superior retinal arcade. There are areas of blocked fluorescence due to vitreous hemorrhage. Temporal to fovea, some small areas of hyper-fluorescence can be seen, corresponding to microaneurysms (b) Left eye FFA image, venous phase, showing microaneurysms and NVD and NVE

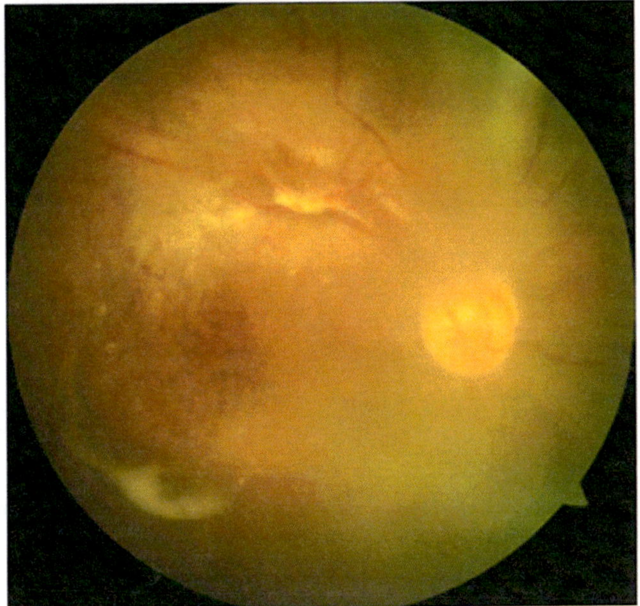

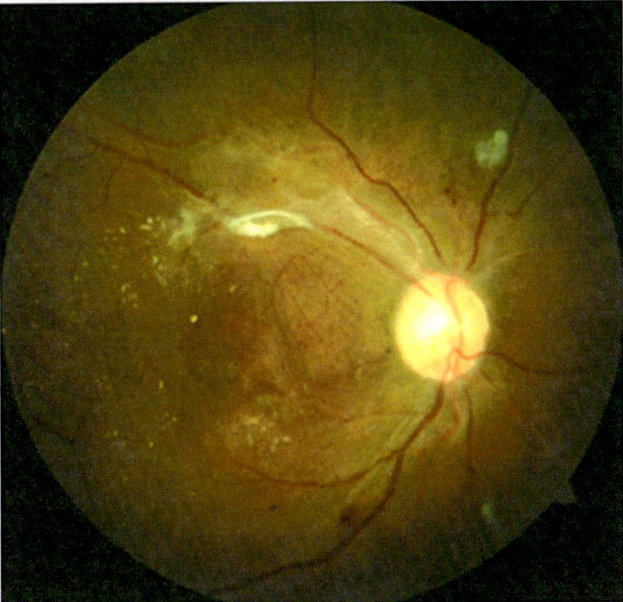

Figure 47.4: Fundus image of the right eye of our case. The post-operative image on the right, shows removal of vitreous hemorrhage and removal of retinal traction along superior arcade

For management of the left eye DME, intra-vitreal dexamethasone implant was injected (Fig. 47.5). At 3 months follow-up, the vision in the left eye improved from 6/60 to 6/12 parts. Left eye DME was assessed using OCT, during each follow up, to look for anatomical resolution of macular edema (Fig. 47.6).

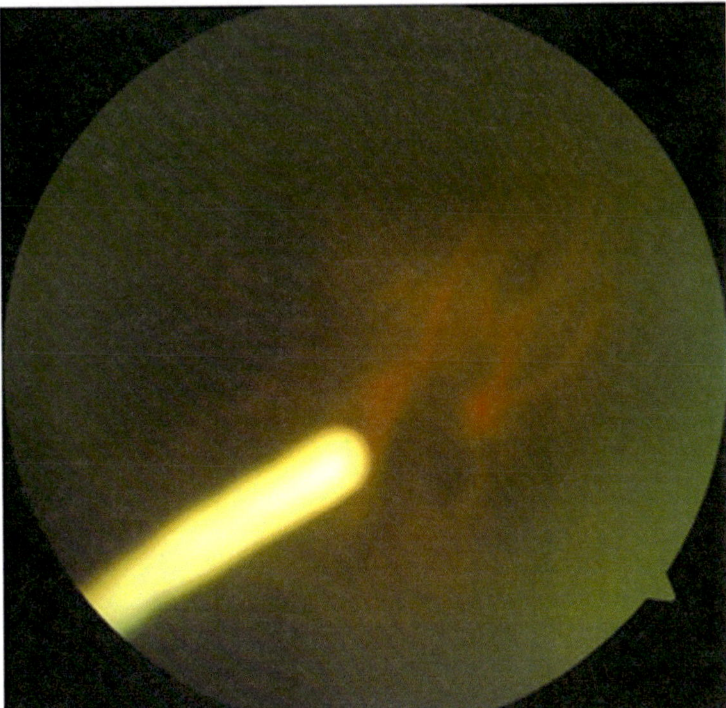

Figure 47.5: Fundus picture of the left eye–showing the intravitreal dexamethasone implant

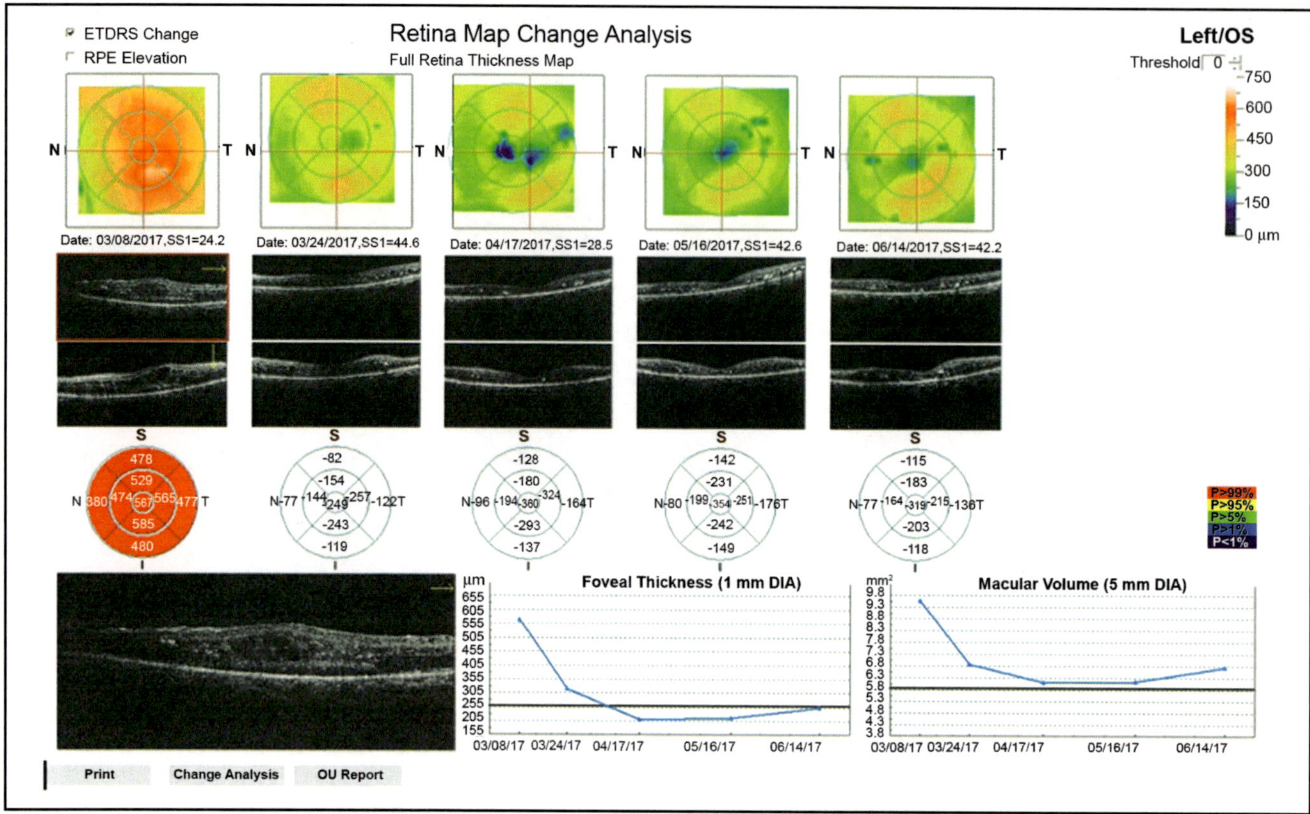

Figure 47.6: The OCT retina map change analysis showing resolution of DME

Diabetic Retinopathy

Diabetic Retinopathy (DR), is a potentially blinding eye condition. However, signs of DR in the retina can be examined, much before vision loss occurs, hence the role of retinal screening.

Screening

All type 2 diabetics, are recommended to undergo retinal screening at the time of diagnosis. For type 1 diabetes, there are various recommendations, of retinal screening from 2 to 5 years from the time of diagnosis of diabetes.

Retinal Examination Techniques

Retinal examination by an ophthalmologist, using slit-lamp biomicroscopy and 90D lens is considered most desirable. Indirect ophthalmoscopy by an ophthalmologist gives a stereoscopic, complete retinal field exam. Direct ophthalmoscope, is easy to carry, and gives a view of the posterior pole, or central areas of the retina.

Retinal Imaging

Retinal imaging has an important role. It helps document and follow-up retinal changes in patients with Diabetic Retinopathy. Ultra-wide field retinal imaging, with a field of view upto 200 degrees, gives most complete view of retina (Fig. 47.7). A dilated 7 field image of retina (modified Airlie House) using a standard 50 degree fundus camera, has been considered standard by most retina specialists for retinal imaging. A non-mydriatic fundus camera with 45 to 50 degrees field of view, for imaging the posterior pole of fundus, is considered more practical for quick screening of retina in high volumes practices.

Clinical Features

For those with most initial changes of Diabetic Retinopathy, retina examination shows, small deep-red dots between 25 and 100 µm in diameter within the retina, called *microaneurysms*. These microaneurysms are outpouchings of retinal capillary walls, caused due to pericyte loss in Diabetes. This stage is called mild non proliferative diabetic retinopathy (NPDR). At this stage, there no vision loss, patient is asymptomatic, is advised systemic control and annual retina review.

With poor glycemic control, there is progression into more severe stages. The next change seen is presence of *intra-retinal hemorrhages*, which can be flame shaped (more-superficial), or dot-blot (deep). With leaking blood vessels, there may be swelling in the retina, specifically the macula – called *Diabetic Macular Edema (DME)*. With DME there is varying degree of vision loss. At this stage, patients are often managed with intra-ocular injection of anti-vascular endothelial growth factor (anti-VEGF) agents, and/or steroids. This fluid may contain lipids,

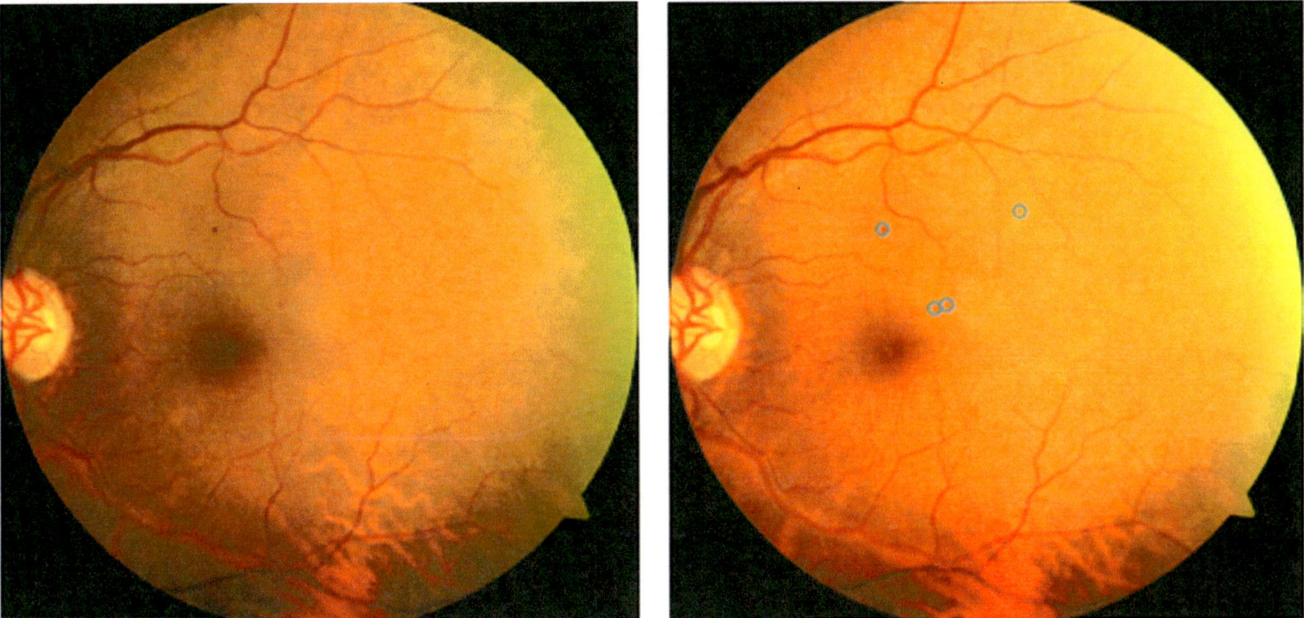

Figure 47.7: On the left is the image of the fundus, showing mild NPDR; the right image is the same fundus picture, with the microaneurysms marked as blue circles

which accumulate and deposit as *hard exudates* in retina. With concomitant vessel occlusion, there is superficial retinal nerve fibre layer infarcts, called *cotton wool spots*, or soft exudates. They appear as yellowish lesions, with indistinct margins. At these stages, the retinopathy is classified as moderate or severe NPDR (Figs. 47.8 and 47.9).[1]

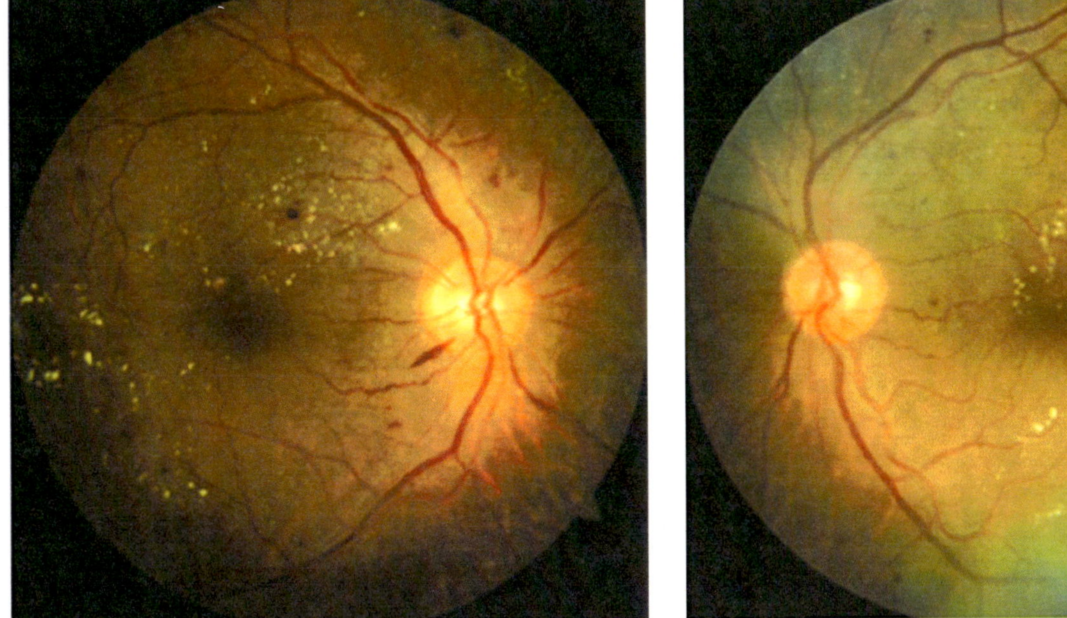

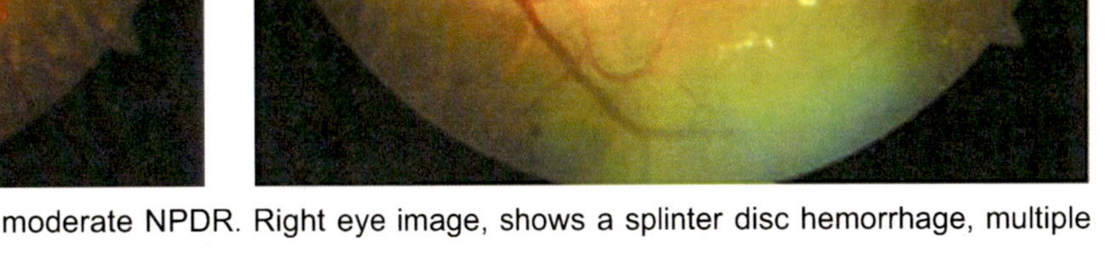

Figure 47.8: Retinal images of a patient with moderate NPDR. Right eye image, shows a splinter disc hemorrhage, multiple dot-blot hemorrhages and hard exudates

With further progression, the ischemic, hypoxic state in the eye, releases Vascular Endothelial Growth Factors (VEGFs), with new vessel formation. At this stage, the retinopathy is classified as *Proliferative Diabetic Retinopathy*

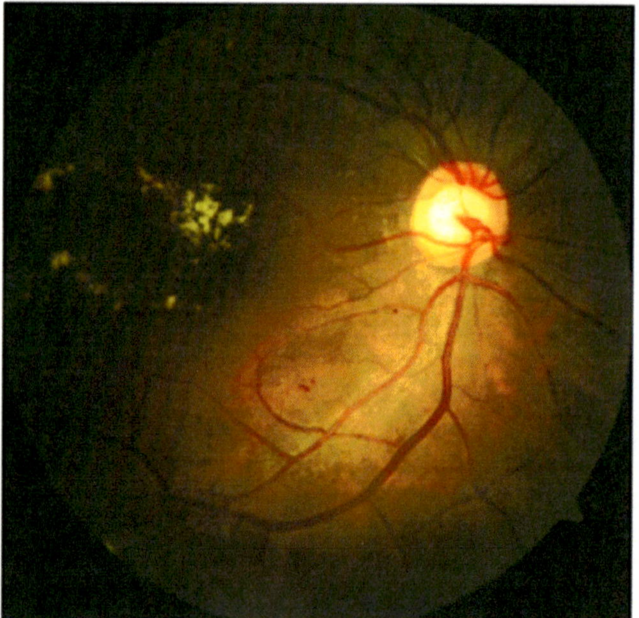

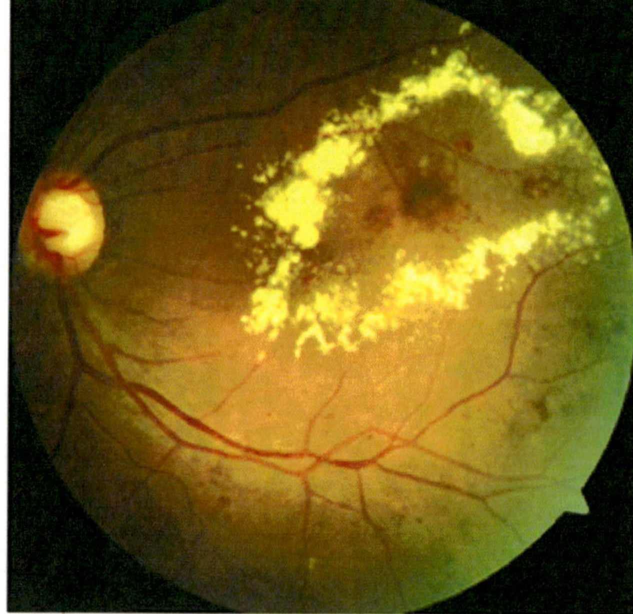

Figure 47.9: Fundus images of a patient with moderate NPDR, with DME, showing *circinate hard exudates*. This circular pattern is seen as the hard exudates accumulate around the leaking microaneurysms. Such a patient is likely to have a DME, which has been rather long standing

(PDR), which is characterised by neovascularization. These new vessels tend to be friable and lead to pre-retinal hemorrhage, as *vitreous haemorrhage*, sub-hyaloid hemorrhage. When non-resolving, present for more than 3 months, and affecting vision, it needs to be surgically removed by performing vitrectomy surgery. These vessels grow towards the vitreous cavity, or on the surface of retina. They lead to *tractional retinal detachment (TRD)*. When involving the macula, it forms an indication for vitrectomy surgery.

CASE 2

Hypertensive Retinopathy

Young, 24-year-old male. Complaining of headaches. Blood pressure – 200/110 mm of Hg. Vision right eye 6/6 and left eye 6/9. Retinal examination shows optic disc edema, with arterio-venous crossing changes – suggestive of malignant hypertensive retinopathy. Systemic, detailed work up revealed co-existing renal damage. Below are the changes seen in severe hypertensive retinopathy (Fig. 47.10).

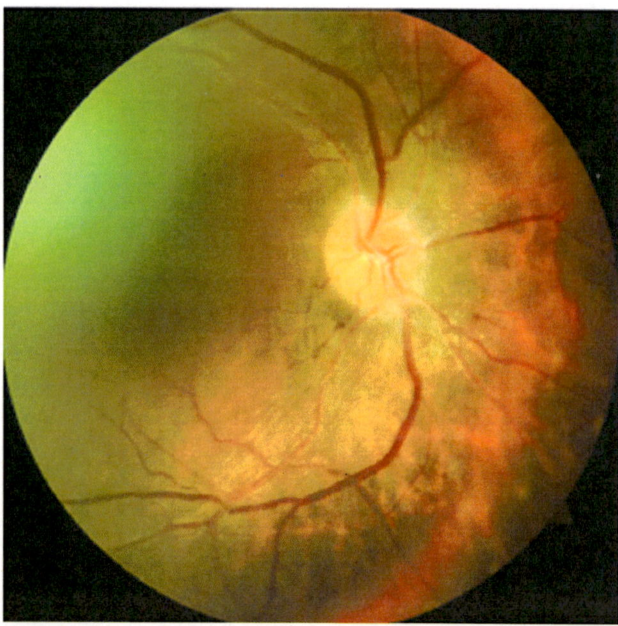

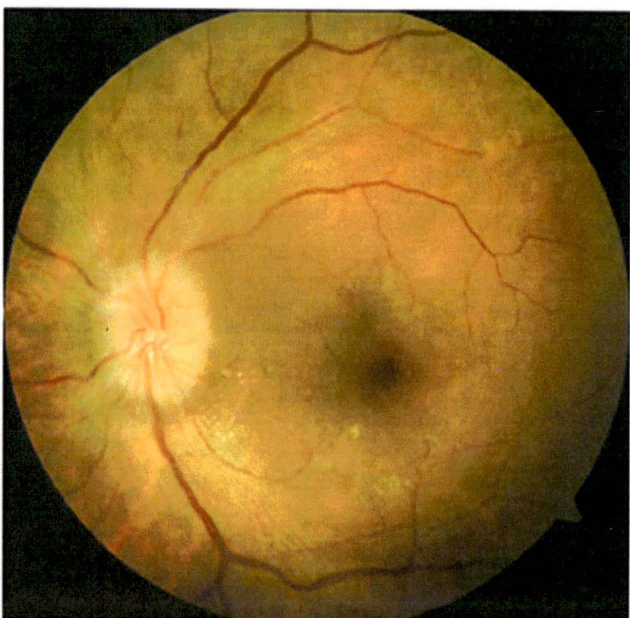

Figure 47.10: Fundus images of patient with Malignant Hypertensive Retinopathy. Note the Optic Disc Edema in both eyes. Also note Arterio-Venous (AV) crossing changes (right eye, inferior arcade). Left eye fundus image also shows exudates (yellow dots)

The ophthalmic management is limited in such cases. Control of blood pressure and treating underlying cause, result in resolution of optic disc edema.

Hypertensive retinopathy is graded as mild, moderate and malignant, as per Wong Mitchell Classification.[2] Mild Retinopathy – has generalized arteriolar narrowing and/or arteriovenous crossing nicking (Fig. 47.11). It is associated with a modest risk of stroke, and coronary heart disease. Moderate retinopathy shows, retinal hemorrhages, with cotton wool spots, hard exudates. It is strongly associated with risk of stroke, cognitive decline, and death from cardiovascular causes. Malignant hypertensive retinopathy – has the above features with optic disc swelling, and a strong association with mortality.

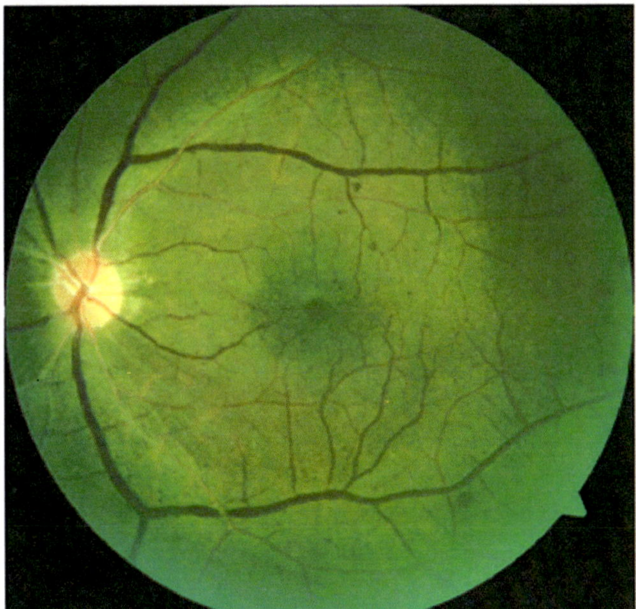

Figure 47.11: Left eye retinal image of a patient with mild hypertensive retinopathy. There is generalized arteriolar narrowing and arteriovenous crossing nicking

In addition, patients with hypertension, are also at a risk of developing retinal vein occlusion, central, or branch retinal vein occlusion.

CASE 3

Retinal Vasculitis in Inflammatory Autoimmune Conditions

50-year-old man presented with complain of sudden loss of vision. Vision was perception of light present, projection of rays inaccurate in left eye; right eye is normal. Retinal examination showed left eye optic disc edema, with marked phlebitis and arteritis. There were severe retinal hemorrhages. The patient was diagnosed to have Wegener's Granulomatosis, with co-existing renal and respiratory involvement. Below is the retinal image (Fig. 47.12).

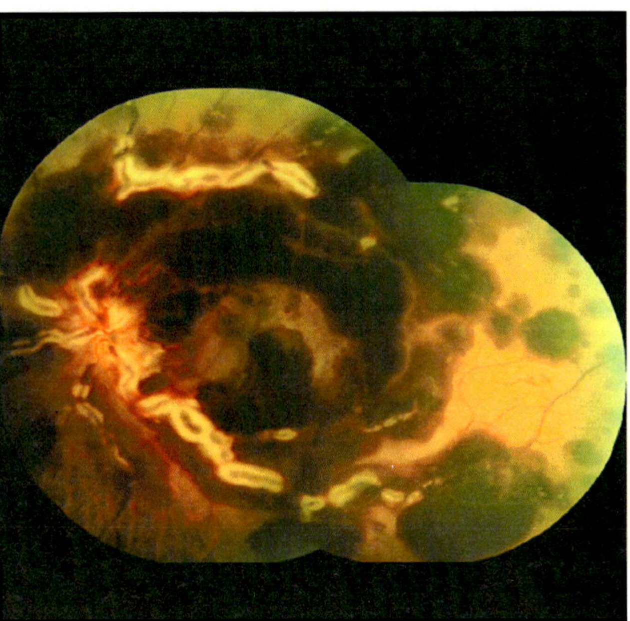

Figure 47.12: Left eye fundus photo of a patient with Wegener's Granulomatosis. There is optic disc edema, marked retinal phlebitis, arteritis and extensive retinal hemorrhages

CASE 4

Retinitis Pigmentosa in Bardet Biedl Syndrome

Parents bring a 12-year-old boy, with complain of gradual progressive dimunition of vision in both eyes, more so in evening and night. The boy had polyuria, polydipsia, truncal obesity, polydactyly and poor intellectual development. Retinal examination showed waxy optic disc pallor, attenuated retinal vessels, and bony spicule pigmentation suggestive of Retinitis Pigmentosa. There were co-existing renal anomalies and a diagnosis of Bardet Biedl Syndrome was made. Below are the retinal images (Figs 47.13).

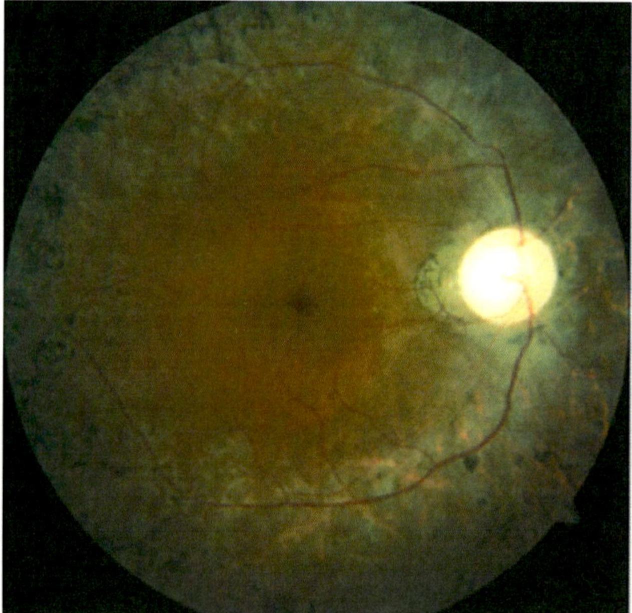
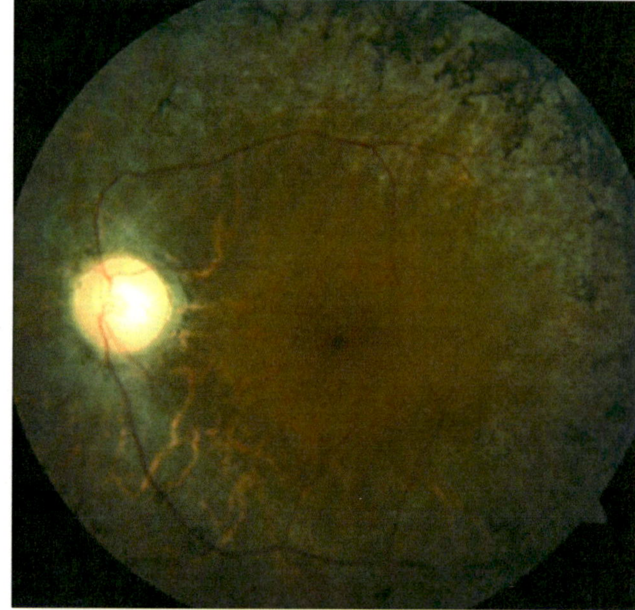

Figure 47.13: Fundus photos of a patient with Bardet Biedl Syndrome, with associated Retinitis Pigmentosa. Note the waxy optic disc pallor, attenuated vessels and retinal pigmentation

Suggested Reading

1. Grading diabetic retinopathy from stereoscopic color fundus photographs–an extension of the modified Airlie House classification. ETDRS report number 10. Early Treatment Diabetic Retinopathy Study Research Group. Ophthalmology 1991 May; 98 (5 Suppl):786-806.
2. Wong TY, Mitchell P. Hypertensive retinopathy. N Engl J Med 2004 Nov 25;351(22):2310-17.

CHAPTER 48

Living Kidney Donor Evaluation

Ajay Kher

Consultant, Nephrologist and Transplant Physician, Max Hospital, Vaishali, Vishwasth Healthcare

End stage renal disease (ESRD) is an increasing burden around the world and especially in India.[1,2] The global burden of disease estimates that there has been an 87% increase in incidence of chronic kidney disease and a doubling of chronic kidney disease deaths over the last two decades.[3] The options for renal replacement therapy (RRT) include dialysis and transplant. In India, many are not able to afford any of these treatments and so die from kidney disease.[2] Kidney transplant is the best modality of RRT as it is associated with mortality benefits, a better quality of life and lower costs over the duration of ESRD.[4-7]

Kidney transplant requires kidney donation, either deceased donor or living donor. In India, currently deceased donor transplants are only limited in nature, though they are increasing, especially in South India. Living donor kidney transplants are associated with better patient and graft outcomes compared to deceased donor transplant.[6] In addition, living donor transplants can be done pre-emptively and hence avoid recipients having to go through the rigors of dialysis. Multiple studies have shown that the longer a recipient has been on dialysis the worse the patient and graft outcomes and that pre-emptive transplant have the best outcomes.[5-7]

The first successful transplant was a living donor transplant between twins.[8,9] Evidence for minimal long-term risks of nephrectomy were initially provided by world war II serviceman who underwent nephrectomy compared to their compatriots who did not undergo nephrectomy[10] and in donors compared to non- donating siblings.[11] Other studies to evaluate donor risks were done by comparing donors to the general population and comparing their risks of death and renal failure.[12,13] These studies found that donors were not at any increased risk of death or renal failure compared to the general population. However, the main critique was that donors are healthier than the general population as they have undergone a screening process and hence their outcomes should be compared to a similar cohort. Recent studies have attempted to do that by taking a general population cohort and removing those with hypertension or other medical or family history that would likely lead to exclusion as a donor and then compared the outcomes.[14,15] These studies have shown an increased relative risk for death and renal failure for donors, though the absolute risk is still small.

These studies highlight the importance of good and through evaluation of donors to minimize their short-term and long-term risks. These studies also highlight the importance of long-term follow-up of donors and need for providing health insurance or coverage for them.

Evaluation

The basic principles of donor selection have remained the same, though the evidence of risks to the donor have changed over the years. The key aspects of donor evaluation are to assess 3 parameters:

1. Donor is in good health and will not face undue perioperative risks (morbidity or mortality).
2. Has good renal function and no significant comorbidities or risk factors that will increase renal risks through the rest of the living donor's life.
3. Has enough renal function that recipient will have good outcome and has no infectious risks for the recipient.

It is important to note that there are no randomized trials that provide data on what or how donor evaluation should be done. The evaluation of living kidney donor is discussed below and has also been discussed in the 2017 Kidney Disease: Improving Global Outcomes (KDIGO) "Clinical Practice Guideline on the Evaluation and Care of Living Kidney Donors".[16]

The usual tests for a donor are presented in Table 48.1. Evaluation of a living kidney donor should include: blood typing, medical evaluation (by a clinician with experience in living donation), surgical evaluation, psychosocial evaluation and human leukocyte antigen (HLA) compatibility.

Table 48.1: Usual tests for donor evaluation
Medical and Family history
Blood Pressure and BMI
Complete Physical Examination
Blood group
HLA typing and Crossmatch
Complete Blood Count
Coagulation Profile
Kidney and Liver Function Tests
Urinalysis and Urine culture
Fasting Glucose and HbA1c
Lipid profile
Pregnancy test (if indicated)
Measured GFR (isotope or creatinine clearance)
Urine albumin excretion (random and timed collection)
Chest X-ray
ECG, other cardiac workup as needed
Renal Anatomy evaluation (CT angio or MR angio)
Age and gender appropriate cancer screening
Infection Screen (HIV, Hep B, HCV, Syphilis, CMV, EBV).
TB and other infection evaluation as per need

Blood typing and crossmatch: Blood group typing and crossmatch compatibility are the primary determinants of biological compatibility between the donor and recipient. If the donor-recipient pair is either blood group or HLA incompatible then benefits, risks and availability of swap (paired donation), incompatible transplant with management of incompatibility or search for an alternate donor should be discussed. HLA matching though still performed is not essential for successful outcomes and allograft survival with unrelated donors are like one haplotype matched living donors.[17-19] Immunological evaluation should be performed, and each centre should develop its protocol of immunological evaluation taking into consideration the immunological risk of the donor-recipient pair and the cost. This is further discussed in the recipient evaluation chapter.

Medical history should focus on any medical conditions and include all organ systems. Donor should also be evaluated for risk factors for kidney and cardiovascular disease and prior episodes of gout. Women should be evaluated with history of any hypertensive disorders during pregnancy (PIH, preeclampsia, eclampsia) and future pregnancy plans. Kidney specific risks should be evaluated with family history and personal history of kidney stones, kidney disease, proteinuria, hematuria or urinary tract infections. Medication history should also be ascertained, current and past, especially chronic pain medicine and any nonsteroidal anti-inflammatory drug use.

Family history of coronary artery disease, cancer (especially kidney cancer), kidney disease, diabetes and hypertension are especially relevant. If family history of kidney disease is present then further details to assess nature and diagnosis, to assess possible risk of disease to the donor currently and more importantly risk for the disease in the future. Social history should include current and past occupation, current health insurance and current social support. History should also include any smoking, alcohol or drug use, presence of any psychiatric illness and any increased infection risk behaviours.

Physical examination should include vital signs, BMI with height and weight, examination of all major organs and blood pressure on 2 separate occasions or a 24-hour ambulatory blood pressure monitoring.

Labs and imaging should include complete blood count (CBC), coagulation profile, kidney and liver function tests, Fasting blood glucose and lipid profile. Risk for diabetes (prediabetes or current diabetes) should be assessed and can be done with Hba1c in all or in those with increased risk. Oral glucose tolerance test may be needed to assess those with borderline results. Urinalysis with microscopy and urine culture (if needed). Proteinuria may be assessed with 24-hour urine protein or albumin excretion (albumin is preferred). Glomerular filtration rate (GFR) should be measured by isotope or 24-hour urine collection for creatinine clearance and be expressed in ml/min/1.73 m^2.

Additional testing may be required depending on findings. Relatives of ADPKD will need a protocol for assessment that will include imaging in those above 30 years of age and either exclusion of those below 30 or genetic testing for mutations. Those with a past history of stone or a stone > 3 mm should have a 24-hour urine calcium, oxalate, uric acid, citrate, creatinine and sodium. Premenopausal females should have a pregnancy test.

All donors should have an electrocardiogram (ECG), chest X-ray (CXR) and some anatomic assessment for equality of kidney size, masses, cysts, and arterial, venous and ureteric anatomy. The anatomic assessment can be done by either CT angiogram or MR angiogram, depending on local expertise or cost.

Infectious disease screening should include Cytomegalovirus (CMV Antibody), Epstein Barr virus (EBV Antibody), Human immunodeficiency virus (HIV Antibody), hepatitis B virus (Hep B surface Antigen, some may add core antibody), hepatitis C virus (HCV Antibody) and syphilis. Each centre should have a screening plan for Tuberculosis and local infections (Strongyloides, Trypanosoma, West nile, Chagas, Ebola, etc).

Cancer screening should be done for all donors and should be based on guidelines for the general public and based on their age and gender. United States Preventive Services Task Force (https://www.

uspreventiveservicestaskforce.org) has published guidelines which are good references to develop protocols for each centre.

Additional tests may be needed based on the individual history or examination findings and may include echocardiography, cardiac stress testing or Apol1 testing.

Psychosocial evaluation should be performed and assess any mental health issues that may complicate the living donor's recovery, increased risk behaviours for HIV, HBV, HCV transmission. If such high-risk behaviours are present, then donor should be informed that there will need to be disclosure of this to the recipient and the donor can withdraw without disclosure or disclose and then proceed with evaluation. Smoking, alcohol and drug use, abuse and dependency also need to be assessed. Donors also must demonstrate that they understand the short-term, long-term medical and psychosocial risks to them and the recipient. They should be assessed whether decision to donate is free of inducement, coercion and other undue pressure. To ensure voluntariness, some portion of the evaluation should be performed in the absence of recipient and any other relatives or family members. There should also be assessment of the ability of the living donor to make informed decision and ability to cope with major surgery and related stress.

Absolute and relative contraindications are listed in Table 48.2 and Table 48.3. It is important to note that each donor should be assessed individually. Many donors may not have an absolute contraindication but may have many relative contraindications that may make their cumulative risk too high to donate. As physician our first principle is "primum non nocere" – First, to do no harm. It is also important to recognize that the younger the donor the more numbers of years they have to develop risk factors that may lead to renal failure.[20] Hence, most transplant programs are stricter with their exclusions in younger donors and are somewhat lenient with older donors.[21] Some of the specific issues and considerations in assessing the donor are discussed below.

Table 48.2: Absolute contraindications
Age < 18
Mentally incapable of making informed decision
GFR <60 ml/min/1.73m^2
Uncontrolled hypertension or hypertension with any end organ damage
Diabetes
Active malignancy or incompletely treated malignancy
Active or persistent infection
Untreated or active psychiatric illness
Kidney stone with likelihood of recurrence
Evidence of donor coercion

Table 48.3: Relative contraindications
Age 18-21
Hypertension in young donor
Prediabetes in young donor or with strong family history
BMI >30
Moderately increased Albuminuria (>30 mg/d)
Bleeding Disorder
History of Thrombosis or Embolism
Nephrolithiasis
History of Malignancy
Significant Cardiovascular Disease

Age

Most programs consider age <18 as absolute contraindication for donation and an age of 18-21 as a relative contraindication. The first consideration is whether the donor at that age would have the ability to fully comprehend the risks and give an informed consent. Another consideration is that the long-term or life long risks of such a young donor would be unknown even if the current evaluation is normal.[20] OPTN data has shown that most donors placed on the list for kidney transplant had donated between the ages of 18-34 and developed ESRD >15 years after donation.[22] There is no upper limit for age in most programs, however the older donors are more likely to have other comorbidities or complex medical histories and lower GFR.

Glomerular Filtration Rate (GFR)

Previously, most programs used a threshold of 80 ml/min or age based GFR criteria.[23] The KDIGO guidelines[16] have acknowledged the lack of good evidence to choose a specific absolute threshold for GFR and hence have recommended a GFR > 90 to accept donors and a GFR <60 to reject donors. They have suggested individualized decision making for those with GFR 60-89 in combination with the transplant programs pre-specified acceptable risk threshold.

Albuminuria

Urinary albumin excretion (measured by urine albumin creatinine ratio UACR and a timed urinary albumin excretion) is more sensitive than urine protein creatinine ratio and hence is the preferred test to assess potential donors as is also recommended for the general population. Albumin excretion 30-300 mg/day is considered moderately increased and > 300 mg/day is severely increased. A meta-analysis from 5 million healthy persons in 7 cohorts has shown that every 10 fold rise in albuminuria is associated with 3 time risk of ESRD over a 4-16 years period.[24] Higher albuminuria has also been associated with higher risk of CKD, CVD and mortality. KDIGO guidelines recommend accepting donors with UACR< 30 and making individualized decision for those with UACR 30-100 mg/day.

Hematuria

Evaluation for hematuria with a urinalysis should be performed for all potential donors. If hematuria is persistent and not related to exercise, trauma, sexual activity or menstruation then it should be evaluated with urine cytology, urine culture, cystoscopy, 24-hour urine stone panel, and kidney biopsy for IgA or alports or thin basement. Those with reversible causes of hematuria can proceed for donation. Other need individualized decision making and those with IgA should be excluded.

Kidney Stones

Donors with current kidney stones or a history of kidney stones need to undergo metabolic workup to assess for cause of nephrolithiasis. Those with metabolic abnormalities, bilateral stones and recurrent stones should be excluded.

Hypertension

Potential donors with hypertension may be considered as donors on an individualized basis if they are well controlled and have no target organ damage. End organ damage would include any of these: cardiovascular event (myocardial infarction or stroke), albumin excretion >30 mg/day, reduced kidney function, hypertensive retinopathy of left ventricular hypertrophy. It is also important to discuss with donors that hypertension worsens with age and that currently available evidence suggests that donation increases blood pressure over and above that caused by ageing.[25,26] They should also be counselled about lifestyle modifications, need for well controlled blood pressure throughout their life to limit impact on the remaining kidney.

Obesity and Metabolic Risks

Obesity is a risk factor for CKD, cardiovascular disease and diabetes.[27] Hence all donors should get their BMI assessed and obese donors (BMI > 30) should be evaluated on their combined risk with other comorbidities. Obesity was also found to be associated with ESRD in the 5 million general population meta-analysis from 7 cohorts.[24] Praga *et al.* found that after uninephrectomy for various indications, those who were obese (BMI >30) were dramatically more likely to develop proteinuria or renal dysfunction.[28] Another study with ~120,000 living kidney donors with follow-up of upto 20 years found that for every 1 rise in BMI above 27 there was a 7% increase in ESRD risk.[29] Donors should be advised to lose weight before donating and then maintain a healthy weight for their lifetime.

Diabetes

Diabetes is the most common cause of ESRD worldwide and hence has been considered an absolute contraindication to donation. The recent KDIGO guidelines[16] and others have noted that diabetes be combined like other risk factors to a comprehensive assessment of the donor to assess the long-term risks. However, with most transplant centres doing a very poor job of following the donors, diabetes should be a contraindication in almost all situations. Prediabetes is a risk factor for future diabetes and cardiovascular disease. The younger the person, the more likely that they may progress to diabetes and then kidney disease in their lifetime.

Malignancy

Past history of cancer with intermediate risk of recurrence (1-10%) or higher risk of recurrence should be excluded. Persons with previous cancers that have a less than 1% risk of recurrence may be considered on a case-by-case basis.

Smokers should quit at least four weeks before surgery to limit perioperative risks of deep vein thrombosis and respiratory complications and should be advised life-long abstinence for decreasing long-term risks.

Counselling and Communication

It is very important to discuss the risks of donation with the potential donor and to accurately reflect the perioperative risks and the long-term risks. It is important to communicate to the donor our current level of understanding of the risks. The risks that must be discussed are:

1. Perioperative pain and other complications, including mortality.
2. Long-term risks, especially of ESRD.
3. Individualized risk discussion based on results of the donor evaluation.

Perioperative risks: Previous studies and current studies have reported the 90-day mortality to be 0.03% (1 in 3000 or 3 in 10,000).[30-32] Perioperative complication and morbidity have been assessed by Norway and US data registries with standardized complication grading with major complications of 2.5-4% and minor complications of 10-18%.[31,33,34] Majority complications are gastrointestinal (4.4%), bleeding (3%), respiratory (2.5%), surgery or anesthesia related (2.4%).[34] Obesity, predonation hematological disorders, psychiatric illness, robotic nephrectomy was associated with higher complications and greater hospital volume with reduced risk.[34]

Long-term risks: The main risk to consider is development of renal disease. As noted above, earlier studies that compared donor outcomes to general population did not show any increase in mortality or kidney disease.[12,13] The 2 more recent studies[14,15] showed that there was an increased risk when compared to a cohort that was selected to be similarly screened. Mjoen *et al.* compared 1901 donors with a median follow-up of 15 years to a selected cohort of ~32000 with a median follow-up of 25 years and found that hazard ratio for death was higher in donors at 1.3 and significantly higher for ESRD at 11. The overall incidence of ESRD in donors was 302 per million (3 per 10,000). Muzzale *et al.* compared 96000 US donors from 1994-2011 with a median follow-up of 7.6 years to 20000 participants in the NHANES cohort with a median follow-up of 15 years. After matching there were only 9364 in the healthy non-donor cohort. 99 donors developed ESRD. The study also found that estimated lifetime risk for ESRD in general population (unscreened) was 326 per 10,000, 14 per 10,000 for screened healthy non-donors and 90 per 10,000 for donors. Hence, the risk for donors is higher than the risk for similar screened healthy population, even though the relative risk is higher, the overall risk is still small. Living donors should be informed of this small but real increase in risk to make a fully informed decision about donation.

References

1. Jha V, Modi GK. Getting to know the enemy better–the global burden of chronic kidney disease. Kidney Int 2018;94(3):462-64.
2. Dare AJ, Fu SH, Patra J, Rodriguez PS, Thakur JS, Jha P, *et al.* Renal failure deaths and their risk factors in India 2001-13: Nationally representative estimates from the Million Death Study. Lancet Glob Health 2017;5(1):e89-e95.
3. Xie Y, Bowe B, Mokdad AH, Xian H, Yan Y, Li T, *et al.* Analysis of the Global Burden of Disease study highlights the global, regional and national trends of chronic kidney disease epidemiology from 1990 to 2016. Kidney Int 2018;94(3):567-81.
4. Wolfe RA, Ashby VB, Milford EL, Ojo AO, Ettenger RE, Agodoa LY, *et al.* Comparison of mortality in all patients on dialysis, patients on dialysis awaiting transplantation, and recipients of a first cadaveric transplant. N Engl J Med 1999;341(23):1725-30.
5. Mange KC, Joffe MM, Feldman HI. Effect of the use or nonuse of long-term dialysis on the subsequent survival of renal transplants from living donors. N Engl J Med 2001;344(10):726-31.
6. Meier-Kriesche HU, Kaplan B. Waiting time on dialysis as the strongest modifiable risk factor for renal transplant outcomes: A paired donor kidney analysis. Transplantation 2002;74(10):1377-81.
7. Meier-Kriesche HU, Port FK, Ojo AO, Rudich SM, Hanson JA, Cibrik DM, *et al.* Effect of waiting time on renal transplant outcome. Kidney Int 2000;58(3):1311-17.
8. Harrison JH, Merrill JP, Murray JE. Renal homotransplantation in identical twins. Surg Forum 1956;6:432-36.
9. Merrill JP, Murray JE, Harrison JH, Guild WR. Successful homotransplantation of the human kidney between identical twins. J Am Med Assoc 1956;160(4):277-82.
10. Narkun-Burgess DM, Nolan CR, Norman JE, Page WF, Miller PL, Meyer TW. Forty-five year follow-up after uninephrectomy. Kidney Int 1993;43(5):1110-15.
11. Najarian JS, Chavers BM, McHugh LE, Matas AJ. 20 years or more of follow-up of living kidney donors. Lancet 1992;340(8823):807-10.
12. Fehrman-Ekholm I, Elinder CG, Stenbeck M, Tyden G, Groth CG. Kidney donors live longer. Transplantation 1997;64(7):976-78.
13. Ibrahim HN, Foley R, Tan L, Rogers T, Bailey RF, Guo H, *et al.* Long-term consequences of kidney donation. N Engl J Med 2009;360(5):459-69.
14. Mjoen G, Hallan S, Hartmann A, Foss A, Midtvedt K, Oyen O, *et al.* Long-term risks for kidney donors. Kidney Int 2014;86(1):162-67.
15. Muzaale AD, Massie AB, Wang MC, Montgomery RA, McBride MA, Wainright JL, *et al.* Risk of end-stage renal disease following live kidney donation. JAMA 2014;311(6):579-86.
16. Lentine KL, Kasiske BL, Levey AS, Adams PL, Alberu J, Bakr MA, *et al.* KDIGO Clinical Practice Guideline on the Evaluation and Care of Living Kidney Donors. Transplantation 2017;101(8S Suppl 1):S1-S109.
17. Delmonico F, Council of the Transplantation S. A Report of the Amsterdam Forum On the Care of the Live Kidney Donor: Data and Medical Guidelines. Transplantation 2005;79(6 Suppl):S53-66.
18. Davis CL. Evaluation of the living kidney donor: Current perspectives. Am J Kidney Dis 2004;43(3):508-30.
19. Port FK, Dykstra DM, Merion RM, Wolfe RA. Trends and results for organ donation and transplantation in the United States, 2004. Am J Transplant 2005;5(4 Pt 2):843-49.
20. Steiner RW. 'Normal for now' or 'at future risk': A double standard for selecting young and older living kidney donors. Am J Transplant 2010;10(4):737-41.
21. Mandelbrot DA, Pavlakis M, Danovitch GM, Johnson SR, Karp SJ, Khwaja K, *et al.* The medical evaluation of living kidney donors: A survey of US transplant centers. Am J Transplant 2007;7(10):2333-43.
22. Gibney EM, King AL, Maluf DG, Garg AX, Parikh CR. Living kidney donors requiring transplantation: Focus on African Americans. Transplantation 2007;84(5):647-49.
23. Kher A, Mandelbrot DA. The living kidney donor evaluation: Focus on renal issues. Clin J Am Soc Nephrol 2012;7(2):366-71.
24. Grams ME, Sang Y, Levey AS, Matsushita K, Ballew S, Chang AR, *et al.* Kidney-Failure Risk Projection for the Living Kidney-Donor Candidate. N Engl J Med 2016;374(5):411-21.
25. Boudville N, Prasad GV, Knoll G, Muirhead N, Thiessen-Philbrook H, Yang RC, *et al.* Meta-analysis: Risk for hypertension in living kidney donors. Ann Intern Med 2006;145(3):185-96.
26. Garg AX, Prasad GV, Thiessen-Philbrook HR, Ping L, Melo M, Gibney EM, *et al.* Cardiovascular disease and hypertension risk in living kidney donors: An analysis of health administrative data in Ontario, Canada. Transplantation 2008;86(3):399-406.
27. Hsu CY, McCulloch CE, Iribarren C, Darbinian J, Go AS. Body mass index and risk for end-stage renal disease. Ann Intern Med 2006;144(1):21-28.
28. Praga M, Hernandez E, Herrero JC, Morales E, Revilla Y, Diaz-Gonzalez R, *et al.* Influence of obesity on the appearance of proteinuria and renal insufficiency after unilateral nephrectomy. Kidney Int 2000;58(5):2111-18.

29. Locke JE, Reed RD, Massie A, MacLennan PA, Sawinski D, Kumar V, *et al.* Obesity increases the risk of end-stage renal disease among living kidney donors. Kidney Int 2017;91(3):699-703.
30. Johnson EM, Remucal MJ, Gillingham KJ, Dahms RA, Najarian JS, Matas AJ. Complications and risks of living donor nephrectomy. Transplantation 1997;64(8):1124-28.
31. Mjoen G, Oyen O, Holdaas H, Midtvedt K, Line PD. Morbidity and mortality in 1022 consecutive living donor nephrectomies: Benefits of a living donor registry. Transplantation 2009;88(11):1273-79.
32. Segev DL, Muzaale AD, Caffo BS, Mehta SH, Singer AL, Taranto SE, *et al.* Perioperative mortality and long-term survival following live kidney donation. JAMA 2010;303(10):959-66.
33. Patel S, Cassuto J, Orloff M, Tsoulfas G, Zand M, Kashyap R, *et al.* Minimizing morbidity of organ donation: Analysis of factors for perioperative complications after living-donor nephrectomy in the United States. Transplantation 2008;85(4):561-65.
34. Lentine KL, Lam NN, Axelrod D, Schnitzler MA, Garg AX, Xiao H, *et al.* Perioperative Complications After Living Kidney Donation: A National Study. Am J Transplant 2016;16(6):1848-57.

CHAPTER

49 Kidney Transplant Recipient Evaluation

Ajay Kher

Consultant, Nephrologist and Transplant Physician, Nephrology, Max Hospital, Vaishali, Vishwasth Healthcare

End stage renal disease (ESRD) is an increasing burden around the world and especially in India.[1,2] The global burden of disease estimates that there has been an 87% increase in incidence of chronic kidney disease and a doubling of chronic kidney disease deaths over the last two decades.[3] The options for renal replacement therapy (RRT) include dialysis and transplant. In India, many are not able to afford any of these treatments and so die from kidney disease.[2] Kidney transplant is the best modality of RRT as it is associated with mortality benefits, a better quality of life and lower costs over the duration of ESRD.[4-7]

Kidney transplant requires kidney donation, either deceased donor or living donor. In India, currently deceased donor transplants are only limited in nature, though they are increasing, especially in South India. Living donor kidney transplants are associated with better patient and graft outcomes compared to deceased donor transplant.[6] In addition, living donor transplants can be done pre-emptively and hence avoid recipients having to go through the rigors of dialysis. Multiple studies have shown that the longer a recipient has been on dialysis the worse the patient and graft outcomes and that pre-emptive transplant have the best outcomes.[5-7]

There is an initial increased mortality risk in the post-operative period.[4] ESRD patients usually have many other comorbidities or coexisting illnesses and these may impact the postoperative morbidity and mortality. Hence, potential kidney transplant recipients need to undergo a thorough evaluation to assess:

1. Candidacy for transplantation (assess for contra-indications).
2. Risks of perioperative complications and management of those to decrease risks.
3. Discussion with patient and family so they understand the risks and benefits of transplant vs initiating dialysis or continuing on dialysis.
4. Discussion of options and process of deceased donor transplantation and living donor transplantation and risks and benefits of both.

Timing of Referral for Transplant

Patients with advanced and irreversible kidney disease should have discussion for transplant options and be referred for kidney transplantation if not done at that centre. Early referral allows patients and their family to first internalize the irreversibility of renal failure and the need for kidney transplant. It also then allows them to understand the process of kidney transplant, the risks and benefits of living and deceased donor transplant and look for family members for living donation. As all of this takes time, it is important to do this early enough to allow patients to be able to receive preemptive kidney transplant which is associated with the best short-term and long-term patient and graft outcomes.[6,7]

Initial Evaluation

It is important to note that there are no randomized controlled clinical trials to guide recipient evaluation and hence the evaluation of potential recipients should be defined by the transplant centre to be thorough yet efficient and cost effective.

The usual tests for a potential recipient are presented in Table 49.1. Evaluation of a potential recipient should include: Medical evaluation (by a clinician with experience in transplantation), surgical evaluation, psychosocial evaluation, detailed examination and human leukocyte antigen (HLA) compatibility. Some of the absolute and relative contraindications are listed in Tables 49.2 and 49.3. If the potential recipient is not a candidate for transplant it is important to assess the patient and determine if some of the contraindications are reversible or treatable. Reassessment after optimization (e.g., non-compliance or severe pulmonary hypertension or cardiomyopathy which may be due to volume overload) may allow some potential recipients to undergo successful transplantation.

Table 49.1: Evaluation of potential kidney transplant recipient
Medical and Family history
Etiology of Renal Failure (Assess risk of recurrence)
Blood pressure and BMI
Complete Physical Examination (Especially cardiac, abdominal and peripheral vascular disease)
Blood group
HLA typing and Crossmatch and Evaluation for sensitization
Complete Blood Count
Coagulation Profile
Kidney and Liver Function Tests and iPTH
Urinalysis and Urine culture
Fasting Glucose and Hba1C
Lipid profile
Pregnancy test (if indicated)
Serum protein electrophoresis +/- Free light chain assay for unexplained renal failure
Urine albumin excretion
Chest X-ray
ECG, Echocardiography, Stress test or Cardiac Angiography as needed
Abdominal Ultrasound (especially for Renal cysts or tumors)
Age and gender appropriate cancer screening
Infection Screen (HIV, Hep B, HCV, Syphilis, CMV, EBV)
TB and other infection evaluation as per need

Table 49.2: Absolute contraindications
Short Expected Life Expectancy
Reversible Renal Failure
Active Infection
Active Malignancy (Recent or Untreatable Malignancy)
Ongoing Noncompliance
Untreated/uncontrolled Psychiatric Disorder or Active Substance Abuse
Primary Oxalosis (consider combined liver and kidney transplant)
Severe Ischemic cardiomyopathy (consider combined heart and kidney transplant)
Severe chronic liver disease (consider combined Liver and Kidney transplant)
Severe bilateral iliac or lower extremity arterial disease not amenable to intervention
Uncorrectable severe pulmonary hypertension
Limited Rehabilitative potential

Table 49.3: Relative contraindications
Active Systemic disease (e.g., lupus or ANCA)
Severe Hyperparathyroidism
Systemic Amyloidosis with cardiac involvement
Angina or severe coronary heart disease with no intervention possible
History of Myocardial infarction within last 3-6 months
Severe peripheral vascular disease
Active hepatitis
Chronic Liver disease
Recent cancer
Severe Pulmonary Hypertension
Severe Chronic Obstructive Pulmonary Disease (COPD)

Medical evaluation should focus on any medical conditions and include all organ systems. It should identify the cause of renal failure and assess the risk of recurrence of disease post-transplant. If the cause is not evident then a kidney biopsy may need to be considered. If a biopsy has previously been performed, then review of the kidney biopsy should be done. They should be evaluated for evidence of any cardiovascular, cerebrovascular, peripheral vascular disease, coagulation (clotted arteriovenous fistula, graft or catheter) or bleeding tendencies. They should also be evaluated for any bladder or urinary tract abnormalities or symptoms, as some potential recipients may be anuric it would be important to assess this from when they had significant residual renal function. Evaluation should also include evaluation of any active systemic disease (e.g., Lupus or ANCA) which may impact the success of the transplant or impact the morbidity or mortality of the perioperative period.

Each transplant program should have a process to assess the immunological risk of transplantation. Blood group and HLA compatibility should both be assessed. If potential donors are either ABO or HLA incompatible then the program should discuss options of alternate donor, swap program and desensitization (ABO-incompatible or HLA-incompatible). These discussions should include discussion of the risks of increased immunosuppression and increased risk of rejection and graft loss with desensitization. For evaluation of immunological risks, the current best method is to use the combination of sensitization history (pregnancy, previous transplant, previous transfusion), complement dependent cytotoxic (CDC) crossmatch, flow crossmatch and single antigen bead testing (SAB) test in each potential donor-recipient pair. However, in situations where cost may be a concern using sensitization history to guide the extent of immunological workup may be a reasonable strategy. Those with history of transplant or pregnancy or multiple transfusions would undergo testing including single antigen bead testing while those with no sensitization history would undergo only crossmatch (CDC and Flow). A donor specific lysate test (also referred to as Luminex crossmatch) is also available and widely used in India. This test has significant false positive and false negative and hence should be avoided. It does not detect HLA C, DQ and DP antibodies[8,9] and hence may miss many sensitized recipients and has also been strongly positive in some patients with no anti-HLA antibodies.[10] HLA typing (A, B, DR) of donor and recipient should be performed for assessment of immunological risk. If single antigen bead test shows HLA C, DQ or DP antibodies then additional typing for those loci should also be performed. As cost of high resolution HLA typing has decreased significantly, it may be appropriate to get high resolution typing of donor and recipient at HLA A, B, C, DQ, DR, DP loci.

Examination should be thorough and cover all organ systems, particular focus should be paid to cardiopulmonary exam, dental examination, peripheral pulses and abdominal examination for any previous surgeries. Surgical evaluation should include evaluation for any issues that may limit technical feasibility of the surgery (e.g., severe peripheral vascular disease, large polycystic kidneys limiting space for placement of transplant kidney).

Cardiovascular Evaluation

Cardiovascular disease is the leading cause of death in CKD and ESRD and is also the leading cause of death after kidney transplantation. Hence, potential transplant recipients need a thorough cardiac evaluation. However, the correct screening protocol has not been yet defined. Minimum evaluation should include history, examination, ECG and Chest X-ray. Further testing depends on the probability of CAD for that individual. Very high risk patients should proceed directly for cardiac angiography (e.g., angina symptoms, diabetic with diabetic nephropathy as cause of ESRD, positive non-invasive test, cardiomyopathy with reduced ejection fraction). Non-invasive testing should be performed in those with multiple risk factors (previous cardiac disease, family history of cardiac disease, age, diabetes, hypertension, smoking, hyperlipidemia, peripheral vascular disease, duration of dialysis). The appropriate testing strategy for those who are asymptomatic and functionally active and with no risk factors is not clear.[11] A risk stratified screening strategy has been shown to reduce the need for additional testing in 40% of potential recipients.[12] Dobutamine stress echocardiogram and thallium myocardial perfusion scan both have moderate sensitivity and specificity in kidney transplant recipients and can be chosen for testing as per center preference or patient characteristics.[13] Those on the waiting list should have repeat testing at some regular intervals due to the high risk of CAD in patients with ESRD.

Patients with risk for left ventricular dysfunction or valvular disease should be evaluated by echocardiography. Non-ischemic cardiomyopathy can be due to uremia and improve after transpant and hence should not be a contraindication for transplant. They may warrant an angiography to confirm that this is not due to an ischemic cause.

Infection

Potential recipients should be screened for HIV, Hepatitis B and Hepatitis C. These infections are no longer contraindications for transplant. However, they do require further evaluation and management. HIV positive patients need to be on a stable HAART regimen (preferably without protease inhibitors, as they significantly inhibit calcineurin metabolism) for atleast 6 months and have an undetectable viral load and CD4 count >200 cell/microl. Potential recipients with Hep B or Hep C infection need evaluation for chronic liver disease and its severity and if they have severe disease then can be considered for combined liver and kidney transplant. CMV and EBV status should be assessed to plan prophylaxis. Those who have lost their first transplant from BK virus need evaluation of BK viremia and viruria and ideally should be free of virus replication prior to retransplant. Vaccination status should be assessed and those who are not immunized can be immunized if there is time prior to transplantation. Influenza, pneumococcus, hepatitis B and varicella vaccinaiton should be considered for all, hemophilus influenza and meningiococcus vaccination should be performed for asplenic or those that may have need for eculizumab (ABO-Incompatible or HLA-Incompatible). If administering live vaccines (measles, mumps, rubella, varicella or zoster) transplant should be postponed atleast 4 weeks from vaccine administration.

Cerebrovascular Disease

Patients at risk for cerebrovascular disease (older patients with hypertension, smoking, diabetes or hyperlipidemia or those with history of transient ischemic attack) should be examined for carotid stenosis and may need carotid doppler studies. A screening magnetic resonance angiogram (MRA) should be performed for all ADPKD patients with family history of aneurysms or headaches, some transplant centres perform MRA for all recipients with ADPKD.

Peripheral Vascular Disease

Peripheral vascular disease is a common complication in ESRD and can present post transplant, especially in diabetics. It is associated with an increased risk of amputation, need for angioplasty or bypass surgery.

Hence, evaluation of all potential recipients should include any history of claudication, examination of bilateral femoral and pedal pulses. Additional testing with doppler vascular studies or noncontrast computed tomography (CT) of abdomen/pelvis to evaluate for iliac calcification may be needed to determine optimal placement of the transplant graft. In addition, severe bilateral iliac or lower extremity arterial disease that are not amenable to intervention are contraindication for transplant.

Pulmonary Disease

There is little evidence or studies to guide the optimal pulmonary evaluation prior to transplantation. However, the evaluation should atleast consist of the preoperative assessment performed for all surgeries. ESRD patients may have symptoms of dyspnea or heart failure due to a multitude of factors and hence evaluation of those symptoms if present should also consist of evaluation for pulmonary hypertension with an echocardiography. If pulmonary hypertension is present then diuresis or dialyzing to lower dry weight should be performed and then the patient reevaluated. All patients should be advised and assisted in quitting smoking. Severe pulmonary disease (severe COPD, severe pulmonary hypertension, home oxygen requirement) not improving with treatment is a contraindication for transplant.

Malignancy

All potential transplant candidates should be screened for malignancy. Transplant immunosuppression is associated with increased risks of some malignancy and increased growth of malignant cells.[14] Age appropriate screening as recommended for the general public should be performed for potential transplant recipients. This includes colonoscopy, mammography and breast examination, pap smear, prostate and testicular examination and serum prostate antigen. In addition, ESRD patients are at increased risk for renal cancers and hence should undergo some imaging modality (renal ultrasound or CT) to assess for cysts and tumors.

For patients who have previously had a malignancy it is important to note that recurrence of cancer post transplant is associated with higher mortality rates. Patients with previous malignancy require thorough evaluation to ensure that there is no recurrence. There is marked variability in the likelihood of recurrence by cancer type and staging of the disease and hence there is variability in the recommendation of duration of waiting time. Depending on the type of cancer and extent of spread prior to treatment a waiting period of 2-5 years may be warranted. These questions are best resolved by a multidisciplinary team in collaboration with the patient and the family. American Society of Transplantation guidelines published in 2001 may be a good starting reference for decision on duration of waiting time required for a particular cancer.[15]

Lower Urinary Tract

Many patients may develop ESRD due to abnormal lower urinary tract and hence these patients need evaluation of their lower urinary tracts to ensure a successful transplant or to decrease their complications post transplant. History should include questions about any lower urinary tract symptoms. Patients may warrant additional testing which may include uroflowmetry with post void residuals, urodynamics or voiding cystourethrogram. As many ESRD patients may be oligo-anuric they may not give history of some of these symptoms at the time of being evaluated for transplant. In addition, some of the interventions needed may need to be delayed till after transplant due to high recurrence rate due to the oligo-anuric state.

Hematology

ESRD patients with recurrent thrombosis of arteriovenous fistulas (AVF), grafts or catheters or recurrent miscarriages, lupus, or abnormal tests need evaluation for hypercoagulability and may need perioperative anticoagulation. Patients with bleeding disorders also need thorough evaluation. Patients with unknown etiology of renal failure or those with monoclonal gammopathy of unknown significance (MGUS) should be carefully evaluated by hematologist to exclude myeloma prior to transplantation.

Psychosocial

Psychosocial evaluation is a critical component of the pretransplant evaluation and should assess the behavioral, social and financial issues that may affect the compliance of the recipient or may affect the outcome post transplant. Current ongoing noncompliance, active alcohol and substance abuse are contraindications to transplant. Ideally social workers and psychologists trained in evaluation of transplant candidates should perform the psychosocial evaluation. Patients with psychiatric disorders should be stable and have a psychiatrist to assist in managing of medications and treatment of side effects of transplant immunosuppression. Financial support (including insurance coverage) should be assessed pretransplant to avoid situations in which patient develops rejection due to inability to afford transplant immunosuppression. Financial barriers should be addressed prior to transplant.

Retransplantation

Recipients who have a failed allograft can be considered for a second transplant. In addition to the evaluation done for transplant as noted above they need to be evaluated for the cause of transplant failure (especially for any noncompliance, or recurrence of disease). Their previous transplant course, presence of any rejections or infections (including BK) should be elicited. Any antibody mediated rejections would be important as this would increase the likelihood of HLA antibodies and increase the risk of antibody rejection for the retransplant. If the graft failed due to recurrence of disease then that will need to be discussed with the patient and the donor. FSGS (focal segmental glomerulosclerosis) for example has a recurrence of ~30% for the first transplant, however if the first transplant has failed due to recurrent FSGS then rate of recurrence in the second transplant is much higher (~75%).[16,17] In such a situation this risk of recurrence and possibility of graft failure should be discussed not only with the potential recipient but also with the donor.

Potential recipients waiting on the deceased donor list should have regular reevaluations to ensure no new issues have developed and no immunological risk changes (sensitization events) have occurred. In addition, it is important to consider the potential recipient holistically rather than individual risks as there may be potential recipients who may have multiple relative contraindications or multiple risk factors none of which are individually absolute contraindications but together may place the patient at an unacceptably high post transplant morbidity or mortality risk.

References

1. Jha V, Modi GK. Getting to know the enemy better–the global burden of chronic kidney disease. Kidney Int 2018;94(3):462-64.
2. Dare AJ, Fu SH, Patra J, Rodriguez PS, Thakur JS, Jha P, *et al.*, Renal failure deaths and their risk factors in India 2001-13: Nationally representative estimates from the Million Death Study. Lancet Glob Health 2017;5(1):e89-e95.
3. Xie Y, Bowe B, Mokdad AH, Xian H, Yan Y, Li T, *et al.* Analysis of the Global Burden of Disease study highlights the global, regional and national trends of chronic kidney disease epidemiology from 1990 to 2016. Kidney Int 2018;94(3):567-81.
4. Wolfe RA, Ashby VB, Milford EL, Ojo AO, Ettenger RE, Agodoa LY, *et al.* Comparison of mortality in all patients on dialysis, patients on dialysis awaiting transplantation, and recipients of a first cadaveric transplant. N Engl J Med 1999;341(23):1725-30.
5. Mange KC, Joffe MM, Feldman HI. Effect of the use or nonuse of long-term dialysis on the subsequent survival of renal transplants from living donors. N Engl J Med 2001;344(10):726-31.
6. Meier-Kriesche HU, Kaplan B. Waiting time on dialysis as the strongest modifiable risk factor for renal transplant outcomes: A paired donor kidney analysis. Transplantation 2002;74(10):1377-81.
7. Meier-Kriesche HU, Port FK, Ojo AO, Rudich SM, Hanson JA, Cibrik DM, *et al.* Effect of waiting time on renal transplant outcome. Kidney Int 2000;58(3):1311-17.
8. Billen EV, Voorter CE, Christiaans MH, van den Berg-Loonen EM. Luminex donor-specific crossmatches. Tissue Antigens 2008;71(6):507-13.
9. Guillaume N, Mazouz H, Piot V, Presne C, Westeel PF. Correlation between Luminex donor-specific crossmatches and levels of donor-specific antibodies in pretransplantation screening. Tissue Antigens 2013;82(1):16-20.
10. Chacko MP, Augustin A, David VG, Valson AT, Daniel D. Nonspecific positivity on the Luminex crossmatch assay for anti-human leukocyte antigen antibodies due to antibodies directed against the antibody coated beads. Indian J Nephrol 2016;26(2):134-37.
11. Hart A, Weir MR, Kasiske BL. Cardiovascular risk assessment in kidney transplantation. Kidney Int 2015; 87(3):527-34.
12. Kasiske BL, Malik MA, Herzog CA. Risk-stratified screening for ischemic heart disease in kidney transplant candidates. Transplantation 2005;80(6):815-20.
13. Pilmore H. Cardiac assessment for renal transplantation. Am J Transplant 2006;6(4):659-65.
14. Engels EA, Pfeiffer RM, Fraumeni JF, Jr., Kasiske BL, Israni AK, Snyder JJ, *et al.* Spectrum of cancer risk among US solid organ transplant recipients. JAMA 2011;306(17):1891-901.
15. Kasiske BL, Cangro CB, Hariharan S, Hricik DE, Kerman RH, Roth D, *et al.* The evaluation of renal transplantation candidates: Clinical practice guidelines. Am J Transplant 2001;1 Suppl 2:3-95.
16. Lewis EJ. Recurrent focal sclerosis after renal transplantation Kidney Int 1982;22(3):315-23.
17. Striegel JE, Sibley RK, Fryd DS, Mauer SM. Recurrence of focal segmental sclerosis in children following renal transplantation Kidney Int Suppl 1986;19:S44-50.

CHAPTER

Peritoneal Dialysis Prescription and Optimization

Tarun Jeloka

Director, Nephrology and Renal Transplant, Aditya Birla Memorial Hospital, Pune

CASE

A 52 years male presented with complaints of anorexia, itching and weakness. He had no swelling, no shortness of breath and normal urine output. He was later diagnosed with chronic kidney disease secondary to autosomal dominant polycystic kidney disease. His calculated glomerular filtration rate (eGFR) was 12 ml/min. There was no obvious acute factor and patient was referred to pre-dialysis clinic for long-term renal replacement therapy. He was waitlisted for kidney transplant. He was explained about the two forms of dialysis. He had several questions:

1. Which of the two modalities are better?
2. Is peritoneal dialysis (PD) reasonable option considering his disease?
3. What determines the frequency in PD and what parameters are evaluated?
4. If PD is selected, does he have to do 3-4 exchanges every day from start?
5. Does his prescription need changes from time to time or remain the same?

These are some typical questions which one would encounter in CKD clinics. Overall, the outcome of both modalities are similar. Polycystic kidneys are also not a contraindication for PD. Here, I will try to address the other three questions.

The concept of adequate dialysis has become synonymous with achieved solute clearance, measured as Kt/V urea. However, adequate dialysis is not just to achieve a number on 'solute clearance' but overall well being of a patient. Clinical assessment of well being includes absence of uremic symptoms, euvolemia, absence of malnutrition, and biochemical balance with 'target' solute clearance. To achieve this, one has to optimize and individualize a prescription. There are various ways to write a prescription and following is one simple method which we follow at our center.

Peritoneal Dialysis (PD) Prescription

Peritoneal Dialysis (PD) prescription can be divided into 2 sets – initial prescription and maintenance prescription. The following guideline is just a rough guide and cannot replace the clinical judgment of modifications needed in individual patient.

Initial Prescription

This should take into account the clinical condition of the patient like presence or absence of swelling, uncontrolled blood pressure, diabetic or proteinuric status, daily urine output, and ultrafiltration during training period. Based on these data, one can plan for either 'incremental dialysis' or conventional dialysis. As ADEMEX has showed no added survival advantage with higher adequacy beyond KT/V of 1.7.[1] Also, it has been shown that residual renal function is the most powerful predictor of survival in PD patients.[2] With this background, 'incremental dialysis' is an option for those who have significant residual renal function. Incremental dialysis has been shown to have several advantages. Without compromising adequacy, it has better survival rates, lower peritonitis rates, preservation of residual renal function and possible better quality of life.[3,4]

Incremental Dialysis

If the patient has significant residual renal function (RRF), incremental dialysis is an option of initiation. The idea is to make up for the difference in 'target clearance' by adding minimum dialysis to RRF. Here, the patient is started either on "Ico alone" single nocturnal exchange or 2 dextrose based dialysate exchanges. For patient selection, we do a urinary Kt/V of the native kidney while the patient is on 'break-in' period and having significant urine output (like ~ 1 l/day). This can be done in similar simple way as we do routine adequacy, except putting 'zero' for dialysate columns. One should note that Kt/V of single Icodextrin bag with a dwell of 10 hours is about 0.6.[5] If the Kt/V of native kidneys (i.e., residual renal function) is > 1, then it is likely that the patient would achieve total adequate clearance with single Icodextrin exchange. One can also do a residual GFR and if > 5 ml/min, can initiate on incremental dialysis as suggested by Guest *et al.*[6] GFR of 1 ml/min adds about 0.25 to the total weekly Kt/Vurea for a 70 kg person.[7] When selecting dextrose dialysate, it is suggested that one should use the lowest concentration bags as possible because of adverse effects of higher concentration of glucose.[8]

With presence of swelling, low daily urine output, and poor ultrafiltration with 2.5% dextrose over 4 hours during training period, one has to choose higher concentration bags. With proteinuric illness, it is noted that patients have more swelling and needs higher concentration of dextrose. Diabetes poses difficult situation as one has to balance for reasonable ultrafiltration with minimum dextrose concentration.

It is advisable to call the patient for review after 1 week of initial prescription so that prescription optimization can be done as per clinical requirement rather than patient presenting with complications after 1 month. At one week follow-up, blood pressure and fluid status is assessed and concentration of bags adjusted as per need. If possible, simple laboratory tests like renal function and electrolytes may help in deciding on the number of exchanges especially in cases of incremental dialysis.

Maintenance Prescription

This should take into account the data of PD done within the first month, peritoneal membrane characteristics, and adequacy (Kt/V). Peritoneal membrane characteristics is determined by Peritoneal Equilibration Test (PET). Both PET and adequacy should be determined by the end of first month. PET helps in optimizing the prescription and determining the dwell period.

PET divides patients into four different categories – *low, low average, high average and high.* Both low and low average can be grouped into slow transporter and high and high average into fast transporter. Slow transporter equilibrates dextrose slowly and hence results in better ultrafiltration but relatively poor solute clearance. Fast transporter equilibrates dextrose fast and has poor ultrafiltration and good clearance. Hence, fast transporter should be advised for short dwells. If there is reasonable residual renal function, 'night dry' may be optimal, at least for initially. If the ultrafiltration is low or inadequate, higher concentration of dextrose or Icodextrin for longer dwell would be useful. Another option for fast transporter would be Automated PD. Slow transporter needs longer dwells for adequate solute clearance. If APD is selected, one should make sure to have longer dwells possible.

Adequacy

Adequacy is calculated by solute clearance of urea–Kt/V. Kt/V target accepted by both national and international bodies is 1.7[1,9] and arbitrary ultrafiltration (UF) goal is 750-1000 ml/day in anuric patient, based on better outcome in studies.[10] If a patient is deficient in achieving any of these targets, then following measures help in management of patient.

Optimization of Prescription

Achieving small solute clearance, i.e., Kt/V – This can be done either by increasing the dialysate fill volume, dwell period, or number of exchanges.[11]

Achieving adequate Ultrafiltration – This can be done by increasing the fill volume, increasing the concentration of dextrose, shortening the dwell period, or use of Icodextrin for long dwell.

Ways for Preservation of Residual Renal Function

Use of Angiotensin concerting enzyme inhibitors/ Angiotensin receptor blockers ACEI/ARB
Avoid dehydration/hypotensive episodes
Prevent peritonitis episodes
Minimize exposure to nephrotoxic drugs like NSAIDs, Radio contrasts, over use of aminoglycosides
Evaluate for urinary tract obstruction
Avoid hypocalcemia

Ways to Influence Solute Clearance or Ultrafiltration

Ways to increase solute clearance	Ways to increase ultrafiltration
Increase dialysate fill volume	Increase dialysate fill volume
Increase number of exchanges	Increasing the concentration of dextrose
Increase dwell period in slow transporters	Decreasing the dwell period in fast transporters
	Use of Icodextrin

Key Points

1. Consider 'incremental' peritoneal dialysis in patients with significant residual renal function.
2. Use lowest concentration of dextrose to prevent metabolic complications and damage to peritoneal membrane.
3. Do PET and adequacy for optimizing maintenance prescription.
4. Increase volume first, before increasing the number of exchanges to increase solute clearance or ultrafiltration.
5. Use of Icodextrin and Automated PD are to be individualized.

References

1. Paniagua R, Amato D, Vonesh E, *et al*. Effects of increased peritoneal clearances on mortality rates in peritoneal dialysis: ADEMEX, a prospective, randomized, controlled trial. J Am Soc Nephrol 2002;13:1307-20.

2. Bargman JM, Golper TA. The importance of residual renal function for patients on dialysis. Nephrol Dial Transplant 2005;20:671-73.

3. Jeloka T, Sanwaria P, Chaudhari L, Periera A. "Ico alone" single nocturnal exchange to initiate peritoneal dialysis in patients with residual renal function–Five year single center experience. Indian J Nephrol 2013;23(4):276-79.

4. Sandrini M, Vizzardi V, Valerio F, Ravera S, Manili L, Zubani R, Lucca BJA, Cancarini G. Incremental peritoneal dialysis: A 10-year single center experience. J Nephrol 2016; 29:871-79.

5. Jeloka T, Pawar S, Periera A, Sanwaria P. What could be the expected solute clearance with single exchange of icodextrin. Indian J Nephrol 2014;24:406-07.

6. Guest S, Leypoldt JK, Cassin M, Schreiber M Kinetic modelling of incremental ambulatory peritoneal dialysis exchanges. Perit Dial International 2017;37:205-11.

7. Li KT, Chow KM, Wong TYH, *et al.* Effects of an angiotensin-converting enzyme inhibitor on residual renal function in patients receiving peritoneal dialysis. Ann Intern Med 2003;139:105-12.

8. Abu-Alfa AK, Burkart J, Piraino B *et al.* Approach to fluid management in peritoneal dialysis: A practical algorithm. Kidney Int 2002;62 (Suppl 81):S8-S16.

9. Lo WK, Ho YW, Li CS *et al.* Effect of Kt/V on survival and clinical outcome in CAPD patients in a randomized prospective study. Kidney Int 2003;64:649-56.

10. Brown EA, Davies SJ, Rutherford P, *et al.* Survival of functionally anuric patients on automated peritoneal dialysis: The European APD outcome study. J Am Soc Nephrol 2003;14:2948-57.

11. Blake P, Burkart JM, Churchill DN, *et al.* Recommended clinical practices for maximizing peritoneal dialysis clearance. Perit Dial Int 1996;16:448-56.

CHAPTER

51 Hemodialysis Prescription

Manoj Singhal

Director, Nephrology and Renal Transplant, Max Superspeciality Hospital, Vaishali, Ghaziabad

Dialysis is a therapy to remove 'uremic solutes/toxins' from blood in a patient with kidney failure. Historically the first solute recognized to be retained in persons with kidney failure was urea, hence the terms; uremia and uremic syndrome. Urea is a low molecular weight solute (60 Daltons) that is water soluble. Its volume of distribution is the total body water. It is produced by the liver and is also the end product of protein catabolism. It is only mildly toxic by itself. However, it is considered an easily measurable surrogate for other small molecular weight uremic toxins. We frequently measure success of dialysis in terms of how effectively we clear the patients blood of urea. This is also called *'urea clearance'*.

Blood is cleared of urea by its movement across the dialysis filter membrane into the dialysate. This occurs via both *diffusion* (diffusive clearance) and *convection* (convective clearance).

Diffusion is the movement of solutes across a semi-permeable membrane along the solute concentration gradient. This movement depends on random contact of the solute with the membrane pore. Diffusion is directly proportionate to solute concentration, solute velocity, temperature which increases solute velocity and surface area of the membrane. Diffusion is inversely proportionate to solute size/molecular weight (Small solutes are <500 Daltons (Da), middle molecules range from 500-60,000 Da, and large molecules are above 60,000 Da), and membrane resistance (increased thickness, low pore size, and low pore number increase membrane resistance). Countercurrent flow delays equilibrium between solutes and maximizes diffusion.

Diffusive clearance of a dialyzer is measured by its coefficient of mass transfer for urea (KoA), a product of membrane mass transfer coefficient (Ko) and area (A). Ko reflects the maximum clearance of solute across the dialysis membrane when blood and dialysate flows are infinite. It is expressed in ml/min. The higher the KoA of a dialyzer, the higher its diffusive clearance and efficiency to clear urea. A high efficiency dialyzer typically has an in vitro KoA of 800-1000 ml/min.

Convection refers to the movement of solutes out of the blood compartment along with movement of water or ultrafiltration. Irrespective of the molecular size, solutes are dragged along with water (i.e., solvent drag) across the dialysis membrane at the same rate as long as the solute can fit through the 'pore' of the membrane. The larger the pore size of the dialysis membrane, and the thinner the membrane, the higher its convective clearance. Such dialyzers are referred to as high-flux dialyzers (Table 51.1).

Table 51.1: High efficiency vs. High flux dialyzers

	High Efficiency Dialyzers	**High Flux Dialyzers**
Membrane Characteristics	Numerous pores, thin membrane, and high surface area allowing high small molecule (urea) clearance	Larger pores allowing better middle molecule (β2 microglobulin) clearance
General Characteristics	High diffusive clearance–Dialyzer urea clearance rate (K) is usually >210 ml/min High KoA urea of the dialyzer (usually > 800-1000) ml/min Kuf is variable Clearance of middle molecular weight molecules (β2 microglobulin) is variable	High convective clearance – Kuf of dialyzer is high (>15-20 ml/h/mm Hg) Clearance of middle molecules (β2 microglobulin) is high (>20 ml/min) High KoA urea of the dialyzer–High efficiency and High Flux

Sieving coefficient describes the membrane passage of a particular solute during convection. The sieving coefficient is determined by dividing the concentration of the solute in the effluent by the concentration in the blood. For example, urea (small molecule) generally will have a sieving coefficient of 1 which indicates that the concentration in the blood is equal to the concentration in the effluent whereas albumin (66,000 Da), will have a sieving coefficient of 0.

Convective clearance of a dialyzer is indicated by coefficient of ultrafiltration (Kuf). This refers to the 'leakiness' or permeability of the membrane to water. The higher the Kuf, the leakier is the membrane. Kuf is expressed in ml/hour/mm Hg, i.e., the volume of fluid (in ml/h) transferred across the membrane per mm Hg of pressure gradient (transmembrane pressure TMP). High flux dialyzers have a Kuf >15-20 ml/h/mm Hg (Fig. 51.1).

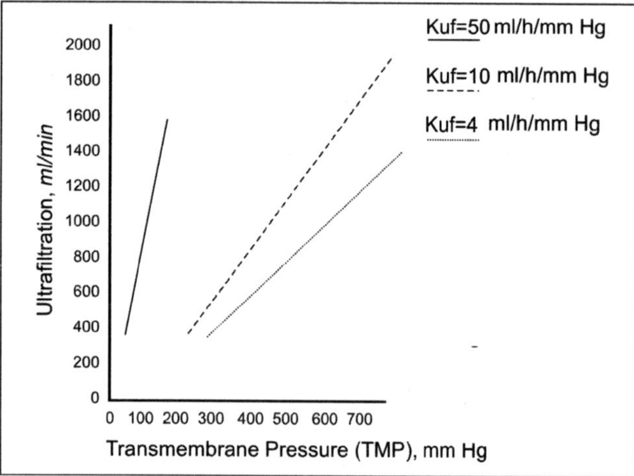

Figure 51.1: Dialyzer coefficient of ultrafiltration (Kuf)

Transmembrane pressure is the hydrostatic pressure gradient which allows for ultrafiltration or convection across a dialyzer membrane, i.e., pulls water from the blood to the dialysate compartment. This is achieved by applying a negative suction pressure at the dialysate compartment relative to the positive hydrostatic pressure in the blood compartment. For a given TMP, the ultrafiltration rate (UF) will depend on the Kuf of the dialyzer membrane. High flux dialyzers need less TMP to achieve same UF.

With older dialysis machines and low flux dialyzers, TMP was manually calculated to achieve a certain level of UF. In modern machines and high flux dialyzers, ultrafiltration is volumetrically controlled. This is because a small change in TMP with a high Kuf dialyzer membrane, can lead to significant changes in UF. Therefore, imprecise TMP calculations can cause massive fluid shifts and hypotension when using high flux dialyzers. Although it is no longer used to control ultrafiltration during hemodialysis, TMP still has value for monitoring dialyzer filter function. A drop in TMP could be due to a leak or filter rupture. A rise in TMP could be due to filter clotting.

Normal kidneys have a urea clearance (K) of around 125 ml/min, stable across various molecular weights up to 50,000-60,000 daltons. High efficiency dialyzers have a urea clearance (K) of >200 ml/min (as long as blood flow and dialysate flow are not limiting) but this decreases significantly with solutes of middle and high molecular weights such as β2 microglobulin (11,800 Da). Dialyzers that are high flux (and typically also high efficiency – high Kuf and KoA) have high small solute (urea) clearance and high middle molecule clearance (Fig. 51.2).

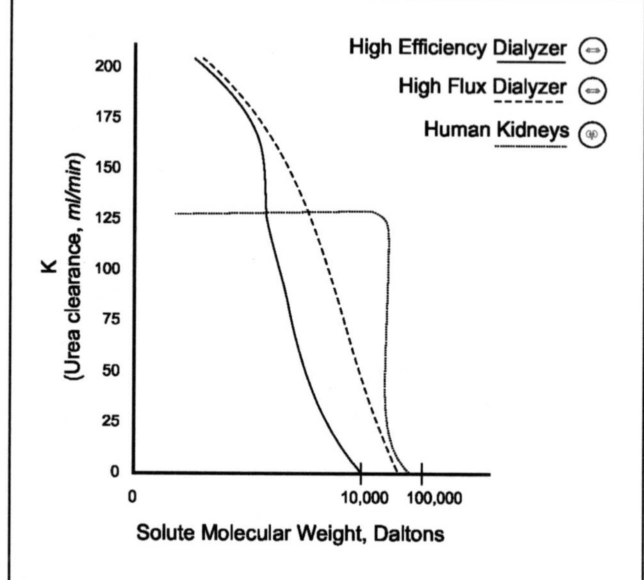

Figure 51.2: Human kidney vs. Dialyzers

HEMO study did not show a mortality benefit between high flux and low flux dialysis. However, the HEMO study, MPO trial, and EGE trial showed a survival benefit (especially cardiovascular) in subset of patients with albumin ≤ 4 mg/dl, dialysis vintage ≥ 3.7 years, diabetes or those with an AV fistula. KDOQI Adequacy Work group (2015) recommends the use of biocompatible, either high or low flux hemodialysis membranes for intermittent hemodialysis.

Adequacy of Solute Clearance

Current methods for evaluating the adequacy of solute clearance focus on urea removal during dialysis. In general, to assess clearance, urea removal during dialysis is estimated and indexed to the volume of distribution of urea (total body water, TBW). The different metrics used to assess urea clearance are described below:

Kt/Vurea

Kt/Vurea is the measurement of solute removal during hemodialysis. Urea is considered a surrogate marker for other uremic toxins because it is easily measured in the serum. Urea clearance is the preferred method to assess hemodialysis dose and adequacy. Sargent and Gotch, in 1985, proposed a mathematical model called Kt/V to quantify dialysis dose and dialytic removal of urea. Kt/V is a dimensionless ratio that reflects volume of plasma cleared of urea (Kt) during a conventional hemodialysis session, relative to volume of distribution of urea (V) (V for urea is the total body water). A Kt/V=1 means that the total volume of blood cleared of urea during a dialysis session is equal to the total body water of the patient.

Daugirdas Mathematical Formula to Calculate Kt/V:

$$Kt/V = -\ln(R - 0.008 \times T) + [(4 - 3.5\,R) \times 0.55\,(UF \div W)]$$

Where…

R= Post HD BUN/pre HD BUN

T = Treatment time in hours

UF= UF volume in l

W= Post dialysis weight in kg

Online calculators and normograms are available to calculate Kt/V using the above formula.

This metric is calculated using urea levels before and immediately after dialysis. It assumes that urea is distributed in a 'single pool or compartment'. It does not account for postdialysis urea rebound. The urea level in plasma is lowest immediately at the end of dialysis. In the 30-60 minutes after dialysis, interstitial and intracellular urea levels equilibrate with the plasma space resulting in a higher plasma level. This phenomenon is called post-dialysis urea rebound and it occurs in phases with equilibration of access recirculation taking place first, followed by equilibration of the cardiopulmonary circuit with the rest of the systemic circulation, and lastly by remote compartment equilibration. This remote compartment is primarily composed of muscle.

eKt/Vurea

The eKt/Vurea attempts to correct the single pool Kt/V by estimating the postdialysis urea rebound. Post dialysis urea levels, drawn 30-60 min after dialysis, would be ideal to assess urea rebound, however, time constraints and additional phlebotomy make it impractical to accomplish. The following equation is recommended for calculating eKt/Vurea in patients undergoing thrice weekly hemodialysis:

$$eKt/Vurea = spKt/Vurea \times t/(t+30)$$

t = duration of dialysis treatment (minutes)

Standard Weekly Kt/Vurea (stdKt/Vurea)

This metric allows comparison of the amount of dialysis urea clearance delivered over the period of a week by different dialysis modalities and by different hemodialysis frequencies and duration (for example, twice weekly, short daily, and nocturnal hemodialysis). The stdKt/Vurea is a hypothetical continuous urea clearance that is comparable across modalities and treatment regimens. This metric also allows for incorporation of dialysis urea clearance and urea clearance from residual kidney function. The following formula is recommend for stdKt/Vurea calculation:

$$std(Kt/V)=1440[0.184(PCRn-0.17)]/Co \text{ daily}$$

$$std(Kt/V)=7*1440[0.184(PCRn-0.17)/Co \text{ weekly}$$

stdKt/Vurea = Residual stdKt/Vurea + Dialysis stdKt/Vurea

Residual stdKt/Vurea = Urea Clearance in ml/min * 10,080/v.

What is the Goal Kt/V?

As per KDOQI Adequacy Work group (2015):

- In patients with minimal residual renal function (<2 ml/min per 1.73 m^2).
  - Minimally delivered dose should be a spKt/V of 1.2.
  - Target recommended dose should be a spKt/V of 1.4 (or eKT/V of 1.2).
- In patients with significant residual native kidney function (Kru), the dose of hemodialysis may be reduced provided Kru is measured periodically to avoid inadequate dialysis.
- This applies to conventional intermittent 3 times a week hemodialysis.
- For hemodialysis schedules other than thrice weekly, guidelines suggest a target standard Kt/V of 2.3 volumes per week with a minimum delivered dose of 2.1 using a method of calculation that includes the contributions of ultrafiltration and residual kidney function.
- There is a lack of randomized studies to support the minimum dialysis dose of spKt/V ≥1.2. However, retrospective studies suggest that a Kt/V <1.0 is associated with poor outcomes and that a Kt/V ≥1.2 is associated with better survival.
- The HEMO study showed that targeting a spKt/V higher than 1.4 did not improve survival or reduce hospitalization rates over 2.8 years.
- Delivered Kt/V is often lower than the prescribed Kt/V. This could be related to multiple reasons such as interrupted treatment due to machine alarms, access recirculation, blood or dialysate pump calibration errors that leads to decreased delivered Qb or Qd etc. Therefore, to achieve a delivered spKt/V of 1.2, a target spKt/V of 1.4 is recommended. This equates to an eKt/V of 1.2.

Limitations of Kt/V

- Kt/V overestimates dialysis adequacy in thin, malnourished patients and elderly females due to sarcopenia and a low 'V'. This may lead to under-dosing of dialysis. Kt corrected for body surface area may be a more accurate measure of dialysis dose in these patients.

- There is a high index of error related to inaccurate post-dialysis BUN measurement.
- Single treatment may not represent other treatments (missed or shortened).
- spKt/V or eKt/V is not applicable to daily or nocturnal dialysis. It is useful only for conventional 3 times a week intermittent hemodialysis (standard Kt/V urea helps to address this issue).
- Kt/V is a marker only of urea clearance and not of other toxic/uremic solutes that exist. Other uremic toxins such as phosphate, β2 microglobulin, guanidino compounds etc. do not follow the same hemodialysis kinetics as urea and therefore their clearances are not accurately reflected by Kt/Vurea.
- A high Kt/V (>1.4) has not been shown to predict better survival in any randomized controlled studies (e.g., HEMO study). This implies that there are other determinants of poor survival in hemodialysis patients besides urea clearance and that despite a high dialysis urea clearance (Kt/V), patients may retain other toxic solutes that ultimately are equally or more important than urea in influencing prognosis on dialysis.

Dialysis Prescription

As we go through this section, let's consider the following scenario:

A 67 years old gentleman with history of diabetes, hypertension, and advanced chronic kidney disease has been initiated on dialysis in the hospital. He has received 5 treatments so far and has done well. He will now be transferred to an outpatient dialysis unit. The patient weighs 70 kg and has a well functioning AV fistula. How would one calculate the initial dialysis prescription in this patient?

Based on clinical practice guidelines, the goal prescribed spKt/V is 1.4.

Calculate V = 60% × TBW. In a 70 kg man, V = 0.60 × 70 = 42 l or 42,000 ml.

Replace known variables for Kt/V: Kt/42,000 = 1.4.

Calculate Kt = 1.4 × 42,000 = 58,800 ml.

Let's assume the dialyzer urea clearance (K) is 250 ml/min (based on choice of dialyzer) and Qb is 400 ml/min to calculate t (treatment duration).

t= 58,800 ml/250 ml/min = 235 minutes or 3.9 hours.

Therefore, this patient will need to be dialyzed for 4 hours to achieve goal single pool Kt/V of 1.4.

The delivered Kt/V often tends to be lower than the prescribed Kt/V, which is why we target a spKt/V of 1.4 to achieve a minimum goal spKt/v of 1.2. When calculating treatment time using manufacturer's provided in vitro K and KoA values, it is important to remember that these values tend to be about 20% higher than actual in vivo values. This is one of the reasons why delivered Kt/V may be lower than prescribed Kt/V.

In smaller patients, determining treatment time using goal spKt/V of 1.4 may lead to under dose dialysis since a low 'V', mathematically increases the ratio spKt/V, hence gives a false sense of reassurance and may prompt one to decrease dialysis time. Smaller patients have higher post dialysis urea rebound, so their eKt/V may be significantly lower than spKt/V. In addition, short dialysis treatments may not be adequate to remove middle molecules and other uremic solutes as well as may result in higher ultrafiltration rates and intra-dialytic hypotension. Therefore, before reducing dialysis time, other variables such as BP, phosphorus and potassium control, ultrafiltration goals etc. need to be considered.

KDOQI Adequacy Work group (2015) recommends a bare minimum of 3 hours per session irrespective of Kt/V. Consider additional hemodialysis sessions or longer hemodialysis treatment times for patients with large weight gains, high ultrafiltration rates (more than 15 ml/kg/hr), poorly controlled blood pressure, difficulty achieving dry weight, or poor metabolic control such as hyperphosphatemia, metabolic acidosis, and/or hyperkalemia.

Impact of Qb, Qd and KoA on K and Kt/V

Dialyzer urea clearance (K) is determined by the lowest of the 3 parameters: Qb, Qd and KoA. Dialyzer blood flow rate (Qb) is a major determinant of K and ultimately Kt/V (Fig. 51.3). At low blood flow (Qb <200 ml/min), K is linear to the Qb and is flow-limited so a high KoA or a high Qd does not matter. A bigger dialyzer or higher dialysate flow are helpful in improving K only at higher Qb (>400 ml/min). Ideally Qb should be set between 400 ml/min and 500 ml/min as tolerated. Dialysis catheters tend to allow lower Qb than AVF and AVG. K can NEVER exceed the Qb. If all the blood entering the dialyzer is cleared of urea in a minute, K is equal to Qb.

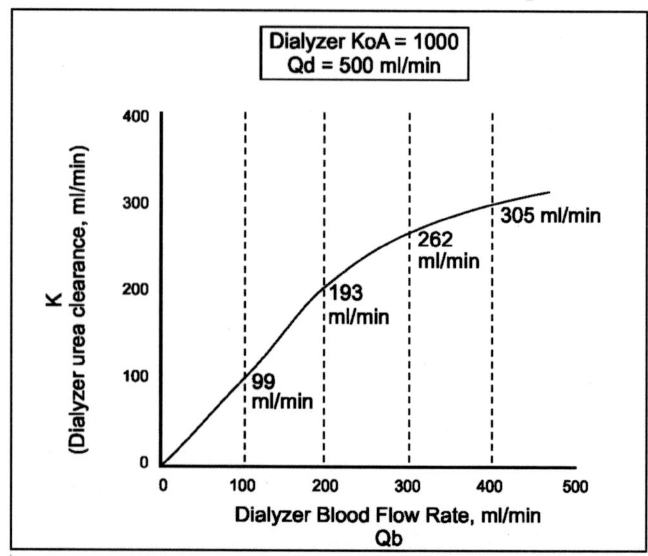

Figure 51.3: Dialyzer urea clearance (K) increases with increase in dialyzer blood flow rate (Qb)

Higher dialysate flow rate (Qd) increases dialyzer urea clearance (K) but as Qb approaches Qd, K starts to plateau (Fig. 51.4). Therefore, Qd should typically be 1.5-2 times the Qb to maximize diffusive clearance. At a Qb of 400-500 ml/min, a Qd of up to 800 ml/min may be enough. An increase of Qd from 500 ml/min to 800 ml/min increases K only by 8-12% when the Qb and KoA are not limiting, i.e., a high efficiency dialyzer is used and the Qb >400 ml/min. Increasing Qd >800 ml/min usually doesn't add to the K or KT/V as the Qb becomes limiting. Qd of 500-600 ml/min is often adequate to achieve target urea clearance with a conventional Qb of 400 ml/min.

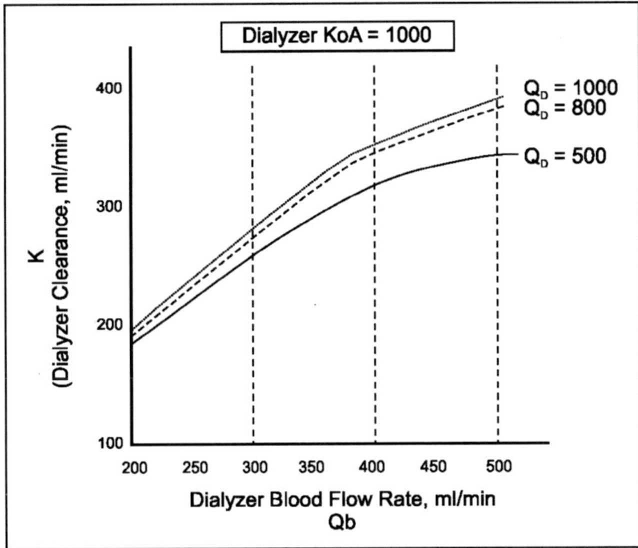

Figure 51.4: Dialyzer urea clearance increases with increase in dialysate flow rate

An additional lesson is that with daily hemodialysis methodologies that have reduced Qd of 150 ml/min or continuous veno-venous hemodialysis (CVVHD) techniques with Qd of 50-100 ml/min, there is no reason to employ higher Qb or to use large dialyzers, as K will be limited by Qd.

K increases with increasing dialyzer efficiency (KoA). However, the increase in K is most pronounced at adequate blood flow. At a Qb of <200 ml/min, despite using a high efficiency dialyzer, K is low (flow limited). At a Qb of >200 ml/min, the curves start to separate and K rises in proportion to the rise in KoA. Rise in K at this point is therefore 'membrane limited' (Fig. 51.5). Hence, if one wants the most benefit out of a high efficiency dialyzer, one needs adequate Qb preferably >400 ml/min. However, KoA >1000 ml/min are of marginal benefit especially with standard Qb of 400-500 ml/min. Qb limits the benefit of dialyzers with excessively high KoA. Qb >500 ml/min are difficult to achieve due to access flow limitations and needle resistance. Also higher Qb may be unphysiologic and increase risk of access recirculation. Most dialyzers that are currently in use have a KoA between 800-1600 ml/min.

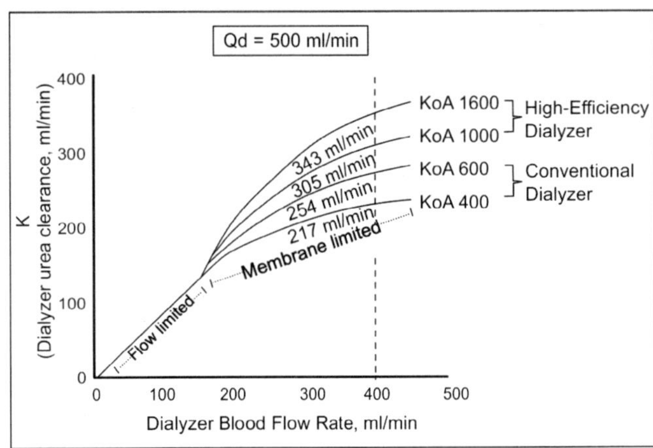

Figure 51.5: Dialyzer urea clearance increases with increase in KoA

Dialysis Disequilibrium Syndrome

Patients are at a risk of dialysis disequilibrium syndrome during first dialysis treatment when they have high BUN, chronic uremic symptoms, severe metabolic acidosis and a history of stroke and alcohol liver disease. The rapidity and magnitude of osmotic shifts associated with dialysis can lead to cerebral swelling and neurologic compromise. The goal here is to avoid abruptly high urea clearance with the first few hemodialysis treatments. Using a low blood flow, low dialysate flow, a small dialyzer with a low KoA, and short treatment duration will avoid high urea clearances. Qb and treatment time can be increased in a step wise manner over the next 3-4 daily treatments.

Access Recirculation

Let's see a 63 years old gentleman with diabetic ESRD on HD via a left radio-cephalic AVF. His dialysis prescription is a dialyzer Fx6, Qb of 350 ml/min, Qd-500 ml/min for a duration of 4 hours. His Kt/V on three times a week hemodialysis has ranged between 1.3-1.4. The most recently checked Kt/V has dropped down to 0.9-1.0 confirmed on 2 different occasions. He has been compliant with his dialysis and has completed the full 4 hours as prescribed. Patient feels fine and his physical exam is unremarkable with normal BP and trace edema.

A drop in Kt/V can be due to multiple factors. Inaccurate post dialysis BUN measurement, shortened dialysis treatment (affecting T), low access blood flow or access recirculation (the latter two affecting K), are some of the common ones. Poor access flow is the most common cause of a drop in Kt/V (40% of cases). In our patient, access flow seems maintained at 350 ml/min and his treatment time has not been reduced. Access recirculation is seen in about 25% of cases of reduced Kt/V. If this is suspected, a fistulogram should be done to evaluate for access stenosis. Increasing treatment time and dialysate flow will likely help improve Kt/V to varying degrees, however access recirculation should be ruled out first if suspected.

Access Recirculation should be suspected when there is a significant discrepancy between prescribed and delivered dialysis dose. Dialyzed blood mixes with the un-dialyzed blood in the extra corporeal circuit rather than returning to the systemic circulation. This decreases dialysis efficiency due to decrease in solute concentration pre-filter (in the arterial circuit). The higher the blood flow rate, the higher the chances of access recirculation. 25% of patients with a drop in Kt/V tend to have access recirculation issues. 20% recirculation happens with reverse needle placements. Usually close needle placements are an uncommon cause for recirculation as long as fistula flow is more than the blood flow rate. Access recirculation is a late marker for access stenosis so it is not the ideal method for AVF monitoring.

Suggested Reading

1. National Kidney Foundation. KDOQI clinical practice guideline for hemodialysis adequacy: 2015 update. Am J Kidney Dis 2015;66(5):884-930.
2. Eknoyan G, Beck GJ Cheung AK, *et al.* Effect of dialysis dose and membrane flux in maintenance hemodialysis. N Engl J Med 2002;347:2010. Hemodialysis study (HEMO).
3. Locatelli, martin-Malo, Hannedouche *et al.* Membrane permeability Outcome (MPO) study group. Effect of membrane permeability on survival of hemodialysis patients. JASN 2009;20(3):645.
4. Asci, Tz, Ozkahya *et al.* EGE study group. The impact of Membrane permeability and dialysate purity on cardiovascular outcomes. JASN 2013 May;24(6):1014-23.

CHAPTER

Vascular Access for Hemodialysis

Dinesh Kumar Yadav[1], Manish Jain[2], Ashish Nandwani[3]

[1] *Senior Consultant, Nephrology, Medanta, The Medicity, Gurugram*

[2] *Director, Nephrology, Medanta, The Medicity, Gurugram*

[3] *Consultant, Nephrology, Manipal Hospital, Delhi*

End stage renal disease patients requiring renal replacement therapy in the form of hemodialysis require the vascular access for the same. There are different types of vascular access, which can be used depending upon, whether the dialysis is required on urgent basis or not. This needs a timely placement of vascular access in CKD stage 4-5 patients to decrease the morbidity associated with these procedures. In this chapter, we will discuss regarding the different types of vascular access, their placement and related complication and their management.

What are Types of Vascular Access?

1. Native arteriovenous fistula (AVF).
2. Arteriovenous graft (AVG).
3. Central venous catheter (CVC).
4. Arteriovenous shunt.

Arteriovenous Fistula (AVF)

James E. Cimino, a physician who earlier was phlebotomist at New York City's Bellevue Hospital in the 1950s observed that drawing blood was very easy from fistula caused by trauma without causing any harm. He discussed the concept with Dr Brescia and Dr Kenneth Appell who created the first AV fistula by anastomoses of the artery and vein. So AV fistula is also called as Cimino fistula, or Cimino-Brescia fistula.

Why Arteriovenous Fistula is Better?

- Less infection rates.
- Less thrombosis.
- Lasts longer.

The Preoperative Assessment

History: It is important to know the dominant hand, previous history of central vein cannulation, heart disease, diabetes mellitus. Patient with severe heart failure may not tolerate the additional cardiac output required to circulate blood through the vascular access.

The physical examination is aimed to investigate arterial and venous system functioning and presence of any edema, surgical scars, radial, ulnar and brachial pulses and superficial venous circles.

The Allen test/Modified Allen's test should be performed to evaluate an abnormal vascularization of the palmar arch.

The original test proposed by Allen is performed as follows–both hand examined at one time.

1. The patient is asked to clench both fists tightly for 1 minute at the same time.
2. Pressure is applied over both radial arteries simultaneously so as to occlude them.
3. The patient then opens the fingers of both hands rapidly, and the examiner compares the colour of both. The initial *pallor* should be replaced quickly by *rubor*.
4. The test may be repeated, this time occluding the ulnar arteries.

Steps of modified Allen's test–One hand is tested at one time.

1. Arm should to extended and palm turned upwards.
2. Ask patient to clench the fist so that hand becomes blanched.
3. Compress both radial and ulnar arteries.
4. Release compression of ulnar artery and watch the palm to become pink.
5. Similar steps are done for radial artery.

If blanching persists for > 5 seconds after pressure release of either artery, then insufficiency of that arterial territory.

Colour Doppler Ultrasound

The gold standard to decide on the type and location of vascular access is the duplex ultrasound scan. It allows the assessment of the arterial and venous diameters; a vein diameter > 2 mm and an artery diameter >1.6 mm are considered adequate. These two parameters are predictive of AVF maturation.

Vein dilatation test: >50% increase in vein diameter on proximal tourniquet application is predictive of good outcome.

Artery dilatation test: Clinch the fist for 2 minutes then release. Hyper thermic response converts normal triphasic arterial pulse to biphasic one.

Venography: Shows exact venous anatomy.

Arteriography: When blood pressure difference between two arms is more than 20 mm Hg.

Timing of AV Fistula Creation

6 months before anticipated dialysis initiation.

Back-up AV Fistula

Made in patients undergoing peritoneal dialysis to avoid catheter use when peritoneal dialysis is to be discontinued.

Preferred Site for AV Fistula

According to the guidelines of the National Kidney Foundation (NKF-K/DOQI), the site order for the surgical intervention of AVF for HD is the following: Forearm (Radio-cephalic or distal AVF), elbow (Brachio-cephalic or proximal AVF), and arm (Brachial-basilic AVF with transposition or proximal AVF).

Snuff box: It is relatively simple to create, and since there is a low incidence of complications, the long-term patency rates are excellent and do not preclude the possibility of future access.

Gracz fistula: Anastomosis between perforating vein of proximal forearm to proximal radial artery.

Lower limb AV fistula: Superficial femoral artery to femoral vein, saphenous vein to popliteal artery.

Type of Anastomosis

Different types of arteriovenous anastomosis are possible:

Side-to-end–Anastomosis between end of vein to side of artery–most common type.

Side-to-side–Risk of venous hypertension.

End-to-end.

Blood Flow Rates in AV Fistula

Flow is increased from 20-30 ml/min to 200-300 ml/min immediately after operation. In well-developed fistulae, flow rates may ultimately reach values of 600 to 1200 ml/min.

Flow increases as a result of both vasodilation and vascular remodelling.

Rule of Six

"Rule of six" in fistula assessment—at six weeks post-creation the diameter of the body of the fistula should be at least 6 mm and the depth no more than 0.6 cm. The blood-flow rate should be 600 ml/min or more by this time. The length of the fistula should be 6 cm to allow for a successful two-needle dialysis.

Cannulation Technique

The needle should be held at a 20- to 35-degree angle for AV fistulas, and at approximately a 45-degree angle for grafts. Once the needle has been advanced through the skin, subcutaneous tissue, and graft or fistula wall, the blood flashback should be visible. Continue to advance the needle no greater than 1/8 of an inch and then rotate the needle 180 degrees. The needle bevel is rotated to help prevent a "back wall" or posterior wall infiltration.

There are three options for cannulation:

(a) **The rope ladder pattern:** The punctures are regularly distributed along the entire length of the arterialized vein. It expands the lifespan of the fistula. Changing cannulation site gives the previous needle site time to heal and prevents aneurysms from forming.

(b) **The area puncture pattern:** Punctures restricted to a small area.

(c) **The buttonhole pattern:** Punctures are performed through the exactly identical spot. More frequently used in Europe and Japan for more than 25 years, although it is becoming more popular in the U.S. It can be used for self cannulation using blunt needle. Increased risk of aneurysm development due to weakening of wall.

Needle Placement

Needle size for cannulation–16-17 G.

Insertion angle–25 degree.

Should be at least 3 cm away from anastomosis and distance between needles should be 5 cm.

Complications of AV Fistula

The most frequent complications related to AVFs are insufficient maturation of the AVF, stenosis, thrombosis, infection, aneurysm, "steal syndrome" due to ischemia, and high-rate flow AVF.

Primary failure: Failure to mature or lack of ability to be cannulated and used successfully for dialysis over a sustained period of 3 weeks.

Primary failure rates range from 30 to 50%, most often secondary to juxta-anastomotic stenosis which is routinely attributed to intimal hyperplasia (IH). IH is caused by the hyperplastic accumulation of myofibroblast-like cells in the venous intima. The aetiology of IH in hemodialysis patients remains poorly understood.

Roy-Chaudhury *et al.* have proposed a group of upstream and downstream events as causes of IH development. The upstream factors include comorbidities, surgical trauma, endothelial dysfunction, inflammation, and abnormal flow conditions after anastomosis. Downstream factors are secondary to upstream events, and mostly include biologic events reflecting the adaptive, and maladaptive, response of the vein to injury and new flow conditions (Fig. 52.1).

AV Fistula Stenosis

Most common cause–neo intimal hyperplasia:

- **AV fistula:** Juxta-anastomotic.
- **Signs of stenosis:** Depends on site of stenosis.
- **Juxta-anastomotic:** Poor thrill, low urea reduction ratio.
- **Central:** Venous hypertension, high venous pressure.
- **Indication of intervention:** > 50% stenosis.

AV Fistula Thrombosis

Most common complication. The causes of thrombosis are:

- Stasis of flow.
- Vascular endothelial injury.
- Hypercoagulable blood–due to high fibrinogen level, reduced protein C and protein S level, factor V Leiden mutation.
- Elevated hematocrit due to erythropoietin therapy.
- Arterial stenosis, hematoma from cannulation injury.

Steal Syndrome

Approximately 75% of the blood flow through distal radiocephalic fistulae is supplied by the proximal radial artery, but 25% comes from a patent ulnar artery via the distal radial artery and palmar arch.

It is caused by excessive retrograde inflow of blood into the access.

Classification of Steal Syndrome

Stage I	Retrograde diastolic flow without complaints; steal phenomenon.
Stage II	Pain on exertion and/or during hemodialysis.
Stage III	Rest pain.
Stage IV	Ulceration/necrosis/gangrene.

Differential Diagnosis

- Carpal tunnel syndrome.
- Peripheral vascular disease.
- Nerve trauma.
- Ischemic monomeric neuropathy dueto loss of blood supply to nerve.

Management

Converting side of artery to end of artery (Fig. 52.2).

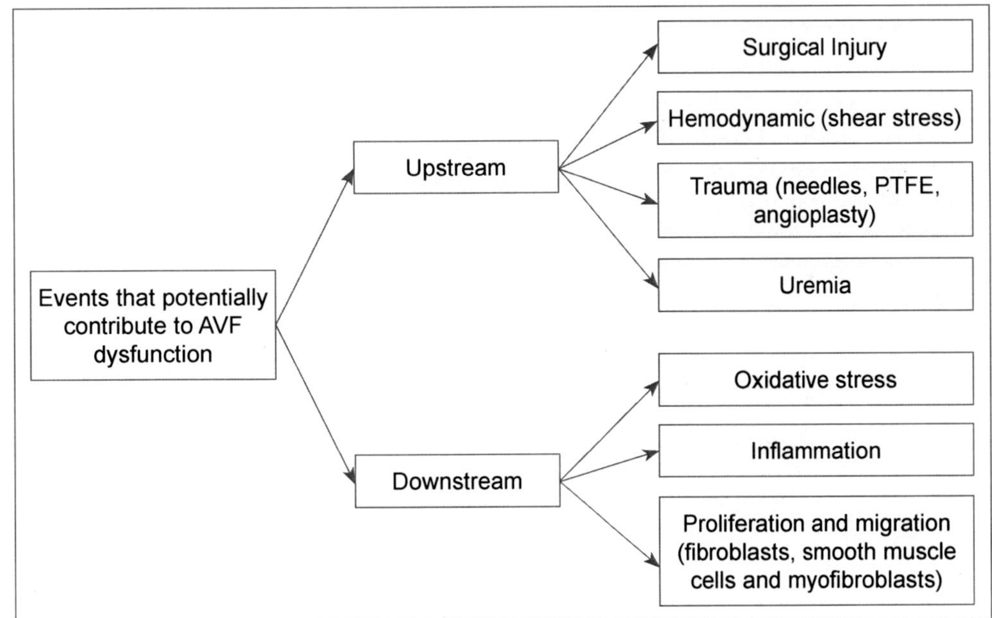

Figure 52.1: Causes of AVF dysfunction

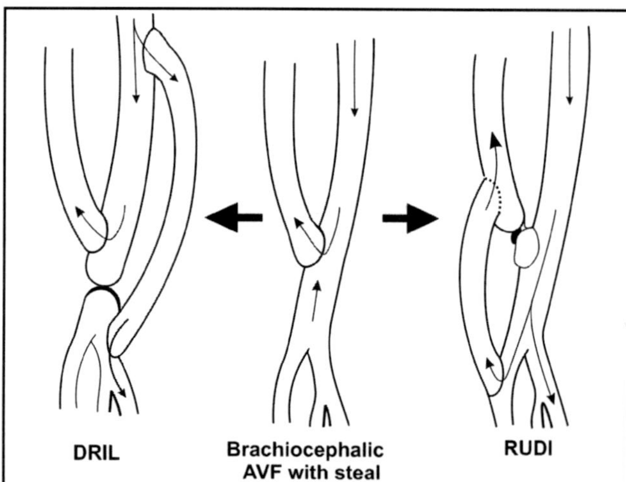

Figure 52.2: Management of brachiocephalic AVF with steal

DRIL (Distal revascularization interval ligation): The technique involves ligation of the brachial artery distal to the AVF inflow and revascularization of the distal arm with a bypass taken from a more proximal inflow source.

RUDI (Revision using distal inflow): In the case of high flow induced cardiac failure due to a brachial AV access, closing the anastomosis in the antecubital fossa and interposing a graft between the forearm ulnar or radial artery has been shown to effectively reduce access flow by more than 50%.

Pseudo Aneurysm

- **AV Fistula:** Glue injection, surgical correction.

Congestive Heart Failure

The creation of an AVF leads to shunting of blood flow from the high resistance arterial system into the low resistance venous system, with a subsequent rise in venous return and cardiac output. Also, the presence of an AVF decreases arterial impedance which lessens the left ventricular afterload. The lowering of arterial impedance may also reduce the effective circulating volume of the systemic circulation, activating arterial baroreceptors, and leading to secondary increase in cardiac sympathetic tone, contractility, and cardiac output. The net effect of AVFs is a significant increase in cardiac output.

Treatment

Banding of access to reduce access flow.

Complications of Percutaneous Interventions

Vessel rupture, pulmonary embolism.

Arteriovenous Graft (AVG)

AV Graft (AVG) is indicated as the first line of treatment for patients with short obese limbs, where the superficial veins are deep in the subcutaneous tissue, patients with extreme vascular fragility (thrombocytopenic purpura), where the simple venous puncture produces wounds and serious hematomas.

Advantage of AV Graft

- Can be used after 1-3 weeks–Multilayered Self-sealing polyurethane graft–can be used within week and Heparin bonded polycarbonate graft–immediately.
- Provide large area for cannulation.
- Easy cannulation.
- Risk of neointimal hyperplasia, occurs at graft-vein anastomosis.

Pre-op Evaluation

A minimal vein diameter of 4 mm was required for a successful polytetrafluoroethylene-vein anastomosis. It is done by duplex ultrasound.

Site for AV Graft

Graft can have a straight, looped, or curved configuration.

- Upper limb.
- Lower limb.
- Axillary loop grafts are indicated when more distal options for VA are exhausted or when the risk of steal syndrome is extremely high.

Material

- **Biological:** Saphenous vein, umbilical vein, bovine heterograft.
- **Synthetic:** PTFE, polyurethane.

Disadvantage

More risk of infection, thrombosis, ischemia and short survival than AVF.

Complications

The common complication of AVG is *thrombosis* due to venous stenosis caused by neointimal hyperplasia. The increased production of smooth muscle cells, myofibroblast, and vascularization within the neointima is the main cause of thrombosis.

Factors causing thrombosis of an AVG are: stenosis, hypotension, and excessive compression for hemostasis, decreasing blood flow.

Infections

The incidence of HD-related bacteremia is more than ten-fold higher in AVGs than AVFs. Treatment involves intravenous antibiotics and total graft excision in septic patients or when the graft is bathed in pus; subtotal, when all of the graft is removed except an over sewn small cuff of prosthetic material on an underlying patent vessel; and partial, when a limited portion of AVG is removed and a new graft is inserted through adjacent sterile tissue.

Ischemia as a result of access placement is more common for AVGs than AVFs. Vascular steal syndrome and ischemic monomeric neuropathy are common manifestation.

This needs endovascular treatment with stent grafts to relieve the stenosis.

Central Venous Catheters (CVC)

Catheter Types

1. Single-lumen catheters–two catheters needed to be inserted for dialysis.
2. Dual-lumen, incorporating both access and return limbs in the one device.
3. Triple-lumen catheters which include a third narrow lumen that can be used for other purposes (such as right atrial pressure monitoring or administering medications) without disrupting the ongoing dialysis.

Catheter Design

1. Non-tunnelled catheters.
2. Tunnelled catheters placed under the skin-two types of tunnelled catheters: cuffed or non-cuffed.

   Tunnelled cuffed catheters, a type recommended by the NKF for temporary access, can be used for longer than 3 weeks when:

   - An AV fistula or graft has been placed but is not yet ready for use.
   - There are no other options for permanent access. For example, when a patient's blood vessels are not good enough for a fistula or graft.

   The cuff ends up under the skin near the entry point and stimulates a local fibroblastic response, leading to ingrowth of the surrounding tissue over time which secures the device more firmly. Together, the cuff and tunnel act as barriers to microbial migration along the outside of the catheter, reducing the risk of catheter-associated bloodstream infections compared to non-tunnelled catheters.

   Catheters have two openings inside; one is a red (arterial) opening to draw blood from your vein and out of your body into the dialysis pathway and the other is a blue (venous) opening that allows cleaned blood to return to your body.
3. Implantable vascular access devices–like chemo port both ports remain subcutaneous.

Tip Design

(a) Quinton step-tip PermCath™ oval catheter with round lumens.

(b) Mahurkar step-tip catheter.

(c) Canaud and Tesio twin catheters (Canaud with subcutaneous grommets rather than Dacron® cuffs).

(d) Ash Splitcath® split-tip catheter.

(e) Tal Palindrome™ symmetrical-tip catheter (with side-holes).

(f) CentrosFlo™ self-centering catheter (with pressure relief holes on the inside surfaces distal limbs are present near the tips). Arrow indicates position of a self-sealing hole to allow the catheter to be threaded over a single guide-wire or stylet.

Length of the Vascath Inserted: Right IJV is typically 15 cm, whilst it should be 17 cm via the left IJV. Femoral – 20 cm in length.

Diameter of vascath–11.5 Fr.

Length of permcath: Length from cuff to tip is called as length of permcath–19 cm (preferred form females due to short height), 23 cm (preferred for males), 27 cm (for left side), 44 cm and 55 cm (for femoral).

Diameter of permcath–14.5 Fr.

Volume of heparin/other lock solution–written on catheter tip, usually 1 to 1.1 ml for each limb in non-tunnelled catheter and 1.6 ml each limb for 19 cm tunnelled cuff, 1.9 ml for 23 cm catheters and 3.3 ml for 55 cm tunnelled catheter.

Preferred Sites

The preferable locations for insertion are the internal jugular and femoral veins. The subclavian vein is considered the third choice because of the high risk of thrombosis and stenosis. The right IJ is preferred because of the lower pleural dome, more direct route to the superior vena cava, and absence of thoracic duct.

Internal Jugular

Advantage: Large vein, easily visualized on ultrasound, straight course to right atrium, more chance of correct placement even with blind approach.

Disadvantage: Uncomfortable socially.

Femoral

Advantage: Suitable for emergency dialysis especially in patients with fluid overload, Hyperkalemia, Lower bleeding risk, No need for post procedure X-ray.

Disadvantage: More risk of bleeding, thrombosis, poor catheter performance when patient sits up, cannot keep for more than seven days.

Subclavian

Advantage: Ease of insertion, lower infection risk.

Disadvantage: More risk of pneumothorax, bleeding, thrombosis and difficulties to create a vascular access in the ipsilateral arm. It cannot be done guided as vein is deep and not visualized properly, risk of central stenosis.

Technique of Insertion

Sedillot's triangle: Used as surface marking for IJ catheter insertion, formed by the junction of the sternal and clavicular insertions of the sternomastoid muscle and the clavicle.

Normally, the vein lays anterolateral to the artery, but in a small percentage of patients, the vein is immediately anterior to the artery or even medial to it. Therefore, for the significant anatomical variation in the vein and its course, percutaneous ultrasound-guided technique for IJV access has become the standard practice.

For the insertion of a CVC into the IJV, the patient should be optimally positioned, with a 10° head-down tilt (Trendelenburg position) to help distend the vein and reduce the risk of air embolism.

A very modest degree of rotation of the head away from the side to be cannulated may be necessary, but extreme rotation is best avoided as it may reduce vein diameter. Indeed, head rotation can cause the IJV to move laterally in relation to surface landmarks and become more difficult to locate.

The common method for direct insertion into the great veins is the Seldinger technique, using a guide wire over the needle.

Tip Position

Ideally, for temporary catheters, the tip should lie outside the right atrium and for tunnelled cuffed catheter, tip should lie inside the right atrium. When correctly placed, the tip of the catheter should rest in the middle of a large central vein away from the vessel wall, so that the opening of the withdrawal lumen–which is under negative pressure–does not become occluded due to the vessel wall being sucked across it.

Type of Catheter Related Infection and Treatment

- Exit site infection.
- Tunnel infection.
- Catheter related bloodstream infection.

Exit site infection: Hyperaemia, induration, and/or tenderness ≤ 2 cm from catheter exit site. It may be associated with fever and purulent drainage from the exit. Treated with topical antibiotics, catheter removal if systemic signs of infection develop.

Tunnel infection: Tenderness, hyperemia, and/or induration that extends >2 cm from the exit site and along the subcutaneous tunnel.

Catheter related bloodstream infection (CRBSI): Blood culture–2 sets are sent–one from catheter hub and other from peripheral vein.

Metastatic infections: Osteomyelitis, endocarditis, meningitis, pneumonitis.

Indications of Catheter Removal

- Septic shock due to CRBSI.
- Metastatic infection.
- Not responding to antibiotics in 72 hours.
- Infection due to S. Aureus, Pseudomonas, Candida.

Duration of Antibiotics

- **S. aureus:** 2-3 weeks.
- **Pseudomonas:** 3 weeks.
- **Endocarditis:** 4-6 weeks.
- **Osteomyelitis:** 6-8 weeks.

What is Antibiotics Lock Solution and Its Uses?

Used for prevention of infections:

- Especially those with repeated CRBSI despite standard aseptic precautions.
- Treatment of CRBSI–in conjugation with systemic antibiotics.

Antibiotic lock is indicated for patients with catheter related bloodstream infections involving long-term catheters with no signs of exit site or tunnel infection for whom catheter salvage is the goal. For CRBSI, antibiotic lock therapy should not be used as monotherapy. It should be used in conjunction with systemic antimicrobial therapy.

Drugs used: Vancomycin, Cefazolin, Ceftazidime, Ciprofloxacin, Gentamicin, Ampicillin.

Disadvantage: Risk of antibiotics resistance.

What is Catheter Dysfunction and Its Management?

Failure to attain and maintain an extracorporeal blood flow of 300 ml/min or greater at a prepump arterial pressure more negative than–250 mm Hg.

Poor Catheter Flow (Catheter Dysfunction)

Early dysfunction: Kinking, compression of catheter due to tunnel edema, malposition of catheter, improper tip placement.

Late dysfunction: Fibrin sheath-produce ball valve effect, treatment–disruption of sheath thrombosis.

Late dysfunction due to thrombosis can be cured with thrombolytic–our practice is to use Urokinase – 25,000 units in each limb and is kept for 4 hours.

What is Arteriovenous Shunt?

Popularly called as Scribner shunt, which consisted of a Teflon tube with a needle at each end.

When dialysis is to be done, the U tube connecting arterial and venous limbs is removed and between treatments, the needles were left in place and the tube allowed blood flow to reduce clotting.

After treatment, U tube is connected, which would shunt the blood from the tube in the artery back to the tube in the vein.

Scribner shunts lasted only a few days to weeks.

It was as used before AV fistula was invented. It can help in vein dilation which later can be used for AV fistula creation.

Suggested Reading

1. Al-Jaishi AA, Liu AR, Lok CE, *et al.* Complications of the Arteriovenous Fistula: A Systematic Review. J Am Soc Nephrol 2017;28:1839.
2. Feldman HI, Kobrin S, Wasserstein A. Hemodialysis vascular access morbidity. J Am Soc Nephrol 1996;7:523.
3. Ascher E, Gade P, Hingorani A, *et al.* Changes in the practice of angioaccess surgery: Impact of dialysis outcome and quality initiative recommendations. J VascSurg 2000; 31:84.
4. Allon M, Robbin ML. Increasing arteriovenous fistulas in hemodialysis patients: Problems and solutions. Kidney Int 2002;62:1109.
5. Mendes RR, Farber MA, Marston WA, Dinwiddie LC, Keagy BA, Burnham SJ. Prediction of wrist arteriovenous fistula maturation with preoperative vein mapping with ultrasonography. J Vasc Surg 2002;36(3):460-63.
6. Lorenzo Sellarés V. Analysis of Emergency Department Frequentation among patients with advanced CKD (chronic kidney disease): Lessons to optimise scheduled renal replacement therapy initiation. Nefrologia 2018 Nov–Dec;38(6):622-29.
7. Effects of the creation of arteriovenous fistula for hemodialysis on cardiac function and natriuretic peptide levels in CRF. Am J Kidney Dis 2002;40:974-82.

CHAPTER 53

Peritoneal Dialysis Access

Amit Kumar Mahapatra

Consultant, Nephrology, Medanta, The Medicity, Gurugram

Peritoneal dialysis (PD) access is the most vital part of success of the Peritoneal Dialysis program. Catheter access designs has been in continuous evolution since early 1920s. The primary goal of an access design is to minimize technique failure which can be peri-catheter leakage, infection, or catheter migration etc. and improve longevity of access and maximize the flow of PD fluid.

Peritoneal dialysis access depends upon the type of dialysis prescribed, which can be intermittent flow or continuous flow, acute or chronic.

Acute Peritoneal Dialysis

For acute peritoneal dialysis, the catheters used should be easy to insert and the dialysis can be started immediately after insertion. In this case, the semi-rigid PD catheter, currently manufactured by Romsons, is inserted percutaneously. This is made of polyamide, and has stainless steel stylet for easy insertion.

Advantages of Semi Rigid Catheters

1. Skill of insertion needs little training.
2. Low cost.

Disadvantages of Semi Rigid Catheters

1. Risk of bowel perforation.
2. Lower diameter–poor flow achieved.
3. Risk of blockage due to fibrin and need repeated flushing.
4. High risk of peritonitis.

Currently flexible catheters like Tenckhoff with double cuff with subcutaneous tunnelling is advocated for patients with likely chance of prolonged AKI. After insertion double cuffed tenckhoff catheter, PD can be started immediately with low volume exchange and in supine position. It requires trained clinicians to able to do this bedside procedure and runs a high risk of peri catheter leakage.

Chronic Intermittent Peritoneal Dialysis

The most common chronic catheters used for intermittent flow peritoneal dialysis is essentially designed by Tenckhoff, followed by swan neck catheters. Other catheters that are used across the world but less frequently are: Missouri catheter, Cruz catheter, Toronto western design, Ash, Valli etc.

Classification

The chronic catheters can be divided into following categories depending upon:

1. **Catheter material:**
   a. Silicon (most common).
   b. Poly urethane silicone rubber (Cruz catheter).
2. **Number of cuffs:**
   a. Single cuff–not advisable.
   b. Dual Dacron Cuff (Polyester).
   c. Disc-shaped deep cuff with a silicone ball within the peritoneum (Missouri Catheter).
   d. Moncrief-Popovich (longer subcutaneous cuff 2.5 cm).
3. **Basic shapes of the subcutaneous portion:**
   a. Straight.
   b. Preformed arc
      i. Swan Neck–150 degree
         1. Swan neck tenckhoff straight or coiled.
         2. Swan neck Missouri straight or coiled.
         3. Swan neck pre-sternal (Extension catheter).
         4. Moncrief-Popovich catheter.
      ii. Pail-handle (Cruz)–90 degree bend.
4. **Intraperitoneal portions of catheter:**
   a. Straight
      i. Classic Tenckhoff.

ii. With inner discs (Toronto Western Hospital).

iii. Self-Locating (12 g of silicone encased in tungsten, Di Paolo).

iv. Short (Vicenza).

b. Coiled.

c. T-Fluted catheters (Ash advantage).

d. Balloon (Valli).

ISPD Guidelines 2019 Update suggest the catheter to be made of silicon rubber, should have double Dacron cuff. The choice of catheter tip can be either straight or coiled and the inter cuff or subcutaneous segment can be either straight or preformed arc. Pre sternal (extended) catheters can be used when optimal pelvic position with satisfactory exit site location cannot be found in abdomen wall.

Parts of Catheter

Catheters with external adapters are divided to following portions in the order from out to in as : Minicap Transfer Set (6 inch) ->Titanium connector -> External segment of catheter ->Superficial cuff ->Subcutaneous segment -> deep cuff -> intraperitoneal segment.

Titanium adapter, containing a double locking double barbed connector and a locking sleeve, is light weight, has longevity and is resistant to corrosion due to use of skin disinfectants.

Intraperitoneal segment in tenckhoff catheter has small side holes which is of 1 mm diameter and is in the distal 10 cm of the straight tip catheter and 20 cm of coiled tip catheter.

Cuff is made of polyester which allows ingrowth of tissue and helps in prevention of bacterial migration. Both the cuffs are of 1 cm length.

Catheter Insertion Techniques

Methods of placement of PD catheters:

- Percutaneous, blind
  - Using the Tenckhoff trocar.
  - Modified Seldinger technique.
- Direct visualization
  - Peritoneoscopic (Y-Tec®).
  - Open, surgical dissection.
  - Laparoscopic.

Percutaneous Needle and Guidewire Technique (Modified Seldinger)

- This technique is similar to split sheath technique used for subclavian or internal jugular HD catheters.
- The technique involves inserting introducer needle or 14G peripheral IV catheter attached to a syringe with 2-3 ml of saline, through the linea alba (infra-umbilical) or the dissected rectus muscle sheath into the peritoneal cavity with the syringe contents being injected after appreciating the "give", indicating entry into the peritoneal cavity. Fluoroscopy can be helpful here, in observing contrast used to push through needle in the peritoneal cavity around bowel loops.
- A guidewire is introduced through the needle, which is then removed. The location of guidewire can be confirmed by bedside ultrasonography.
- A tapered dilator with surrounding scored sheath is passed caudally over the wire which in turn removed.

Merits

- Quick and convenient.
- Small incision.
- Low risk of late hernia.
- Low cost of procedure.

Shortcomings

- Blind procedure and higher risk of early solution leakage.
- Inadequate homeostasis results in minor hemorrhages.
- Higher incidence of catheter malfunction (poor flow).
- Precise location of inner segment may be difficult.

- The Tenckhoff catheter is then inserted through the guide and the sheath is split to allow the cuff to reach the outer surface of the fascia.
- With the catheter held in place, the catheter guide is stripped away.

Moncrief-Popovich Technique

- This technique incorporates 2 modifications of the conventional technique. The external portion of the catheter that would be ordinarily be brought out through the skin in the standard technique is completely buried under the skin in a subcutaneous tunnel.
- The entire wound is then closed with no exit site.
- Healing and tissue growth occurs into the cuffs in a sterile environment.
- At a subsequent date of 8 weeks later a small incision is made 2 cm distal to the subcutaneous cuff and the distal segment of the catheter is exteriorized and brought out through the skin.
- **Merits:** No break in period.

Surgical Insertion Technique

- Under local, regional or general anesthesia.
- General anesthesia required in:
  - In patients with obesity.
  - Previous abdominal surgery with possibility of intraperitoneal adhesions.

- Implantation must be done by a competent and experienced operator in a planned manner. (The person doing the implantation should have assisted in 5 patients and independently inserted under supervision in 5 patients).
- Peritoneal entry should be lateral (deep cuff in or below the rectus musculature over posterior rectus sheath), or para-median (deep cuff at the medial edge of the rectus muscle), to give good deep cuff fixation and minimise herniation and fluid leaks.
- After proper positioning of the catheter tip the peritoneum is closed tightly around the catheter below the level of the deep cuff using a purse string suture.
- The subcutaneous cuff should be located near the skin surface and at a distance of at least 2-4 cm from the exit site.
- Care should be taken to avoid mechanically stressing the cuff material.
- Check for catheter patency to ensure adequate inflow and outflow without leakage by infusing 1 litre of PD fluid over 5 minutes and allowing it to drain out in an equal time.
- The exit site should be facing downwards or be directed laterally.
- Upward directed exit sites should be avoided.
- No sutures should be placed at the exit site.
- The intra peritoneal portion of the catheter should be placed between the visceral and parietal peritoneum towards the pouch of Douglas and should not be placed within the loops of the bowel or directly in omental tissues.

Merits

- Good hemostasis and low risk of bleeding.
- Tissue injury or viscus perforation is completely eliminated.
- Precise positioning of the inner segment is possible.
- All types of catheters can be inserted.
- Low risk of dialysate solution leaks.

Shortcomings

- Larger incision may predispose to late hernias.
- Immediate use is not recommended due to risk of dialysis solution leak.
- High cost of surgical procedure (dependence on surgeon's availability, OR time).

Peritoneoscopic Insertion Technique

- This technique would require specialised equipment (Y-TEC; Merit Medical, South Jordan, UT, USA) and the operator needs to be experienced and comfortable using the peritoneoscope.
- This technique has the advantage that the insertion of the catheter is done under direct vision, under local anesthesia and can be used in patients who are likely to have intra abdominal adhesions.
- Like the blind insertion it is performed through single abdominal puncture.
- No fluid is instilled before insertion of the cannula and trocar into the abdomen.
- After trocar is introduced through the medial or lateral border of rectus, it is removed and the peritoneoscope is inserted through cannula.
- After assuring the intra-peritoneal location by observing motion of the glistening surfaces, scope is removed and 600-1500 cm^2 of air is placed in the peritoneal cavity in trendlenberg position.
- The scope is reinserted and during continuous observation, scope, quill and the cannula are advanced into the clearest space and the most open direction between the viscera and the parietal peritoneum.
- Following this, the scope and the cannula are removed and the quill catheter guide is left in place.

Merits

- Quick and convenient.
- Small incision.
- Immediate use possible.
- Adequate homeostasis; low risk of bleeding.
- Low risk of tissue injury.
- Precise positioning of inner segment possible.

Shortcomings

- Need for special equipment.
- Expertise in using the peritoneoscope.

- After the next procedure is the dilatation of quill and musculature to 0.5 cm.
- Then the catheter is inserted through rectus muscle and cuff is advanced into the muscle.
- The catheter follows the path as directed by the Quill guide and is on a stylet.
- After the catheter has reached the desired position and the deep cuff is in the place the quill guide is removed.
- Subsequently a subcutaneous tunnel is made as in the surgical insertion technique.

Laparoscopic Insertion Technique

- Require general anesthesia.
- Laparoscopic port wounds should be away from exit and entry sites.

- Can be extremely useful if advanced implanting techniques used to minimise technique failure.
- Catheter can be immobilised by tunnelling in rectus sheath so the catheter stays in craniocaudal position or a suture sling can be placed around the tubing in lower abdominal wall.
- Omentopexy and adhesiolysis can be done simultaneously.

Break-in Period (for percutaneous inserted catheters)

Day of Operation	:	Day 0
Change of Dressing	:	Day 3
Flushing	:	Day 7
Initiation	:	Day 10 (start with low volume)
Stitch Removal	:	Day 14 (Complete training with patient able to do night dwell)

Exit Site Care

- The surgical dressing should not be changed for 72 hours unless there is obvious bleedings or signs of infection.
- Patients should avoid taking a bath until the exit site has fully healed (when exit site can be labeled as good or equivocal as per Twardowski's classification).
- **Cleansing agents:** Povidone iodine and hydrogen peroxide should not be used for cleaning the exit site–cytotoxic causing tissue damage and delaying clean wound healing.
- The newer cleansing agents recommended in the early post operative period are normal saline, or a nonionic surfactant agent (20% polaxamer) and pure soap.
- Proper immobilisation of external segment catheter should be done with tape or dressing to allow proper tissue in growth to cuff.

Continuous Flow Peritoneal Dialysis (CFPD)

Continuous flow peritoneal dialysis which was first introduced by Rosenak and Siwon in 1925 in animal and later on in humans by Ballads and Rosenak in 1934, has gained interest in recent past. It depends on continuous infusion of peritoneal dialysis solution through one peritoneal access, and simultaneous drainage by another. The intra-peritoneal tips should be away from each other to avoid recirculation but at the same time should allow maximum exposure to peritoneal surface.

There are two double lumen catheters developed recently, one by Jose A. Diaz-Buxo from Fresenius Medical Care North America, Lexington, Maryland, USA and the other with diffuser by Ronco and Dell'Aquila from St. Bortolo Hospital, Vicenza, Italy, Gloukhoff Wentling from Medcomp, Medical Components, Inc., Harleysville, Pennsylvania, USA and Amerling, Cruz and Levin from Beth Israel Medical Center, New York, USA.

Advantages of CFPD are shorter sessions, better clearances and ultrafiltration, leading to lower glucose concentration use. The disadvantages are primarily cost and recirculation. The other issues would be to see long term effects of dialysis regeneration system (synthetic membrane) and membrane damage due to high flow of dialysate. CFPD can be useful for patients with losing RRF, specifically before planning to shift to hemodialysis due to poor clearances. The concept CFPD has been utilised to make wearable artificial kidney.

Suggested Reading

1. Crabtree JH, Shrestha BM, Chow M *et al.* Creating and maintaining optimal peritoneal dialysis access in the adult patient: 2019 update. Peritoneal Dialysis International 2019; Vol. 39,414-36.
2. Twardowski ZJ. Peritoneal Access: The Past, Present and the Future. Contrib Nephrol. Basel, Karger 2006;Vol 150, 195-201.
3. Hagen SM, Lafranca JA, Ijzermans JN, *et al.* Systematic review and meta-analysis of the influence of peritoneal dialysis catheter type on complication rate and catheter survival. Kid Int 2014;Vol. 85, Issue 4,920-32.
4. Gallieni M, Giordano A, Pinerolo C, Cariati M. Type of peritoneal dialysis catheter and outcomes. J Vasc Access 2015;Vol. 16,Issue 9,S68-S72.
5. Ash SR. Chronic Peritoneal Dialysis Catheters: Overview of Design, Placement and Removal Procedures. Seminars in Dialysis 2003;Vol. 16,Issue 4,323-34.

CHAPTER

Plasmapheresis – Indications and Procedure

PN Gupta[1], Hemanth Kumar MK[2]

[1] *Senior Consultant, Nephrology, Paras Hospital, Gurugram*

[2] *Consultant, Nephrology, Paras Hospital, Gurugram*

Definition and Rationale

Plasmapheresis involves the removal of a portion or most of the patient's plasma by passing venous blood through an extracorporeal device that separates blood into its components (i.e., red blood cells, white blood cells and plasma), shunts some or most of the plasma into a discard container, and returns most of the remaining blood to the patient, along with a short-acting anticoagulant.[1]

The major mode of action of plasmapheresis is rapid depletion of specific disease associated factors. The pathogenic factors may be in the form of:

1. Antibody (Anti-GBM disease, Myasthenia gravis, Guillain-Barré Syndrome).
2. Monoclonal protein (Waldenstrom macroglobulinemia, Myeloma protein).
3. Circulating immune complexes (Cryoglobulinemia, SLE).
4. Lipoproteins and Endotoxins.

Plasmapheresis also has some immune-modulatory actions like:

1. Alterations in idiotypic/anti-idiotypic antibody balance.
2. Shift in antibody to antigen ratio to more soluble forms of immune complexes (facilitating their clearance).
3. Stimulation of lymphocyte clones to enhance cytotoxic therapy.
4. Removal of high molecular weight inflammatory mediators (cytokines, activated complement components).
5. Plasmapheresis also allows for replacement of deficient plasma components with infusion of normal plasma as in HUS and TTP.

At least one of the following conditions must be present for therapeutic plasma exchange (TPE) to be a rational therapeutic choice:

1. The substance to be removed should be sufficiently large (molecular weight greater than 15,000) so that it cannot be easily removed by less expensive purification techniques such as hemofiltration or high-flux hemodialysis.
2. The substance to be removed must have a sufficiently long half-life so that extracorporeal removal is much more rapid than endogenous clearance pathways.
3. The substance to be removed must be acutely toxic and/or resistant to conventional therapy so that the rapid elimination from the extracellular fluid by TPE is indicated.

Indications[2]

A collaborative survey by the AABB (formerly the American Association of Blood Banks) and the American Society for Apheresis (ASFA) found that more than one-half of all procedures were performed for neurologic conditions such as Guillain-Barré syndrome or myasthenia gravis. The various indications are summerized in Table 54.1.

1. **Anti-GBM Disease:** It is a rapidly progressive glomerulonephritis characterised by antibodies against NC1 domain of $\alpha3$ chain of Type IV collagen, frequently accompanied by pulmonary hemorrhage.

   Couser *et al.*,[4] reviewed 22 published uncontrolled studies involving 186 patients, and reported a favourable effect of plasmapheresis on pulmonary disease in around 90% of patients, and a favourable effect of plasmapheresis on renal disease in about 40% of patients. In a retrospective analysis involving 221 patients Beijing,[5] it was demonstrated that, in comparison with corticosteroids alone and corticosteroids plus cyclophosphamide, the combination of plasma exchange, corticosteroids and cyclophosphamide has an overall beneficial effect on patient and kidney survival. Particular benefit was seen for patients with pulmonary hemorrhage and, in relation to kidney survival, for those with anti-GBM nephritis and initial SCr higher than 6.8 mg/dl (600 μmol/l) (Cui *et al.*, 2011a).

Table 54.1: ASFA therapeutic categories[3]		
ASFA category	**Recommendation**	**Pathologic conditions**
Category I	Apheresis is accepted as **first-line therapy,** either as primary stand-alone treatment or in conjunction with other modes of treatment	1. GB Syndrome (AIDP)/CIDP 2. Myasthenia Gravis 3. ANCA vasculitis–Dialysis Dependent and/or DAH 4. Recurrent FSGS 5. Anti-GBM Disease–Dialysis Independent and/or DAH 6. Monoclonal Gammopathy with Hyper Viscosity 7. Desensitisation of ABO-I Kidney Transplantation 8. Acute ABMR in Renal Transplantation 9. Acquired Autoimmune TTP
Category II	Apheresis is accepted as **second-line therapy,** either as primary stand-alone treatment or in conjunction with other modes of treatment	1. Myeloma Cast Nephropathy 2. Catastrophic APS 3. Severe/Symptomatic Cryoglobulinaemia 4. Severe SLE
Category III	Optimum role of apheresis therapy is **not established**	1. Aplastic Anemia 2. Drug overdose/Envenomation 3. Acute Liver Failure 4. ANCA vasculitis–Dialysis Independent 5. Anti-GBM Disease–Dialysis Dependent and no DAH 6. HSP 7. ITP 8. IgA Nephropathy 9. Sepsis with MODS
Category IV	Apheresis to be **ineffective or harmful**	1. Active Rheumatoid Arthritis 2. Dermatomyositis/Polymyositis 3. Lupus Nephritis

In a large retrospective study of anti-GBM disease from Hammersmith Hospital (Levy *et al.*, 2001),[6] including 85 patients seen over 25 years, the kidney outcome was strongly influenced by kidney function at presentation. Patients who had an initial serum creatinine (SCr) < 5.7 mg/dl (500 µmol/l) had 1-year overall survival of 100% and kidney survival of 95%. If the initial SCr was > 5.7 mg/dl (500 µmol/l) but dialysis was not required immediately, the patient and kidney survivals were 83% and 82% at 1 year, respectively. However, among patients who needed dialysis at presentation, patient and kidney survival were reduced to 65% and 8% at 1 year, respectively. The treatment consisted of high-dose prednisone (1 mg/kg/day) tapered over 6–9 months, oral cyclophosphamide for 2–3 months, and daily plasmapheresis (approx. 1.5 plasma volumes each day) for 14 days, or until anti-GBM antibody was no longer detectable.

In oliguric dialysis dependent patients with 100% crescents on biopsy, plasmapheresis should be probably reserved to only those with pulmonary hemorrhage as the renal functions are unlikely to recover.[7]

Usually 5% albumin is used for replacement and if the patient is fluid overloaded, the amount of albumin can be reduced to 85% (but not less) of the removed plasma volume.

Citrate anticoagulation and use of FFP in the last litre is preferred in presence of lung hemorrhage and after renal biopsy.

2. **Thrombotic Thrombocytopenic Purpura (TTP)/ Hemolytic Uremic Syndrome (HUS):** TTP is caused by deficiency of ADAMTS13 which is a protease that cleaves large vWF polymers or antibodies to ADAMTS13. HUS is caused by abnormal complement activation due to genetic deficiency of regulators or inhibitors of complement activation or due to antibodies against it.

   Plasmapheresis will replace normal plasma constituents and also remove autoantibodies if present.

   In severe TTP, daily plasmapheresis of at least one plasma volume should be performed daily for 7-10 days. Treatment is continued until platelet count normalizes and hemolysis has ceased (LDH <400 IU/l). Relapse may occur once treatment is stopped and if platelet count declines to <1 lac/ cumm, alternate day plasma exchange must be recommenced until platelet count stabilizes.[8]

   Providing sufficient ADAMTS13 to achieve 5% normal enzymatic activity may be sufficient to degrade large vWF multimers, which may be relevant to induce remission of the microangiopathic process and this effect is sustained over time due to the relatively long half-life of the protease. Infused ADAMTS13 has a plasma half-life of 2–3 days *in vivo*, and although plasma levels fall below 5% within 3–7 after fresh FFP administration, the effect on platelet count and clinical parameters may last up to 3 weeks, suggesting that ADAMTS13 remains available, for example, on platelets and endothelial cells.[9]

   Two RCTs[10,11] have shown the benefit of plasmapheresis with FFP compared to FFP infusion alone. A recent meta-analysis of RCTs[12] showed plasmapheresis with FFP is the most effective approach in TTP.

   D+ HUS in children is a self-limiting disease and no role of plasmapheresis but reports of benefit with plasmapheresis in adults with severe D+ HUS has been seen. Similarly in atypical HUS, there are reports of benefit seen with plasmapheresis.

   In atypical HUS, Typically 1-2 volume plasma exchange is undertaken daily initially, the duration and frequency of treatment is then determined by the clinical response. Patients with abnormalities in soluble regulators such as factor H respond better to plasma exchange than patients with abnormalities in the transmembrane regulator MCP (Noris *et al.*, 2010). Despite treatment with plasma therapy the majority of patients progress to end-stage renal failure within 3 years of presentation.[13,14]

   Removed plasma is replaced with same volume of FFP as it provides deficient plasma components.

3. **Cryoglobulinemia:** Cryoglobulinemia is a pathological condition in which the blood contains immunoglobulins that have the property of reversible precipitation from human serum cooled to 4°C. Patients are considered to have a significant cryoglobulin level when it is > 0.05 g/l on two determinations.

   Although the main treatment involves antiviral treatment in HCV associated cases of mixed cryoglobulinemias and B cell depletion with rituximab and non-specific immunosuppression with corticosteroids. Plasmapheresis is used in cases of hyper viscosity syndromes and in patients about to undergo surgery requiring hypothermia.

   Although there are no controlled trials regarding the efficacy of PLEX, there are multiple reports demonstrating the efficacy of PLEX in patients with acute vasculitis and renal involvement. Generally, exchange of one plasma volume daily for 7 days is recommended.[15] Replacement fluid must be 5% albumin which must be warmed to avoid precipitation of cryoglobulins. Centrifugal device are preferred as cryoglobulins may block the membrane filter as they cool and precipitate.

4. **ANCA Associated Vasculitis:** There is increasing evidence for the pathogenic involvement of ANCA in AAV (which consists of GPA, EGPA and MPA) which provides for rationale for removal of these pathogenic antibodies in using plasmapheresis.

   A large European Trial (MEPEX) confirmed the beneficial therapeutic role of addition of plasmapheresis in patients with AAV with a Serum Creatinine of > 5.7 mg/dl (500 µmol/l) as compared to 3000 mg of intravenous methylprednisolone to standard therapy of oral cyclophosphamide and oral prednisolone in renal recovery (independent of dialysis) at 3 months and reduced risk of progression to ESRD at 12 months.[16]

   The recommended regimen based on this study is daily exchange of 1.5 plasma volumes for 7 days. FFP must be used for the last litre of exchange for those with lung hemorrhage and recent renal biopsy.[16]

   However, a long-term follow-up study of the patients of MEPEX trial with a median follow-up of 3.95 years failed to show benefit of PLEX over IV methyl prednisolone in primary outcome of death and ESRD.[17]

   Also the recent PEXIVAS trial which evaluated the effect of PLEX in patients with new or relapsing severe AAV including lung hemorrhage and/or eGFR <50 ml/min/1.73 m^2 on 7 years follow-up for primary end point of death or ESRD failed to show any benefit of PLEX over no PLEX in these conditions.[18]

5. **Multiple Myeloma:** Various studies[19] have shown benefit of plasmapheresis in proven myeloma cast nephropathy where the level of light chains were high and patient had severe renal impairment. Five consecutive plasma exchanges with 5% albumin in patients with acute light chain cast nephropathy with longer course may be needed on the basis of clinical course and paraprotein levels.

   Alternative approach to the plasmapheresis that has gained importance is the removal of light chains by hemodialysis using high cut-off dialyzers. High-cut off dialyzers have high permeability for substances in the molecular weight range of 15-45 kDa and such membranes can effectively clear both κ and λ free light chain (FLC). As compared to conventional high-flux dialysers have a molecular weight cut-off around 15–20 kDa.

   A multicentre RCT, MYRE trial compared the effect of intensive dialysis (eight 5-hour sessions over 10 days) with either high cut off (HCO) dialyzer or a conventional high flux dialyzer in addition to bortezomib based chemotherapy on dialysis independence at 3, 6 and 12 months in patients with myeloma cast nephropathy. This study did not find any beneficial effect of HCO dialysis over high flux dialysis at 3 months but did show statistically significant benefit with HCO dialysis at 6 and 12 months.[20]

   Similarly another multicentre Trial, EuLITE trial which compared the effect of HCO Dialysis with High Flux dialysis in patients with myeloma cast nephropathy and severe AKI due to myeloma in patients on bortezomib based chemotherapy on renal recovery at 90 days failed to show any difference.[21]

6. **Systemic Lupus Erythematosus:** In Lupus Nephritis, plasmapheresis has not shown to be consistently beneficial. However, plasmapheresis should be considered in patients with life threatening manifestations of SLE like Refractory Lupus Nephritis, CNS Lupus, Pulmonary hemorrhage, Hyper Viscosity Syndrome, TTP or Catastrophic Antiphosholipid Antibody Syndrome.[22]

   Initial course of 1-1.5 plasma volume exchange daily for 7 days with 5% albumin replacement to be adopted in patients with life threatening disease. FFP replacement for last litre in patients with lung hemorrhage and after renal biopsy to be considered.

7. **Recurrent FSGS Post Transplant:** Relapse of nephrotic syndrome and glomerular lesions are observed in approximately 30% of patients undergoing renal transplantation.[23] Repeated sessions of plasmapheresis are carried out alone or with increased immunosuppression but the efficacy is not clear as there are no large RCTs.[24] Consider one plasma volume exchange for 5 consecutive days with 5% albumin replacement or longer depending on clinical response.

   Pre-emptive plasmapheresis[25] can be repeated over days and weeks in case of transplantation with a living donor and thus achieve substantial removal of the glomerular permeability factor, whereas in case of deceased donor transplantation there may be no sufficient time for performing plasma exchanges before grafting.

8. **Hyperviscosity Syndrome:** Most commonly caused by Waldenstrom's macroglobulinemia (50%) and occasionally with myeloma and cryoglobulinemia. Hyperviscosity leads to reduced blood flow and ischemia of organs.

   Even though there are no controlled trials on benefit of plasmapheresis, one plasma exchange daily for 3-5 days with 5% albumin replacement or until patient is clinically stable and blood viscosity normalizes can be adopted.[26]

9. **Renal Transplantation:** Plasmapheresis has been used in treating acute antibody mediated rejection (ABMR) and also in desensitization protocols for ABO-i and highly sensitized patients.

   In acute ABMR concurrent IVIg along with PLEX has been the standard of care but there is no apparent benefit of PLEX in chronic ABMR.

   In desensitisation of ABO-i renal transplantation, concurrent Rituximab along with IVIg and CNI/ Mycophenolate has been the standard of care to reduce the antibody to acceptable levels.[27]

10. **Acute Inflammatory Demyelinating Polyneuropathy (GBS):** In protocol of North American trial a total of 200-250 ml/kg was exchanged over 7-10 days. At least 2 PE are needed to significantly reduce the circulating immunoglobulin complexes. In India small volume PE was used by Tharakan *et al.* with comparable results. They used 15 ml/kg body weight/day to be continued till the progression of the disease got arrested or recovery started.

    PE is more beneficial when started within 7 days after disease onset rather than later, but was still beneficial in patients treated up to 30 days after disease onset.

    All patients with mild, moderate, and severe GBS benefit from treatment. Patients who need even minimum assistance for walking, who are steadily progressing and those who are bed- and ventilator-bound should be advised PE.[28]

11. **Myasthenia Gravis:** Plasmapheresis directly removes acetylcholine receptor (AChR) antibodies from the circulation. Clinical improvement with plasmapheresis roughly correlates with the reduction in antibody levels and the beneficial clinical effect of plasmapheresis is usually seen within days, but the benefit typically lasts only three to six weeks unless concurrent immunosuppression is started.

The main indications for plasmapheresis in MG include:

- Acute exacerbations, including myasthenic crisis.
- Preoperatively, before thymectomy or other surgery.
- As a "bridge" to slower-acting immunosuppressive therapies for patients in whom it is especially desirable to avoid or minimize glucocorticoid use.

Procedure

Kinetics of Immunoglobulin[1]

The Immunoglobulins have a relatively long half life with that of IgG- 21 days and IgM- 5 days. The extent of extravascular distribution determines how effectively they can be removed in the single plasmapheresis session. Intravascular to extravascular equilibration is approx. 1-2% per hour whereas the reverse is little faster (Table 54.2).

Table 54.2: Characteristic of various substances

Substance	Molecular weight (Da)	% Intra-vascular	Half-life (days)	Normal serum conc. (mg/dl)
Albumin	69000	40%	19	3500-4500
IgG	180000	45%	21	640-1430
IgA	150000	50%	6	30-300
IgM	900000	80%	5	60-350
LDL-Cholesterol	1300000	100%	3-5	140-200

Plasma Volume=TBV * (1-Hematocrit).

Total Blood Volume (TBV) is assumed to be 70 ml/kg body weight in males and 65 ml/kg body weight in females.

For example, In a 70 kg man with hematocrit of 45%, the TBV is 4900 ml. Then the Plasma Volume is 2700 ml.

In simpler words, one Plasma volume is 35-40 ml/kg body weight when hematocrit is normal. The plasma volumes will be higher when hematocrit is lower (in anemia).

The kinetics of Ig removal by TPE follows an exponential relationship:

$$C_t=C_0\, e^{-Ve/Vp}$$

Where C_0=the initial plasma concentration of macromolecule, C_t= its concentration at time t, V_e= volume of plasma exchanged at time t, Vp= estimated total plasma volume.

The Macromolecular Reduction Ratio (MRR) is expressed as:

$$MRR= 100 * (1-C_t/C_0) \text{ or } MRR= 100 * (1-e^{-Ve/Vp})$$

If we substitute Ve from 1400 ml to 8400 ml and if we assume V_p is 2800 ml, we get values of V_e/V_p from 0.5 to 3.0. So MRR ranges from 39% to 95% (Table 54.3).

Table 54.3: Macromolecular reduction ratio

Portion of plasma volume exchanged (V_e/V_p)	Volume exchanged (V_e, ml)	Ig or other substances removed (MRR)
0.5	1400	39%
1.0	2800	63%
1.5	4200	78%
2.0	5600	86%
2.5	7000	92%
3.0	8400	95%

The largest decrease occurs with removal of first plasma volumes and subsequent plasma volume removal during same session becomes less effective in removing macromolecule. This effectiveness is reduced by further by dilution by exchange fluid. For this reason, 1.0-1.5 plasma volume equivalents are exchanged during a plasmapheresis session.

Also there is reaccumulation of Ig into the vascular space by two processes: Re-synthesis and redistribution from extravascular space via lymphatic drainage and diffusion from interstitial space.

If the macromolecule in question is IgM which has a relatively short half-life of 5-7 days, then there may be a role for more extended period of TPE as the endogenous rate of synthesis is higher for IgM than IgG. In addition, IgM is predominantly intravascular. So while removing IgM or paraproteins, daily PLEX is recommended.

If the macromolecule is IgG which has a half-life of 21 days, then PLEX must be done every other day as a majority of it is in extravascular space and must be given adequate time to redistribute.

If the substance removed is measurable by quantitative measures, then treatment schedule can be designed based on its pharmacokinetics.

Methods[1]

PLEX is done using one of the either methods (Table 54.4, Figs. 54.1 and 54.2):

1. Membrane Plasma Separation using Hollow Fibers (separation based on hemofiltration procedure without dialysate).
2. Centrifugation blood cell separators using apheresis machines (separation based on gravity according to its density).

The Membrane Plasma Separators have a molecular weight cut-off of 3 million Daltons and is sufficient to allow passage of immune complexes. The membrane has a sieving coefficient (ratio of concentration in filtrate to blood) between 0.8-0.9 for albumin, IgG, IgA, IgM, C3,

Table 54.4: Methods of plasmapheresis

	Advantages	**Disadvantages**
Membrane Plasma Separation	Faster and smaller	Removal of substances limited by sieving coefficient of membrane
	No citrate	Reduced efficiency in hyper viscosity syndromes (WM) and cryoglobulinemia
	Can be adapted for cascade filtration	No cytapheresis
		Requires high blood flow and central venous access
		Requires heparin (limited use in bleeding disorders)
Centrifugal Apheresis	Cytapheresis can be done	Large and heavy
	No heparin	Requires citrate
	More efficient removal of all plasma components	
	Peripheral line can be used as needs low blood flow rate	

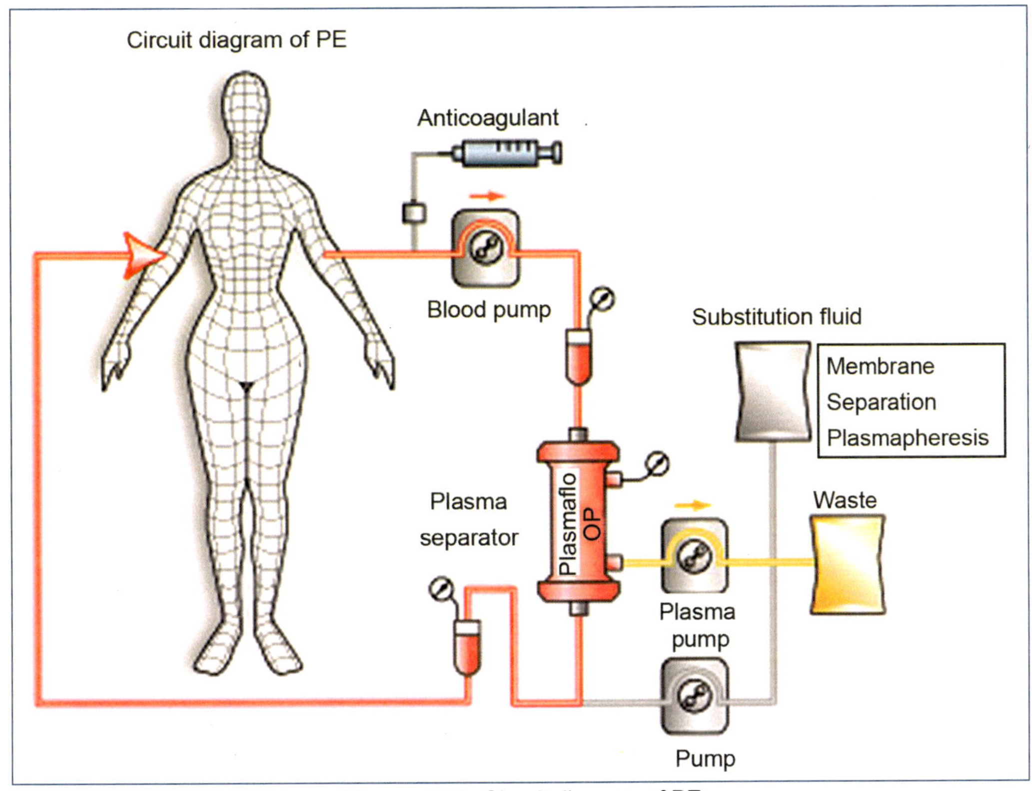

Figure 54.1: Circuit diagram of PE

C4, fibrinogen, Cholesterol and TG. A sieving coefficient of 1 implies that the substance can freely pass through and 0 implies that it cannot pass through the membrane.

MPS must be performed at low TMP (<100 mm Hg) to avoid hemolysis. The blood flow must exceed 50 ml/min to avoid clotting with an average blood flow of 100-150 ml/min.

With blood flow rate of 100 ml/min, a plasma removal rate of 30-50 ml/min can be expected and thus the time to perform a typical membrane filtration (V_e=2800 ml) is < 2 hours.

Centrifugal devices operate at a lower speed of 40-50 ml/min and such flows can be obtained with a large peripheral needle.

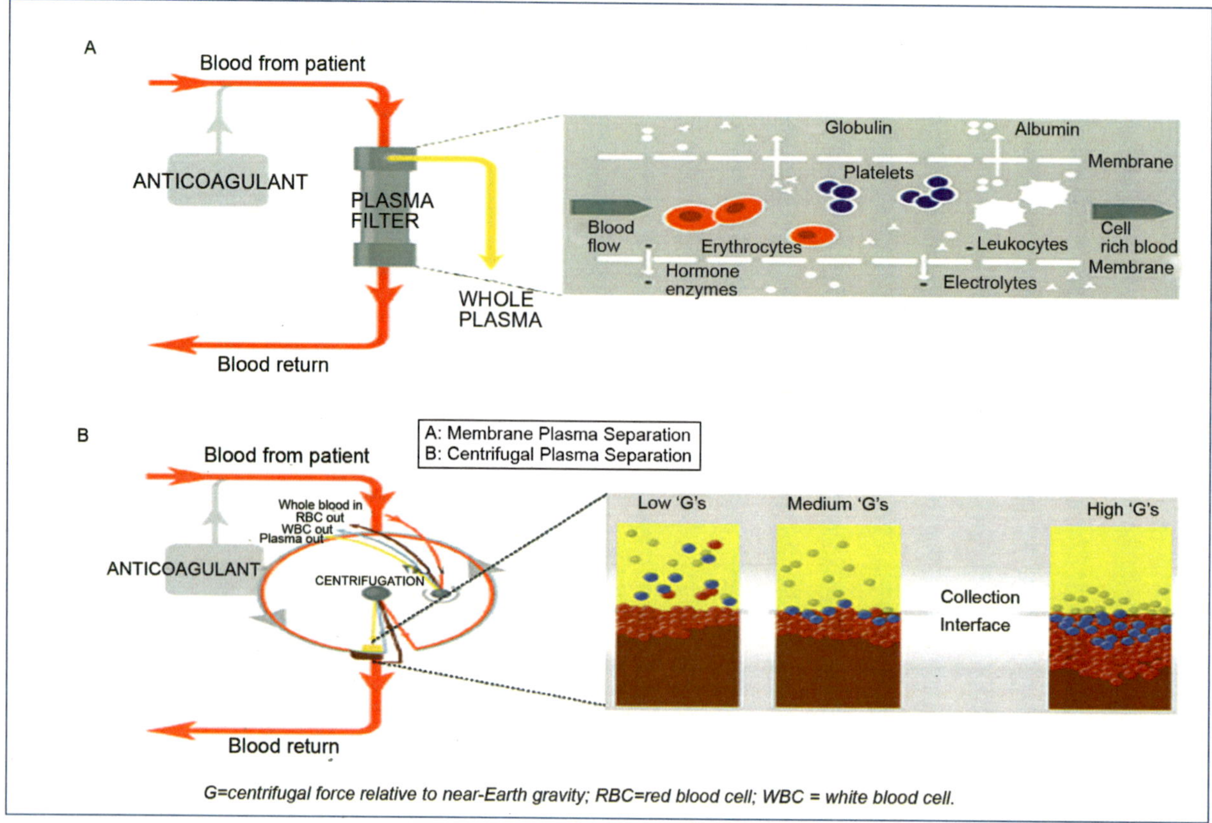

Figure 54.2: PLEX methods A. Membrane plasma separation; B. Centrifugation blood cell separators

Anticoagulation[1]

Anticoagulation is mandatory for plasmapheresis. Usually centrifugal machines require citrate and MPS require heparin.

Heparin dose needs to be increased in patients with low Hct (increased volume of distribution) and when plasma filtration rate is high (high plasma filtration rate results in increased net removal of heparin which has a sieving coefficient 1.0).

Citrate anticoagulation can cause low plasma ionized calcium levels which may cause perioral parasthesias, twitching, tremors, muscular contractions, tetany, myocardial depression, arrhythmias and seizures. FFP used as replacement solution also contains 14% citrate by volume. So delivery of citrate has to be carefully monitored. Moreover in patients with renal and liver insufficiency, the metabolism of citrate is impaired.

Additional calcium as continuous IV infusion of 10 ml 10% calcium gluconate per litre of replacement fluid can be given to reduce risk of hypocalcemia.

Also citrate can cause alkalosis in the patient as it is converted to bicarbonate in liver.

Replacement Solution[1]

The selection of type and amount of replacement solution depends on the basic disease and the condition of the patient. The most common replacement solutions are Isonatric 5% Albumin and FFP (Table 54.5).

Table 54.5: Replacement solutions

	Advantages	**Disadvantages**
Albumin	No risk of hepatitis	Expensive
	Room temperature storage	No coagulation factors
	Allergic reactions rare	No Ig
	No concern about ABO blood group	
	Depletes inflammation mediators	
Fresh frozen Plasma (FFP)	**Provides coagulation factors**	**Risk of hepatitis, HIV**
	Provides Ig with beneficial effects	**Allergic reactions**
	Similar in composition to the filtrate removed	Must be thawed
	Provides deficient complement components	**Must be ABO compatible**
		Citrate load

The use of FFP may sometimes make the measurement of the pathogenic Ig levels difficult and also it may replenish some of the factors which were removed during plasmapheresis and then reduce the efficacy of the procedure.

Specific indications for replacing some or all of the removed plasma with FFP are:

1. TTP-HUS.
2. Preexisting defect in hemostasis or low pre-treatment fibrinogen levels.
3. Patient at risk of bleeding or those with active bleeding including pulmonary hemorrhage.

When albumin is used as replacement solution, 5% albumin in every litre of normal saline can be infused at rate equal to that of plasma removed. Another economical approach is to replace initial 20-30% of removed plasma with crystalloid and the balance with above mentioned albumin solution.

Complications[1]

The incidence of hypotension is 2% and causes include intravascular volume depletion, vasovagal episodes, use of hypo-oncotic fluid replacement, inadequate volume replacement, anaphylaxis, cardiac arrhythmias and cardiovascular collapse.

After a single plasma exchange, serum fibrinogen levels decrease by 80%, prothrombin and many other clotting factor levels fall by 50-70% and APTT increases by 100%.

Recovery of coagulation factors is biphasic with a rapid increase up to 4 hours postapheresis followed by a slower rise 4-24 hours postapheresis. 24 hours after treatment, fibrinogen levels are approx 50% and ATIII levels are 85% of initial levels; both need 48-72 hours for complete recovery. One day following treatment, prothrombin levels are 75% and FX levels are 30% and all other factors would have recovered completely to normal levels.

Depletion of clotting factors is more pronounced when multiple treatments are performed over a short time.

There is also risk of 25% reduction in serum potassium levels which can be reduced by adding 4 meq of potassium per litre of replacement solution.

Anaphylactic reaction may be noted in persons taking ACEI during plasmapheresis due to the presence of prekallikrein activating factor present in albumin solution. So short acting ACEI should be stopped 24 hours prior and long acting ACEI be stopped 48 hours prior to plasmapheresis with membrane devices.

If severe infection develops in the immediate postapheresis period, single infusion of IVIg (100-400 mg/kg IV) be used.

Double Filtration Plasmapheresis/Cascade Filtration

There is primary membrane plasma separator followed by a secondary plasma fractionator to remove target solutes based on molecular size and weight. This is more selective than the conventional plasmapheresis and can reduce loss of albumin (Fig. 54.3).

Immunoadsorption Columns

These are membrane plasma separators which are selectively designed to bind the target molecule and remove from ciculation. These columns contain either SPA or immobilized antibody bound to an inert and insoluble matrix in a column of gel beads. SPA has high affinity for Fc portion of IgG1, IgG2 and IgG4 and depletes them or immune complexes containing them.

The Glycosorb ABO column contains terminal trisaccharide A or B blood group antigen immobilized

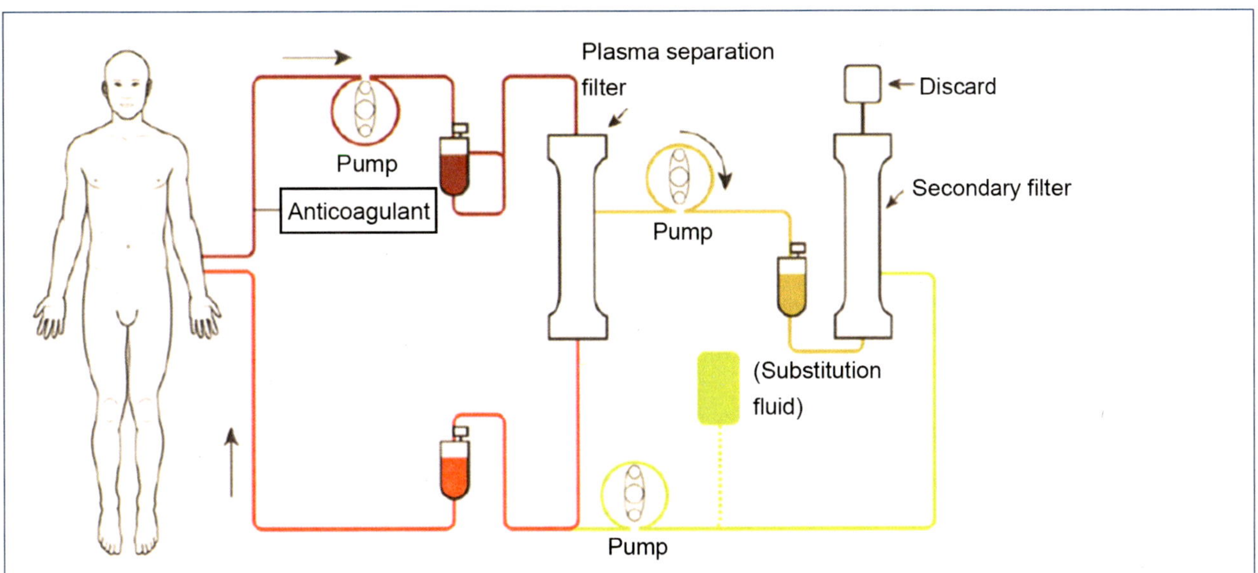

Figure 54.3: Double filtration plasmapheresis

on sepharose which binds circulating anti-A or anti-B antibodies and used for desensitization in ABO-I renal transplantation.

References

1. Daugirdas John T Blake, Peter G and Ing, Todd S. "Handbook of Dialysis (5th ed.)" (2015).
2. Turner Neil, Goldsmith David, Winearls Christopher, Lamiere Norbert, Himmelfarb Jonathan, Remuzzi Giuseppe. "Oxford Textbook of Clinical Nephrology (4th ed.)" (2015).
3. Schwartz J, Padmanabhan A, Aqui N, *et al.* Guidelines on the use of therapeutic apheresis in clinical practice–Evidence-based approach from the Writing Committee of the American Society for Apheresis: The seventh special issue. J Clin Apher 2016;31:149.
4. Couser WG. Rapidly progressive glomerulonephritis: Classification, pathogenetic mechanisms and therapy. Am J Kidney Dis 1988;11:449-64.
5. Cui Z, Zhao J, Jia XY, *et al.* Anti-glomerular basement membrane disease: Outcomes of different therapeutic regimens in a large single-center Chinese Cohort study. Medicine (Baltimore) 2011a;90:303-11.
6. Levy JB, Turner AN and Rees AJ. Long-term outcome of anti-glomerular basement membrane antibody disease treated with plasma exchange and immunosuppression. Ann Intern Med 2001;134:1033-42.
7. Flores JC, Taube D, Savage CO, *et al.* Clinical and immunological evolution of oligoanuric anti-GBM nephritis treated by hemodialysis Lancet 1986;1:5-8.
8. Scott EA, Puca KE, Pietz BC, *et al.* Comparison and stability of ADAMTS13 activity in therapeutic plasma products. Transfusion 2007;47:120-25.
9. Furlan M, Robles R, Morselli B, *et al.* Recovery and half-life of von Willebrand factor–cleaving protease after plasma therapy in patients with thrombotic thrombocytopenic purpura. Thromb Haemost 1999;81:8-13.
10. Henon P. Thrombotic thrombocytopenic purpura: Clinical results of a French controlled trial. Transfusion Science 1992;13:63-72.
11. Rock GA, Shumak KH, Buskard NA, Blanchette VS, Kelton JG, Nair RC, Spasoff RA and the Canadian Apheresis Study Group. Comparison of plasma exchange with plasma infusion in the treatment of thrombotic thrombocytopenic purpura. New England Journal of Medicine 1991;325: 393-97.
12. Brunskill SJ, Tusold A, Benjamin S, Stanworth SJ and Murphy MF. A systematic review of randomized controlled trials for plasma exchange in the treatment of thrombotic thrombocytopenic purpura. Transfusion Medicine 2007;17(1):17-35.
13. Noris M, Caprioli J, Bresin E, *et al.* Relative role of genetic complement abnormalities in sporadic and familial aHUS and their impact on clinical phenotype. Clin J Am Soc Nephrol 2010;5:1844-59.
14. Noris M and Remuzzi G. Atypical hemolytic-uremic syndrome. N Engl J Med 2009;361:1676-87.
15. Rockx MA and Clark WF. Plasma exchange for treating cryoglobulinemia: A descriptive analysis. Transfusion and Apheresis Science 2010;42(3):247-51.
16. Jayne DRW, Gaskin G, Rasmussen N, Abramowicz D, Ferrario, F Guillevin L. Randomized Trial of Plasma Exchange or High-Dosage Methylprednisolone as Adjunctive Therapy for Severe Renal Vasculitis. Journal of the American Society of Nephrology 2007;18(7):2180-88.
17. Walsh M, Casian A, Flossmann O, Westman K, Höglund, P Pusey C and Jayne DRW. Long-term follow-up of patients with severe ANCA-associated vasculitis comparing plasma exchange to intravenous methylprednisolone treatment is unclear. Kidney International 2013;84(2):397-402.
18. Walsh M, Merkel PA, Jayne D. The Effects of Plasma Exchange and Reduced-Dose Glucocorticoids during Remission-Induction for Treatment of Severe ANCA-Associated Vasculitis [abstract]. Arthritis Rheumatol 2018; 70 (suppl 10).
19. Gupta D, Bachegowda L, Phadke G, Boren S, Johnson D and Misra M. Role of plasmapheresis in the management of myeloma kidney: A systematic review. Hemodialysis International 2010;14(4):355-63.
20. Bridoux F, Carron PL, Pegourie B, Alamartine E, Augeul-Meunier K, Karras A. Effect of High-Cutoff Hemodialysis vs Conventional Hemodialysis on Hemodialysis Independence Among Patients With Myeloma Cast Nephropathy. JAMA 2017;318(21):2099.
21. Hutchison CA, Cockwell P, Moroz V, Bradwell AR, Fifer L, Gillmore JD, Cook M (2019). High cutoff versus high-flux haemodialysis for myeloma cast nephropathy in patients receiving bortezomib-based chemotherapy (EuLITE): A phase 2 randomised controlled trial. The Lancet Haematology.
22. Pagnoux C, Korach JM and Guillevin L. Indications for plasma exchange in systemic lupus erythematosus in 2005. Lupus 2005;14(11):871-77.
23. Ponticelli C. Recurrence of focal segmental glomerular sclerosis (FSGS) after renal transplantation. Nephrol Dial Transplant 2010;25:25-31.
24. Artero ML, Sharma R, Savin VJ, *et al.* Plasmapheresis reduces proteinuria and serum capacity to injure glomeruli in patients with recurrent focal glomerulosclerosis. Am J Kidney Dis 1994;23:574-81.
25. Gohh RY, Yango AF, Morrissey PE, *et al.* Preemptive plasmapheresis and recurrence of FSGS in high-risk renal transplant recipients. Am J Transplant 2005;5:2907-12.
26. Correction of Hyperviscosity by Apheresis. Seminars in Thrombosis and Hemostasis 2003;29(5):535-42. doi:10.1055/s-2003-44560.
27. Pusey CD and Levy JB. Plasmapheresis in Immunologic Renal Disease. Blood Purification 2012;33(1-3):190-98. doi:10.1159/000334155.
28. Meena AK, Khadilkar S V, Murthy J. Treatment guidelines for Guillain-Barré Syndrome. Ann Indian Acad Neurol 2011;14,Suppl S1:73-81.